A PRIMER OF **DRUG ACTION**

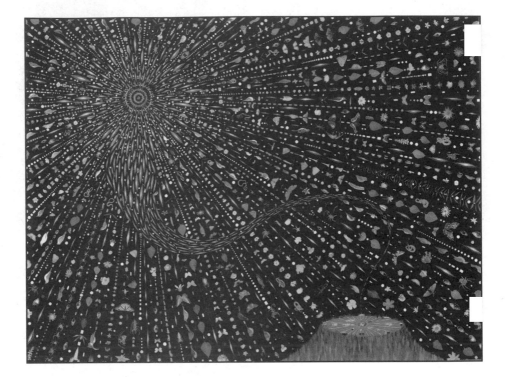

Fred Tomaselli
Ectoplasmic Event over New Jerusalem, 2001
Pills, leaves, insects, photocollage, acrylic, and resin on wood panel
72" × 96"
Copyright the artist
Courtesy James Cohan Gallery, New York.

Fred Tomaselli (born in 1956 in Santa Monica, California) has exhibited widely in the United States and abroad. His work is included in many private and public collections, including the Sintra Museum of Modern Art in Sintra, Portugal, and the Whitney Museum of American Art and the Museum of Modern Art in New York City. In the 1990s Tomaselli first gained attention for his collage-based paintings composed of painted lines and various forms of psychoactive drugs, pills, and marijuana leaves. He lives and works in Brooklyn, New York.

A PRIMER OF **DRUG ACTION**

A comprehensive guide to the actions, uses, and side effects of psychoactive drugs

TWELFTH EDITION

ROBERT M. JULIEN, M.D., PH.D.
Portland, Oregon

CLAIRE D. ADVOKAT, PH.D.
Louisiana State University

JOSEPH E. COMATY, PH.D., M.P.
Louisiana State Office of Behavioral Health

WORTH PUBLISHERS

Senior Publisher: Catherine Woods
Acquisitions Editor: Erik Gilg
Executive Marketing Manager: Katherine Nurre
Art Director and Cover Designer: Barbara Reingold
Associate Managing Editor: Tracey Kuehn
Project Editor: Penelope Hull
Illustration Coordinator: Bill Page
Illustrations: Matt Holt, Lyndall Culbertson, Dragonfly Graphics, TSI Graphics
Photo Editor: Ted Szczepanski
Production Manager: Barbara Anne Seixas
Composition: TSI Graphics
Printing and Binding: RR Donnelley

Library of Congress Control Number: 2010933047

ISBN-13: 978-1-4292-3343-9
ISBN-10: 1-4292-3343-5

© 2001, 2005, 2008, 2011 by Worth Publishers

Printed in the United States of America

Fourth printing

Worth Publishers
41 Madison Avenue
New York, NY 10010
www.worthpublishers.com

Contents

Preface

The twelfth edition of *A Primer of Drug Action* marks 36 years of continuous publication of this now classic textbook. In these years, *A Primer of Drug Action* has documented the dramatic advances made in the psychopharmacological treatment of mental illness and substance abuse. These years have seen a revolution in the development of psychoactive drugs and in our understanding of the psychological disorders for which they are used. From the initial discoveries that certain chemical compounds could help people who suffer from psychosis, depression, anxiety, mania and other neurological and psychological conditions, medications have been developed that greatly improved our treatment of these devastating disorders. There has been an explosion in our knowledge of the physiological and neurological substrates, the receptors and enzymes that are affected by these drugs, and an appreciation that they can be most effective when integrated with appropriate behavioral therapy. Comparable advances have been made in understanding the neurobiological consequences of substance abuse and dependence, which have opened new avenues for pharmacological approaches to addiction.

Each of the prior eleven editions of *A Primer of Drug Action* sought to present these developments in a clear, concise, and timely manner. We have strived to maintain this quality in the twelfth edition, describing the general principles of each class of psychoactive drug, as well as providing specific information about the individual agents. Each chapter includes an overview of the mechanisms of action of the drugs, current models of the disorders, rationales for drug treatment, and the limitations of psychopharmacology in patient care. Chapters are included on drugs of abuse as well as medications for psychiatric disorders. Addiction is not only a significant behavioral disorder but, in many cases, the same drugs may have addictive properties as well as therapeutic applications.

FEATURES OF THE TWELFTH EDITION

In its 36 years of publication, *A Primer of Drug Action* has been the classic psychopharmacology textbook, thanks to the dedication of the long-time author, Robert Julien, who for over three decades single-handedly accomplished the herculean tasks of revising each edition and maintaining a succinct yet comprehensive and clear review of the most up-to-date advances in psychopharmacology. The book was the premier text for anyone interested in accessing this expanding and important body of science.

For the twelfth edition, Dr. Julien sought major contributions from Claire Advokat and Joseph Comaty. Dr. Advokat is a professor in the Department of Psychology at Louisiana State University in Baton Rouge, and she holds an adjunct faculty appointment with the Alliant International University/California School of Professional Psychology. Dr. Comaty is chief psychologist, HIPAA privacy officer, and director of the Division of Policy, Standards, and Quality Assurance of the Louisiana State Office of Behavioral Health, Department of Health and Hospitals, in Baton Rouge, Louisiana. He holds adjunct faculty appointments in the Department of Psychology, Louisiana State University, and the Alliant International University/California School of Professional Psychology. Dr. Comaty is a clinical and medical psychologist, licensed to prescribe psychotherapeutic drugs in the state of Louisiana. Dr. Julien retired as staff anesthesiologist at St. Vincent Hospital and Medical Center in Portland, Oregon. He is an active consultant and lecturer on pharmacology and anesthesiology.

We three authors have worked closely on the eleventh and twelfth editions to maintain the qualities exemplified by the previous editions of the textbook, namely, concise description and analysis, clarity of writing, and inclusion of the most current information available. As in earlier editions, each chapter of the twelfth edition has been updated to reflect the latest developments in the field. Presentations, specific medications, and literature citations are updated in each chapter, and a broad overview of these changes since the last edition suggests two prominent themes.

First, there has been a dramatic expansion in the clinical application of the major therapeutic drug classes. Medications (such as antipsychotics), historically prescribed primarily for one category of disorder (such as schizophrenia), are now approved for use with numerous conditions (such as major depression and bipolar disorder). Distinctions among the accepted indications of major psychotropic drugs are becoming more diffuse. A parallel reconsideration of the diagnostic categories themselves is also in progress in the forthcoming new version of the American Psychiatric Association's *Diagnostic and Statistical Manual* (DSM). An important result is the continued expansion and refinement of psychiatric diagnoses and prescriptions of powerful drugs for children and adolescents. The long-term consequences of this shift to the health of the next generation bears watching. These issues are addressed as we discuss the use of psychoactive medications during pregnancy, in preschool-age children, and in older children and adolescents.

Second, it is becoming apparent that newer medications may not represent better medications. Initial optimism for the most recent (and most expensive) drugs has been tempered by findings that they may not be more effective than the older agents, although they may present a different side effect profile. This realization has revived interest in the classic agents and in comparisons of therapeutic effectiveness not only among psychiatric medications but also between pharmacological and nonpharmacological treatments.

These developments signal a period of maturation in the field of psychopharmacology. It is perhaps to be expected that the rapid discovery of the major psychiatric medications will be followed by a more measured analysis of the progress and an appreciation of how much is yet to be accomplished. We are optimistic that this examination will result in new insights into the etiology of mental illness and that the future will bring even more effective treatments for these devastating disorders. Future editions of this text will parallel the progress.

MEDIA AND SUPPLEMENTS

A free companion Web site for *A Primer of Drug Action*, Twelfth Edition, is located at www.worthpublishers.com/Julien. This free Web site contains resources for both instructors and students and does not require any special access codes or passwords.

Also available is the *Computerized Test Bank* by Peter E. Simson, Miami University of Ohio. The *Test Bank* contains approximately 850 items in multiple-choice, true/false, and short-answer formats. Each question is keyed to the page in the book on which the answer is located. If you are an instructor and would like to order the *Test Bank*, contact your Worth Publishers sales representative.

Robert M. Julien, M.D., Ph.D.
Lake Oswego, Oregon
drsjulien@comcast.net

Claire Advokat, Ph.D.
Baton Rouge, Louisiana
cadvoka@lsu.edu

Joseph Comaty, Ph.D., M.P.
Baton Rouge, Louisiana
joseph.comaty@la.gov

A PRIMER OF **DRUG ACTION**

PART 1

Introduction to Psychopharmacology: How Drugs Interact with the Body and the Brain

Pharmacology is the science of how drugs affect the body. *Psychopharmacology*, a subdivision of pharmacology, is the study of how drugs specifically affect the brain and behavior. To understand the actions, behavioral uses, therapeutic uses, and abuse potentials of psychoactive drugs, we must necessarily understand how the body responds to the taking of a drug. This understanding involves the basic principles of drug absorption, distribution, metabolism, and excretion (collectively termed *pharmacokinetics*) as well as the interactions of a drug with its "receptor," or the structure with which the drug interacts to produce its effects (the area of study termed *pharmacodynamics*).

This book is specifically oriented to drugs that affect the brain and behavior. Therefore, it is an introduction to psychopharmacology, presenting not only drugs useful in treating psychological disorders but also drugs prone to compulsive use and abuse. The book begins with three chapters devoted to the fundamentals of drug action. Chapter 1 explores the area of pharmacokinetics, the movement of drug molecules into, through, and out of the body. It addresses such questions as the following: Once a drug arrives in the stomach (if taken orally), how and why does it gain access to the bloodstream? Once in the bloodstream, how is it distributed throughout the body? Is it distributed evenly? How is distribution reflected in the actions of the drug? Finally, how does the body eventually get rid of the drug?

Chapter 2 explores the area of pharmacodynamics. It examines the interaction between drugs and the receptors to which the drugs attach as well as how the attachment results in alterations in cell function and behavior. Receptors are described both structurally and functionally, and how drugs alter receptor structure and function is discussed. Finally, the ways in which such actions underlie the therapeutic effects and the side effects of drugs are illustrated.

Chapter 3 applies knowledge about basic pharmacology to the specifics of drug action on the brain and behavior. For readers without a background in neuroscience, the structure and function of the neuron are explained because psychoactive drugs produce their effects on various parts of neurons. We focus on the point of connection between two different neurons, an area called the *synapse*. By studying the process of synaptic transmission and specific neurotransmitters, we begin to understand the mode of action of psychoactive drugs as well as the complexity of brain functioning in both health and disease. Furthermore, this process of synaptic transmission is not a static process; rather, neurons have the ability to continually remodel themselves, a process called *synaptic plasticity*. Such a process is involved in learning and memory as well as in such disorders as anxiety and depression. A healthy, functioning brain is one that through this process of synaptic plasticity is continually remodeling itself in response to the environment. Healthy neurons continually form new synaptic contacts, maintaining the beautiful architecture that exists through healthy interactions with millions of other neurons.

Chapter 1

Pharmacokinetics: How Drugs Are Handled by the Body

When we have a headache, we take it for granted that after taking some aspirin our headache will probably disappear within 15 to 30 minutes. We also take it for granted that, unless we take more aspirin later, the headache may recur within 3 or 4 hours. This familiar scenario illustrates four basic processes in the branch of pharmacology called *pharmacokinetics*. Using the aspirin example, the four processes are as follows:

1. *Absorption* of the aspirin into the body from the swallowed tablet
2. *Distribution* of the aspirin throughout the body, including into a fetus if a female patient is pregnant at the time the drug is taken
3. *Metabolism* (detoxification or breakdown) of the drug as the aspirin that has exerted its analgesic effect is broken down into metabolites (by-products or waste products) that no longer exert any effect
4. *Elimination* of the metabolic waste products, usually in the urine

These four processes are sometimes abbreviated as ADME. In concert, they determine the *bioavailability* of a drug, that is, how much of the drug that is administered actually reaches its target.

The goal of this chapter is to introduce these processes of pharmacokinetics, concluding with discussion about how pharmacokinetics can be used to determine the time course of action for drugs. Because many drugs need to be taken chronically, for various periods of time, the chapter also explores the steady-state maintenance of therapeutic blood levels of drugs in the body and the usefulness of therapeutic drug monitoring. Finally, the chapter introduces the concepts of drug *tolerance* and drug *dependence*.

The understanding of pharmacokinetics, along with knowledge about the *dosage* taken, allows determination of the concentration of a drug at its *receptors* (sites of action) and the *intensity* of drug effect on the receptors as a function of time. Thus, pharmacokinetics in its simplest form describes the time course of a particular drug's actions—the time to onset and the duration of effect. Usually, the time course simply reflects the amount of *time* required for the rise and fall of the drug's concentration at the target site. Figure 1.1 illustrates the complexity of drug movement through the body and its equilibrium at its site of action.

The root *kinetics* in the word *pharmacokinetics* implies movement and time. As each of the drugs in this book is discussed, the focus is first on the time course of the drug's movement through the body, particularly its *half-life* and any complications that arise from alterations in its

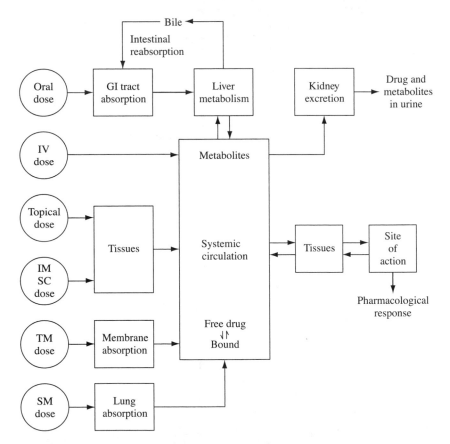

FIGURE 1.1 Schematic representation of the fate of a drug in the body. IM = intramuscular; IV = intravenous; TM = transmembrane; SC = subcutaneous; SM = smoked.

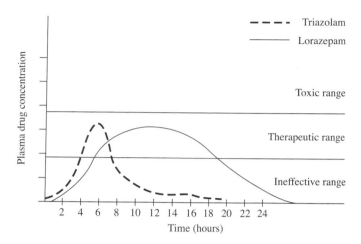

FIGURE 1.2 Theoretical blood levels of triazolam (a short-acting benzodiazepine) and lorazepam (a longer-acting benzodiazepine) over time following oral administration. Approximations for ineffective, therapeutic, and toxic blood levels are shown.

rate of metabolism. Knowledge of movement and time offers significant insight into the action of a drug. At the very least, it helps distinguish a particular drug from other related drugs. For example, the main difference between the two benzodiazepines (Chapter 7) lorazepam (Ativan) and triazolam (Halcion) is in their pharmacokinetics. Both these drugs depress the functioning of the brain, causing sedative and antianxiety effects. However, lorazepam persists for at least 24 hours in the body, while triazolam persists for only about 6 to 8 hours. If lorazepam is administered at bedtime for treatment of insomnia, daytime sedation the next day can be a problem, since lorazepam persists in the body through the next day. However, for longer, steady action (as might be useful in treating anxiety), lorazepam would be the superior agent to use.[1]

The kinetic differences between lorazepam and triazolam are illustrated in Figure 1.2, which shows three ranges: an ineffective range

---

[1]Most drugs used in medicine are known by two or even three names. The most complicated name for a drug is its *structural name*, which accurately describes its chemical structure in words. In this book, the chemical names for drugs are not used. The second name for a drug is its *generic name*, a somewhat easier-to-remember name, often derived from the structural name, given to the drug by its discoverer or manufacturer. After a drug's patent protection runs out (usually 17 years after the date of its patent registration by the manufacturer), any other generic drug manufacturer may legitimately sell the drug under this name. The third name is the drug's *trade name*, a unique name given to the drug by its original patent holder. Only that manufacturer can ever sell the drug under that name, even after the patent runs out and others sell the drug under its generic name. For example, many companies sell aspirin, a generic name for acetylsalicylic acid, the structural name. However, only Bayer Pharmaceuticals (the original company that patented acetylsalicylic acid) can call it Bayer Aspirin. In this book, when a drug is introduced, the generic name is given first and is not capitalized. The trade name follows in parentheses, is capitalized, and usually is not given again.

(where not enough drug is present to produce either sedative or antianxiety effects), a therapeutic range, and a toxic range (where sedation becomes excessive). Triazolam reaches peak blood level rapidly and is of short duration. Lorazepam, on the other hand, reaches peak blood level later and persists longer in the therapeutic range. In essence, pharmacokinetic differences account for these results and allow two similar drugs to be used to achieve quite different therapeutic goals.

Drug Absorption

The term *drug absorption* refers to processes and mechanisms by which drugs pass from the external world into the bloodstream. For any drug, a route of administration, a dose of the drug, and a dosage form (liquid, tablet, capsule, injection, patch, spray, or gum) must be selected that will both place the drug at its site of action in a pharmacologically effective concentration and maintain the concentration for an adequate period of time. Drugs are most commonly administered in one of six ways, which may be divided into two categories:

1. *Enteral* routes refer to administration involving the gastrointestinal (GI) tract:
   a. Orally (swallowed when taken by mouth)
   b. Rectally (embedded in a suppository, which is placed in the rectum)
2. *Parenteral* routes refer to administration that does not involve the GI tract:
   a. Injected (given in liquid form with a needle and syringe)
   b. Inhaled through the lungs as gases, as vapors, or as particles carried in smoke or in an aerosol
   c. Absorbed through the skin (usually as a drug-containing skin patch)
   d. Absorbed through mucous membranes (from "snorting," or sniffing, the drug, with the drug depositing on the oral or nasal mucosa)

Oral Administration

To be effective when administered orally, a drug must be soluble (able to dissolve) and stable in stomach fluid (not destroyed by gastric acids), enter the intestine, penetrate the lining of the stomach or intestine, and pass into the bloodstream. Because they are already in solution, drugs that are administered in liquid form tend to be absorbed more rapidly than those given in tablet or capsule form. When a drug is taken in solid form, both the rate at which it dissolves and its chemistry limit the rate of absorption. In some cases, rather than the active drug itself, the oral formulation contains a precursor (forerunner) of a drug, called a *prodrug*. A prodrug must undergo chemical conversion by metabolic processes before becoming an active pharmacological agent. An example of this type of medication is the drug lisdexamfetamine (Vyvanse), recently approved for the treatment of attention deficit/hyperactivity disorder (ADHD; Chapter 18).

After a tablet dissolves, the drug molecules contained within it are carried into the upper intestine, where they are absorbed across the intestinal mucosa by a process of *passive diffusion*, passing from an area of high concentration into an area of lower concentration. This process necessitates that the drug molecules, at least to some degree, be soluble in fat (be *lipid soluble*). In reality, even a small amount of lipid solubility allows for absorption after oral administration; the most lipid-soluble drugs are merely absorbed faster than less lipid-soluble drugs. In general, most psychoactive drugs have good solubility in the lipid linings of the stomach and intestine; therefore, about 75 percent (or more) of the amount of an orally administered psychoactive drug is absorbed into the bloodstream within about 1 to 3 hours after its administration.

There are only rare exceptions to this general rule. One involves the antidepressant/antianxiety drug buspirone (BuSpar; Chapter 7). This drug has limited clinical efficacy, primarily because most of it is rapidly broken down (metabolized) by a drug-metabolizing enzyme located in the walls of the stomach lining. This enzyme (called CYP-3A4, discussed later) reduces the oral absorption of buspirone by over 90 percent. However, should buspirone be taken with grapefruit juice, a component in the juice (furanocoumarin) inhibits the buspirone-metabolizing enzyme, allowing the drug to be more completely absorbed (Figure 1.3) and increasing its therapeutic utility (Lilja et al., 1998; Rheeders et al., 2006; Paine et al., 2006). Greenblatt and coworkers (2003) demonstrated increases in the absorption of the antianxiety drug diazepam (Valium) when taken with grapefruit juice, although the increase in diazepam absorption is not as great when it is taken with grapefruit juice as is the increase of absorption when buspirone is taken with grapefruit juice.

Although oral administration of drugs is common, it does have disadvantages. First, it may occasionally lead to vomiting and stomach distress. Second, although the amount of a drug that is put into a tablet or capsule can be calculated, how much of it will be absorbed into the bloodstream cannot always be accurately predicted because of genetic differences between individual people and because of differences in the manufacture of the drugs. Finally, the acid in the stomach destroys some orally administered drugs, such as the local anesthetics and insulin, before they can be absorbed. To be effective, those drugs must be administered by injection.

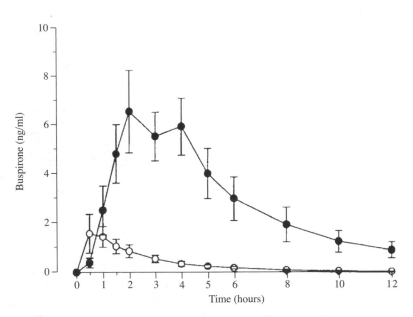

FIGURE 1.3 Plasma concentrations (mean and SEM) of buspirone (in nanograms per milliliter of plasma) in ten healthy volunteers after a single oral dose of 10 mg buspirone, after ingestion of 200 ml (about 7 oz) grapefruit juice (*solid circles*) or water (*open circles*) three times a day for two days, and on day 3 with buspirone administration 30 and 90 minutes later. [Data from Lilja et al. (1998).]

Rectal Administration

Although the primary route of drug administration is oral, some drugs are administered rectally (usually in suppository form) if the patient is vomiting, unconscious, or unable to swallow. However, absorption is often irregular, unpredictable, and incomplete, and many drugs irritate the membranes that line the rectum.

Administration by Inhalation

In recreational drug misuse and abuse, inhalation of drugs is a popular method of administration. Examples of drugs taken by this route include nicotine in tobacco cigarettes and tetrahydrocannabinol in marijuana, as well as smoked heroin, crack cocaine, crank methamphetamine, and the various inhalants of abuse, all of which are discussed at length later in the book. The popularity of inhalation as a route of administration follows from two observations:

1. Lung tissues have a large surface area through which large amounts of blood flow, allowing for rapid absorption of drugs from the lung into the blood (often within seconds).

2. Drugs absorbed into pulmonary (lung) capillaries are carried in the pulmonary veins directly to the left (arterial) side of the heart

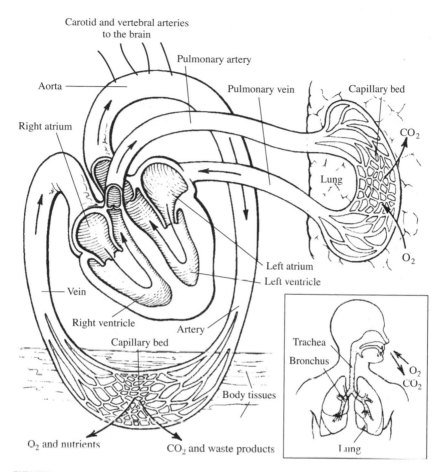

FIGURE 1.4 Heart and circulatory system. Blood returning from the systemic venous circulation to the heart enters the right atrium and flows into the right ventricle. With contraction of the heart, this blood is pumped into the pulmonary arteries leading to the lungs. Once in the pulmonary capillaries, carbon dioxide (CO_2) is lost and replaced by oxygen. The oxygenated blood returns to the heart in the pulmonary veins, which empty into the left atrium. With heart contraction, the oxygenated blood is pumped from the left ventricle into the aorta and is carried to the body tissues and brain, where oxygen and nutrients are exchanged in the systemic capillary beds. Oxygen and nutrients are supplied to the body tissues through the walls of the capillaries; CO_2 and other waste products are returned to the blood. The CO_2 is eliminated through the lungs, and the other waste products are metabolized in the liver and excreted in the urine.

(Figure 1.4) and from there directly into the aorta and the arteries carrying blood to the brain. As a result, drugs administered by inhalation may have an even faster onset of effect than drugs administered intravenously. If drugs administered in this fashion are behaviorally reinforcing, intoxicating, and subject to compulsive abuse, the rapid onset of effect can be intense, to say the least.

Administration Through Mucous Membranes

Occasionally, drugs are administered through the mucous membranes of the mouth or nose. A few examples:

- A heart patient taking nitroglycerine places the tablet under the tongue, where the drug is absorbed into the bloodstream rapidly and directly.
- Cocaine powder, when sniffed, adheres to the membranes on the inside of the nose and is absorbed directly into the bloodstream. (Cocaine is discussed in Chapter 12).
- Nasal decongestants are sprayed directly onto mucous membranes from which they are both absorbed and act locally to constrict the mucous membranes, relieving nasal congestion.
- Nicotine (Chapter 11) in snuff, nasal spray, or chewing-gum formulations is absorbed through the mucosal membranes directly into the bloodstream.
- Caffeine (Chapter 11) became available in 1999 in chewing-gum form; the caffeine is rapidly absorbed as the gum is chewed.
- For use before and after surgery on children, the opioid narcotic fentanyl (Sublimase; Chapter 10) became available in 1998 in lollipop form, so this pain-relieving drug can be provided without subjecting a child to a painful injection. As the lollipop is sucked, the drug is released and absorbed through the mucous membranes of the mouth. This form of administering fentanyl has also become popular for patients with disabling pain when orally administered pain relievers are insufficient and injection of opioid narcotics is too painful.
- A sublingual (placed under the tongue) combination of buprenorphine (an opioid narcotic) and naloxone (an opioid antagonist) for the office-based treatment of opioid dependency has recently been introduced. The combination product, called Suboxone, is discussed in Chapter 10. The buprenorphine is absorbed through the mucous membranes, but the antagonist, naloxone, is not. When the pill is administered sublingually, the desired narcotic effect is achieved. However, should the pill be crushed, dissolved, and injected, the antagonist, naloxone, precipitates drug withdrawal. This effect tends to discourage abuse of the buprenorphine and reduce illicit use, providing yet another example of how knowledge of pharmacokinetics can be used to therapeutic benefit in special circumstances.

Administration Through the Skin

Over the past several years, several prescribed medications have been incorporated into *transdermal patches* that adhere to the skin. A transdermal patch is a unique bandagelike therapeutic system that provides continuous, controlled release of a drug from a reservoir through a semipermeable membrane. The drug is slowly absorbed into the bloodstream at the area of contact. Following are some examples of drug-containing patches.

- Nicotine (used to deter smoking behaviors)
- Fentanyl (used to treat chronic pain)
- Nitroglycerine (used to prevent the symptoms of angina pectoris in patients with coronary artery disease)
- Clonidine (used to treat hypertension)
- Estrogen or other hormones (used to replace reduced hormones in postmenopausal women or for contraception).
- Scopolamine (used to prevent motion sickness)
- Selegiline (Emsam; used to treat depression; Chapter 5)
- Methylphenidate (Daytrana, a 9-hour patch used to treat attention-deficit/hyperactivity disorder in children; Chapter 18)

All these transdermal skin patches allow for slow, continuous absorption of the drug over hours or even days, potentially minimizing side effects associated with rapid rises and falls in plasma concentrations of the drug contained in the patch. In all cases, the drug is slowly, predictably, and continuously released from the liquid in the patch and absorbed into the systemic circulation, allowing the levels of drug in the plasma to remain relatively constant over the time of absorption.

Administration by Injection

Administration of drugs by injection can be *intravenous* (directly into a vein), *intramuscular* (directly into a muscle), or *subcutaneous* (just under the skin). Each of these routes of administration has its advantages and disadvantages (Table 1.1), but all share some features. In general, administration by injection produces a more prompt response than does oral administration because absorption is faster. Also, injection permits a more accurate dose because the unpredictable processes of absorption through the stomach and intestine are bypassed.

Administration of drugs by injection, however, has several drawbacks. First, the rapid rate of absorption leaves little time to respond to an unexpected drug reaction or accidental overdose. Second, administration by injection requires the use of sterile techniques. Hepatitis and AIDS are examples of diseases that can be transmitted as a drastic consequence of unsterile injection techniques. Third, once a drug is administered by injection, it cannot be recalled.

TABLE 1.1 Some characteristics of drug administration by injection

Route	Absorption pattern	Special utility	Limitations and precautions
Intravenous	Absorption circumvented Potentially immediate effects	Valuable for emergency use Permits titration of dosage Can administer large volumes and irritating substances when diluted	Increased risk of adverse effects Must inject solutions slowly as a rule Not suitable for oily solutions or insoluble substances
Intramuscular	Prompt action from aqueous solution Slow and sustained action from repository preparations	Suitable for moderate volumes, oily vehicles, and some irritating substances	Precluded during anticoagulant medication May interfere with interpretation of certain diagnostic tests (e.g., creatine phosphokinase)
Subcutaneous	Prompt action from aqueous solution Slow and sustained action from repository preparations	Suitable for some insoluble suspensions and for implantation of solid pellets	Not suitable for large volumes Possible pain or necrosis from irritating substance

Intravenous Administration. In an intravenous injection, a drug is introduced directly into the bloodstream. This technique avoids all the variables related to oral absorption. The injection can be made slowly, and it can be stopped instantaneously if untoward effects develop. In addition, the dosage can be extremely precise, and the practitioner can dilute and administer in large volumes drugs that at higher concentrations would be irritants to the muscles or blood vessels.

The intravenous route is the most dangerous of all routes of administration because it has the fastest speed of onset of pharmacological action. Too-rapid injection can be catastrophic, producing life-threatening reactions (such as collapse of respiration or of heart function). Also, allergic reactions, should they occur, may be extremely severe. Finally, drugs that are not completely solubilized before injection cannot usually be given intravenously because of the danger of blood clots or emboli forming. Infection and transmission of infectious diseases are an ever-present danger when sterile techniques are not employed.

Intramuscular Administration. Drugs that are injected into skeletal muscle (usually in the arm, thigh, or buttock) are generally absorbed fairly rapidly. Absorption of a drug from muscle is more rapid than absorption of the same drug from the stomach but slower than absorption of the drug administered intravenously. The absolute rate of absorption of a drug from muscle varies, depending on the rate of blood flow to the muscle, the solubility of the drug, the volume of the injection, and the solution in which the drug is dissolved and injected.

Intramuscular injections are of two types: (1) fairly rapid onset and short duration of action and (2) slow onset and prolonged action. In the former situation, the drug is dissolved in an aqueous (water) solution. Following injection, the water and dissolved drug are quite rapidly absorbed, with complete absorption occurring over a very few hours. In the latter situation, classically the drug is suspended in an oily solution. The oil and dissolved drug solution is only slowly absorbed, and complete absorption can take days or weeks. More recently, space-age manufacturing techniques have allowed the drug to be placed in bioabsorbable polymer microspheres, and a constant amount of drug is released each day for a period of a week or more (Risperdol Consta; Chapter 4). Similarly, the opioid narcotic antagonist naltrexone suspended in injected microcapsules releases a constant amount of drug into blood over a period of several weeks. This new product is marketed under the trade name Vivitrol and is indicated in the treatment of opioid-dependent patients (Chapter 10).

Subcutaneous Administration. Absorption of drugs that have been injected under the skin (subcutaneously) is rapid. The exact rate depends mainly on the ease of blood vessel penetration and the rate of blood flow through the skin. Irritating drugs should not be injected subcutaneously because they may cause severe pain and damage to local tissue. The usual precautions to maintain sterility should be applied.

Drug Distribution

Once absorbed into the bloodstream, a drug is distributed throughout the body by the circulating blood, passing across various barriers to reach its target, that is, its site of action (its receptors). At any given time, only a very small portion of the total amount of a drug that is in the body is actually in contact with its receptors (see Figure 1.1). Most of the administered drug is found in areas of the body that are remote from the drug's site of action. For example, in the case of a psychoactive drug, most of the drug circulates outside the brain and therefore does not contribute directly to its pharmacological effect. This wide distribution often accounts for many of the side effects of a drug. *Side effects* are results that are different from the primary, or therapeutic, effect for which a drug is taken.

Action of the Bloodstream

Every minute in the average-size adult, the heart pumps a volume of blood that is roughly equal to the total amount of blood in the circulatory system. Thus, the entire blood volume circulates in the body about once every minute. Once absorbed into the bloodstream, a drug is rapidly (usually within the 1-minute circulation time) distributed throughout the circulatory system.

A schematic diagram of the circulatory system is presented in Figure 1.4. Blood returning to the heart through the veins is first pumped into the pulmonary (lung) circulation system, where carbon dioxide is removed and replaced by oxygen. The oxygenated blood then returns to the heart and is pumped into the great artery (the aorta). From there blood flows into the smaller arteries and finally into the capillaries, where nutrients (and drugs) are exchanged between the blood and the cells of the body. After blood passes through the capillaries, it is collected by the veins and returned to the heart to circulate again. Psychoactive drugs quite quickly become evenly distributed throughout the bloodstream, diluted not only by blood but also by the total amount of water in the body.

If a drug is taken orally, it passes through the cells lining the GI tract and then through the liver; from there the drug enters the central circulation and is carried to the heart to be distributed throughout the body. Occasionally, drug-metabolizing enzymes in the cells of either the GI tract or the liver can markedly reduce the amount of drug that reaches the bloodstream. This process is called *first-pass metabolism*. Examples of first-pass metabolism of the drugs buspirone and diazepam were presented earlier in this chapter. Another example involves ethyl alcohol and the enzyme that metabolizes the alcohol. This enzyme is called *alcohol dehydrogenase*. It is found in the cells lining the GI tract and in cells of the liver. As we will see in Chapter 13, women have less of this enzyme in the GI tract cells and therefore exhibit higher blood alcohol levels for a given amount of alcohol ingested (corrected for body weight) than do men.

When injected (by whatever route), absorbed transdermally, or absorbed from mucous membranes, a drug bypasses intestinal absorption, rapidly enters veins, and is carried in blood to the right side of the heart (with minimal amounts passing initially through the liver). The drug then circulates through the pulmonary vessels, returns to the left side of the heart, and finally travels through the aorta to the brain and the body. Sodium pentothal is an example of an injected general anesthetic. Injected intravenously, it circulates to the heart, then the lungs, and then the brain (see Figure 1.4). After injection, consciousness is lost within about 30 seconds.

Inhaled drugs are absorbed from the lungs and carried in pulmonary veins directly to the left side of the heart and, from there, rapidly to the brain. The effects of smoked tobacco or smoked marijuana are felt within a breath or two.

Body Membranes That Affect Drug Distribution

Four types of membranes in the body affect drug distribution: (1) cell membranes, (2) walls of the capillary vessels in the circulatory system, (3) blood-brain barrier, and (4) placental barrier.

Cell Membranes. To be absorbed from the intestine or to gain access to the interior of a cell, a drug must penetrate the cell membranes. The structure and properties of cell membranes determine their permeability to drugs. In Figure 1.5, the two layers of ovals represent the water-soluble head groups of complex lipid

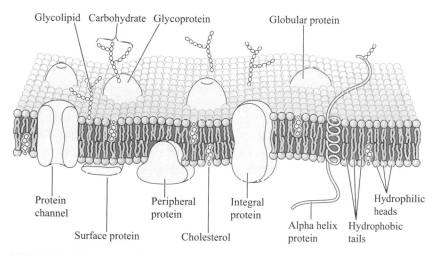

FIGURE 1.5 Diagrammatic representation of a cell membrane, a phospholipid bilayer in which cholesterol and protein molecules are embedded. Both globular and helical kinds of protein traverse the bilayer. Cholesterol molecules tend to keep the tails of the phospholipids relatively fixed and orderly in the regions closest to the hydrophilic phospholipid heads; the parts of the tails closer to the core of the membrane move about freely.

molecules called *phospholipids*. The phospholipid heads form a rather continuous layer on both the inside and the outside of the cell membrane. The wavy lines that extend from the heads into the membrane are the lipid chains of the phospholipid molecules. Therefore, for our present purposes, the interior of the cell membrane can be considered to consist of a sea of lipid in which large proteins are suspended.

Cell membranes, consisting of protein and fat, provide a physical barrier that is permeable to small, lipid-soluble drug molecules but is impermeable to large, lipid-insoluble drug molecules. Cell membranes (as barriers to the absorption and distribution of drugs) are important for the passage of drugs (1) from the stomach and intestine into the bloodstream, (2) from the fluid that closely surrounds tissue cells into the interior of cells, (3) from the interior of cells back into the body water, and (4) from the kidneys back into the bloodstream.

Capillaries. Within a minute or so of entering the bloodstream, a drug is distributed fairly evenly throughout the entire blood volume. From there, drugs leave the bloodstream and are exchanged (in equilibrium) between blood capillaries and body tissues. Figure 1.6 shows a cross-sectional diagram and a schematic of a capillary. Capillaries are tiny, cylindrical blood vessels with walls that are formed by a thin, single layer of cells packed tightly together. Between the cells are small pores (fenestra) that allow passage of small molecules between blood and the body tissues. The diameter of these pores is between 90 and 150 angstroms (Å), which is larger than most drug molecules. Thus, most drugs freely leave the blood through these pores in the capillary membranes, passing along their concentration gradient until equilibrium is

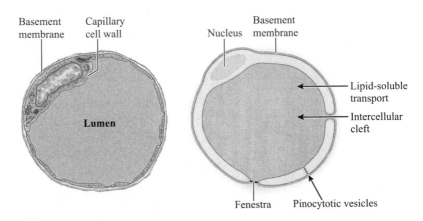

FIGURE 1.6 Cross section of a typical capillary (*left*) and the schematic (*right*), showing the pores (fenestra) and indicating that lipid-soluble substances can pass through the cell wall.

established between the concentrations of drug in the blood and in body tissues and water.

The transport of drug molecules between plasma and body tissues is independent of lipid solubility because the membrane pores are large enough for even fat-insoluble drug molecules to penetrate. However, the pores in the capillary membrane are not large enough to permit the red blood cells and the plasma proteins to leave the bloodstream. Thus, the only drugs that do not readily penetrate capillary pores are drugs that bind to plasma proteins. The rate at which drug molecules enter specific body tissues depends on two factors: the rate of blood flow through the tissue and the ease with which drug molecules pass through the capillary membranes.

Because blood flow is greatest to the brain and much less to the bones, joints, and fat deposits, drug distribution generally follows a similar pattern (Figure 1.7). An example might be appropriate. When marijuana is smoked, the active drug, tetrahydrocannabinol (THC; Chapter 14), achieves plasma concentrations of about 10 to 20 nanograms of drug per milliliter of plasma (ng/ml) soon after initiation of smoking. Within about 30 minutes, it achieves levels of about 50 to 100 ng/ml, which fall off within 1 hour to less than 5 to 10 ng/ml because the drug is rapidly taken up into body fat. From there, it slowly returns to plasma and is metabolized to an inactive metabolite (carboxy-THC) that is excreted in the urine.

Blood-Brain Barrier. The brain requires a protected environment to function normally, and a specialized structural barrier, called the

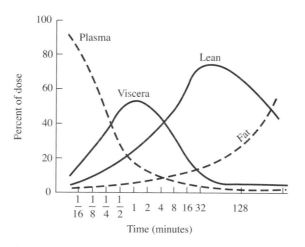

FIGURE 1.7 Diagrammatic representation of the distribution of a lipid-soluble drug (thiopental, a barbiturate discussed in Chapter 7) in blood plasma, body fat, lean body mass (muscle), and visceral tissues at various times after intravenous injection of the drug.

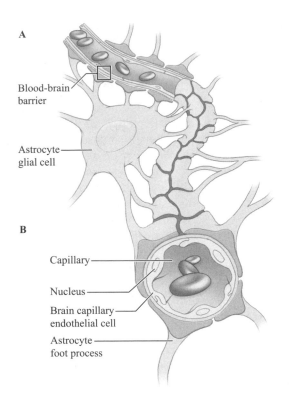

FIGURE 1.8   Cellular basis of the blood-brain barrier. **A.** Blood and brain are separated by capillary cells packed tightly together and by a fatty barrier called the glial sheath, which is made up of extensions (glial feet) from nearby astrocyte cells. A drug diffusing from blood to brain must move through the cells of the capillary wall because there are tight junctions rather than pores between the cells; the drug must then move through the fatty glial sheath. **B.** Cross section of a brain capillary.

blood-brain barrier (BBB), plays a key role in maintaining this environment (Figure 1.8). In contrast to capillaries in most of the body, the capillary walls in the brain do not have pores. The endothelial cells that make up the capillary walls are tightly joined together and covered on the outside by a fatty barrier called the *glial sheath*, which arises from nearby astrocyte cells.

Thus, to reach the neurons, a drug leaving the capillaries in the brain has to traverse both the wall of the capillary itself (because there are no pores to pass through) and the membranes of the astrocytes. Therefore, the rate of passage of a drug into the brain is generally determined by two factors: (1) the size of the drug molecule and (2) its lipid (fat) solubility. Large drugs penetrate poorly, while small, fat-soluble drugs penetrate rapidly. Oxygen is small enough and most psychoactive drugs are both small enough and sufficiently lipid soluble to cross the BBB. Drugs that cannot cross the BBB are restricted to structures outside the central nervous system (CNS). Penicillin is an example of such a drug. It does not cross the BBB, and its effectiveness as an antibiotic is restricted to infections located outside the brain.

Unfortunately, some other lipid-soluble drugs, like steroids and beta blockers, are also unable to pass through capillary walls, because they are detected as foreign and expelled by cellular export pumps (of which at least 15 are known), which protect the brain from toxins. Larger molecules, such as glucose, amino acids, and vitamins, reach the brain because they are carried by special transport systems out of the capillaries. Even larger substances like iron and insulin can be transported across the capillary wall by a process called *transcytosis*. In this situation, the substances attach to a receptor that is located in the cell wall membrane. A small segment of this membrane then forms a vesicle, which crosses over to, and fuses with, the membrane on the opposite side of the capillary wall, after which the receptor releases the substance into the brain.

Unfortunately, according to Pardridge (2003) only a few diseases, such as depression and mania, schizophrenia, chronic pain, and epilepsy, consistently respond to molecules that can cross the BBB. In contrast, 98 percent of drugs that would have some effect on the nervous system cannot cross the BBB. Many serious brain disorders do not respond to the conventional lipid-soluble small-molecule model, including Alzheimer's disease, stroke, brain and spinal cord injury, brain cancer, HIV infections of the brain, various ataxia-producing disorders, amyotrophic lateral sclerosis, multiple sclerosis, Huntington's disease, and childhood inborn genetic errors of the brain. Researchers are trying to develop ways in which to "trick" the BBB and "sneak" therapeutic drugs into the brain. Efforts are being made to inhibit specific export pumps or to devise lipid vesicles that could carry drug molecules inside their hollow cores and slide through the capillary walls. Perhaps someday we might be able to overcome the constraints of the BBB and deliver medications for all types of brain disorders.

Chapter 12 discusses amphetamine- and cocaine-induced disruptions of the BBB, a mechanism now thought to be responsible for their neurotoxic effect.

Placental Barrier. Among all the membrane systems of the body, the placental membranes are unique, separating two distinct human beings with differing genetic compositions and differing sensitivities to drugs. The fetus obtains essential nutrients and eliminates metabolic waste products through the placenta without depending on its own organs, many of which are not yet functioning. The dependence of the fetus on the mother places the fetus at the mercy of the placenta when foreign substances (such as drugs or toxins) appear in the mother's blood (Gilstrap and Little, 1998). The placental barrier is discussed further in the discussions of individual drugs.

A schematic representation of the placental network, which transfers substances between the mother and the fetus, is shown in Figure 1.9. In general, the mature placenta consists of a network of vessels and pools of maternal blood into which protrude treelike or fingerlike villi (projections) that contain the blood capillaries of the fetus. Oxygen and nutrients travel from the mother's blood to that of the fetus, while carbon dioxide and other waste products travel from the blood of the fetus to the mother's blood.

The membranes that separate fetal blood from maternal blood in the intervillous space resemble, in their general permeability, the cell membranes that are found elsewhere in the body. In other words, drugs cross the placenta primarily by passive diffusion. Fat-soluble substances (including all psychoactive drugs) diffuse readily, rapidly, and without limitation. The view that the placenta is a barrier to drugs is inaccurate. A more appropriate approximation is that the fetus is to at least some extent exposed to essentially all drugs taken by the mother.

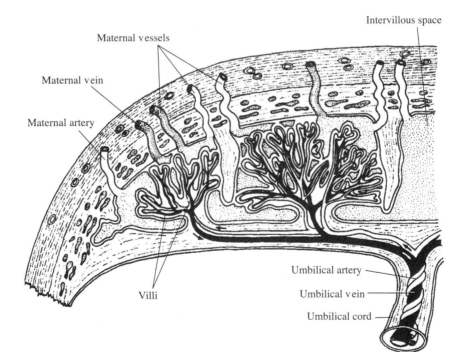

FIGURE 1.9 Placental network separating the blood of mother and fetus. Note the close relationship between fetal and maternal blood in the villus.

As a general rule, all psychoactive drugs (and all those discussed in this book) will be present in the fetus at a concentration quite similar to that in the mother's bloodstream. However, the presence of the drug in the fetus is not necessarily detrimental to the fetus. Some drugs certainly are detrimental, and their use should be avoided in women who are or might become pregnant. Ethyl alcohol is an obvious example. Many psychoactive medicines have been shown to be relatively safe to fetal growth and development when taken by a pregnant female. The effects of specific psychoactive drugs on the fetus is presented in Chapter 18.

Termination of Drug Action

Routes through which drugs can leave the body include (1) the kidneys, (2) the lungs, (3) the bile, and (4) the skin. Excretion through the lungs occurs only with highly volatile or gaseous agents, such as the general anesthetics and, in small amounts, alcohol ("alcohol breath"). Drugs that are passed through the bile and into the intestine are usually reabsorbed into the bloodstream from the intestine. Also, small amounts of a few drugs can pass through the skin and be excreted in sweat (perhaps 10 to 15 percent of the total amount of the drugs). However, most drugs leave the body in urine, either as the unchanged molecule or as a broken-down *metabolite* of the original drug. More correctly, *the major route of drug elimination from the body is renal (urinary) excretion of drug metabolites produced by the hepatic (liver) biodegradation of the drug.*[2]

Psychoactive drugs are usually too lipid soluble to be excreted passively with the excretion of urine. They have to be transformed into metabolites that are more water soluble, bulkier, less lipid soluble, and (usually) less biologically active (even inactive) when compared with the parent molecule (the molecule that was originally ingested and absorbed).[3]

Thus, for a lipid-soluble drug to be eliminated, it must be metabolically transformed (by enzymes located in the liver) into a form that can

[2]When evaluating urine for the presence of drugs of abuse, inactive drug metabolites rather than active drug are found in the urine. It is often unclear whether there is a correlation between the presence of the metabolite in urine and active drug in plasma *at the time the urine sample was taken.*

[3]Some drugs are exceptions: an administered drug may be metabolized into an "active" metabolite, which is at least as active and possibly more active and may have a longer duration of action than the parent drug. Examples in psychopharmacology include diazepam (Valium; Chapter 7), which is metabolized to nordiazepam, and fluoxetine (Prozac; Chapter 5), which is metabolized to norfluoxetine. In both cases, the parent drug has an effect that lasts for two or three days, while the metabolite is active for over a week, until it is eventually biotransformed to an inactive compound that can be excreted.

be excreted rapidly and reliably. This biotransformation relieves the body of the burden of foreign chemicals and is essential to our survival. Such mechanisms are not new. Biotransformation of foreign substances probably originated millions of years ago when humans invented fire and began to eat the char of barbecued meat, ingesting and absorbing substances that were foreign and potentially toxic to the body.

Role of the Kidneys in Drug Elimination

Physiologically, our kidneys perform two major functions. First, they excrete most of the products of body metabolism; second, they closely regulate the levels of most of the substances found in body fluids. The kidneys are a pair of bean-shaped organs that lie at the rear of the abdominal cavity at the level of the lower ribs. The outer portion of the kidney is made up of more than a million functional units, called *nephrons* (Figure 1.10). Each nephron consists of a knot of capillaries (the *glomerulus*) through which blood flows from the renal artery to the renal vein. The glomerulus is surrounded by the opening of the

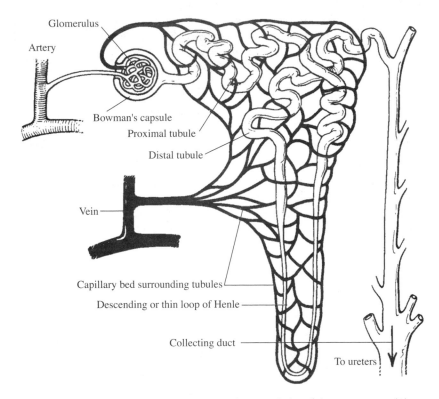

FIGURE 1.10 Nephron within a kidney. Note the complexity of the structure and the intimate relation between the blood supply and the nephron. Each kidney is composed of more than a million nephrons.

nephron (*Bowman's capsule*), into which fluid flows as it filters out of the capillaries. Pressure of the blood in the glomerulus causes fluid to leave the capillaries and flow into the Bowman's capsule, from which it flows through the tubules of the nephrons into a duct that collects fluid from several nephrons. The fluid from the collecting ducts is eventually passed through the ureters and into the urinary bladder, which is emptied periodically.

In an adult, about 1 liter (1000 cubic centimeters) of plasma is filtered into the nephrons of the kidneys each minute. Left behind in the bloodstream are blood cells, plasma proteins, and the remaining plasma. As the filtered fluid (water) flows through the nephrons, most of it is reabsorbed into the plasma. By the time fluid reaches the collecting ducts and bladder, only 0.1 percent remains to be excreted. Because about 1 cubic centimeter per minute of urine is formed, 99.9 percent of filtered fluid is therefore reabsorbed.

Lipid-soluble drugs can easily cross the membranes of renal tubular cells, and they are reabsorbed along with the 99.9 percent of reabsorbed water. Drug reabsorption occurs passively, along a developing concentration gradient—the drug becomes concentrated inside the nephrons (as a result of water reabsorption), and the drugs are themselves reabsorbed with water back into plasma. Thus, the kidneys alone are not capable of eliminating psychoactive drugs from the body; some other mechanism must overcome this process of passive renal reabsorption of the drug.

Role of the Liver in Drug Metabolism

Since the kidneys are not capable of ridding the body of drugs, the reabsorbed drug is eventually picked up by liver cells (*hepatocytes*) and enzymatically biotransformed (by enzymes located in these hepatocytes) into metabolites that are usually less fat soluble, less capable of being reabsorbed, and therefore capable of being excreted in urine. As the drug is carried to the liver (by blood flowing in the hepatic artery and portal vein), a portion is cleared from blood by the hepatocytes and metabolized to by-products that are then returned to the bloodstream (Figure 1.11). The metabolites are then carried in the bloodstream to the kidneys, are filtered into the renal tubules, and are poorly reabsorbed, remaining in the urine for excretion. Mechanisms involved in drug metabolism by hepatocytes are complex, but they have gained increased importance in psychopharmacology because of recently described drug interactions involving certain antidepressant drugs (Chapter 5) (Greenblatt et al., 1999).

The *cytochrome P450 enzyme family,* physically located in hepatocytes (with a few located in the cells lining the GI tract), is the major system involved in drug metabolism. This gene family originated more than 3.5 billion years ago and has diversified to accomplish the

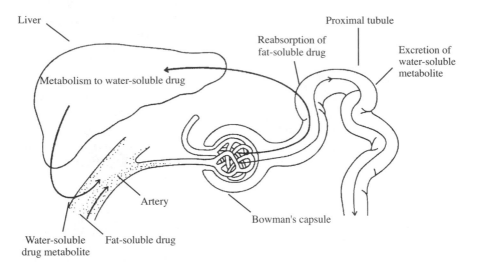

FIGURE 1.11 How the liver and kidneys interact to eliminate drugs from the body. Drugs may be filtered into the kidney, reabsorbed into the bloodstream, and carried to the liver for metabolic transformation to a more water-soluble compound that, having been filtered into the kidney, cannot be reabsorbed and is therefore excreted in urine.

metabolism (detoxification) of environmental chemicals, food toxins, and drugs—all foreign to our needs. Thus, the cytochrome P450 enzyme system (of which hundreds exist and about 50 of which are functionally active in humans) can detoxify a chemically diverse group of foreign substances. Several P450 enzyme families can be found within any given hepatocyte.

A few of these enzyme families, particularly cytochrome families 1, 2, and 3 (designated *CYP-1*, *CYP-2*, and *CYP-3*), encode enzymes involved in most drug biotransformations. By definition, since these three families promote the breakdown of numerous drugs and toxins, enzyme specificity is low (the enzymes are nonspecific in action). Thus, the body is enzymatically capable of metabolizing multiple different drugs. CYP-3A4 (a subfamily of CYP-3) catalyzes about 50 percent of drug biotransformations (Figure 1.12); this variant is found not only in the liver but also in the GI tract, as we saw with the metabolism of buspirone. CYP-2D6 catalyzes about 20 percent of drugs, and CYP-2C variants catalyze an additional 20 percent. Other CYP enzyme variants are responsible for metabolizing the remaining 10 percent of drugs.

Factors Affecting Drug Biotransformation

Several different factors can alter the rate at which drugs are metabolized, either increasing or decreasing the rate of drug elimination from the body. In general, *genetic, environmental, cultural,* and *physiological factors* can be involved (Lin et al., 2001).

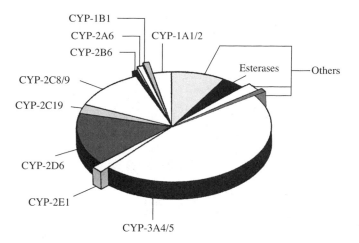

CYP-1B1
CYP-2A6
CYP-2B6
CYP-1A1/2
CYP-2C8/9
Esterases — Others
CYP-2C19
CYP-2D6
CYP-2E1
CYP-3A4/5

FIGURE 1.12 The approximate proportion of drugs metabolized by the major hepatic CYP enzymes. The relative size of each pie section indicates the estimated percentage of metabolism that each enzyme contributes to the metabolism of drugs.

First, it is now becoming apparent that genetic variations may affect how different people respond to medications. Psychogenetic testing allows prescribers to consider genetic information from patients in selecting medications and doses for certain psychiatric disorders. As one example, the AmpliChip CYP-450 test screens for variations of two genes, CYP-2D6 and CYP-2C19 (deLeon et al., 2006; deLeon, 2009). A recent study examining clinicians' experiences with this system in psychiatric practice found it had a supporting role in decisions about drug doses (Dunbar et al., 2009).

A simple example may be in order. Genetic DNA testing can now identify how a person may metabolize several drugs of different therapeutic classes, including antidepressants, analgesics, and antipsychotics. In general, DNA testing using a simple mouth swab can identify whether a person is a normal metabolizer of a specific drug, a slow metabolizer, or a fast metabolizer. Results provide a scientific basis for understanding why a person might have an unexpectedly toxic reaction after therapeutic doses of a drug or, on the other hand, might fail to respond to what was thought to be a therapeutic dose (Table 1.2).[4]

Second, if more than one drug is present in the body, the drugs may interact with one another either in a therapeutically beneficial way or in a way that can adversely affect the patient. Beneficially, two drugs can have additive therapeutic effects; for example, improving antidepressant or antianxiety treatment. In the liver, however, one drug

[4]For a Web-based introduction to genetic DNA testing for drug metabolism, see www.genemedrx.com.

TABLE 1.2 Significance of genetic testing in the determination of drug dosage for an antidepressant

	Normal metabolizer	Slow metabolizer	Fast metabolizer
Genetic variation	Your genes produce a typical amount of enzyme.	Your genes produce too little enzyme.	Your genes produce too much enzyme.
Effects on you	The antidepressant helps your depression and causes few side effects.	The antidepressant builds up in your body, causing intolerable side effects.	The antidepressant is eliminated too quickly, providing little or no improvement in depression.
Treatment options	Follow the recommended dosage.	Switch anti-depressants or reduce your dosage.	Switch anti-depressants or increase your dosage.

can either increase or reduce the rate of metabolism of a second drug, reducing or increasing the blood level of the second drug. For example, *carbamazepine* (Tegretol; Chapter 6) is particularly effective in stimulating the production of the drug-metabolizing enzyme CYP-3A3/4 in the liver (a process called *enzyme induction*), inducing an apparent *metabolic tolerance* to other drugs metabolized by CYP-3A3/4. In essence, in the presence of carbamazepine, the rate at which all drugs metabolized by the CYP-3A3/4 enzymes increases. Therefore, metabolic drug *tolerance* develops as the blood level of drug for a given amount taken falls more rapidly than would be expected if tolerance had not developed. Thus, increasing doses of a drug must be administered to maintain the same level of drug in the plasma and to produce the same effect produced by previously administered smaller doses. In essence, the second drug becomes less effective because it is metabolized more rapidly as a result of the increased amount of metabolic enzyme. One consequence of this development of *metabolic tolerance* is that any other drug that is metabolized by the same enzyme will also be broken down more rapidly. As a result, those drugs will also exert less of an effect, a phenomenon termed *cross-tolerance*.

In contrast to carbamazepine (which increases the rate of metabolism of other drugs), some psychoactive drugs *depress* the activity of the CYP enzyme that metabolizes other drugs metabolized by the same enzyme. This process *increases* the blood level of the other drugs and unexpectedly increases their toxicity. For example, antidepressants that are selective serotonin reuptake inhibitors (SSRIs), such as fluoxetine (Prozac; Chapter 5), inhibit the enzyme CYP-2D6, increasing the toxicity of several other types of antidepressants and certain antipsychotic drugs.

Similarly, the antibipolar drug *valproic acid* (Chapter 6) inhibits the metabolism of lamotrigine (Lamictal, another antibipolar drug), increasing the plasma level of lamotrigine and thus potentially increasing its toxicity. Such drug interactions are potentially severe and have been known to produce fatalities. As an interesting aside, the pain-relieving drug codeine (Chapter 10) needs to be metabolized by CYP-2D6 into morphine, which is codeine's active metabolite responsible for its analgesic effect. Some SSRIs (for example, fluoxetine and paroxetine) block this metabolic conversion of codeine to morphine, and for patients taking SSRIs codeine is ineffective as a pain-relieving agent.

Preskorn and Flockhart (2009) present a recent review of psychiatric drug interactions. Spina and Perucca (2002) discuss the pharmacokinetic interactions between widely used psychotropic medications. DeVane (2006) and Preskorn and Werder (2006) debate the significance of drug interactions involving antidepressant drugs.

Other Routes of Drug Elimination

Other routes for excreting drugs include the air we exhale, bile, sweat, saliva, and breast milk. Many drugs and drug metabolites may be found in these secretions, but their concentrations are usually low, and these routes are not usually considered primary paths of drug elimination. Perhaps clinically significant, however, is the transfer of psychoactive drugs (such as nicotine) from mothers to their breast-fed babies (Chapter 18).

Time Course of Drug Distribution and Elimination: Concept of Drug Half-Life

Knowledge about the relationship between the time course of drug action in the body and its pharmacological effects is essential for (1) predicting the optimal dosages and dose intervals needed to reach a therapeutic effect, (2) maintaining a therapeutic drug level for the desired period of time, and (3) determining the time needed to eliminate the drug. The relationship between the pharmacological response to a drug and its concentration in blood is fundamental to pharmacology. With psychoactive drugs, the level of drug in the blood closely approximates the level of drug at the drug's site of action in the brain.

Figure 1.13 illustrates the time-concentration relationship for a drug that is injected intravenously and therefore reaches peak plasma concentration immediately. For our purposes here, intravenous injection removes the variability involved with oral absorption and slow

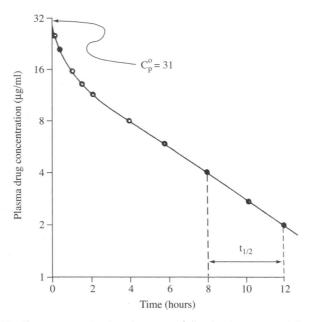

FIGURE 1.13 Plasma concentration time curve following intravenous injection of a drug. In this example, drug concentrations are measured in plasma every 30 minutes for the first 2 hours following drug injection, then every 2 hours until 12 hours after injection. Over the first 2 hours, redistribution exists as the drug leaves plasma and enters body tissues and equilibrates with those tissues. After redistribution, the fall in plasma level is linear, exhibiting a metabolic half-life of 4 hours, regardless of the plasma concentration of the drug.

attainment of peak blood levels. Note that after the immediate peak in the plasma concentration, the concentration appears to fall very rapidly, followed by a slower decline in concentration. The rapid fall reflects the rapid redistribution of the drug out of the bloodstream into body tissues. This process of *redistribution* takes only minutes to spread a drug nearly equally throughout the major tissues of the body. The upper left portion of the curve in Figure 1.13 represents the rapid-distribution phase, which lasts only a few minutes. The shallower part of the curve represents the slower, prolonged decrease in the level of drug in the blood required for the body to detoxify the drug by hepatic metabolism. (The plasma concentration of the drug metabolites is not illustrated.) The calculated elimination half-life is a measure of this process, and it allows the time course of drug action to be determined.

Figure 1.13 shows that the elimination half-life of the drug is about 4 hours (the time for the blood level to fall from 4 μg/ml to 2 μg/ml). The 4-hour half-life then remains constant over time. In other words, it takes the same amount of time for the blood level to fall from 8 μg/ml to 4 μg/ml as it does to fall from 4 μg/ml to 2 μg/ml or

TABLE 1.3 Half-life calculations

Number of half-lives	Amount of drug in the body	
	Percent eliminated	Percent remaining
0	0	100
1	50	50
2	75	25
3	87.5	12.5
4	93.8	6.2
5	96.9	3.1
6	98.4	1.6

from 2 μg/ml to 1 μg/ml. Thus, a different absolute amount of drug is metabolized within each half-life; the time interval remains constant.

The knowledge of a drug's half-life is important because it tells us how long a drug remains in the body. As shown in Table 1.3, it takes four half-lives for 94 percent of a drug to be eliminated by the body and six half-lives for 98 percent of the drug to be eliminated. At that point, a person is, for most practical purposes, drug free. It is important to remember that even though the blood level of the drug is reduced by 75 percent after two half-lives, the drug persists in the body at low levels for at least six half-lives. The so-called drug hangover is a result.

Throughout this book, drug half-lives are cited to describe the duration of action of psychoactive drugs in the body and allow comparisons between drugs with similar actions but differing half-lives. Most drug half-lives are measured in hours; others are measured in days, and recovery from the drug may take a week or more. For example, the elimination half-life of diazepam (Valium; Chapter 7) is about 30 hours in a healthy young adult (Figure 1.14), much longer in the elderly. The half-life of its active metabolite (nordiazepam, not illustrated in Figure 1.14) is even longer, on the order of several days to a week. The elderly exhibit even more prolongation of the half-lives of both diazepam and nordiazepam; the duration of action can be 4 weeks or even longer.

Note that drug half-life is the *time* for the plasma level of drug to fall by 50 percent. Thus, half-life is independent of the absolute level of drug in blood: the level falls by 50 percent every half-life, regardless of how many molecules of drug were actually metabolized during that time. In such cases, called *first-order elimination* (or *kinetics*), the metabolism rate of the drug is a constant fraction of the drug remaining in the body, rather than a constant amount of drug per hour. Therefore, a varying amount of drug is metabolized with each half-life

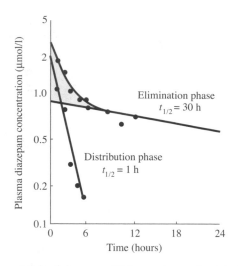

FIGURE 1.14 Plasma levels of diazepam (Valium, a benzodiazepine) following a single intravenous dose. The fast (distribution) phase has a half-life of about 1 hour. The slower, metabolic elimination phase shows a half-life of 30 hours. The long half-life of the active diazepam metabolite nordiazepam is not shown.

(fewer actual molecules are metabolized per half-life as the plasma level of drug falls).

One of the rare exceptions to this concept is the metabolism of ethyl alcohol by the enzyme alcohol dehydrogenase. Here, a constant amount of alcohol is metabolized per hour, regardless of the absolute amount of alcohol present in blood, and the blood level falls in a straight line. (The metabolism of alcohol is discussed in Chapter 13.)[5]

Drug Half-Life, Accumulation, and Steady State

The biological half-life of a drug is not only the time required for the drug concentration in blood to fall by one-half; it is also the determinant of the length of time necessary to reach a steady-state concentration (Figure 1.15). If a second full dose of drug is administered before the body has eliminated the first dose, the total amount of drug in the body and the peak level of the drug in the blood will be greater than the total amount and peak level produced by the first dose. For example, if 100 milligrams (mg) of a drug with a 4-hour half-life were administered at 12 noon, 50 mg of drug would remain in the body at 4 P.M. If an additional 100 mg of the drug were then taken at 4 P.M.,

---

[5]Usually, about 10 cubic centimeters (cc) of absolute alcohol are metabolized per hour, regardless of blood level. This relationship is termed *zero-order* kinetics and is discussed in Chapter 13.

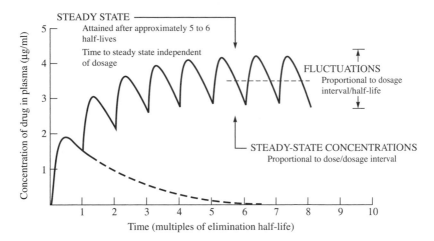

FIGURE 1.15 Plasma drug concentrations during repeated oral administration of a drug at intervals equal to its elimination half-life. The heavy dashed curve illustrates elimination if only a single dose is given. Because only 50 percent of each dose is eliminated before the next dose is given, the drug accumulates, reaching steady-state concentration in five to six half-lives. The sinusoidal curve shows the maximal and minimal drug concentrations at the beginning and end of each dosage interval, respectively. The light dashed line illustrates the average concentration achieved at steady state.

75 mg of drug would remain in the body at 8 P.M. (25 mg of the first dose and 50 mg of the second). If this administration schedule were continued, the amount of drug in the body would continue to increase until a plateau (steady-state) concentration was reached.

In general, the time to reach *steady-state concentration* (the level of drug achieved in the blood with repeated, regular-interval dosing) is about six times the drug's elimination half-life and is independent of the actual dosage of the drug. In one half-life, a drug reaches 50 percent of the concentration that will eventually be achieved. After two half-lives, the drug achieves 75 percent concentration; at three half-lives, the drug achieves the initial 50 percent of the third dose, the next 25 percent from the second dose, plus half of the remaining 25 percent from the first dose. At 98.4 percent (the concentration achieved after six half-lives), the drug concentration is essentially at steady state. This is the rationale behind the general rule. The steady-state concentration is achieved when the amount administered per unit time equals the amount eliminated per unit time. The interdependent variables that determine the ultimate concentration (or steady-state blood level of drug) are the dose (which determines the blood level but not the time to steady state), the dose interval, the half-life of the drug, and other more complex factors that can affect drug elimination.

In summary, steady, regular-interval dosing leads to a predictable accumulation, with a steady-state concentration reached after about six half-lives; the magnitude of the concentration is proportional to dose and dosage interval. Clinically, these factors guide drug therapy when blood levels of the drug are monitored and correlated with therapeutic results.

Therapeutic Drug Monitoring

Therapeutic drug monitoring (TDM) can aid a clinician in making critical decisions in therapeutic applications. In psychopharmacology, TDM can dramatically improve the prognosis of psychological disorders, making previously difficult-to-treat disorders much more treatable. The basic principle underlying TDM is that a threshold plasma concentration of a drug is needed at the receptor site to initiate and maintain a pharmacological response. Critically important is that plasma concentrations of psychoactive drugs correlate well with tissue or receptor concentrations. Therefore, TDM is an indirect, although usually quite accurate, measurement of drug concentration at the receptor site. To make the correlation between TDM, dosage, and therapeutic response, large-scale clinical trials are performed, and blood samples are drawn at several time periods during both acute (short-term) and chronic (long-term) therapy. Statistical correlation is made between the level of drug in plasma and the degree of therapeutic response. A dosage regimen can then be designed to achieve the appropriate blood level of a drug.

The goals of TDM are many. One goal is to assess whether a patient is taking medication as prescribed; if plasma levels of the drug are below the therapeutic level because the patient has not been taking the required medication, therapeutic results will be poor. Another goal is to avoid toxicity; if plasma levels of the drug are above the therapeutic level, the dosage can be lowered, effectiveness maintained, and toxicity minimized. A third goal is to enhance therapeutic response by focusing not on the amount of drug taken but on the measured amount of drug in the plasma. Other goals include possible reductions in the cost of therapy (since a patient's illness is better controlled) and the substantiation of the need for unusually high doses in patients who require higher-than-normal intake of prescribed medication to maintain a therapeutic blood level of a drug.

Winek and coworkers (2001) and Baselt (2008) present blood level data for numerous medications. Sparshatt and coworkers (2010) related the dose, plasma concentrations, receptor binding, and clinical response for the antipsychotic aripiprazole (Chapter 4).

Drug Tolerance and Dependence

Drug tolerance is defined as a state of progressively decreasing responsiveness to a drug. A person who develops tolerance requires a larger dose of the drug to achieve the effect originally obtained by a smaller dose. At least three mechanisms are involved in the development of drug tolerance—two are pharmacological mechanisms; one is a behavioral mechanism.

In *metabolic tolerance,* the first of the two classically described types of pharmacological tolerance, more enzyme is available to metabolize a drug and, as a result, more drug must be administered to maintain the same level of drug in the body. *Cellular-adaptive,* or *pharmacodynamic, tolerance* is the second type of pharmacological tolerance. Receptors in the brain adapt to the continued presence of the drug, with neurons adapting to excess drug either by reducing the number of receptors available to the drug or by reducing their sensitivity to the drug. Such reduction in numbers or sensitivity is termed *down regulation,* and higher levels of drug are necessary to maintain the same biological effect.

Behavioral conditioning processes are the third type of drug tolerance. The exposure of drugs to receptors does not account for the substantial degree of tolerance that many people acquire to opioids, barbiturates, ethyl alcohol, and other drugs. Instead, tolerance can be demonstrated when a drug is administered in the context of usual predrug cues but not in the context of alternative cues. Poulos and Cappell (1991) proposed a *homeostatic theory* of drug tolerance. They found that, with morphine analgesia, testing in an environment in which tolerance had developed affected the manifestation of tolerance, and an environmental cue could maintain the tolerance. This *contingent tolerance* is pervasive and represents a general process underlying the development of all forms of systemic tolerance.

The environmental cues routinely paired with drug administration will become conditioned stimuli that elicit a conditioned response that is opposite in direction to or compensation for the direct effects of the drug. Over conditioning trials, the compensatory conditioned response grows in magnitude and counteracts the direct drug effects; that is, tolerance develops.

Physical dependence is an entirely different phenomenon from tolerance, even though the two are often associated temporally. A person who is physically dependent needs the drug to avoid the withdrawal symptoms that occur if the drug is not taken. The state is revealed by withdrawing the drug and noting the occurrence of physical and/or psychological changes (withdrawal symptoms). These changes are referred to as an *abstinence syndrome.* Readministering the drug can relieve the symptoms of withdrawal.

Because physical dependence is often manifested following cessation of use of drugs of abuse such as alcohol and heroin, the term has been linked with "addiction," implying that withdrawal signs are "bad" and observed only with drugs of abuse. This conclusion is far from the truth; rather, severe withdrawal signs can follow cessation of such therapeutic drugs as the SSRI type of clinical antidepressants (Chapter 5).[6] Therefore, the occurrence of withdrawal signs after drug removal is not necessarily a sign of the drug "addiction" that is usually associated with "bad" drugs such as heroin. Rather, physical dependence is an indication that brain and body functions were altered by the presence of a drug and that a different homeostatic state must be initiated at drug withdrawal. It takes time (from a few days to about two weeks) for the brain and the body to adapt to the new state of equilibrium where the drug is absent.

STUDY QUESTIONS

1. What is meant by the term *pharmacokinetics*?

2. Why must a psychoactive drug be altered metabolically in the body before it can be excreted?

3. Discuss the advantages and disadvantages of the various methods of administering drugs.

4. List the various membrane barriers that may affect drug distribution.

5. Discuss the blood-brain barrier as a limitation to drug transport.

6. Discuss the placental barrier as it affects the distribution of psychoactive drugs. What are the cautions for the use of psychotropic medication during pregnancy?

7. If a drug has an elimination half-life of 6 hours, how long does it take for the drug to be effectively eliminated from the body after administration of a single dose?

8. What are the various routes through the body whereby a drug can be eliminated?

9. Define *half-life*. How does *half-life* apply to steady state?

10. What is meant by the term *therapeutic drug monitoring*? In what instances might it be of value?

11. What is drug tolerance and why does it occur?

---

[6]Discontinuation of SSRI-type antidepressants is followed in many patients by withdrawal signs that can be organized into five symptom categories: (1) disequilibrium (dizziness, vertigo, ataxia), (2) GI symptoms (nausea, vomiting), (3) flu-like symptoms (fatigue, lethargy, myalgias, chills), (4) sensory disturbances (paresthesias, sensation of electric shocks), and (5) sleep disturbances (insomnia, vivid dreams).

REFERENCES

Baselt, R. C. (2008). *Disposition of Toxic Drugs and Chemicals in Man,*. 8th ed. Foster City, CA: Biomedical Publications.

deLeon, J. (2009). "Pharmacogenomics: The Promise of Personalized Medicine for CNS Disorders." *Neuropsychopharmacology* 34: 159–172.

deLeon, J., et al. (2006). "The AmpliChip CYP450 Genotype Test: Integrating a New Clinical Tool." *Molecular Diagnostic Therapeutics* 10: 135–151.

DeVane, C. L. (2006). "Antidepressant-Drug Interactions Are Potentially but Rarely Clinically Significant." *Neuropsychopharmacology* 31: 1594–1604.

Dunbar, L., et al. (2009). "Clinician Experiences of Employing the AmpliChip CYP450 Test in Routine Psychiatric Practice." *Journal of Psychopharmacology* doi:10.1177/0269881109106957.

Gilstrap, L. C., and Little, B. B. (1998). *Drugs and Pregnancy,* 2nd ed. New York: Chapman & Hall.

Greenblatt, D. J., et al. (1999). "Human Cytochromes and Some Newer Antidepressants: Kinetics, Metabolism, and Drug Interactions." *Journal of Clinical Psychopharmacology* 19, Supplement 1: 23S–35S.

Greenblatt, D. J., et al. (2003). "Time Course of Recovery of Cytochrome P450 3A Function After Single Doses of Grapefruit Juice." *Clinical Pharmacology and Therapeutics* 74: 121–129.

Lilja, J. J., et al. (1998). "Grapefruit Juice Substantially Increases Plasma Concentrations of Buspirone." *Clinical Pharmacology and Therapeutics* 64: 655–660.

Lin, K. M., et al. (2001). "Culture and Psychopharmacology." *Psychiatric Clinics of North America* 24: 523–538.

Paine, M. F., et al. (2006). "A Furanocoumarin-Free Grapefruit Juice Establishes Furanocoumarins as the Mediators of the Grapefruit Juice-Felodipine Interaction." *American Journal of Clinical Nutrition* 84: 1097–1105.

Pardridge, W. M. (2003). "Blood-Brain Barrier Drug Targeting: The Future of Brain Drug Development." *Molecular Interventions* 3: 90–105.

Poulos, C. X., and Cappell, H. (1991). "Homeostatic Theory of Drug Tolerance: A General Model of Physiological Adaptation." *Psychological Reviews* 98: 390–408.

Preskorn, S. H., and Flockhart, D. (2009). "2010 Guide to Psychiatric Drug Interactions." *Primary Psychiatry* 16: 45–74.

Preskorn, S. H., and Werder, S. (2006). "Detrimental Antidepressant Drug-Drug Interactions: Are They Clinically Relevant?" *Neuropsychopharmacology* 31: 1605–1612.

Rheeders, M., et al. (2006). "Drug-Drug Interactions After Single Oral Doses of the Furanocoumarin Methoxsalen and Cyclosporine." *Journal of Clinical Pharmacology* 46: 768–775.

Sparshatt, A., et al. (2010) "A Systematic Review of Aripiprazole—Dose, Plasma Concentration, Receptor Occupancy, and Response: Implications for Therapeutic Drug Monitoring." *Journal of Clinical Psychiatry,* in press.

Spina, E., and Perucca, E. (2002). "Clinical Significance of Pharmacokinetic Interactions Between Antiepileptic and Psychotropic Drugs." *Epilepsia* 43, Supplement 2: 37–44.

Winek, C. L., et al. (2001). "Winek's Drug & Chemical Blood Level Data 2001." *Forensic Science International* 122: 107–123.

Chapter 2

Pharmacodynamics:
How Drugs Act

While the body is trying to rid itself of an ingested psychoactive drug, the drug is exerting effects by attaching to receptors in cells in both the brain and the body. As a result of the interactions, the body experiences effects that are characteristic for the drug. *It is a basic principle of pharmacology that the pharmacological, physiological, or behavioral effects induced by a drug follow from their interaction with receptors.*

The study of the interactions, termed *pharmacodynamics*, involves exploring the mechanisms of drug action that occur at the molecular level. While *pharmacokinetics* is the study of what the body does to a drug, *pharmacodynamics* is the study of what the drug does to the body. The two studies provide the basis for both the rational therapeutic use of a drug and the design of new and superior therapeutic agents.

To produce an effect, a drug must bind to and interact with specialized receptors, usually located on cell membranes. In the case of psychoactive drugs, these receptors are usually located on the surface of neurons in the brain. The occupation of a receptor by a drug (*drug-receptor binding*) leads to a change in the functional properties of the neuron, resulting in the drug's characteristic pharmacological response. In most instances, drug-receptor binding is both *ionic* and *reversible* in nature, with positive and negative charges on various portions of the drug molecule and the receptor protein attracting one to the other. The strength of ionic attachment is determined by the fit of the three-dimensional structure of the drug to the three-dimensional site on the receptor.[1]

Importantly, when a psychoactive drug binds to a receptor and thereby alters (activates or blocks) the normal functions of that receptor, the neuronal response to the drug is one of two types: (1) an immediate response to the presence of the drug on the receptor or (2) when the drug is given over a longer period of time, long-term changes in the properties of the receptors resulting in long-term changes in neuronal, brain, and behavioral functioning.

Immediate responses follow from the acute binding of a drug to its receptor with initiation of an immediate neuronal (and behavioral) response. For example, smoking a cigarette (containing nicotine) or smoking illicit cocaine or methamphetamine results in release of the neurotransmitter dopamine; dopamine activates our reward system, and a stimulant or pleasurable feeling can follow. With respect to medications, ingestion of methylphenidate (Ritalin) can rapidly relieve the symptoms of attention deficit/hyperactivity disorder (ADHD), potent opioid analgesia can rapidly relieve severe pain, and certain sedatives can rapidly induce drowsiness and be used in the treatment of insomnia. Such actions are all thought to follow an acute agonist action at specific receptors. Similarly, many of the side effects of drugs (such as dry mouth, unwanted sedation, blurred vision, and so on) follow from acute actions at other receptors, often distinct from those responsible for the desired drug action.

Longer-term responses to a drug require that a drug be taken continually over a period of time. Here, the drug is in contact with its receptors for days to months. As a result, neurons "adapt" to the presence of drug, resulting in long-term changes in neuronal functioning. In the case of long-term antidepressant drug therapy, neuronal adaptation may be followed by relief of depression (Chapter 5). The same principle probably applies to medication therapy for bipolar illness and various anxiety disorders. Some long-term adaptations to the presence of drug can be harmful. For example, drug "dependency" can follow long-term use of certain sedatives, stimulants, opioid narcotics, and even (although this is debated) antidepressants. In all these cases, withdrawal symptoms are observed after drug discontinuation. The exact responses vary with each type of drug and are discussed in the appropriate chapter of this book.

---

[1] Reversible ionic binding is contrasted with the formation of a permanent, irreversible, covalent bond between a drug and a receptor. One of the rare instances in psychopharmacology where an irreversible covalent bond forms is between certain antidepressant drugs and the enzyme monoamine oxidase (Chapter 5).

Receptors for Drug Action

Drugs exert their effects by forming reversible ionic bonds with specific receptors. A *receptor* is a fairly large molecule (usually a protein[2]) on the surface of or within a cell that is the site (or sites) where biologically active, naturally occurring endogenous compounds (called *transmitters* or *modulators)* produce their normal biological effects. Literally hundreds of different types of receptors are known (each being a unique protein molecule), and the ability to recognize one specific neurotransmitter characterizes each one. Thus, only one neurotransmitter might be specific enough to fit or bind to a specific receptor protein. For example, if only serotonin binds to a specific receptor, that protein is called a serotonin receptor. But although the receptor is specific for serotonin, serotonin (as a neurotransmitter) also binds to other, structurally different receptors.

To date, more than 15 different serotonin receptor proteins have been identified.[3] This diversity makes it possible to develop closely related drugs, each with a slightly different degree of affinity (strength of attachment) for the different serotonin receptors. For example, a specific drug might have affinity for a serotonin 1 receptor but not for any other serotonin receptor. Until recently, it was not possible to develop such a drug. However, with the understanding that drug receptors are proteins, it became possible to isolate a specific receptor protein from the rest of the brain, purify it, determine its amino acid sequence, isolate the portion of DNA responsible for making the protein, and clone the protein receptor to produce sufficient quantities of receptor against which drugs could be screened for affinity and activity.

A given drug may be more specific for a given set of receptors than is the endogenous neurotransmitter. Serotonin, for example, must necessarily attach to all its more than 15 different serotonin receptors (it has to because it is the endogenous neurotransmitter at each receptor). However, a given drug might attach to only one receptor. For example, buspirone (BuSpar) attaches to 5-HT$_{1A}$ receptors, which results in antianxiety and antidepressant actions. It

---

[2] A protein is a complex chain of various amino acids. Proteins are essential to life, functioning, among other things, as metabolic enzymes and receptors.

[3] Each receptor protein that binds serotonin, for example, has a slightly different amino acid composition; nevertheless, their three-dimensional structures are similar enough that serotonin, for example, still fits a "slot" (like a lock-and-key arrangement) and ionically binds to the protein. Pharmacologists have named these different protein receptors serotonin 1, serotonin 2, serotonin 3, and so on; in earlier years, multiple receptors for a single neurotransmitter were given more exotic names (for example, muscarinic and nicotinic for acetylcholine receptors; alpha and beta for adrenergic receptors; and mu, delta, and kappa for opioid receptors).

has no affinity for other serotonin receptors. Binding of a drug to a receptor results in one of three actions:

- Binding to a receptor site normally occupied by the endogenous neurotransmitter can initiate a cellular response similar or identical to that exerted by the transmitter; the drug thus mimics the action of the transmitter. This is called an *agonistic action,* and the drug is termed an *agonist* for that transmitter.

- Binding to a site near the binding site for the endogenous transmitter can facilitate transmitter binding. This is also an agonistic action. Such a facilitative effect is termed an *allosteric action.*

- Binding to a receptor site normally occupied by a neurotransmitter, but not initiating a transmitterlike action, blocks access of the transmitter to its binding site, which inhibits the normal physiological action of the transmitter. This is called an *antagonistic action,* and the drug is termed an *antagonist* for that neurotransmitter or receptor site.

It is also a general rule of psychopharmacology that drugs do not create any unique effects; they merely modulate normal neuronal functioning, mimicking or antagonizing the actions of a specific neurotransmitter. Binding that produces mimicry or facilitation of neurotransmitter action is an agonistic action. For example, buspirone attaches to the 5-HT$_{1A}$ receptor and activates it, mimicking serotonin's action on the receptor, which results in an antianxiety action of clinical significance. Drug occupation of a receptor that blocks the access of the neurotransmitter to that receptor is an antagonistic action. For example, all the drugs developed to treat schizophrenia (antipsychotic drugs; Chapter 4) are antagonists at D$_2$ receptors. By attaching to this subtype of dopamine receptor, they prevent endogenous dopamine molecules from attaching, activating, and producing an effect at these sites.

Receptor Structure

What does a receptor look like? Although there are several different configurations of proteins that may serve a receptor function, the following is a brief summary of the major types most relevant to the action of drugs.

Ion Channel Receptors. (Ion channel receptors are also called *ionotropic receptors.*) The first type of membrane-spanning receptor is the kind that forms an *ion channel.* That is, the central portion of the receptor forms a pore that spans the membrane of the neuron, which enlarges in size when either an endogenous neurotransmitter or exogenous drug attaches to the receptor-binding site. The attachment allows flow of a specific *ion* (such as chloride ions) through the enlarged pore (Figure 2.1A). (It should be noted that, in some cases, the pore is normally open, and the attachment of a

A

1. Neurotransmitter binds directly to the channel protein.

Outside cell

Inside cell

2. Channel opens immediately.   **3.** Ions flow across membrane for a brief time.

B

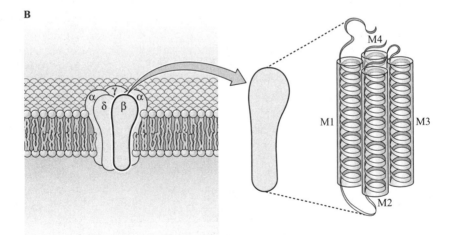

FIGURE 2.1 A. Schematic of neurotransmitter activation of an ionotropic receptor that contains an ion channel. **B.** Detailed schematic representation of the individual subunits of an ion channel (ionotropic) receptor, showing the helical coils of which they are composed. [Part A from Breedlove et al. (2007), p. 79, Figure 3.13a. Part B from M. Bear et al. (2007). *Neuroscience: Exploring the Brain*, 3rd ed. New York: Lippincott, Williams and Wilkins, p. 153, Figure 6.18a.]

drug or transmitter will close it. Although such situations are beyond the scope of this text, the general phenomenon is the same.)

As shown in Figure 2.1B, the ionotropic receptor is composed of five sections, or subunits, each of which crosses the cell membraine. Each of these sections is labeled, usually with a Greek letter. (If they are very similar in composition, two subunits may be given the same Greek letter.) Each of these subunits is, in turn, made up of four helical coils, which also cross the membrane and are also labeled, usually M_1 through M_4. It is the arrangement of these five transmembrane subunits that forms the channel of the ionotropic receptor, as seen in Figure 2.2.

Figures 2.2 and 2.3 illustrate how the neurotransmitter gamma aminobutyric acid (GABA) and various drugs (benzodiazepines, barbiturates) bind to the GABA receptor and affect the inward flow of chloride ions. Benzodiazepines (Chapter 7) serve as agonists by binding to a site near the GABA-binding site and by facilitating the action of GABA in increasing the flow of chloride ions into the neuron. Because

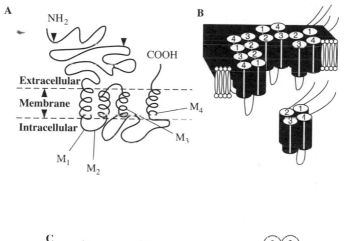

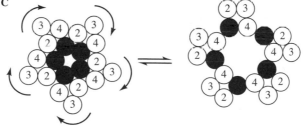

FIGURE 2.2 Presumed topology of the GABA$_A$ receptor. **A.** Single subunit with its large extracellular terminal part and four transmembrane helical coils. **B.** Arrangement of the transmembrane domains of five subunits to form a central channel. **C.** Transmembrane domain in a transverse section through the membrane when the channel is closed (*left*) and open (*right*).

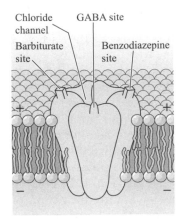

Chloride   GABA site
channel

Barbiturate   Benzodiazepine
site   site

FIGURE 2.3 Schematic of the GABA$_A$ receptor, with its binding sites for GABA, benzodiazepines, and barbiturates.

chloride ions are negative, their inward flow hyperpolarizes the neuron and inhibits neuronal function. This action underlies the use of benzodiazepines as sedative, antianxiety, amnestic, and antiepileptic agents.

In contrast, the drug flumazenil (Romazicon) attaches to the benzodiazepine-binding site but does not facilitate the action of GABA. It does, however, compete with any benzodiazepine that is present, displacing the benzodiazepine from the receptor and reversing the actions of the benzodiazepine. Flumazenil is classified pharmacologically as a benzodiazepine antagonist and is used clinically to diagnose and treat benzodiazepine overdoses.[4]

G-Protein-Coupled Receptors.   The second type of membrane-spanning receptor protein is called a *G-protein-coupled receptor*. These receptors are also called *metabotropic* receptors (Figure 2.4). The activation of these receptors induces the release of an attached intracellular protein (a *G protein*) that, in turn, controls enzymatic function within the postsynaptic neuron.

G-protein-coupled receptors (sometimes abbreviated as GPCRs) are discussed throughout this book because they are involved in the synaptic effects of many neurotransmitters, such as acetylcholine, norepinephrine, dopamine, serotonin, and opioid endorphins, all of which are involved in the action of psychoactive drugs. The molecular structure of G-protein-coupled receptors consists of a single protein chain

---

[4] Several other substances, such as barbiturates, also have binding sites on the GABA receptor complex, shown in Figure 2.3. Barbiturates (Chapter 7) act like benzodiazepines in increasing the effect of GABA on the chloride channel within the GABA receptor. Thus, with a site and mechanism of action similar to that exerted by benzodiazepines, the two classes of drugs might be expected to demonstrate similar clinical and behavioral effects. In general, they do.

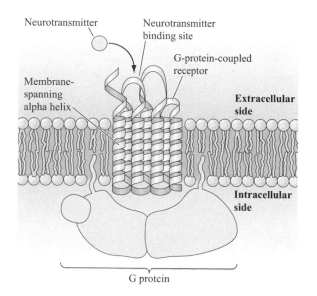

FIGURE 2.4 Schematic of a G-protein-coupled (metabotropic) receptor, showing the 7-helical, membrane-spanning coils. [From M. Bear et al. (2007). *Neuroscience: Exploring the Brain*, 3rd ed. New York: Lippincott, Williams and Wilkins, p. 158, Figure 6.23.]

of 400 to 500 amino acids possessing seven transmembrane alpha helices (see Figures 2.4 and 2.5). The endogenous neurotransmitter (and presumably drugs also) attaches inside the space between these coils (Figure 2.5) and is held in place by ionic attractions.

G-protein-coupled receptors constitute a large and diverse family of proteins whose primary function is to change extracellular stimuli (transmitters and drugs) into intracellular signals (Figure 2.6). Unlike ionotropic receptors, metabotropic receptors do not form a membrane-spanning pore that can allow the direct passage of ions. Instead, when a neurotransmitter associates with the extracellular recognition site, an intermediate molecule within the postsynaptic cell, the G protein, is activated and, either *directly* or *indirectly*, through a series of enzymatic reactions, *opens or closes ion channels located at other places on the cell membrane*. Because the effect of metabotropic receptors is not as immediate as that of ionotropic receptors, their action is slower.

The process starts when a receptor binds to its proper hormone or neurotransmitter, such as adrenaline. This changes the shape of the receptor, which then binds to the three-chain G protein inside the cell membrane and activates it. The G protein can then *directly* activate an ion channel, or it can trigger several biochemical reactions that will cause the G protein to move along the membrane until it finds and then *(indirectly)* activates the enzyme adenylyl cyclase. The activated adenylyl cyclase then produces lots of cyclic AMP, which spreads the signal through the cell and, in turn, affects many ion channels. The cyclic AMP is called the second messenger (the first being the neurotransmitter). One major

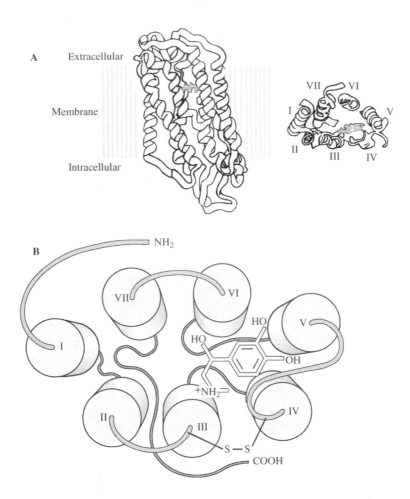

FIGURE 2.5 Schematic representation of a G-protein-coupled transmembrane receptor, with a molecule of neurotransmitter (norepinephrine) lying in its binding site. Note the arrangement of the 7-transmembrane helical coils and the site of the transmitter attachment deep within the structure. The ionic interactions between the transmitter and particular amino acid side chains are not illustrated. **A.** The membrane and continuous coils. **B.** The helical coils are represented as cylinders with the molecule of norepinephrine interacting with four of the coils.

advantage of this approach is that it allows the signal to be amplified; that is, a single molecule of adrenaline can stimulate the production of many molecules of cyclic AMP. By incorporating an enzyme (such as adenylyl cyclase) into the chain, a weak signal from outside the cell can be translated into a strong signal throughout the inside of the cell.

G-protein-coupled receptors are the middlemen, able to effect communication between the neurotransmitter-receptor complex and intracellular enzymes (the *second messenger*) or adjacent ion channels.

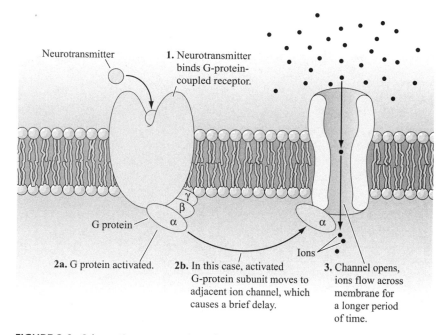

Neurotransmitter

1. Neurotransmitter binds G-protein-coupled receptor.

G protein

γ

β

α

α

Ions

2a. G protein activated.

2b. In this case, activated G-protein subunit moves to adjacent ion channel, which causes a brief delay.

3. Channel opens, ions flow across membrane for a longer period of time.

FIGURE 2.6 Schematic representation of G-protein-receptor function. [From Breedlove et al. (2007), p. 79, Figure 3.13b.]

Metabotropic receptors control many cellular processes, such as ion channel function, energy metabolism, cell division and differentiation, and neuronal excitability.

Furthermore, cyclic AMP is not the only second messenger known to mediate the effects of neurotransmitters. Figure 2.7 summarizes a general model of transmitter-receptor interactions and the resulting cascade of effects produced by second and, in some cases, third messengers (not shown here). Cyclic AMP is shown, associated with its enzyme, adenylyl cyclase; other second messengers are similarly indicated.

Ionotropic and (direct and indirect) metabotropic receptors are not the only receptor types important for understanding drug action. There are additional receptors that mediate the effect of hormones (steroids) and neurotrophic substances (a generic term for any of a family of substances with roles in the maintenance and survival of neurons, for example, secretory proteins or nerve growth factors, such as brain-derived growth factor). Two other types of proteins are also crucial to understanding psychoactive drug mechanisms; they are described below.

Carrier Proteins. The third type of membrane-spanning protein is a *carrier* (or *transport*) *protein*. This type of receptor transports small organic molecules (such as neurotransmitters) across cell

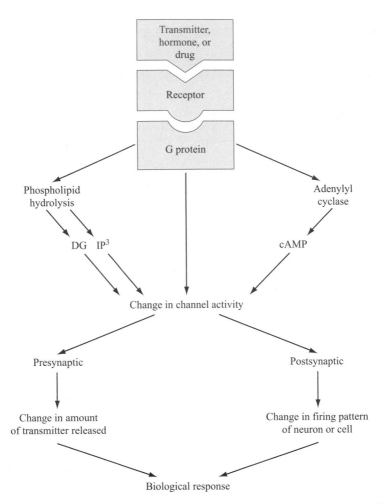

FIGURE 2.7 Major pathways for modulation of synaptic transmission. cAMP = cyclic adenosine monophosphate; IP₃ = inositol triphosphate; DG = diacylglycerol (all three substances are second messengers). [Adapted and modified from Iverson et al. (2009), p. 74, Figure 4.6.]

membranes against concentration gradients. Most important in psychopharmacology are the *presynaptic* carrier proteins that bind dopamine, norepinephrine, or serotonin (and other neurotransmitters) in the synaptic cleft and transport them back into the presynaptic nerve terminal, terminating the synaptic transmitter action of these neurotransmitters. Many drugs discussed in this book (both therapeutic and abused) exert their actions by blocking the carrier protein that is specific for transporting a specific neurotransmitter. Until recently, little was known about these transporters except that they genetically encoded chains of amino acids (proteins) arranged as 12 helical arrays of amino acids embedded in the membrane of the presynaptic nerve terminal.

Work by Gouaux and coworkers (Yernool et al., 2004; Gouaux and MacKinnon, 2005; Armstrong et al., 2006) has added considerably to our knowledge of these transporters. They carry molecules of neurotransmitter across membranes of presynaptic nerve terminals, even against a concentration gradient (therefore more than passive diffusion). To do so, the transporters must exist in at least three ionic states: open to the synapse, occluded with the transmitter "trapped" inside, and open to the cytoplasm of the presynaptic neuron (Figure 2.8). It now appears that the transporter is a bowl-shaped structure with a fluid-filled basin (open to the synaptic cleft) extending halfway across the membrane of the presynaptic nerve terminal (Figure 2.9). At the bottom of the basin are three binding sites for the neurotransmitter, each cradled by two helical "hairpins" reaching from opposite sides of the membrane. In the resting state, the bowl is open to the synaptic cleft. It traps one or more molecules of released transmitter per "cycle," allowing floods of molecules to move from the synaptic cleft into the presynaptic terminal and become available for rerelease. It seems that the transport of transmitter is achieved by movements of the hairpins that allow alternating access to either side of the membrane (for example, the outer layer closes,

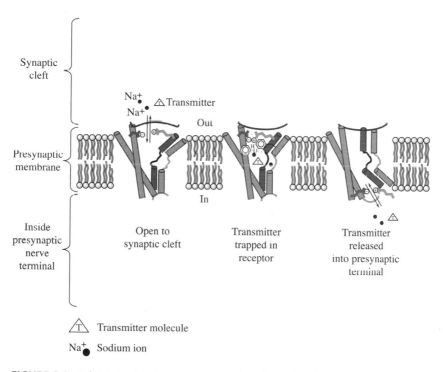

FIGURE 2.8 Schematic drawing of a proposed conformational change involving transport of transmitter and sodium ions across the membrane of the presynaptic nerve terminal. *Left:* Transporter open to the synaptic cleft. *Center:* Transmitter "trapped" inside the transporter. *Right:* Inward-facing state with transmitter "released" into the cytoplasm of the neuron. [From A. Yamashita et al., "Crystal Structure of a Bacterial Homologue of Na+/Cl-Dependent Neurotransmitter Transporters," *Nature* 437 (2005): 221, Figure 6.]

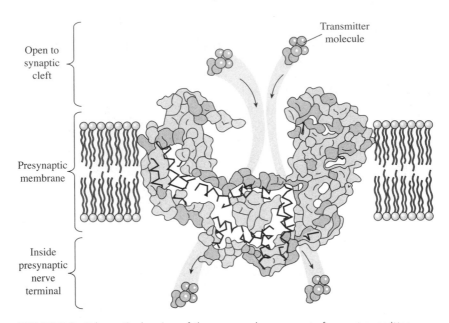

Open to synaptic cleft

Transmitter molecule

Presynaptic membrane

Inside presynaptic nerve terminal

FIGURE 2.9 Schematic drawing of the proposed movement of neurotransmitter molecules through a transporter protein and into the presynaptic nerve terminal. The drawing illustrates the total movement and summarizes the three-step outline in Figure 2.8. The deep aqueous basin reaches halfway across the membrane. [Adapted from Yernool et al. (2004), Figure 2, p. 813.]

trapping the transmitter, and then the inner layer opens, ejecting the transmitter into the cytoplasm of the presynaptic terminal).

Enzymes. The fourth type of receptor protein for psychoactive drugs is *enzymes*—in particular, enzymes that regulate the synaptic availability of certain neurotransmitters. These enzymes break down neurotransmitters, and their inhibition by drugs increases transmitter availability. Two examples are *acetylcholine esterase*, the enzyme that breaks down acetylcholine within the synaptic cleft (Chapter 3), and *monoamine oxidase*, the enzyme that breaks down norepinephrine and dopamine in presynaptic nerve terminals, controlling the amount available for release (Chapters 3 and 5).

Drugs known as *irreversible acetylcholine esterase inhibitors* form covalent bonds with the enzyme, preventing it from functioning, and have been used as insecticides and as lethal "nerve gases." Drugs that *reversibly* inhibit the enzyme *acetylcholine esterase* are used clinically as cognitive enhancers, delaying the onset of Alzheimer's disease (Chapter 19). Drugs that irreversibly inhibit the enzyme *monoamine oxidase* are called monoamine oxidase inhibitors (MAOIs) and are used primarily as antidepressants (Chapter 5). [For more advanced discussions of receptor structure and function, see Iverson and coworkers (2009) and Nestler and coworkers (2009).]

Drug-Receptor Specificity

Receptors exhibit high specificity both for one particular neurotransmitter and for certain drug molecules. Making only modest variations in the chemical structure of a drug may greatly alter the intensity of a receptor's response to it. For example, amphetamine and methamphetamine (Chapter 12) are both powerful psychostimulants. Although their chemical structures are very close, they differ by the simple addition of a methyl ($-CH_3$) group to amphetamine, forming methamphetamine. Methamphetamine produces much greater behavioral stimulation at the same milligram dosage. Both drugs attach to the same receptors in the brain, but methamphetamine exerts a much more powerful action on them, at least in milligrams. The drug molecule with the "best fit" to the receptor (methamphetamine, in this example) elicits the greatest response from the cell. In pharmacological terms, methamphetamine is more *potent* than amphetamine because a lower absolute dose achieves the same level of response as a higher dose of amphetamine. But as we will see next, a more *potent* drug is not necessarily a more *effective* drug. It merely produces its effects at a somewhat lower dose.

One important concept in regard to drug specificity is the phenomenon of optical isomers. *Isomers* are molecules formed around a carbon atom that have the same molecular formula but have a different arrangement of their atoms in space. Simple substances that show optical isomerism exist as two (or more) isomers known as *enantiomers*. Isomers represent forms of a molecule that are mirror images of each other.

The difference in the spatial arrangement of the two molecules means that they rotate a beam of polarized light in equal but opposite directions. The isomer that rotates the light in a clockwise direction is designated as the (+) isomer; conversely, the isomer that rotates the light in a counterclockwise direction has the (−) designation. Sometimes the designation is made as D (*dextrorotatory*—"to the right") and L (*levorotatory*—"to the left"). Yet another system uses the letters R and S, based on the atomic numbers of molecules, and is not equivalent to the (+) and (−) nomenclatures.

Only one of these optical isomers is biologically active. Therefore, when these molecules interact with a receptor, only one of the isomers would be effective. In other words, optical isomers behave the same way chemically but not biologically.

When optically active substances are made in the laboratory, and eventually become medications, they are often produced as a 50/50 mixture of the two enantiomers. In the laboratory, it takes more work to separate the two, so it is the mixture (50 percent active and 50 percent inactive) that is marketed. This is known as a *racemic mixture* or *racemate*. Thus, only the (−) half of the medicine will be biologically active in the body. Most medicines are manufacturesd as racemates. However, sometimes an isomer is also produced. An example is the antidepressant citalopram. This is the racemate version, marketed as the antidepressant Celexa. When the patent on the racemate expired, the active isomer was separated out and is marketed as escitalopram, or Lexapro. As a result, escitalopram doses are approximately half of the clinically comparable citalopram doses (Chapter 5).[5]

As a consequence of a drug binding to a receptor, cellular function is altered, resulting in observable effects on physiological or psychological functioning. The total action of the drug in the body results from drug actions either (1) on one specific type of receptor or (2) at different types of receptors. In either case, whether the drug is used for therapeutic or recreational purposes, the total action will produce additional responses, called *side effects*.

As an example of the side effects produced by the first mechanism, fluoxetine-induced blockade of presynaptic serotonin reuptake increases serotonin availability at all postsynaptic serotonin receptors. This single action results not only in relief of depression but also in such side effects as anxiety, insomnia, and sexual dysfunction (Chapter 5). As an example of the side effects produced by the second mechanism, certain other antidepressants (the tricyclic antidepressants; Chapter 5) increase both serotonin and norepinephrine availability (reducing depression). But, in addition, they also produce sedation, dry mouth, and blurred vision as a result of their blocking acetylcholinergic receptors. A balance between therapeutic effects and inevitable but unwanted side effects is always the most desirable outcome.

Dose-Response Relationships

One way of quantifying drug-receptor interactions is to use *dose-response curves*. In Figure 2.10, two different types of dose-response curves are illustrated. In graph A, the dose is plotted against the percentage of people (from a given population) who exhibit a characteristic effect at a given dosage. In graph B, the dose is plotted against the intensity, or magnitude, of the response in a single person. These curves indicate that a dose exists that is low enough to produce little or no effect; at the opposite extreme, a dose exists beyond which no

---

[5] Other drugs discussed in this book that have isomeric formulations include amphetamine and methylphenidate, stimulant drugs used in the treatment of ADHD (Chapter 18), and modafinil, used in the treatment of narcolepsy (Chapter 7). Both isomers of amphetamine are active; the D-isomer is familiar as dexadrine. The L-isomer of methylphenidate is metabolized much faster than the D-isomer, which is marketed separately as Focalin. The racemic mixture of modafinil is marketed as Provigil; the R-isomer is marketed as Nuvigil, which is more soluble in water.

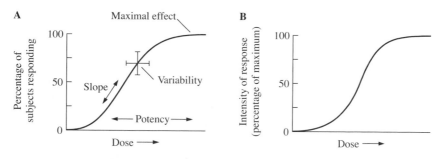

FIGURE 2.10 Two types of dose-response curves. **A.** Curve obtained by plotting the dose of drug against the percentage of subjects showing a given response at any given dose. **B.** Curve obtained by plotting the dose of drug against the intensity of response observed in any single person at a given dose. The intensity of response is plotted as a percentage of the maximum obtainable response.

greater response can be elicited. Dose-response curves demonstrate several important characteristics:

- *Potency* refers to the absolute number of molecules of drug required to elicit a response, a measurement of the dose required.
- *Efficacy* refers to the maximum effect obtainable, with additional doses producing no more effect.
- *Variability* and *slope* refer to individual differences in drug response; some patients respond at very low doses and some require much more drug.

The location of the dose-response curve along the horizontal axis reflects the potency of the drug. If two drugs produce an equal degree of stimulation, but one exerts this action at half the dose level of the other, the first drug is considered to be *twice* as *potent* as the second drug (Figure 2.11). As stated, however, potency is a relatively unimportant characteristic of a drug, because it makes little difference whether the effective dose of a drug is 1.0 milligram or 100 milligrams as long as the drug is administered in an appropriate dose with no undue toxicity.

Slope refers to the more or less linear central portion of the dose-response curve. A steep slope on a dose-response curve implies that there is only a small difference between the dose that produces a barely discernible effect and the dose that causes a maximal effect. The steeper the slope, the smaller is the increase in dose required to go from a minimum response to a maximum effect. This can be good because it may indicate that there is little biological variation in the response to the drug. Conversely, it may be a disadvantage if it indicates that even a small increase in dose will produce a toxic reaction.

The *peak* of the dose-response curve indicates the maximum effect, or efficacy, that can be produced by a drug, regardless of further

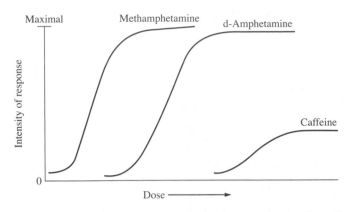

FIGURE 2.11   Theoretical dose-response curves for three psychostimulants illustrates equal efficacy of methamphetamine and dextroamphetamine, increased potency of methamphetamine, and reduced potency and efficacy of caffeine.

increases in dose. Not all psychoactive drugs can exert the same level of effect. For example, caffeine, even in massive doses, cannot exert the same intensity of central nervous system (CNS) stimulation as amphetamine (see Figure 2.11). Similarly, aspirin can never achieve the greater analgesic effect of morphine. Thus, the maximum effect is an inherent property of a drug and is one measure of a drug's efficacy.

Most psychoactive drugs are not used to the point of their maximum effect because side effects and toxicities limit the upper range of dosage, regardless of whether the drug is administered for a therapeutic purpose or taken for recreational use. Therefore, the usefulness of a compound is correspondingly limited, even though the drug may be inherently capable of producing a greater or more intense effect.

Drug Safety and Effectiveness

For a drug to be approved by the federal Food and Drug Administration (FDA), its manufacturer must demonstrate both that the drug is *effective* for the claimed therapeutic use and that it is *safe* to use in a wide population. Effectiveness is determined in animal experiments and in human trials. Effectiveness is further assessed as the drug undergoes wider use in the general population. Safety refers to the potential for the drug to cause adverse effects, effects that vary from predictable and tolerable side effects to serious and unpredictable toxicities such as unrecognized allergic reactions. Also, when a drug is introduced into a general population, there is variability in response because of genetic or other population variances. Drug-drug interactions are also a common and important type of adverse effect, often predictable and often underappreciated during clinical trials (Jurrlink et al., 2003; al-Khatib et al., 2003).

Variability in Drug Responsiveness

The dose of a drug that produces a specific response varies considerably among patients. Variability among patients can result from differences in rates of drug absorption and metabolism; previous experience with drug use; various physical, psychological, and emotional states; and so on. Despite the etiology of the variability, any population will have a few subjects who are remarkably sensitive to the effects (and side effects) of a drug and a few who will exhibit remarkable drug tolerance, requiring quite large doses to produce therapeutic results. The variability, however, usually follows a predictable pattern, resembling a Gaussian distribution (Figure 2.12). In a few instances, however, a specific population (following a genetically predetermined pattern) will skew this distribution by exhibiting a unique pattern of responsiveness, usually due to genetic alterations in drug metabolism.

From Figure 2.12, it is obvious that, although the average dose required to elicit a given response can be calculated easily, some people respond at very much lower doses than the average and others respond only at very much higher doses. Thus, it is extremely important that the dose of any drug be individualized. Generalizations about "average doses" are risky at best.

The dose of a drug that produces the desired effect in 50 percent of the subjects is called the ED_{50}, and the lethal dose for 50 percent of the subjects is called the LD_{50}. The LD_{50} is calculated in exactly the same way as the ED_{50}, except that the dose of the drug is plotted against the number of experimental animals that die after being administered various doses of the compound. Both the ED_{50} and the LD_{50} are determined

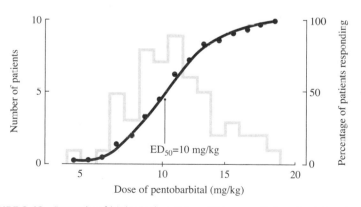

FIGURE 2.12 Example of biological variation. Histogram (*left ordinate*) and cumulative frequency histogram (*right ordinate*) following intravenous administration of pentobarbital, used to cause drowsiness in hospitalized patients. An ED_{50} of about 10 mg/kg body weight is shown. Note, however, that some patients exhibited sedation at about 4 mg/kg, while others required a dose of about 18 mg/kg The stair-step bars illustrate the data behind the dose-response curve.

in several species of animals to prevent accidental drug-induced toxicity in humans. The ratio of the LD_{50} to the ED_{50} is used as an index of the relative safety of the drug and is called the *therapeutic index.*

To illustrate, two dose-response curves are shown in Figure 2.13. The curve at the left illustrates the dose of drug necessary to induce sleep in a population of mice, and the one at the right illustrates the dose of drug necessary to kill a similar population. In this example, the LD_{50}:ED_{50} ratio is seen to be 100:10, or 10. This may seem like a rather large margin, but note that at a dose of 50 milligrams, 95 percent of the mice sleep while 5 percent of the mice die. This overlap demonstrates both the difficulty in assessing the relative safety of drugs for use in large populations and the biological variation in individual responses to drugs. With this particular compound, a dose cannot be administered that will guarantee that 100 percent of the mice will sleep and none will die. Thus, a more useful indication of the margin of safety is a ratio of the lethal dose for 1 percent of the population to the effective dose for 99 percent of the population (LD_1:ED_{99}). A sedative drug with an LD_1:ED_{99} of 1 would be a safer compound than the drug shown in Figure 2.13. Note that the clinical usefulness of indices obtained from laboratory animals is limited because these indices do not reflect the occasional unexpected response (from the causes listed earlier) that can seriously harm a patient.

Drug Interactions

The effects of one drug can be modified by the concurrent administration of another drug. Understanding drug interactions is vital to understanding psychopharmacology as well as psychotherapeutics (the use of drugs to treat psychological disorders). First, it is important to state that some drug interactions are "good" and some are "bad." Interactions are beneficial when two drugs used together achieve therapeutic benefit when a single drug alone is insufficient. For example, combining two drugs with antidepressant properties may afford relief from depression

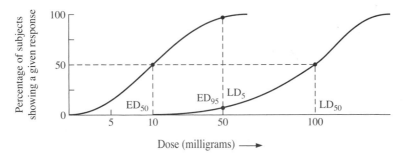

FIGURE 2.13   Illustration of therapeutic index. *Left:* Dose of drug required to induce a given response. *Right:* Lethal dose of the compound. See text for discussion.

that was unattainable with either drug alone (Blier et al., 2010). On the other hand, drug interaction can be detrimental. Detrimental actions can have either a pharmacokinetic or a pharmacodynamic basis.

Chapter 1 explained how certain drugs might either increase or decrease the rate of hepatic metabolism of other drugs and how this interaction can affect the plasma levels of other drugs metabolized by the same enzymes. For example, carbamazepine increases the rate of metabolism of certain other medicines, reducing the blood concentration of the second drug and its effectiveness. Conversely, valproic acid can inhibit the metabolism of other drugs, such as lamotrigine, increasing its blood concentrations and potentially increasing its toxicity or side effects.

In a pharmacodynamic interaction, drugs can interact through an adverse *additive mechanism,* where the effects of one drug potentiate the side effects of a second drug. For example, alcohol taken after ingesting a benzodiazepine tranquilizer or smoking marijuana increases sedation and loss of coordination. This action may have little consequence if the doses of each drug are low, but higher doses of either or both drugs can be dangerous both to the user and to others. Even though a person may normally be able to ingest a limited amount of alcohol and still drive a car without significant loss of control or coordination, the concurrent use of tranquilizers or marijuana may profoundly impair driving performance, endangering the driver, passengers, and other motorists. Ramaekers and coworkers (2000) document the adverse interaction between alcohol and marijuana on driving performance.

Drug Toxicity

All drugs can produce harmful effects as well as beneficial ones. Unwanted effects fall into one of two categories:

1. Effects that are related to the principal and predictable pharmacological actions of a drug (for example, the sedation caused by drinking alcohol or the dry mouth experienced while taking certain antidepressants)
2. Effects that are unrelated to the expected actions of a drug (for example, a severe allergic reaction to a drug)

It is important to categorize harmful effects of drugs in terms of their severity and to distinguish between effects that cause temporary inconvenience or discomfort and effects that can lead to organ damage, permanent disability, or even death.

Most drugs exert effects on several different body functions. To achieve the desired therapeutic effect or effects, some side effects often must be tolerated. Toleration is possible if the side effects are minor, but if they are more serious, they may be a limiting factor in the use of the drug. The distinction between therapeutic effects and side effects is relative and depends on the purpose for which the drug is administered: one person's side effect may be another person's therapeutic effect. For example, in one patient receiving morphine for its pain-relieving properties, the intestinal constipation that morphine induces may be an undesirable side effect that must be tolerated. For a second patient, however, morphine may be used to treat severe diarrhea, in which case the constipation induced is the desired therapeutic effect and relief of pain is a side effect.

In addition to side effects that are merely irritating, some drugs may cause reactions that are very serious, including serious allergies, blood disorders, liver or kidney toxicity, or abnormalities in fetal development. Fortunately, the incidence of serious toxic effects is quite low. As specific drugs are discussed in later chapters, both side effects and more serious toxicities are presented for each drug.

Allergies to drugs may take many forms, from mild skin rashes to fatal shock. Allergies differ from normal side effects, which can often be eliminated or at least made tolerable by a simple reduction in dosage. However, a reduction in the dose of a drug may have no effect on a drug allergy because exposure to any amount of the drug can be hazardous and possibly catastrophic for the patient.

Damage to the liver and kidneys results from the role of these organs in concentrating, metabolizing, and excreting toxic drugs. Examples of drug-induced liver damage include damage caused by alcohol and damage caused by certain inhalants of abuse (Chapter 13). Some of the antipsychotics (for example, the phenothiazines) may induce jaundice by increasing the viscosity of bile in the liver (Chapter 4).

Data quite clearly show the adverse effects of nicotine and ethyl alcohol on the fetus. Similarly, the effects of cocaine and other stimulant drug abuse on the fetus have received much attention. These drugs are responsible for a majority of preventable fetal toxicities and are some of the major health hazards in the country today.

Placebo Effects: Powerful or Problematic?

Placebos have a long history in medicine. Translated from the Latin, the word means "I will please," and, in fact, the first modern definition, appearing in 1811, described placebos as "any medicine adopted more to please than to benefit the patient." (Scheindlin, 2009, p. 108). Since then, the extent to which, or even whether, placebos are beneficial for patients has been the subject of much research and controversy.

Among the first to scientifically study the placebo response were Louis Lasagna and colleagues, who attempted to determine experimentally whether certain subgroups of patients were more likely to be placebo responders and, if so, whether they could be differentiated from nonresponders (Lasagna et al., 1954). Using a measure of postoperative pain, the researchers recorded the consistency of the placebo response and conducted thorough psychological evaluations of the patients. They concluded that their subjects could be divided into three groups: those who sometimes responded to placebo treatment (55 percent), those who always responded (16 percent), and those who never responded (29 percent). A colleague of Lasagna's, Henry Beecher, after further analyzing the data from 15 studies, reported that placebo reactions generally occurred in 30 to 40 percent of all patients (Beecher, 1955). Although placebo responders occurred in both sexes and across all ages, there was no clearly defined set of traits that differentiated them from nonresponders.

Support for the classic Beecher-Lasagna studies was provided more recently by Ernst and Resch (1995), who analyzed the results of studies in which placebo effects were compared with that of "no treatment." They appreciated the fact that, even without placebo treatment, patients may improve for many reasons, such as spontaneous recovery, waxing and waning of symptoms, decrease in anxiety, or other, nondrug, interventions, such as rest or exercise, diet, hot baths, and meditation or other relaxation techniques. Of the six papers that included sufficient information, all of which used a pain rating as the clinical measure, Ernst and Resch (1995) found that four reported a substantial placebo response, one showed a borderline effect, and only one showed no effect.

Since then, however, the validity of the placebo response has been questioned. In their analysis of 32 clinical trials, Hrobjartsson and Gotzsche (2001) argued that there was little support for placebo treatment, except for a small beneficial effect in pain conditions. They concluded that only in the clinical trial setting was placebo treatment justified.

The *double-blind, randomized, placebo-controlled clinical trial* is currently the gold standard for studying the effectiveness and safety of drugs in humans. First reported in 1937 (Scheindlin, 2009) and accepted as the standard by the 1950s, controlled trials were intended to remove the bias, expectations, and even fraud associated with clinical studies in which uncontrolled variables led to much subjective and presumably biased outcomes (Lakoff, 2002).

Even in double-blind, randomized, controlled trials, placebo effects may be substantial. As summarized by Walsh and coworkers (2002) in an analysis of clinical trials of drugs used to treat depression, about 28 percent of patients treated with placebo respond positively and significantly. This compares with 50 percent of patients who responded similarly when treated with active medication, illustrating that placebo effects contributed significantly (perhaps half or more) to the clinical response. Recently, evidence was presented that suggests a possible biological cause for the large placebo effect in antidepressant drug studies. Leuchter and colleagues (2009) report that there may be a genetic basis for the placebo response in people suffering from major depressive disorder.

The large placebo response in clinical trials of antidepressants also illustrates the usefulness of including a "no treatment" condition in addition to comparisons between placebo and active comparators. If there is little or no separation between the placebo and the experimental treatment, then it is not clear whether the placebo response was especially powerful, or the experimental treatment was ineffective, or both. A comprehensive review of the placebo response was recently published by Finniss and coworkers (2010).

Nevertheless, there are situations in which placebo treatment is not required by the FDA to be included, even in clinical trials. Antipsychotic drugs may be approved on the basis of a comparison between the new agent and an antipsychotic that is already approved. Orphan drugs (drugs that treat rare diseases—that is, diseases that occur in fewer than 200,000 people in the United States) may be approved on the basis of comparisons with historical controls, derived from what is known about the course of the disorder in the absence of treatment. Moreover, if other effective treatments are available, placebo treatment may be unethical.

Clearly, at the bicentennial of the first placebo definition, provided in 1811, there is still much to learn about the mechanisms responsible for placebo reactions and whether they can, or should, be part of clinical drug evaluations.

STUDY QUESTIONS

1. What is meant by the term *pharmacodynamics*?

2. What is a drug receptor? What are the major types and how do they differ in structure?

3. Distinguish between *agonist* and *antagonist* as they relate to drug-receptor interactions.

4. Discuss drug-receptor specificity. Can a drug ever be more specific for a receptor than is the endogenous neurotransmitter? Explain.

5. What is meant by a dose-response relationship? Draw a hypothetical example of a dose-response relationship.

6. Discuss how two drugs might interact with each other in the body.

7. Which factors contribute to the intensity, safety, and toxicity of drug effects?

8. Discuss the placebo response.

REFERENCES

Armstrong, N., et al. (2006). "Measurement of Conformational Changes Accompanying Desensitization in an Ionotropic Glutamate Receptor." *Cell* 127: 85–97.

Beecher, H. K. (1955). "The Powerful Placebo." *Journal of the American Medical Association* 159: 1602–1606.

Blier, P., et al. (2010). "Combination of Antidepressant Medications from Treatment Initiation for Major Depressive Disorder: A Double-Blind Randomized Study." *American Journal of Psychiatry* 167: 281–288.

Breedlove, M., et al. (2007). *Biological Psychology: An Introduction to Behavioral, Cognitive and Clinical Neuroscience*, 5th ed. Sunderland, MA: Sinauer.

Ernst, E., and Resch, K. L. (1995). "Concept of True and Perceived Placebo Effects." *British Medical Journal* 311: 551–553.

Finniss, D. G., et al. (2010). "Biological, Clinical and Ethical Advances of Placebo Effects." *Lancet* 375: 686–695.

Gouaux, E., and MacKinnon, R. (2005). "Principles of Selective Ion Transport in Channels and Pumps." *Science* 310: 1461–1465.

Hrobjartsson, A., and Gotzsche, P. C. (2001). "Is the Placebo Powerless? An Analysis of Clinical Trials Comparing Placebo with No Treatment." *New England Journal of Medicine* 344: 1594–1602.

Iverson, L. L., Iverson, S. D., Bloom, F. E., and Roth, R. H. (2009). *Introduction to Neuropsychopharmacology*. New York: Oxford University Press.

Jurrlink, D. N., et al. (2003). "Drug-Drug Interactions Among Elderly Patients Hospitalized for Drug Toxicity." *Journal of the American Medical Association* 289: 1652–1658.

Khatib, S. M. al-, et al. (2003). "What Clinicians Should Know About the QT Interval." *Journal of the American Medical Association* 289: 2120–2127.

Lakoff, A. (2002). "The Mousetrap: Managing the Placebo Effect in Antidepressant Trials." *Molecular Interventions* 2: 72–76.

Lasagna, L., et al. (1954). "A Study of the Placebo Response." *American Journal of Medicine* 16: 770–779.

Leuchter, A. F., et al. (2009). "Monoamine Oxidase A and Catechol-O-Methyltransferase Functional Polymorphisms and the Placebo Response in Major Depressive Disorder." *Journal of Clinical Psychopharmacology* 29: 372–377.

Nestler, E. J., Hyman, S. E., and Malenka, R. C. (2009). *Molecular Pharmacology. A Foundation for Clinical Neuroscience*, 2nd ed. New York: McGraw Hill Medical.

Ramaekers, J. G. (2000). "Marijuana, Alcohol, and Actual Driving Performance." *Human Psychopharmacology* 15: 551–558.

Scheindlin, S. (2009). "The Problematic Placebo." *Molecular Interventions* 9: 108–113.

Walsh, B. T., et al. (2002). "Placebo Response in Studies of Major Depression: Variable, Substantial, and Growing." *Journal of the American Medical Association* 287: 1840–1847.

Yernool, D., et al. (2004). "Structure of a Glutamate Transporter Homologue from *Pyrococcus horikoshii*." *Nature* 431: 811–818.

Chapter 3

The Neuron, Synaptic Transmission, and Neurotransmitters

All our thoughts, actions, memories, and behaviors result from biochemical interactions that take place in and between *neurons*. Drugs that affect these processes are, in general, called *psychoactive drugs*. In essence, psychoactive drugs are chemicals that alter (mimic, potentiate, disrupt, or inhibit) the normal processes associated with neuronal function or communication between neurons. To understand the actions of psychoactive drugs, therefore, it is necessary to have some idea of how the brain is organized, what a neuron is, and how neurons interact with each other.

Overall Organization of the Brain

The human nervous system consists of two divisions, the central nervous system (CNS) and the peripheral nervous system (PNS). The CNS includes the brain and the spinal cord; the PNS includes the nerves that originate in the spinal cord and that connect the spinal cord to the organs of the body. The drugs discussed in this book exert their primary actions and some of their side effects by acting in the brain. However, many of their side effects are produced by their actions in the PNS, that is, at various organ systems, such as the digestive system and the cardiovascular system, as described in subsequent chapters.

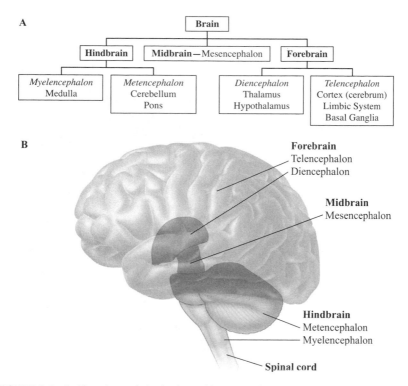

FIGURE 3.1 **A.** Flowchart of the brain and its major divisions. **B.** Drawing of the human brain and its primary divisions.

The human brain consists of perhaps 90 billion individual neurons located in the skull and the spinal cord. Part A of Figure 3.1 shows the organization of the brain, with the various divisions indicated. There are three primary divisions: the hindbrain, the midbrain, and the forebrain. The hindbrain and the forebrain are further divided, each into two sub-divisions, which results in five major sections. Part B of Figure 3.1 shows the anatomical arrangement of these structures.

The *spinal cord* extends from the bottom of the brain, from the medulla to the sacrum. The spinal cord consists of neurons and fiber tracts involved in the following activities:

- Carrying sensory information from the skin, muscles, joints, and internal body organs to the brain
- Organizing and modulating the motor outflow to the muscles (to produce coordinated movement)
- Modulating sensory input (including pain impulses)
- Providing autonomic (involuntary) control of vital body functions

The lower part of the brain, attached to the upper part of the spinal cord, is the *brain stem* (Figure 3.2). It is divided into three parts:

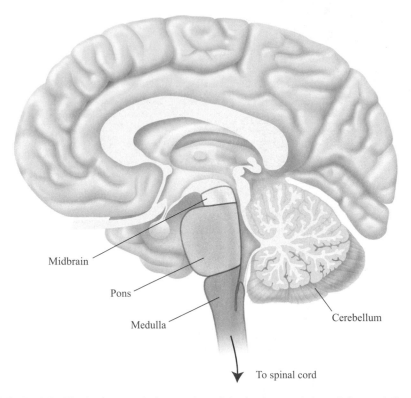

Midbrain

Pons

Medulla

Cerebellum

To spinal cord

FIGURE 3.2 The brain stem is the portion of the brain, consisting of the medulla oblongata, pons, and midbrain, that connects the spinal cord to the forebrain and cerebrum.

the *medulla*, the *pons*, and the *midbrain*. All impulses that are conducted in either direction between the spinal cord and the brain pass through the brain stem, which is also important in the regulation of vital body functions, such as respiration, blood pressure, heart rate, gastrointestinal functioning, and the states of sleep and wakefulness. The brain stem is also involved in behavioral alerting, attention, and arousal responses. Depressant drugs, such as the barbiturates (Chapter 7), depress the brain-stem activating system, which probably underlies much of their hypnotic action.

Behind the brain stem is a large, bulbous structure—the *cerebellum*. A highly convoluted structure, the cerebellum is connected to the brain stem by large fiber tracts. The cerebellum is necessary for the proper integration of movement and posture. Drunkenness, which is characterized by ataxia (loss of coordination and balance, staggering, and other deficits), is caused largely by an alcohol-induced depression of cerebellar function. Together, the brain stem and the cerebellum make up two of the five brain sections, the hindbrain and midbrain.

The area immediately above the brain stem and covered by the cerebral hemispheres (cerebrum; see Figure 3.1) is the fourth major brain division, the *diencephalon* (Figure 3.3). In addition to the thalamus and hypothalamus, this area includes the subthalamus, pituitary

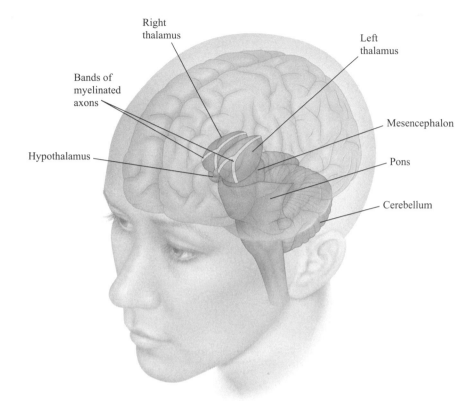

Right thalamus

Left thalamus

Bands of myelinated axons

Mesencephalon

Hypothalamus

Pons

Cerebellum

FIGURE 3.3 The diencephalon. [From Pinel (2007), p. 53, Figure 2.23.]

gland, and various fiber tracts (bundles of axons that travel as a group from one area to another), which are not shown in Figure 3.3.

The *subthalamus* is a small area underneath the thalamus. It contains a variety of small structures that, together with the *substantia nigra* (SN) in the midbrain (see Figure 3.1) and the basal ganglia (Figure 3.4) in the telencephalon (see Figure 3.1), constitute one of our motor systems, the *extrapyramidal system*. The major structures of the basal ganglia are the caudate, putamen, and globus pallidus. Patients who have Parkinson's disease (Chapter 19) have a deficiency of the neurotransmitter dopamine in the terminals of their nerve axons, which originate in cell bodies in the substantia nigra (see Figure 3.13). As a result, the amount of dopamine that is released by the SN onto the structures of the basal ganglia is substantially reduced. This deficiency produces the symptoms of Parkinson's disease. Treatment, described in Chapter 19, involves efforts to restore dopaminergic function.

The *hypothalamus* is a collection of neurons in the lower portion of the brain near the junction of the midbrain and the thalamus. It is located near the base of the skull, just above the pituitary gland (whose function it modulates). The hypothalamus is the principal center in the

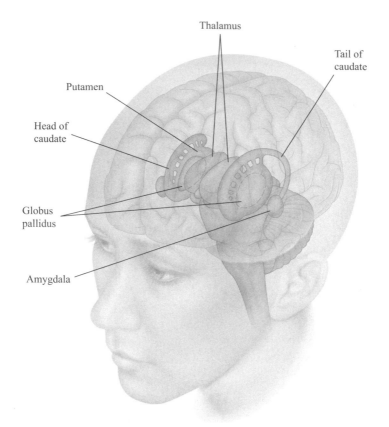

Thalamus

Tail of
caudate

Putamen

Head of
caudate

Globus
pallidus

Amygdala

FIGURE 3.4 The basal ganglia (caudate, putamen, and globus pallidus). [From Pinel (2007), p. 57, Figure 2.28.]

brain responsible for the integration of our entire autonomic (involuntary or vegetative) nervous system. Thus, it helps control such vegetative functions as eating, drinking, sleeping, regulation of body temperature, sexual behavior, blood pressure, emotion, and water balance. In addition, the hypothalamus closely controls the hormonal output of the pituitary gland. Neurons in the hypothalamus produce substances called *releasing factors*, which travel to the nearby pituitary gland, inducing the secretion of hormones that regulate fertility in females and sperm formation in males. The hypothalamus is a site of action for many psychoactive drugs, either a site for the primary action of the drug or a site responsible for side effects associated with the use of a drug.

Closely associated with the hypothalamus (see Figure 3.3) is the *limbic system* (Figure 3.5A), the major components of which are the *amygdala* and the *hippocampus*. These structures integrate memory (hippocampus), emotion (amygdala), and reward with behavioral, motor, and autonomic functions. Because the limbic system and the

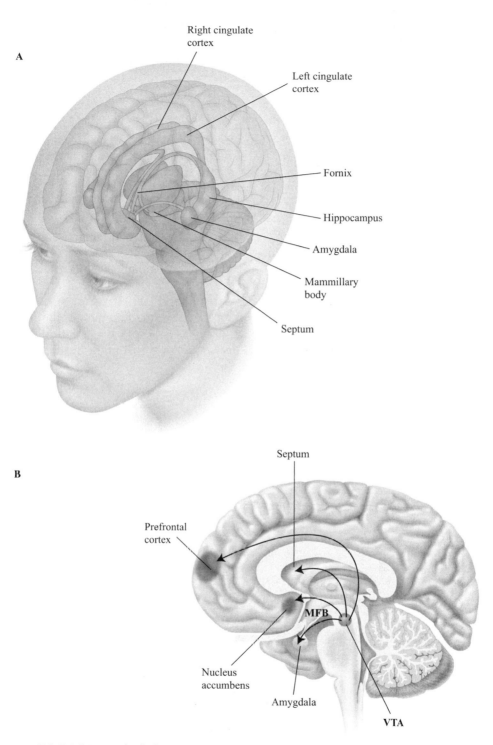

FIGURE 3.5 A. The limbic system. **B.** The reward circuit: major structures of the reward system. VTA = ventral tegmental area; MFB = medial forebrain bundle. [From Pinel (2007), p. 57, Figure 2.27.]

hypothalamus interact to regulate emotion and emotional expression, these structures are logical sites for the study of psychoactive drugs that alter mood, affect, emotion, or responses to emotional experiences.

The hypothalamic and limbic areas also contain structures important in psychopharmacology and the abuse potential of drugs. Included here are the dopamine-rich reward centers (Figure 3.5B) that involve the *ventral tegmental area,* the *medial forebrain bundle,* and the *nucleus accumbens.* Throughout this text, this reward system is discussed as a site of the behavior-reinforcing action of psychoactive drugs that are subject to compulsive abuse (Chapter 17).

Almost completely covering the brain stem and the diencephalon is the *cerebrum* (Figure 3.6). In humans the cerebrum is the largest part of the brain. It is separated into two distinct hemispheres, left and right, with numerous fiber tracts connecting the two. Because skull size is limited and the cerebrum is so large, the outer layer of the cerebrum, the *cerebral cortex,* is deeply convoluted and fissured. Like other parts of the brain, the cerebral cortex is subdivided; it consists of four major lobes, each of which has areas that are responsible for specific functions, such

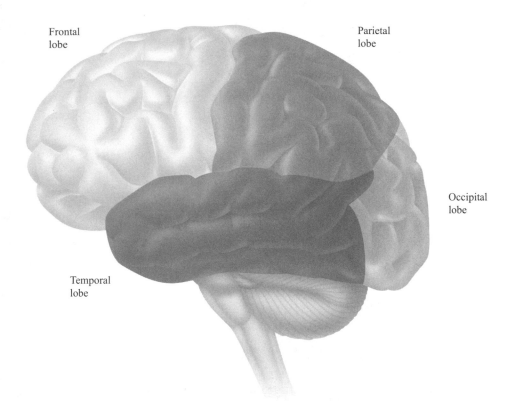

Frontal lobe

Parietal lobe

Occipital lobe

Temporal lobe

FIGURE 3.6 The cerebrum. The four major lobes of the human brain.

as vision (occipital lobe), hearing (temporal lobe), sensory perception (parietal lobe), and higher-level cognitive functions (frontal lobe).

The Neuron

The neuron is the basic unit of the central nervous system (CNS), and each neuron shares common structural and functional characteristics (Figure 3.7). A typical neuron has a *soma* (cell body), which contains the nucleus (within which is the genetic material of the cell). Extending from the soma in one direction are many short fibers, called *dendrites* (hundreds of widely branched extensions), that receive input from other neurons through *receptors* located on the dendritic membrane. On receipt of a signal from another cell, current is generated and travels down the dendrite to the soma. Extending in another direction from the soma is a single elongated process called an *axon,* which varies in length from as short as a few millimeters to as long as a meter (meter-length examples are the axons that run from the motor neurons of the spinal cord out to the muscles that they innervate). The axon, in essence, transmits electrical activity (in the form of *action potentials)* from the soma to other neurons or to muscles, organs, or glands of the body. Normally, the axon conducts impulses in only one direction—from the soma down the axon to a specialized structure that, together with one or more dendrites from another neuron, forms a complex microspace called *a synapse* (see Figure 3.7).

A given neuron in the brain may receive several thousand synaptic connections from other neurons (Hyman, 2005). The number of possible different combinations of synaptic connections among the neurons in a single human brain is larger than the total number of atomic particles that make up the known universe. Hence the diversity of the interconnections in a human brain seems almost without limit.

It was once thought that the brain has the maximal number of neurons at birth; once a neuron dies, it is not replaced. This concept has been debunked because we now realize that new neurons form every day (a process called *neurogenesis)* and existing neurons need to be maintained in a state of health (Kempermann et al., 2004; Schaffer and Gage, 2004). The synaptic connections appear to form the anatomical basis of memory and the maintenance of a normal state of mood (Sutton and Schuman, 2006; Ashraf and Kunes, 2006). This continual reshaping and remodeling of neurons is associated with the process of synaptic plasticity (Thomas and Davies, 2005). The synaptic contacts between neurons are continually being reshaped, and the axon terminals as well as the dendrites are continually reforming new synaptic connections while losing old ones. This remodeling probably begins even before birth and continues all our lives. The relationship between neuronal "health" and various psychological disorders, such as depression, bipolar disorder, and drug addiction, is discussed in subsequent chapters in this book.

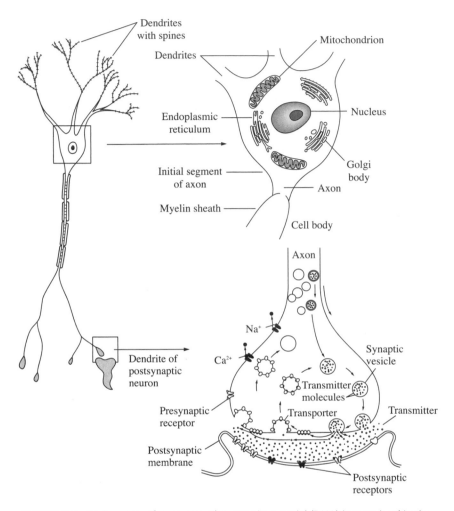

FIGURE 3.7 Major parts of a neuron. The genetic material (DNA) is contained in the nucleus, and several specialized organelles are present in the cytoplasm, the material of the cell outside the nucleus. The cell is enclosed by a thin wall, or membrane. Mitochondria are present in the cell body, the fibers, and the terminals. The terminals also contain small, round vesicles that contain neurotransmitter chemicals. Synaptic connections from the fibers of other neurons cover the cell body and dendrites. In many neurons the synapses on dendrites can be seen as little spines. The axon itself has no synapses on it except sometimes at its synaptic terminals, where other neuron axon terminals may form synapses on synapses.

A synapse is the point of functional contact between an axon termi-nal and another cell. A synapse consists of a minute space (the *synaptic cleft*) between the presynaptic membrane (which is the axon terminal) of one neuron and the postsynaptic membrane of the receiving neuron. The presynaptic terminal contains numerous structural elements, the most important of which (for our purposes) are the small synaptic vesicles, each of which contains several thousand molecules of neuro-transmitter chemical (the *first messenger*) that transmits information from one neuron to another. These vesicles store the transmitter, which is available for release. Through a process called *exocytosis* and under the influence of calcium ions, vesicles fuse with the presynaptic membrane and molecules of transmitter are released into the synaptic cleft. The transmitter substance diffuses across the synaptic cleft and attaches to various types of receptors on the postsynaptic membrane of the next neuron, transmitting information chemically from one neuron to another. The neurons do not physically touch each other; synaptic transmission is a chemical rather than an electrical process.

The process of synaptic transmission takes a remarkably short time; the entire process may occur over a time span as short as a millisecond for transmitter release (from presynaptic vesicles), diffusion (across the cleft), receptor attachment, and activation. The nature of the response produced by synaptic transmission depends on the characteristics of the receptor that is activated (Chapter 2). Receptors may respond quickly, within milliseconds, or they may produce responses that last hundreds of milliseconds. The ultimate outcome of receptor activation is a function of the organ or tissue in which it is located.

Termination of Synaptic Transmission

The arrival of an action potential at the synapse induces release of a neurotransmitter into the synaptic cleft, and the transmitter then reversibly binds to its receptors. However, there must be mechanisms available to get rid of neurotransmitter; otherwise transmitter would stay in the synaptic cleft and continually bind to the postsynaptic receptors. In most cases, transmitter removal occurs through one of three mechanisms:

1. An enzyme present in the synaptic cleft breaks down any neurotransmitter remaining in the synapse.
2. The transmitter is taken back into the presynaptic cell through the reuptake transporter present on the presynaptic membrane.
3. In the case of glutamate neurotransmission, after release, the glutamate is taken up into an adjacent glial cell, reprocessed, and returned to the presynaptic nerve terminal.

Following are some of the neurotransmitters removed by presynaptic reuptake and examples of drugs that block the process:

- Norepinephrine, presynaptic reuptake of which is blocked by the *tricyclic antidepressants* and *atomoxetine* (Strattera)
- Serotonin, presynaptic reuptake of which is blocked by the *selective serotonin reuptake inhibitor* (SSRI) *antidepressants*
- Dopamine, presynaptic reuptake of which is blocked by *bupropion* (Wellbutrin) and by *cocaine*

In the case of the neurotransmitter acetylcholine, processes 1 and 2 are involved. The enzyme *acetylcholine esterase* breaks down the transmitter into acetate and choline in the synaptic cleft, after which they are taken up into the nerve terminal to be resynthesized into acetylcholine.

Receptor Specificity

It would be nice if there were a single receptor type for each specific neurotransmitter. In actuality, virtually every transmitter binds to several distinct receptor subtypes. For example, norepinephrine, serotonin, and dopamine bind to multiple presynaptic and postsynaptic receptors as well as their specific presynaptic transporter. For example, for serotonin receptors, at least 15 different subtypes of receptors have been described. All this leads to immense opportunity for the development of drugs with incredible specificity—for example, for blocking one specific subtype of postsynaptic serotonin receptor, reducing or eliminating the side effects that limit the clinical usefulness of existing psychotherapeutic agents. Table 3.1 lists a few of the commonly recognized neurotransmitters, some of the receptor subtypes that have been identified, and some of the brain functions thought to be under the control of each transmitter. Besides these substances, many lipids and proteins (peptides) have also been implicated in synaptic transmission (Hyman, 2005).

TABLE 3.1 Classification of the major neurotransmitter families with selected neurotransmitters

Family and subfamily	Transmitters
AMINES	
Quaternary amines	Acetylcholine (ACH)
Monoamines	*Catecholamines:* Norepinephrine (NE), epinephrine (adrenaline), dopamine (DA)
	Indoleamines: Serotonin (5-hydroxytryptamine: 5-HT)
AMINO ACIDS	Gamma-aminobutyric acid (GABA), glutamate, glycine
NEUROPEPTIDES	
Opioid peptides	*Enkephalins:* Met-enkephalin, leu-enkephalin
	Endorphins: β-endorphin
	Dynorphins: Dynorphin A
PEPTIDES	Oxytocin, substance P, cholecystokinin (CCK), vasopressin, hypothalamic-releasing hormones
GASES	Nitric oxide, carbon monoxide

From Breedlove et al. (2007), Table 4.1, p. 90

The Soma

Present in all cells of the body (except red blood cells), the soma has a *nucleus* that contains the basic genetic material (the DNA) for the cell (Figure 3.8). Because the neuron is a specialized type of cell, its DNA expresses a subset of genes that encode the special structural and enzymatic proteins that determine its size, shape, location, and other functional characteristics (Cooper et al., 2003). Also located in the soma are the *mitochondria*, which provide the biological energy for the neuron. This energy, in the form of *adenosine triphosphate* (ATP), is made available for all the various chemical reactions carried out in the cell (such as neurotransmitter synthesis, storage, release, and reuptake).

In response to stimuli, the DNA in the nucleus is transcribed into a second similar molecular form as strands of ribonucleic acid (hnRNA), which is then "edited" by several rapid steps and exported from the nucleus to the cytoplasm of the soma. The edited RNA is called *messenger RNA*, and this nuclear material is then translated from the nucleic acid code of the RNA into the amino acid sequence of the protein that is to be expressed (see Figure 3.8). Expression, or translation, occurs on the *endoplasmic reticulum*, where the neurotransmitters are synthesized

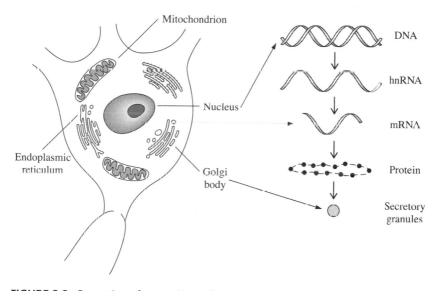

FIGURE 3.8 Formation of transmitter substances and "packaging" in vesicles from genetic material in the nucleus. DNA-encoded information is transcribed in the nucleus to a primary transcript form (hnRNA), which is edited and exported from the nucleus to the cytoplasm as messenger RNA (mRNA). The information is then translated from the genetic nucleic acid code of RNA into the amino acid sequence of the protein that is to be expressed. Within the Golgi body portion of the endoplasmic reticulum, the transmitter is packaged into secretory organelles for transport down the axon to the neuron terminals.

and then "packaged" into vesicles that are then transported in specialized *microtubules* down the axon to the synaptic terminals, where they await release. Even presynaptic components (such as transporters) are made in the soma and carried down the axon, embedding in the cell membrane where they exert their synaptic functions.

Specific Neurotransmitters

Neurons release specific chemical substances from their presynaptic nerve terminals, and it is the interaction between psychoactive drugs and the receptors on which the natural transmitters act that underlies the actions of the drugs. The earliest chemicals identified as CNS neurotransmitters were acetylcholine and norepinephrine, largely because of their established roles in the peripheral nervous system. In the 1960s, serotonin, epinephrine, and dopamine were added. In the 1970s, gamma aminobutyric acid (GABA), glycine, glutamate, and certain neuropeptides (such as the endorphins) were identified. In the late 1980s, the lipid amide anandamide was identified as the endogenous transmitter for the tetrahydrocannabinol receptor. For a personal account of this history, see Snyder (2002).

Acetylcholine

Acetylcholine (ACh) was identified as a transmitter chemical first in the peripheral nervous system and later in brain tissue. Deficiencies in acetylcholine-secreting neurons have classically been associated with the dysfunctions seen in Alzheimer's disease. Certainly drugs that either potentiate or inhibit the central action of acetylcholine exert profound effects on memory. For example, scopolamine is a psychedelic drug (Chapter 15) that blocks central cholinergic receptors and as a result produces amnesia. Conversely, drugs that increase the amount of acetylcholine in the brain appear to improve memory function and are used to delay the onset of Alzheimer's disease (Chapter 19).

ACh is synthesized in a one-step reaction from two precursors (choline and acetyl CoA) and is then stored within synaptic vesicles for later release. This reaction and the dynamics of ACh release, metabolism, and resynthesis are shown in Figure 3.9. Like other neurotransmitters, ACh is released into the synaptic cleft, rapidly diffuses across the cleft, and reversibly binds to postsynaptic receptors. Once ACh has exerted its effect on postsynaptic receptors, its action is terminated by *acetylcholinesterase* (AChE).

The enzymatic reaction that degrades ACh is important not only in the treatment of Alzheimer's disease but also in agriculture and in the military. Drugs that inhibit the action of AChE, referred to as *AChE inhibitors,* include both "reversible" and "irreversible" AChE inhibitors.

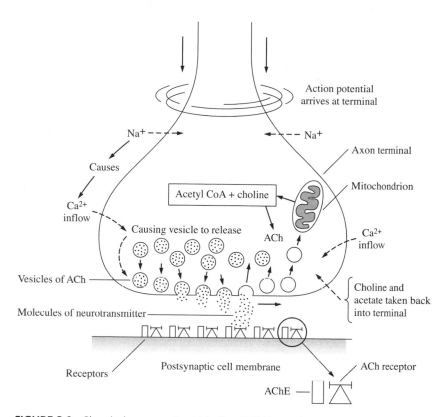

FIGURE 3.9 Chemical synapse. Acetylcholine (ACh) is used as the example. It is made in the axon terminal from acetyl coenzyme A (acetyl CoA) and choline, stored in vesicles, and released. When the action potential arrives at the terminal, closed calcium channels in the terminal are opened and Ca^{2+} rushes into the terminal, triggering vesicles to fuse with the membrane and release ACh molecules into the synaptic cleft. They attach to ACh receptors on the postsynaptic membrane and trigger the opening of Na^+ channels. ACh is immediately broken down at the receptors by acetylcholinesterase (AChE) into choline and acetate, which are taken back up by the terminal and reused.

Irreversible AChE inhibitors form a permanent covalent bond with the enzyme and totally inhibit enzyme function. They are usually administered in "toxic" doses, and the result is usually fatal. Some of these toxic drugs (such as *malathion* and *parathion)* are exploited in gardening and agriculture as insecticides because they kill insects on contact. Other irreversible AChe inhibitors (such as *Sarin* and *Soman)* have been used in the military as lethal nerve gases.

Less toxic and shorter acting are the *reversible AChE inhibitors,* used to more modestly increase ACh levels in the brain. They are used clinically as cognitive enhancers, delaying the decline in cognitive function in patients with Alzheimer's disease. Individual agents are discussed in Chapter 19.

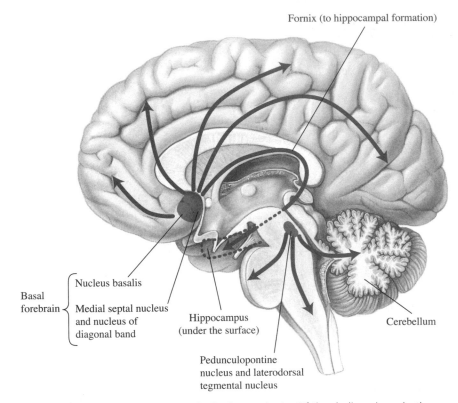

Fornix (to hippocampal formation)

Nucleus basalis

Basal forebrain

Medial septal nucleus and nucleus of diagonal band

Hippocampus (under the surface)

Cerebellum

Pedunculopontine nucleus and laterodorsal tegmental nucleus

FIGURE 3.10 Cholinergic systems in the human brain. Of the cholinergic projection neurons that interconnect central structures, two major subconstellations have been identified: (1) the forebrain cholinergic complex composed of neurons in the medial septal nucleus and nucleus basalis and projecting to the telencephalon; (2) the pontomesencephalotegmental cholinergic complex, composed of cells in the pedunculopontine and laterodorsal tegmental nuclei and projecting ascendingly to the thalamus and other diencephalic loci and descendingly to the pontine and medullary reticular formation (RF), cerebellum, and cranial nerve nuclei. [Modified from Breedlove et al. (2007), p. 92, Figure 4.2.]

ACh is distributed widely in the brain (Figure 3.10). The cell bodies of cholinergic neurons in the brain lie in two closely related regions. One involves the *septal nuclei* and the *nucleus basalis*. The axons of these neurons project to forebrain regions, particularly the hippocampus and cerebral cortex. The second originates in the midbrain region and projects anteriorly (forward) to the thalamus, basal ganglia, and diencephalon and posteriorly (backward) to the medulla, pons, cerebellum, and cranial nerve nuclei. In addition to its generally accepted role in learning and memory, the diffuse distribution of ACh is consistent with suggestions that ACh is involved in circuits that modulate sensory reception; in mechanisms related to behavioral arousal, attention, energy conservation, and mood; and in REM activity during sleep.

Catecholamine Neurotransmitters: Dopamine and Norepinephrine

The term *catecholamine* refers to compounds that contain a catechol nucleus (a benzene ring with two attached hydroxyl groups) to which is attached an amine group (Figure 3.11). In the CNS, the term usually refers to the transmitters *dopamine* (DA) and *norepinephrine* (NE). In the peripheral nervous system, *epinephrine* ("adrenaline") is a third catecholamine transmitter. In the brain, a large number of psychoactive drugs (both licit and illicit, therapeutic and abused) exert their effects by altering the synaptic action of NE and DA.

The chemical synthesis of DA is illustrated in Figure 3.11. NE is produced by an additional step that involves oxidation of the proximal carbon of the ethyl side chain. Biosynthesis of the catecholamines begins with the amino acid tyrosine and is a complicated process involving genetic and enzymatic regulation. Following synthesis, the transmitter is stored in vesicles for release into the synaptic space. This release is controlled by *presynaptic receptors* (autoreceptors) that serve as a negative feedback mechanism. When stimulated by transmitter, these receptors reduce the synthesis and release of transmitter. Thus, when large amounts of transmitter are present in the synaptic cleft, excess transmitter acts on the autoreceptors to reduce further production and release. Conversely, if an autoreceptor is blocked by an antagonist, synthesis and release of transmitter is increased.

After release, NE and DA also attach to postsynaptic receptors. As discussed earlier, inactivation in the synaptic cleft occurs primarily by reuptake of the transmitter from the synaptic cleft into the presynaptic nerve terminal. Within the nerve terminal, catecholamines can be inactivated by enzymes, such as monoamine oxidase (MAO). The products of inactivation are further metabolized and eliminated from the body through the urine. The class of antidepressants referred to as MAO inhibitors (Chapter 5) acts by inhibiting MAO, thereby increasing the amounts of DA and NE available for synaptic release.

Postsynaptic Catecholamine Receptors. Postsynaptic binding of DA or NE triggers a sequence of chemical events in the postsynaptic cell membrane, eventually affecting either ion channels or intracellular metabolic activity. It is possible that the slow onset of action of antidepressant drugs (several weeks to achieve a therapeutic effect) follows the down regulation of postsynaptic catecholamine receptors as an adaptation to the presence of increased amounts of transmitter present in the synaptic cleft (because the reuptake elimination of the transmitter was blocked by the drug).

Each catecholamine transmitter exerts effects on a number of different postsynaptic receptors. Norepinephrine and epinephrine act at two primary types of receptors (alpha and beta), each of

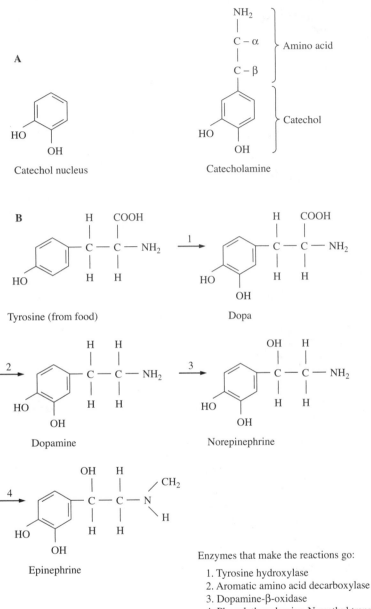

FIGURE 3.11   A. Catechol and catecholamine structure. All catecholamines share the catechol nucleus, a benzene ring with two adjacent hydroxyl (OH) groups. **B.** Structures and synthesis of the catecholamines. Tyrosine, an amino acid found in foods, is converted into dopa, then into dopamine, next into norepinephrine, and finally (in the peripheral nervous system) into epinephrine, depending on which enzymes (1–4) are present in the cell.

which has at least two subtypes. Dopamine exerts postsynaptic effects on at least six receptors, divided into two families (D_1 type and D_2 type). Confusingly, D_1 receptors are subdivided into two subtypes—D_1 and D_5—and D_2 receptors into four subtypes—D_{2A}, D_{2B}, D_3, and D_4. Postsynaptic dopamine receptors of the D_2 family are responsible for at least part of the antipsychotic activity of the drugs discussed in Chapter 4. Alterations in dopamine receptor function have been implicated in numerous diseases and behavioral states, including schizophrenia, parkinsonism, Huntington's chorea, affective disorders, sexual activity, reward, attention deficit/hyperactivity disorder, and others.

Norepinephrine Pathways.   The cell bodies of NE neurons are located in the brain stem, mainly in the locus coeruleus (Figure 3.12). From there, axons project widely throughout the brain to nerve terminals in the cerebral cortex, the limbic system, the hypothalamus,

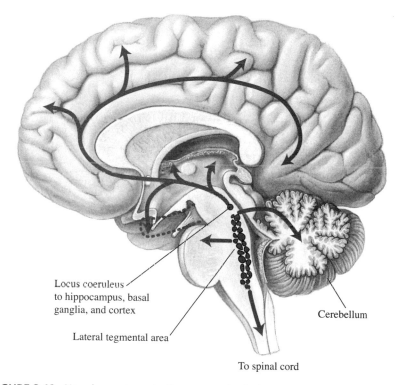

FIGURE 3.12 Noradrenergic projection systems in the human brain. The cell bodies are in the locus coeruleus and adjacent regions of the brain stem and project widely to the forebrain and cerebellum and to the brain stem and spinal cord. [Modified from Breedlove et al. (2007), p. 93, Figure 4.4.]

and the cerebellum. Axonal projections also travel to the dorsal horns of the spinal cord, where they exert an analgesic action. The release of NE produces an alerting, focusing, orienting response, positive feelings of reward, and analgesia. NE release may also be involved in basic instinctual behaviors, such as hunger, thirst, emotion, and sex.

Dopamine Pathways.   Dopamine pathways in the brain originate in the brain stem, sending axons both rostral (forward) to the brain and caudal (backward) to the spinal cord (Figure 3.13). Three dopamine circuits are most relevant for our purposes:

1. Neurons in the hypothalamus send short axons to the pituitary gland (not shown in Figure 3.13). These neurons regulate certain hormones. Alterations in hormone function are commonly seen in

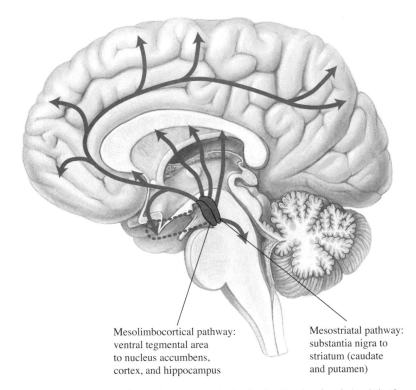

Mesolimbocortical pathway: ventral tegmental area to nucleus accumbens, cortex, and hippocampus

Mesostriatal pathway: substantia nigra to striatum (caudate and putamen)

FIGURE 3.13   The three dopamine systems in the brain. One is a local circuit in the hypothalamus (not shown); another is the pathway from the substantia nigra to the caudate nucleus of the basal ganglia, which is involved in motor functions and Parkinson's disease; the third consists of cell bodies in the brain stem and midbrain (tegmentum) that project widely to the cerebral cortex and forebrain limbic system. [Modified from Breedlove et al. (2007), p. 93, Figure 4.3.]

people with schizophrenia taking various antipsychotics, which block these dopamine receptors (Chapter 4).

2. Neurons in the substantia nigra (see Figure 3.13) that project to the basal ganglia (see Figure 3.4) play a major role in the regulation of movement. As noted earlier, parkinsonism, its treatment with L-dopa (Chapter 19), and extrapyramidal side effects produced by antipsychotic drugs, which block these receptors, all involve this pathway.

3. Cell bodies in the midbrain (ventral tegmentum), next to the substantia nigra, project to higher brain regions (see Figure 3.13). One branch, called the mesocortical, projects to the frontal cortex, and a second branch, called the mesolimbic, projects to the limbic system. Alterations in the development of this pathway may be involved in the pathogenesis of schizophrenia and its amelioration by antipsychotic drugs. In addition, this dopaminergic pathway also involves the ventral tegmentum, nucleus accumbens, and frontal cortex, which constitute our "central reward pathway" (see Figure 3.5B), which is involved in addiction to most drugs of abuse (Chapter 17).

Serotonin

Serotonin (5-hydroxytryptamine, 5-HT) was first investigated as a CNS neurotransmitter in the 1950s when lysergic acid diethylamide (LSD) was found to structurally resemble serotonin and block the contractile effect of serotonin on the gastrointestinal tract. At that time, it was hypothesized that LSD-induced hallucinations might be caused by alterations in the functioning of serotonin neurons and that serotonin might be involved in abnormal behavioral functioning. Today, drugs that potentiate the synaptic actions of serotonin are widely used as antidepressants and as antianxiety agents useful in treating such disorders as obsessive-compulsive disorder, panic disorder, and phobias. Some of these *serotonergic drugs* fall under the category of *selective serotonin reuptake inhibitors* (SSRIs; Chapter 5). Serotonin plays a role in depression and other affective states, sleep, sex, and the regulation of body temperature; use of an SSRI to treat depression can be associated with such side effects as insomnia, anxiety, and loss of libido.

Significant amounts of serotonin are found in the upper brain stem, particularly in the pons and the medulla (areas that are collectively called the *raphe nuclei*). Rostral projections from the brain stem terminate diffusely throughout the cerebral cortex, hippocampus, hypothalamus, and limbic system (Figure 3.14). Serotonin projections largely parallel those of DA, although they are not as widespread. Axons of serotonin neurons projecting to the spinal cord from cell

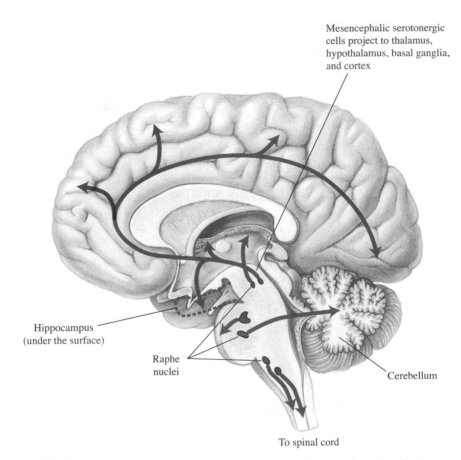

Mesencephalic serotonergic cells project to thalamus, hypothalamus, basal ganglia, and cortex

Hippocampus (under the surface)

Raphe nuclei

Cerebellum

To spinal cord

FIGURE 3.14 Serotonin pathways in the human brain. [Modified from Breedlove et al. (2007), p. 94, Figure 4.5.]

bodies located in the raphe nuclei may be involved in the modulation of both pain (Chapter 10) and spinal reflexes.

In addition to the presynaptic serotonin transporter (blocked by SSRIs), several chemically distinct postsynaptic serotonin (5-HT) receptors have been identified.[1] They have been classified in families (designated by a number) and subtypes within a family (designated by a letter). Note that this is a different type of designation than the one for dopamine. The main families of 5-HT receptors are designated 5-HT_1, 5-HT_2, 5-HT_3, and 5-HT_4. The 5-HT_3 receptor is an ion channel; the others use a G-protein-coupled second-messenger system (Chapter 2).

[1]The symbol *5-HT* refers to 5-hydroxytryptamine, the structural name for serotonin. The terms *5-HT* and *serotonin* are used interchangeably.

Amino Acid Neurotransmitters

The "classical" neurotransmitters (ACh, NE, DA, and serotonin), although important in behavioral regulation and in the actions of psychotropic drugs, are nevertheless used by only a small proportion of the neurons in the brain (Snyder, 2002). Dozens, if not hundreds, of other neurotransmitters exist in the brain, and many of them have been implicated in the actions of psychoactive drugs. Examples include *endorphins* and their receptors, involved in the action of opioid narcotics (Chapter 10), and *anandamide* and its receptors, involved in the action of tetrahydrocannabinol (Chapter 14).

Here we introduce two amino acid neurotransmitters that are widely distributed in the brain. The first, *glutamic acid* (or *glutamate*), is the major universally excitatory neurotransmitter, present on virtually all neurons within the brain. The second is *gamma aminobutyric acid* (GABA), which is the major inhibitory neurotransmitter in the brain. Most other amino acids in the brain do not serve as neurotransmitters (with the exception of aspartate and glycine) but function as precursor molecules for the biosynthesis of other transmitters (for example, tyrosine for catecholamines and tryptophan for serotonin).

Both glutamate and GABA function to modulate a number of receptors, maintaining a balance between excitation and inhibition in the brain. The following sections focus on glutamate and GABA because they are involved in the actions of several psychoactive drugs ranging from the benzodiazepine antianxiety agents (Chapter 7) to the mood stabilizers (Chapter 6).

Glutamate.   Glutamate is a major excitatory neurotransmitter in the brain. Glutamate receptors are found on the surface of virtually all neurons. Glutamate is also the precursor for the major inhibitory neurotransmitter GABA. GABA is formed from glutamate under control of the enzyme *glutamic acid decarboxylase*.

Glutamate neurotransmission plays a critical role in cortical and hippocampal cognitive function, motor function, cerebellar function, and sensory function. Research is focusing on the importance of glutamate dysfunction in the pathogenesis of schizophrenia, especially the negative symptoms, and the cognitive dysfunction associated with the disorder (Chapter 4). Glutamate also plays an important role in "synaptic plasticity" and is involved in the molecular processes that underlie learning and memory. However, glutamate excesses can be a potent neuronal "excitotoxin," triggering either rapid or delayed death of neurons. This excitotoxicity may play a role in the neuronal injury that accompanies alcoholism (Chapter 13), Alzheimer's disease (Chapter 19), head injury, and a variety of other disorders, as reviewed by Weeber and coworkers (2002).

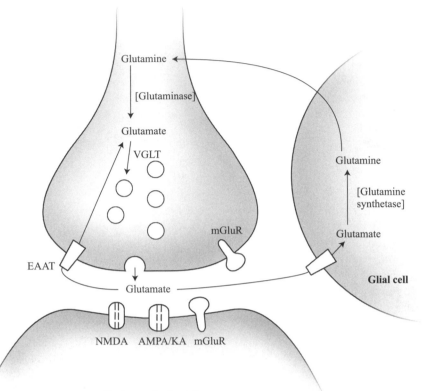

Neuron axon terminal

Postsynaptic dendrite

FIGURE 3.15 Pathways for glutamine release, reuptake, and reutilization. Glutamate (Glu) is released into the synapse and recaptured by a glutamate transporter located on adjacent glial cells. Within the glial cells, glutamate is converted to glutamine (Gln) by the enzyme *glutamine synthetase.* Gln then returns to the cerebrospinal fluid, where it is present in high concentrations. It diffuses into neuronal terminals to replenish the Glu after conversion to Glu from Gln by the enzyme *glutaminase.* [From Cooper et al. (2003), p. 133.]

Glutamate is a nonessential amino acid, meaning that it is easily synthesized in the body and is not required in the diet. It does not readily penetrate the blood-brain barrier, and it is produced locally by specialized neuronal mechanisms (Figure 3.15). It can be synthesized by a number of different chemical reactions, among which is the normal breakdown of glucose. A second reaction is synthesis from glutamine. In this mechanism (which might be the more important for neuronal glutamate), there is a glutamine cycle in which synaptically inactive glutamine serves as a reservoir of glutamate. In this cycle, after glutamate is released from a neuron and exerts its excitatory effect, it is transported (taken up) into astrocytes (neighboring, nonneuronal support cells in the brain) and converted to glutamine, which is stored in the astrocytes. Eventually, the glutamine diffuses out of the astrocytes and enters the presynaptic nerve terminals, where it is converted to glutamate, the active neurotransmitter (Iverson et al., 2009).

There are several different types of glutamate receptors: *ionotropic receptors* (which respond quickly; Chapter 2) and *metabotropic receptors* (which respond more slowly; Chapter 2). The ionotropic receptor subtypes can be further divided into three: NMDA, kainate, and AMPA (the latter two are sometimes referred to as non-NMDA receptors; see Figure 3.15). In the adult human brain, NMDA and AMPA receptors are colocalized in about 70 percent of their synapses. These receptors mediate rapid excitation of postsynaptic neurons, with especially high concentrations in the cerebral cortex, hippocampus, basal ganglia, septum, and amygdala.

NMDA receptors are activated by glutamate in the presence of another amino acid, either glycine or serine. At resting potential, the NMDA ion channel is blocked by magnesium ions (Mg^+). Only when the membrane is depolarized (by the activation of AMPA or kainate receptors on the same postsynaptic neuron) is the Mg^+ blockade of the ion channel relieved. Then the NMDA receptor channel opens and permits the entry of both sodium and calcium ions (Figure 3.16). Within the NMDA receptor ion channel is a binding site for phencyclidine

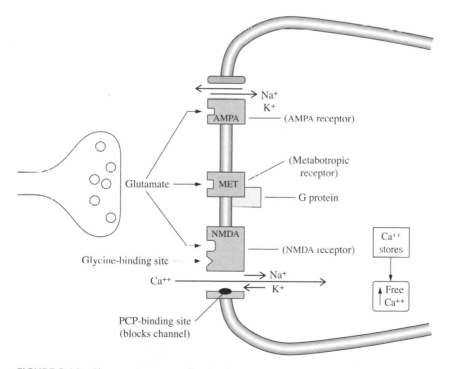

FIGURE 3.16   Glutamate receptor family. The AMPA receptor controls fast sodium and potassium channels; the NMDA receptor controls calcium channels; the metabotropic receptor controls a second-messenger system via a G protein that acts on the intracellular machinery of the cell (described in Chapter 2). (PCP is discussed in Chapter 15.)

(PCP) and ketamine (two "psychedelic" drugs discussed in Chapter 15). These two drugs are noncompetitive antagonists at this NMDA receptor: they inhibit NMDA functioning.

NMDA receptors also play a critical role in regulating synaptic plasticity, that is, in learning, memory, and cognitive ability. To form memory, high-frequency presynaptic activity in cerebral cortical and limbic neurons leads to the presynaptic release of glutamate, which activates a host of glutamate receptors on the postsynaptic dendritic spines. This activity produces a large postsynaptic depolarization, which then activates NMDA receptors, allowing calcium ions into the neuron. The high levels of glutamate also activate non-NMDA (metabotropic) receptors, which activate a cascade of signal transduction pathways, terminating in activation of a cyclic AMP response-element-binding protein (CREB). This action initiates transcription of new proteins involved in the formation of long-term memory. These new "memory" proteins are carried out of the nucleus and translated into functional proteins that effect lasting changes in synaptic strength. The "memory proteins" do so by "increasing the responsiveness to neurotransmitter, and even changing the number and size of synapses" (Weeber et al., 2002, pp. 377–378). Disruption of this process can be deleterious, producing depression or deficits in memory formation.

Although NMDA activity plays an important role in synaptic plasticity (neuronal "health"), excessive glutaminergic signaling is also involved in neuronal toxicity. For example, ethanol (Chapter 13) reduces glutamate activity, and alcohol withdrawal markedly increases glutamate release from neurons. Excesses of glutamate can lead to neuronal destruction through overactivity of NMDA receptors. Traumatic head injury also results in massive release of glutamate, and attempts to provide "brain protection" after head injury are aimed at preventing glutaminergic overactivity. Anoxia and hypoglycemia are other glutamate-releasing events that can lead to neuronal damage. Apparently, the entry of large excesses of calcium ions into cells via the NMDA receptors is an important step in the rapid cell death that occurs with excitotoxicity. Finally, new treatments to prevent the progression of Alzheimer's disease and other dementias are aimed at protecting neurons through blockage of NMDA receptor activity. In 2004, the first anti-Alzheimer's drug that acts through a glutaminergic mechanism became available for clinical use (Chapter 19).

Gamma Aminobutyric Acid. Gamma aminobutyric acid (GABA), a universally inhibitory transmitter, is found in high concentrations in the brain and spinal cord. Two different types of GABA receptors are categorized as $GABA_A$ and $GABA_B$ (Figure 3.17). *$GABA_A$ receptors*

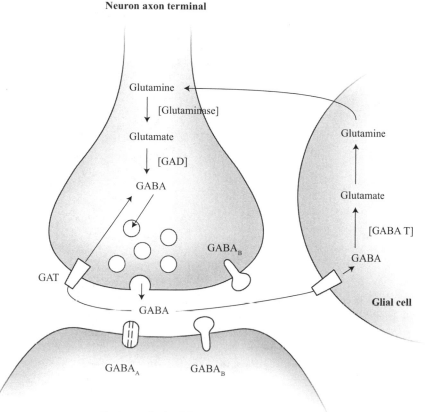

Neuron axon terminal

Glutamine

[Glutaminase]

Glutamate

[GAD]

GABA

GAT

GABA$_B$

GABA

Glutamine

Glutamate

[GABA T]

GABA

Glial cell

GABA$_A$ GABA$_B$

Postsynaptic dendrite

FIGURE 3.17 Schematic of GABA receptor release, reuptake, and reutilization. GABA$_A$ receptors are fast receptors (ionotropic; Chapter 2) and found on the postsynaptic membrane. GABA$_B$ receptors are metabotropic and found on both pre- and postsynaptic membranes. GAT is the GABA transporter; GAD is glutamic acid decarboxylase, which converts L-glutamic acid to GABA; GABA T is the enzyme that metabolizes GABA.

are fast receptors. Activation of this receptor by **GABA** opens an ion channel and leads to an influx of chloride into the cell, hyperpolarizing the cell and reducing its excitability. Barbiturate and benzodiazepine binding to this receptor facilitates the action of **GABA** (Chapter 7). This action is associated with the anxiolytic, amnestic, and anesthetic effects of these sedative drugs (Tomlin et al., 1999). **GABA$_A$** receptors are found in high density in the cerebral cortex, hippocampus, and cerebellum.

Numerous subtypes of the **GABA$_A$** receptors occur, allowing for the development of agonists and antagonists of specific **GABA$_A$** receptor subtypes (Chapter 7). Such drugs might be novel antianxiety agents, anticonvulsants, or cognitive enhancers.

GABA$_B$ receptors are slow-response receptors. Activation of **GABA$_B$** receptors in the amygdala is associated with the membrane-stabilizing, antiaggressive properties of valproic acid, a drug widely used to treat bipolar disorder (Chapter 6).

Peptide Neurotransmitters

Most of the newly identified neurotransmitters are peptides, which are small proteins (chains of amino acid molecules attached in a specific order). Peptide transmitters can be classified into several groups; one important group is the opioid-type peptides. Other groups include the hypothalamic-releasing hormones, the pituitary hormones, and the so-called gut-brain peptides. Feldman and colleagues (1997) and Cooper and colleagues (2003) discuss these peptides and their possible implications in psychopharmacology.

In this book, one peptide transmitter of interest is the type involved in the actions of the opiates, such as morphine. *Opioid peptides* include the *endorphins* (about 16 to 30 amino acids in length) and the shorter-chain *enkephalins* (5 amino acids in length). These substances are formed from a larger protein produced elsewhere in the body. The endorphins may be involved in a wide variety of emotional states, including pain perception, reward, emotional stability, and energy "highs," and in acupuncture. Opiates such as morphine, codeine, and heroin activate (are agonists at) receptors for endorphins and enkephalins (Chapter 10). Opioid receptors are termed *mu, kappa,* and *delta;* the mu receptor mediates the analgesic and reinforcing properties of morphine and other opiates (see Cooper et al., 2003).

Another peptide transmitter of interest in this book is *substance P,* a *gut-brain peptide* (11 amino acids in length) that plays an important role as a sensory transmitter, especially for pain impulses that enter the spinal cord and brain from a peripheral site of tissue injury. Opioids, serotonin agonists, and norepinephrine agonists exert much of their analgesic effect by acting on substance P nerve terminals to limit the release of this pain-inducing peptide. Substance P antagonists are also being developed as antidepressant drugs. The role of substance P in pain transmission is discussed in Chapter 10.

Table 3.1 (page 70) provides a selective summary of the major neurotransmitter classes and some of their members. It can be seen that there are some additional transmitter substances that have not been mentioned here, as well as at least one family, the neurotransmitter gases, that have also not been described. These agents do not play a major role in the action of the drugs described in this text.

STUDY QUESTIONS

1. Define a psychoactive drug.

2. What is a neuron? Describe the following parts of a neuron: dendrites, soma, axon, synaptic terminal.

3. What is a synapse? How does it function?

4. How is the synaptic transmitter action of a released chemical terminated? Give two examples.

5. Name a drug that blocks the action of acetylcholine as a neurotransmitter. What are the consequences of the blockade? Name a drug that potentiates the action of acetylcholine as a transmitter. What might such a drug be used for?

6. Name three catecholamine neurotransmitters. How is their neurotransmitter action terminated? What drugs block this process?

7. Describe the various types of serotonin receptors. What drugs might either stimulate or block them? How might these drugs be applied for therapeutic benefit?

8. Name two amino acid neurotransmitters. Describe any drugs that might potentiate or block the actions of each one. How might these drugs be used therapeutically?

9. What is substance P? How does it relate to psychopharmacology?

REFERENCES

Ashraf, S. I., and Kunes, S. (2006). "A Trace of Silence: Memory and MicroRNA at the Synapse." *Current Opinions in Neurobiology* 16. 535–539.

Breedlove, M., et al. (2007). *Biological Psychology: An Introduction to Behavioral, Cognitive and Clinical Neuroscience*, 5th ed. Sunderland, MA: Sinauer.

Cooper, J. R., et al. (2003). *The Biochemical Basis of Neuropharmacology*, 8th ed. New York: Oxford University Press.

Feldman, R. S., et al. (1997). *Principles of Neuropsychopharmacology*. Sunderland, MA: Sinauer.

Hyman, S. E. (2005). "Neurotransmitters." *Current Biology* 15: R154–R158.

Iverson, L. L., Iverson, S. D., Bloom F. E., and Roth, R. H. (2009). *Introduction to Neuropsychopharmacology*. New York: Oxford University Press.

Kempermann, G., et al. (2004). "Functional Significance of Adult Neurogenesis." *Current Opinions in Neurobiology* 14: 186–191.

Pinel, J. (2007). *Basics of Biopsychology*. New York: Pearson Education.

Schaffer, D. V., and Gage, F. H. (2004). "Neurogenesis and Neuroadaptation." *Neuromolecular Medicine* 5: 1–9.

Snyder, S. H. (2002). "Forty Years of Neurotransmitters: A Personal Account." *Archives of General Psychiatry* 59: 983–994.

Sutton, M. A., and Schuman, E. M. (2006). "Dendritic Protein Synthesis, Synaptic Plasticity, and Memory." *Cell* 127: 49–58.

Thomas, K., and Davies, A. (2005). "Neurotropins: A Ticket to Ride for BDNF." *Current Biology* 15: R262–R264.

Tomlin, S. L., et al. (1999). "Preparation of Barbiturate Optical Isomers and Their Effects on GABA$_A$ Receptors." *Anesthesiology* 90: 1714–1722.

Weeber, E. J., et al. (2002). "Molecular Genetics of Human Cognition." *Molecular Interventions* 2: 376–390.

PART 2

Drugs Used to Treat Psychological Disorders

Now that we have covered the basic principles of pharmacology (pharmacokinetics and pharmacodynamics) and basic physiology of the nervous system and synaptic transmission, the chapters in this part introduce the drugs that are used to treat psychological disorders. These medications include the traditional and "atypical" antipsychotics (Chapter 4), the antidepressants (Chapter 5), the "mood stabilizers" for treating bipolar disorder (Chapter 6), and the medications used classically to treat anxiety and insomnia (Chapter 7). Chapter 8 discusses herbal and other natural products (for example, omega-3 fatty acids) used in the treatment of psychological disorders. Later in this book (Part 5), we will discuss these medications in special populations (the young and the elderly) as well as in the overall principles of management of mental health disorders.

Today, remarkable advances are being made in the pharmacological treatment of psychological disorders, allowing affected people to lead much more "normal" lives than they have ever been able to before in human history. The goals of these five chapters are to impart a sense of the historical development of therapeutics of each disorder, to cover the pharmacology of drugs currently being used to treat these disorders, and to convey a sense of excitement about the promise of even better therapies. The drugs are compartmentalized in these chapters under descriptive headings (antidepressants, mood stabilizers, antipsychotics, and so forth), but the headings do not adequately describe or define the drugs. For example, besides being used to relieve major depression, antidepressants are used as antianxiety drugs, as analgesics, and as antidysthymic agents. Many of the mood stabilizers, besides being used to treat bipolar disorder, are used to treat chronic pain syndromes, psychological disorders associated with agitation and aggression, and even substance abuse. Antipsychotic drugs, besides being used to treat schizophrenia, are now being used to treat bipolar disorder, explosive and aggressive disorders, autism, and other pervasive developmental disorders. Newer antipsychotic agents are even being used to treat depression and dysthymia. Nevertheless, the artificial distinctions are maintained to present the pharmacology of the drugs in a logical manner.

Chapter 4

Antipsychotic Drugs: Major Tranquilizers to Thymic Stabilizers

Schizophrenia

Schizophrenia is a debilitating neuropsychiatric illness that typically strikes young people just when they are maturing into adulthood (Freedman, 2003). Affecting approximately 1 percent of the population, the disorder is associated with marked social and/or occupational dysfunction, and its course and outcome vary greatly. In the premorbid phase of the illness, subtle motor, cognitive, or social impairments are often observed but are not severe enough to place affected people outside the normal range of functioning (Miyamoto et al., 2003). In the prodromal phase, mood symptoms, cognitive symptoms, social withdrawal, or obsessive behaviors may develop. Onset of the full syndrome leads to substantial functional deterioration in self-care, work, and interpersonal relationships, especially during the first 5 to 10 years, after which clinical deterioration reaches a plateau and, in some situations, function may actually improve. Nevertheless, schizophrenia is associated with an increased risk of suicide; approximately 10 to 15 percent of people with this disorder take their own lives, usually within the first 10 years of developing the illness (Sadock and Sadock, 2007; Keltner and Folks, 2005). With regard to violent offenses, however, a recent population-based study found that the association was weak. There was only a minimal link between violent crime and schizophrenia in the absence of substance abuse (Fazel et al., 2009).

Schizophrenia is thought to be a neurodevelopmental disease, associated with significant abnormalities in brain structure and function. Because these abnormalities can be observed in patients who have never been treated with antipsychotic medications, they are considered to be inherent in the disease, not medication related (Torrey, 2002). The illness is presently viewed as a misconnection syndrome, reflecting a basic disorder in neural circuits, caused by many factors that affect brain development (Javitt and Coyle, 2004; Miyamoto et al., 2003).

The symptoms of schizophrenia have classically been divided into positive and negative clusters. The positive symptoms are the symptoms typical of psychosis and include abnormalities in perception (hallucinations) and inferential thinking (delusions) as well as disorganized, incoherent, and illogical speech (thought disorder). The negative symptoms reflect the absence of some normal human quality and include blunting of emotional expression (flattened affect), impoverishment of speech and mental creativity (alogia), loss of motivation and interest (avolition) and the ability to experience pleasure (anhedonia), and social withdrawal. This differentiation of symptomatology is important because the classical agents affect primarily the positive symptoms, while there is less benefit for negative symptoms. Patients with schizophrenia also have impairments in many different cognitive systems, such as memory, attention, and executive function. Therefore, treatment is now aimed at more than reducing abnormal perceptions and thought processes; efforts are also being directed to improving cognitive functioning and quality of life so that patients with severe and persistent mental illness can successfully reintegrate into the community (American Psychiatric Association, 2004; Janicak et al., 2006; Weickert et al., 2003).

Dopamine Involvement

Early scientific evidence supported a specific *dopamine theory* of schizophrenia, which proposed that the disorder developed from dysregulation of dopaminergic brain pathways, resulting in overactivity of dopaminergic function (McGowan et al., 2004). This conclusion was derived from two known facts. (1) Abuse of stimulant drugs that are known to increase synaptic dopamine concentration, such as amphetamine, produce a syndrome indistinguishable from the paranoid type of schizophrenia. (2) Antipsychotic drugs are *dopamine receptor antagonists* that block dopamine receptors in the brain. Dopamine receptors can be classified as either D_1 (of which there are two subtypes, D_1 and D_5) or D_2 (which has three subtypes, D_2, D_3, and D_4). It is now appreciated not only that all antipsychotic drugs have an affinity for the D_2 receptor but that this affinity remains the single best predictor of the effective clinical dose of an antipsychotic (Figure 4.1).

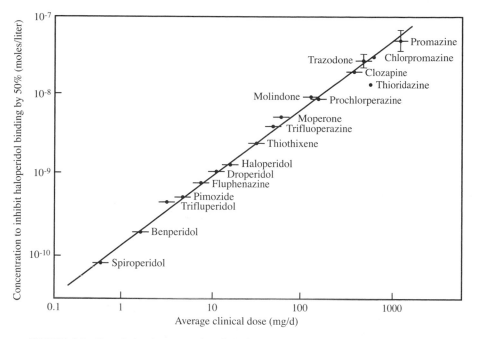

FIGURE 4.1 Correlation between the clinical potency and receptor-binding activities of neuroleptic drugs. Clinical potency is expressed as the daily dose used in treating schizophrenia, and binding activity is expressed as the concentration needed to produce 50 percent inhibition of haloperidol binding. Haloperidol binds to dopamine-2 receptors; other antipsychotic drugs compete for the same receptors. Thus, measuring the competitive inhibition of haloperidol binding correlates with potency of an antipsychotic drug.

Unfortunately, dopamine, released by neurons in the basal ganglia of the brain, is crucial for maintaining normal coordination of movement. In fact, the loss of these neurons is responsible for the neurological disorder Parkinson's disease. Similarly, by blocking dopamine receptors, antipsychotic drugs produce the neurological side effect of parkinsonian symptoms (also known as extrapyramidal symptoms— EPS). Long-term, chronic antipsychotic administration may also elicit other syndromes of abnormal motor function such as tardive dyskinesia (TD), which may be irreversible.

It has been generally assumed that the risk of these neurological symptoms was an unavoidable consequence of antipsychotic drug therapy. However, the discovery of the second-generation antipsychotics (SGAs) has shown that this assumption is incorrect and that antipsychotic efficacy can be obtained with little or no EPS or TD (Correll et al., 2004; Janicak et al., 2006). This is the primary advantage of the newer agents relative to the first-generation drugs.

Serotonin Involvement

As with dopamine, early investigations into the possible role of serotonin (5-HT) in schizophrenia followed from observations of the actions of psychoactive drugs. Because the psychedelic drug LSD produces hallucinations, it was initially proposed to be involved in the clinical syndrome seen in schizophrenia. LSD is one of a group of hallucinogenic drugs that are thought to exert their psychedelic effect as agonists at 5-HT_{2A} receptors. For this reason, it was hypothesized that *5-HT$_2$ receptor antagonism* might be responsible for some of the beneficial actions of antipsychotics. Although it has since been concluded that serotonin does not play an important role in the etiology of schizophrenia, antagonism of this transmitter at 5-HT_2 receptors may be involved in the improved neurological side effect profile of the newer antipsychotic medications. Meltzer (2002) discusses the history of this concept.

Glutamate Involvement

In addition to amphetamine and LSD, the two psychedelic drugs *phencyclidine* (PCP) and *ketamine* (Chapter 15) have also provided insight into the neurochemistry of schizophrenia. These drugs also produce some schizophrenialike symptoms, such as hallucinations, out-of-body experiences, negative symptomatology, and cognitive deficits. The mechanism responsible for these effects is a potent blockade of NMDA-type glutamate receptors. This relationship suggests that there may be a glutamatergic dysfunction in the etiology of schizophrenia, which has prompted a glutamate-NMDA hypothesis of schizophrenia. This theory proposes that NMDA hypofunction results in excessive release of the excitatory neurotransmitters glutamate and acetylcholine in the frontal cortex, damaging cortical neurons and triggering the deterioration seen in patients with schizophrenia (Farber, 2003; Laruelle et al., 2003; Moghaddam, 2003; Rujescu et al., 2006).

Historical Background and Classification of Antipsychotic Drugs

Prior to 1950, there were no effective drugs for treating psychotic patients; these patients were usually permanently or chronically hospitalized. By 1955, more than half a million psychotic patients in the United States were residing in mental hospitals. A dramatic and steady reversal in this trend began in 1956, and by 1983 fewer than 220,000 patients were institutionalized despite a doubling in the number of admissions to state hospitals. By the early 1990s, people with schizophrenia were routinely stabilized on medication and rapidly discharged from institutions.[1] What accounted for this dramatic shift was a class of drugs called phenothiazines, the first category of antipsychotic agents.

Phenothiazines were initially developed as antihistamines and were first studied for their mildly sedating action. The sedative properties led the French anesthesiologist and surgeon H. Laborit to use *promethazine*, the first phenothiazine, to deepen anesthesia. This drug was administered in a "lytic cocktail" to patients the night before surgery to allay their fears and anxieties. Promethazine was soon followed by a second phenothiazine, *chlorpromazine* (Thorazine), which was found to reduce the amount of anesthetic drugs a patient needed without making the patient unconscious; rather, this treatment produced a state characterized by calmness, conscious sedation, and lack of interest in and detachment from external stimuli. This condition was termed a *neuroleptic state,* and chlorpromazine was the first neuroleptic drug.

Laborit persuaded many clinicians to try chlorpromazine, and later the same year the French research psychiatrists Delay and Deniker studied its effect in schizophrenic patients. Although it did not provide a permanent cure, chlorpromazine was found to be remarkably effective in alleviating the clinical manifestations of psychosis (López-Muñoz et al., 2005). In conjunction with supportive therapy, its use allowed thousands of patients who otherwise would have been permanently hospitalized to return to their communities, albeit in a less than satisfactory state.

In the continuing search for more effective drugs with fewer side effects, alternatives to the phenothiazines have been developed. The second class of neuroleptics was the *butyrophenones,* developed in Belgium in the mid-1960s. Two butyrophenones are currently available, *haloperidol* (Haldol) and *droperidol* (Inapsine). Haloperidol is used in the treatment of schizophrenia, droperidol in the treatment of nausea and vomiting associated with surgery.

These first-generation antipsychotics (FGAs) are most effective against the positive symptoms of schizophrenia, and, as noted, the doses required for clinical improvement were significantly correlated with their ability to block D_2 dopamine receptors.

Unfortunately, D_2 antagonism also produced undesirable neurological side effects, which included acute movement disorders, such as extrapyramidal symptoms similar to the symptoms of Parkinson's disease, and, in some cases, involuntary movement disorders resulting from chronic antipsychotic exposure, such as tardive dyskinesia.

---

[1] Although the discharge rate of schizophrenics from institutions is high, there is concern about their ultimate functioning in society. Many patients who were discharged on phenothiazines failed to continue their medication, and they functioned poorly as a result. It has been estimated that about 50 percent of the adult homeless population in the United States may suffer from inadequately controlled schizophrenia.

Therefore, for the FGAs, binding to D_2 receptors not only resulted in clinical efficacy but also increased the likelihood of EPS. Indeed, the antipsychotic and EPS effects of neuroleptics were generally thought to be linked and inseparable. This idea led to a *neuroleptic threshold concept* of treatment, which held that the neuroleptic dose should be gradually increased until EPS was produced. Thus, the "right" dose was the one that caused some degree of motor side effects.

Beginning in the late 1980s, breakthroughs occurred that seemed to offer improvements in regard to such side effects. These developments began with the discovery of the first second-generation antipsychotic, clozapine (Clozaril). Clozapine was a major advance because it was effective for many patients (about 30 percent) who did not respond to standard treatment and because it produced little or no symptoms of movement disorders such as EPS or TD (and, in fact, may even reduce TD caused by other antipsychotics).

Unfortunately, clozapine itself had some serious side effects, which limited its use to patients who had not responded to conventional treatment. However, it prompted the development of other SGAs, collectively referred to as "atypical" antipsychotics. In addition to clozapine (Clozaril), they include risperidone (Risperdal), olanzapine (Zyprexa), quetiapine (Seroquel), ziprasidone (Geodon), and aripiprazole (Abilify), which may actually be the first of a new, third generation of antipsychotics (TGAs) because of a unique mechanism of action.

All the SGAs differ pharmacologically from the FGAs by having relatively less affinity for D_2 receptors (Grunder et al., 2003) and greater affinity for 5-HT (serotonergic) receptors. For some reason, this allows a separation between antipsychotic efficacy and induction of EPS or other movement disorders (with the exception of risperidone at higher doses) (Horacek et al., 2006; Kapur and Remington, 2001; Kapur and Seeman, 2001). Although none of the others share clozapine's superior efficacy for treatment of schizophrenic patients who are refractory to treatment, these drugs have shown that it is possible to separate therapeutic benefit from parkinsonian side effects (Advokat, 2005).[2]

---

[2] Several possible mechanisms might account for this property. First, 5-HT is known to inhibit dopamine release in the nigrostriatal but not the mesolimbic dopamine pathway. By blocking this action (either through 5-HT$_2$ receptor antagonism at the dopamine terminal or by 5-HT$_{1A}$ antagonism at the cell body), SGAs selectively enhance dopamine release in the striatum, which mitigates neuroleptic-induced EPS. Second, clozapine and quetiapine have a low affinity for the D_2 receptor and do not attach very tightly to these binding sites. Because the natural amount of dopamine in the nigrostriatal pathway is greater than that in the mesolimbic pathway, clozapine and quetiapine may be more easily displaced from the striatal dopamine receptors by the higher concentration of the endogenous transmitter. This occurrence would normalize dopaminergic activity in the nigrostriatal system and reduce pseudoparkinsonian side effects.

Initially, the SGAs also appeared to be more effective than FGAs against negative symptoms. However, it is now appreciated that an apparent improvement in negative symptoms may be secondary to the absence of EPS or to other indirect causes, such as improvement in socialization and cognition, rather than a direct therapeutic effect (Rosenheck et al., 2003). Negative symptoms, especially social and emotional withdrawal, poor rapport, and blunted affect are still prominent, even in patients treated in routine clinical practice. Their presence was associated with being male, older, and single/unmarried; having greater illness severity and fewer positive symptoms; and receiving a high antipsychotic dose (Bobes et al., 2010). Unfortunately, recent efforts to alleviate negative symptoms with the wakefulness/antifatigue drug modafinil have not proven successful (Freudenreich et al., 2009).

Criticisms of the comparative efficacy, safety, and cost-benefit ratio of the SGAs have been discussed in several meta-analyses and comparative studies of the first- and second-generation agents (Davis et al., 2003; Davis and Chen, 2004; Leucht et al., 2003). The largest meta-analysis combined results from 124 clinical trials, including some unpublished data from the U.S. Food and Drug Administration (FDA; Davis et al., 2003). There were two conclusions. The first, not surprising, was that clozapine was superior to FGAs. The second was that, among the other SGAs, only olanzapine and risperidone appeared to be better than FGAs. But there were two major criticisms of this conclusion. First, it was suggested that some SGAs didn't separate from FGAs because the doses may have been too low. Second, it was argued that patient recruitment might now be more difficult. With more patients experiencing some improvement, perhaps the population of participants is less responsive to standard treatment. A smaller meta-analysis, appearing around the same time (Leucht et al., 2003), concluded that there were no meaningful differences among the SGAs. To address these issues, the National Institute of Mental Health (NIMH) conducted a large, double-blind, active control clinical trial, designed to directly compare the relative effectiveness of SGAs with the effectiveness of the FGA perphenazine. This was the largest, longest, and most comprehensive independent trial ever done to examine existing therapies for this disease.

CATIE and CUtLASS Studies

The Clinical Antipsychotic Trials of Intervention Effectiveness (CATIE) study was conducted in the United States between January 2001 and December 2004 at 57 clinical sites for up to 18 months or until treatment was discontinued for any reason. In the first of three phases, 1493 patients were randomly assigned to receive either one of three SGAs (olanzapine, risperidone, or quetiapine) or perphenazine under double-blind conditions. Ziprasidone was added later following its FDA approval. Results showed that patients discontinued antipsychotic medications at a high rate, 64 to 82 percent across all the drugs, primarily because of lack of efficacy or intolerable side effects (EPS in the case of perphenazine and weight gain or metabolic changes from olanzapine). There was no overall difference in the rate of discontinuation between the SGAs and the FGA, perphenazine (Lieberman et al., 2005).

Of the 1493 patients enrolled in the study, 1052 were eligible for phase 2. This part of the study provided two treatment pathways. Patients who had not shown optimal improvement on one of the SGAs in the first phase or who had stopped treatment for any other reason were offered the option of random assignment to clozapine or to an SGA other than the one they had received in phase 1. A total of 99 patients entered this "efficacy" pathway. Patients who discontinued treatment for intolerability were offered the opportunity to receive treatment with an SGA other than the one they had previously received—excluding clozapine. A total of 444 patients entered this "tolerability" pathway. The remaining 509 patients (48 percent) did not enter phase 2.

In the "efficacy" pathway, clozapine treatment was found to be more effective than the other SGAs; patients receiving clozapine were less likely to discontinue therapy because of lack of therapeutic response than patients receiving any of the other newer agents. In the "tolerability" pathway, olanzapine and risperidone were more effective than quetiapine or ziprasidone in "time until discontinuation" for any reason. Neither of the phase 2 pathways included either aripiprazole or any first-generation antipsychotic (McEvoy et al., 2006; Stroup et al., 2006).

A British comparison between SGAs and FGAs—Cost Utility of the Latest Antipsychotic Drugs in Schizophrenia Studies (CUtLASS 1)—was reported in October 2006 (Jones et al., 2006). It evaluated 227 people with a diagnosis of schizophrenia who had an inadequate response or adverse reaction to their previous medication. Prescriptions for either an FGA or an SGA (excluding clozapine) were monitored for 1 year, with blind assessments at 12, 26, and 56 weeks. The primary outcomes were a measure of quality of life, symptoms, adverse effects, participant satisfaction, and costs of care. Like the CATIE trial, the results of this study showed that patients with schizophrenia did just as well on antipsychotic drugs from either category, with patients taking FGAs actually showing a trend toward greater improvement on the quality-of-life scale and symptom scores. Participants expressed no clear preference, and the costs were similar.

Although antipsychotic drugs remain the "cornerstone of treatment for schizophrenia" (Lieberman et. al., 2005), the results of the CATIE and CUtLASS 1 trials have prompted a reassessment of the perceived advantages of the second-generation antipsychotics. The initial optimism generated by these new, "atypical" neuroleptics has been tempered by evidence that they do not improve clinical outcome as much as anticipated and are much more expensive than the older drugs.

This perspective was supported by the most recent meta-analysis of SGAs versus FGAs (Leucht et al., 2009), which included 150 studies and more than 21,500 patients. In 95 of the 150 studies, haloperidol was the comparator. In this case, amisulpride, clozapine, olanzapine, and risperidone were significantly more effective at reducing overall symptoms than the FGAs, whereas aripiprazole, quetiapine, sertindole, ziprasidone, and zotepine (not available in the United States) were not more effective than FGAs. All SGAs produced significantly fewer EPS than haloperidol. Even though some differences were statistically significant, they were not absolutely very large. Essentially, it is now understood that not all SGAs are the same (Komossa et al., 2009a, 2009b); they don't all produce better outcomes than FGAs, even in cases of acute toxic ingestion (Ciranni et al., 2009); and the merits of each drug have to be determined independently, taking into account side effects and cost benefits (Rosenheck and Sernyak, 2009). In situations where EPS may preclude the use of FGAs, such as autism, bipolar disorder, borderline personality disorder, and aggressive disorders, SGAs may be the first choice. The imminent generic status of some SGAs (reducing their cost) will most likely affect such considerations as well.

First-Generation Antipsychotic Drugs: Phenothiazines

Historically, the phenothiazines (Figure 4.2; Table 4.1) were the most widely used drugs for treating schizophrenia. They were also used for other purposes, such as to treat nausea and vomiting, to sedate patients before anesthesia, to delay ejaculation, to relieve severe itching, to manage the psychotic component that may accompany acute manic attacks, to treat alcoholic hallucinosis, and to manage the hallucinations caused by psychedelic agents. Today, treatment of most of these conditions now involves the use of newer drugs.

Pharmacokinetics

The phenothiazines are absorbed erratically and unpredictably from the gastrointestinal tract. However, because patients usually take these drugs for long periods of time, the oral route of administration is effective and commonly used. Intramuscular injection of phenothiazines is even more effective: it increases the effectiveness of the drugs about four to ten times that achieved with oral administration. Once these

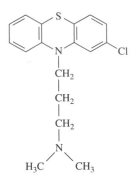

Chlorpromazine (Thorazine)

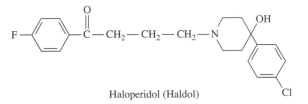

Haloperidol (Haldol)

FIGURE 4.2 Structural formulas of a phenothiazine (chlorpromazine) and a butyrophenone (haloperidol). Both are traditional antipsychotic drugs.

drugs are in the bloodstream, they are rapidly distributed throughout the body. The levels of phenothiazines that are found in the brain are low compared with the levels found in other body tissues; the highest concentrations are found in the lungs, liver, adrenal glands, and spleen.

The phenothiazines have half-lives of 24 to 48 hours, and they are slowly metabolized in the liver. The clinical effects of a single dose persist for at least 24 hours. Thus, taking the daily dose at bedtime often minimizes certain side effects (such as excessive sedation). The phenothiazines become extensively bound to body tissues, which partially accounts for their slow rate of elimination. Metabolites of some of the phenothiazines can be detected for several months after the drug has been discontinued. Slow elimination may also contribute to the slow rate of recurrence of psychotic episodes following cessation of drug therapy.

Pharmacological Effects

In addition to blocking D_2 receptors, the phenothiazines also block acetylcholine (muscarinic), histamine, and norepinephrine receptors. Cholinergic blockade results in dry mouth, dilated pupils, blurred vision, cognitive impairments, constipation, urinary retention, and tachycardia. Noradrenergic blockade can result in hypotension and sedation. Histaminergic blockade has sedating as well as antiemetic effects.

TABLE 4.1 Antipsychotic drugs

Chemical classification	Drug name: Generic (Trade)	Dose equivalent (mg)	Sedation	Autonomic side effects[a]	Involuntary movement
Phenothiazine	Chlorpromazine (Thorazine)	100	High	High	Moderate
	Prochlorperazine (Compazine)	15	Moderate	Low	High
	Fluphenazine (Prolixin)	2	Low	Low	High
	Trifluoperazine (Stelazine)	5	Moderate	Low	High
	Perphenazine (Trilafon)	8	Low	Low	High
	Acetophenazine (Tindal)	20	Moderate	Low	High
	Carphenazine (Proketazine)	25	Moderate	Low	High
	Triflupromazine (Vesprin)	25	High	Moderate	Moderate
	Mesoridazine (Serentil)	50	High	Moderate	Low
	Thioridazine (Mellaril)	100	High	Moderate	Low
Thioxanthene	Thiothixene (Navane)	4	Low	Low	High
	Chlorprothixene (Taractan)	100	High	High	Moderate
Butyrophenone	Haloperidol (Haldol)	2	Low	Low	Very high
Miscellaneous	Loxapine (Loxitane)	10	Moderate	Low	Moderate
	Molindone (Moban)	10	Moderate	Moderate	Moderate
	Pimozide (Orap)	2	Low	Low	Moderate
New generation	Clozapine (Clozaril)	50	Moderate	Moderate	Low
	Risperidone (Risperdal)	1	Low	Low	Low-Moderate
	Olanzapine (Zyprexa)	1.5	Moderate	Low	Low
	Quetiapine (Seroquel)	40	Low	Low	Low
	Ziprasidone (Geodon)	15	Low	Low	Low
	Aripiprazole (Abilify)	3	Low	Low	Low
	Amisulpride (Solian)	NA	Low	Low	Low
	Iloperidone (Fanapt)	NA	Moderate	Moderate	Low
	Asenapine (Saphris)	NA	Moderate	Low	Low

[a]Autonomic side effects include dry mouth, blurred vision, constipation, urinary retention, and reduced blood pressure.

Brain Stem. Through actions on the brain stem, phenothiazines suppress the centers involved in behavioral arousal (the ascending reticular activating center) and vomiting (the chemoreceptor trigger zone). By suppressing these medullary functions, the phenothiazines produce an indifference to external stimuli, reducing sensory input that would otherwise reach higher brain centers.

Hypothalamus-Pituitary. Dopaminergic pathways extend from the hypothalamus to the pituitary gland. Because the hypothalamus is intimately involved in vegetative and motivational processes, suppression of these functions by phenothiazines may produce changes in appetite and food intake, wide fluctuations in body temperature with changes in ambient temperature, and alterations in pituitary gland functions. The pituitary gland is responsible for regulating the secretion of sex hormones; therefore, dopaminergic blockade increases the release of the hormone prolactin, which can produce breast enlargement in males and lactation in females. Phenothiazines also reduce the release of other hormones. In men, ejaculation may be blocked; in women, libido may be decreased, ovulation may be blocked, and normal menstrual cycles may be suppressed, resulting in infertility.

Basal Ganglia. By blocking dopamine receptors in the basal ganglia, phenothiazines produce two main kinds of motor (neurologic) disturbances, which comprise the most bothersome and potentially serious side effects associated with the use of these agents. The two syndromes are (1) acute extrapyramidal reactions, which develop early in treatment in up to 90 percent of patients, and (2) tardive ("tardy," or late) dyskinesia, which occurs much later, during and even after cessation of chronic neuroleptic treatment. Acute extrapyramidal side effects include the following:

- Akathisia, a syndrome characterized by the subjective feeling of anxiety, manifested by restlessness, pacing, constant rocking back and forth, and other repetitive, purposeless, actions. Because it can be extremely upsetting to the patient, akathisia is a common cause of nonadherence to psychotropic treatment. Although its cause is not well established, a decrease in dopaminergic activity appears to be an important etiological factor. In addition to reducing the dose, the most effective treatment of akathisia includes either a beta-adrenergic antagonist (for example, propranolol) or a serotonergic, 5-HT$_2$, receptor antagonist (for example, ritanserin). Emerging evidence suggests that the likelihood of eliciting akathisia may be increased when antipsychotic drugs (particularly the antipsychotic aripiprazole; Abilify) and antidepressant drugs (especially the serotonergic agents) are combined, such as in the treatment of bipolar disorder (Advokat, 2010).

- Dystonia, which presents as involuntary muscle contractions and sustained abnormal, bizarre postures of the limbs, trunk, head, and tongue.

- Neuroleptic-induced (pseudo) parkinsonism, which resembles idiopathic (of unknown etiology) Parkinson's disease. (Drugs used to treat parkinsonism are discussed in Chapter 19).

Neuroleptic-induced parkinsonism is characterized by tremor at rest, "cogwheel type" rigidity of the limbs, and slowing of movement, with a reduction in spontaneous activity. In idiopathic parkinsonism, these symptoms occur when the concentration of dopamine in the nuclei of the basal ganglia (caudate nucleus, putamen, and globus pallidus) decreases to about 20 percent of normal. The same symptoms are produced when neuroleptic drug-induced blockade of dopamine receptors reaches 80 or greater percent. If necessary, antiparkinsonian agents can be administered to control these symptoms, although tolerance may eventually develop to neuroleptic-induced parkinsonism.

Tardive dyskinesia (TD) is a much more puzzling and serious form of movement disorder. Victims exhibit involuntary hyperkinetic movements, often of the face and tongue but also of the trunk and limbs, which can be severely disabling. More characteristic are sucking and smacking of the lips; lateral jaw movements; and darting, pushing, or twisting of the tongue. Choreiform (dancelike) movements of the extremities are frequent. The syndrome appears a few months to several years after the beginning of neuroleptic treatment and is sometimes (~20 percent of the time) irreversible. The incidence of tardive dyskinesia has been estimated at about 20 percent of patients who are treated with phenothiazines, increasing about 4 percent annually for the first 5 years, but this side effect depends greatly on the particular drug, the dosage, and the age of the patient (it is most common in patients older than 50, with approximately 50 percent of the elderly affected after 5 years). Although the incidence of TD is much less with the SGAs, it is not zero. One recent study found an incidence of 0.74 percent (Tenback et al., 2010). Unfortunately, there is no adequate treatment for this condition, except perhaps clozapine or another SGA, although it is not clear if some SGAs are more effective than others or what mediates this phenomenon (Peritogiannis and Tsouli, 2010). Although dyskinesia may be controlled by restarting or increasing the dose of neuroleptic, in the short run parkinsonian side effects may be elicited, and eventually the intensity of the abnormal movements may increase.

A novel approach to treating movement disorders, whether in schizophrenia or other neurological conditions, is being developed by Neurocrine Biosciences, Inc. This company is developing a drug (NBI-98854) that selectively blocks the transporter for the storage vesicles in dopamine neurons, called the vesicular monoamine transporter 2 (VMAT2). By blocking the transporter, the drug would prevent dopamine from being repackaged. The aim is to provide sustained, low levels of dopamine to minimize side effects associated with excessive dopamine depletion. The company is conducting safety trials in humans, which it hopes will lead to approval for an Investigational New Drug Application in the United States, to test for the treatment of tardive dyskinesia.

Limbic System. Dopaminergic neurons of the central midbrain portion of the brain stem project to limbic structures, which regulate emotional expression, as well as to forebrain areas, where emotion and cognition are integrated. Increased sensitivity of dopamine receptors in these areas may be responsible for the positive symptoms of schizophrenia. Thus, a phenothiazine reduces the intensity of schizophrenic delusions and hallucinations, which are particularly sensitive to treatment. It decreases paranoia, fear, hostility, and agitation, and it may dramatically relieve the restlessness and hyperactivity associated with an acute schizophrenic episode.

Side Effects and Toxicity

Much of the art of treating schizophrenic patients with antipsychotics lies in diagnosing and managing side effects. In general, the high-potency agents—agents that block dopamine receptors most strongly and require lower doses—produce more extrapyramidal side effects but less sedation, fewer anticholinergic actions, and less postural hypotension than the low-potency neuroleptics (Table 4.2). The choice of drug depends on the specific situation. When sedation is desired, a low-potency agent may be sufficient or a high-potency drug may be combined with a benzodiazepine. If anticholinergic side effects limit adherence, a high-potency drug may be more appropriate, and drug-induced movement disorders, if elicited, may be controlled with antiparkinsonian agents.

It has long been recognized that cognitive disturbances are evident in 40 to 60 percent of patients with schizophrenia. Neuropsychological tests show deficits in numerous "executive" functions, including attention, memory, problem solving, judgment, concept formation, planning, and language, which appear in the very first episode. Measured IQ and other cognitive abilities decline the most just before symptoms appear and the first episode occurs but then stabilize (Mesholam-Gately, 2009).

TABLE 4.2 Major adverse effects of receptor blockade by neuroleptics

Receptor	Effects
D_2 dopamine	Extrapyramidal symptoms; prolactin increase
α_1 norepinephrine	Postural hypotension
H_1 histamine	Sedation/drowsiness; weight gain
M_1 muscarinic acetylcholine	Memory deficits; constipation/urinary retention; tachycardia; blurred vision; dry mouth

Although it is generally agreed that antipsychotic drugs improve schizophrenic symptomatology, anticholinergic and antihistaminergic actions of the antipsychotics produce memory impairment and sedation, respectively. If these effects are responsible for producing or worsening cognitive dysfunction, then agents without these side effects appear to improve cognition (Carpenter and Gold, 2002; Weiss et al., 2002).

Recent efforts have been especially directed toward novel pharmacological approaches to treat cognitive deficits and negative symptoms. These have focused on the cholinergic and glutamatergic systems, both of which may be involved in cognitive function. The two cholinergic receptor types are nicotinic and muscarinic. In 2008, a trial of one compound, a partial agonist of the alpha-7 nicotinic receptor subtype, named anabaseine (DMXB-A), was conducted in 31 schizophrenic patients. DMXB-A was added to the patients' antipsychotic medications, mostly nonclozapine SGAs. Unfortunately, neither of the two DMXB-A doses differentiated from placebo on the battery of cognitive tests, although there was some evidence for effectiveness against negative symptoms. Atomoxetine (Strattera), a selective norepinephrine (NE) uptake blocker, was also found to be ineffective for improving cognitive function in schizophrenia (Kelly et al., 2009).

The NIMH has recently sponsored two initiatives to develop assessments for cognition in schizophrenia and evaluate new medicines: Measurement and Treatment Research to Improve Cognition in Schizophrenia (MATRICS) and Treatment Units for Research on Neurocognition and Schizophrenia (TURNS). Results are not yet available.

Other potentially serious but less common side effects of phenothiazines include altered pigmentation of the skin, pigment deposits in the retina, permanently impaired vision, allergic (hypersensitivity) reactions, which include liver dysfunction and blood disorders, as well as the previously noted hormonal impairments. Although rare, one potentially lethal reaction to phenothiazines is the neuroleptic malignant syndrome (NMS). The NMS is an acute reaction that may occur in response to a variety of agents that increase dopaminergic tone. Its incidence in FGA-treated patients is 0.02 to 2.4 percent, and it has been reported to occur in response to the SGAs clozapine, risperidone, and olanzapine. The most common symptoms include fever, severe muscle rigidity of the "lead pipe" type, autonomic changes (such as fluctuating blood pressure), and altered consciousness that may progress to stupor or coma. The most important aspect of effective treatment is early recognition, immediate withdrawal of the responsible agent, and initiation of supportive measures.

Tolerance and Dependence

One of the positive attributes of the phenothiazines is that they are not prone to compulsive abuse. They do not produce tolerance or physical or psychological dependence. Psychotic patients may take phenothiazines for years without increasing their dose because of tolerance; if a dose is increased, it is usually to increase control of psychotic episodes.

Alternative First-Generation Antipsychotics

Following the introduction of chlorpromazine and the other phenothiazines during the late 1950s and early 1960s, the limitations of these agents soon became apparent. Pharmaceutical manufacturers therefore attempted to find drugs with novel chemical structures that might exert antipsychotic efficacy without the accompanying side effects, especially the movement disorders. Although this goal was not realized until the mid-1990s, a few nonphenothiazine antipsychotic agents were developed in the 1960s and early 1970s.

Haloperidol

In 1967, haloperidol (Haldol; see Figure 4.2) was introduced as the first therapeutic alternative to the phenothiazines. A related compound, *droperidol* (Inapsine), was subsequently introduced into anesthesia for the treatment of postoperative nausea and vomiting. Although haloperidol is structurally different, its pharmacological efficacy and side effects are comparable to that of the phenothiazines. It produces sedation and an indifference to external stimuli, and it reduces initiative, anxiety, and activity. It is well absorbed orally and has a moderately slow rate of metabolism and excretion; stable blood levels can be seen for up to three days after the drug is discontinued.

It takes approximately five days for 40 percent of a single dose to be excreted by the kidneys.

Haloperidol's mechanism of antipsychotic action is the same as that of the phenothiazines—it competitively blocks D_2 receptors. It does not produce some of the serious side effects occasionally seen in patients taking phenothiazines (such as jaundice and blood abnormalities). But because it is a high-potency D_2 antagonist, it causes parkinsonism and other motor disorders comparable to those induced by high-potency phenothiazines, and it may require adjunctive prophylactic antiparkinsonian medication. In general, however, haloperidol is effective for treating acutely psychotic patients, as it has a rapid onset, especially when given by injection.

Molindone

The two alternative medications molindone (Moban) and loxapine (Loxitane) were introduced in the early 1970s (Figure 4.3). Molindone is a structurally unique molecule resembling the neurotransmitter serotonin. Whether this similarity is relevant to its antipsychotic action is unknown. Molindone is comparable to the traditional antipsychotic drugs in dopamine receptor occupancy, therapeutic efficacy, and side effects, except that it has been shown to produce weight loss. It produces moderate sedation, although it has also been reported to increase motor activity and possibly induce a euphoric effect in rare cases. Both effects may be related to its reported block of the enzyme monoamine oxidase. Molindone may also produce parkinsonian movements similar to those seen in patients taking phenothiazines.

Loxapine

Loxapine (Loxitane) structurally resembles the atypical antipsychotic clozapine, and like the newer SGAs, it binds strongly to both dopaminergic and serotonergic receptors. Nevertheless, its actions differ little from those of the traditional antipsychotic drugs. It has antipsychotic, antiemetic, and sedative properties and causes abnormal motor movements. It lowers convulsive thresholds somewhat more than the phenothiazines. Taken orally, loxapine is well absorbed, and it is metabolized and excreted within about 24 hours.

Alexza Pharmaceuticals, Inc., is developing AZ 004 (Staccato) loxapine, an inhalation formulation to treat acute agitation in patients with schizophrenia or bipolar disorder. Currently, the available treatments are either intramuscular injection, which requires restraint, or rapidly dissolving or standard tablets, which are slower in onset than the inhalation product. The inhaled drug is quickly absorbed through the lungs into the bloodstream, which is as therapeutically rapid as intravenous administration.

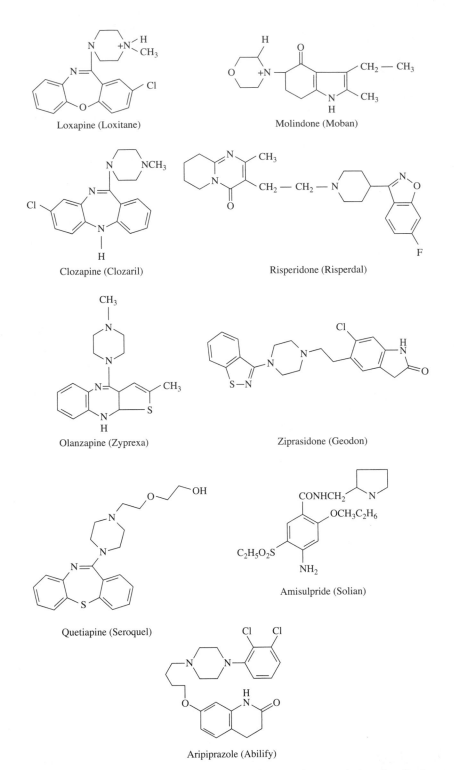

FIGURE 4.3 Structural formulas of some second-generation, atypical, antipsychotic drugs.

Pimozide

Although pimozide (Orap) is an antipsychotic drug, it is currently marketed in the United States for the treatment of motor and phonic tics in patients with Tourette's disorder who are unresponsive to other medications. In Europe and South America, it is more widely used as a neuroleptic antipsychotic drug. Besides the usual movement disorders of EPS and TD, the side effects that most limit the use of pimozide are electrocardiographic abnormalities (called QT prolongation) that are potentially dangerous. QT prolongation is discussed later in this chapter.

The discovery and development of the first-generation antipsychotics was a major advance in the treatment of schizophrenia. Nevertheless, it is recognized that there are three types of unsatisfactory outcomes for schizophrenic patients treated with phenothiazines and other FGAs. The first category includes patients who are treatment-resistant and refractory to medication, despite an adequate trial of an antipsychotic. The second consists of patients who have persistent negative symptoms, despite successful control of positive symptoms. The third consists of patients who are unable to tolerate the side effects of the antipsychotics. Current evidence suggests that, at the very least, SGAs may provide better options for patients in the third category.

Second-Generation (Atypical) Antipsychotic Agents

From 1975 to 1989, not a single new antipsychotic was marketed in the United States. Since then, clozapine (1989), risperidone (1994), olanzapine (1996), sertindole (1997), quetiapine (1997), ziprasidone (2001), aripiprazole (2002), paliperidone (2006), iloperidone (2009), and asenapine (2009) have been introduced. Amisulpride (Solian) is available in Europe and Australia but not yet in the United States.

Clozapine

Clozapine (Clozaril; see Figure 4.3), the first atypical antipsychotic, has been demonstrated to be clinically superior to traditional antipsychotics, first, because it is effective in about one-third of patients who are resistant to conventional medications, and second, because it lacks the extrapyramidal side effects associated with the traditional neuroleptics (Volavka et al., 2002). In fact, for patients with primary parkinsonism who demonstrate psychotic symptoms (such as hallucinations and delusions), clozapine can effectively treat their psychosis without exacerbating the movement disorder (Comaty and Advokat, 2001; Parkinson Study Group, 1999).

Background. Synthesized in 1959, clozapine was introduced into clinical practice in Europe in the early 1970s. Its lack of extrapyramidal effects was immediately appreciated. However, in 1975 several schizophrenic patients in Finland died of severe infectious diseases after developing agranulocytosis (loss of white blood cells in the blood) while taking clozapine. As a result, clinical testing ceased and the drug was withdrawn from unrestricted use in Europe. Later, clozapine was reexamined for two major reasons: (1) the agranulocytosis was found to be reversible when the drug was discontinued, and (2) the drug was found to be therapeutically beneficial in patients who had failed to respond to the traditional antipsychotic medications.

In 1986 a large, multicenter trial of the drug in the United States found improvement in 30 percent of severely psychotic patients who were unresponsive to other drugs; only 1 to 2 percent developed agranulocytosis. More recent studies show that the rate of improvement may approach 60 percent with longer therapy. In some patients the improvements are striking; they are able to be discharged from hospitals or to participate meaningfully in rehabilitation. Other clozapine responders do not improve substantially in their positive symptoms but report that their mood and sense of well-being are improved and their quality of life is better. These clinical data are confirmed by real-world improvements (Wheeler et al., 2009).

A compelling amount of evidence suggests that clozapine reduces the risk of suicide in schizophrenia relative to other antipsychotics. This observation led to the International Suicide Prevention Trial (InterSePT) study, which compared clozapine with another SGA, olanzapine, in patients with schizophrenia or schizoaffective disorder at risk for suicide (Meltzer et al., 2003). Clozapine was better at reducing suicidal behaviors and has been approved by the FDA for reduction of suicide risk in patients with schizophrenia or schizoaffective disorder.

Pharmacokinetics. Clozapine is well absorbed orally, and plasma levels of the drug peak in about 1 to 4 hours. The drug has two major metabolites, both of which are pharmacologically inactive. Its metabolic half-life varies from 9 to 30 hours. A reasonable daily dose of clozapine is about 200 to 400 milligrams, although dosage must be individualized and may be as high as 900 milligrams per day, if clinically warranted. Monitoring plasma levels may be useful in optimizing treatment, for example, to determine whether noncompliance with therapy or abrupt discontinuation of the drug might be at fault when psychotic symptoms recur (Tollefson et al., 1999). A once-daily clozapine formulation is currently in development.

Pharmacodynamics. As noted, clozapine has a receptor profile that differs from that of the FGAs. It antagonizes D_2 receptors less strongly than D_1 receptors and substantially less than 5-HT_2 receptors. Other receptor types antagonized by clozapine include D_3 and D_4 receptors and 5-HT_{1A}, histaminergic, cholinergic (muscarinic), and adrenergic receptors.

Side Effects and Toxicity. Although clozapine's efficacy is well documented, its use is severely limited by its side effects and potential for serious toxicity. Common side effects include sedation, extreme weight gain, decrease in seizure threshold, sialorrhea (hypersalivation), and constipation, with rare instances of agranulocytosis.

Sedation occurs in about 40 percent of patients taking clozapine; it may be dose limiting and have a negative impact on compliance. The sedation appears to be an antihistaminic effect. Taking the drug at bedtime may help improve compliance. Weight gain is a problem for up to 80 percent of patients; it can be severe, with gains of 20 pounds or more not unusual. Seizures occur at a greater rate with clozapine than with other antipsychotics, especially at high doses (600 to 900 milligrams per day), and it has a specific warning for this adverse event.

Sialorrhea (increased saliva production) occurs in one-third to one-half of patients, not only during the day but often much more extensively at night, with patients complaining of waking up with a wet pillow. The mechanism is believed to be due to an impaired ability to swallow, which causes saliva to accumulate. It may be severe and difficult to treat, although it can disappear over time. Constipation occurs in about 30 percent of patients and can be quite bothersome.

The greatest concern with clozapine is the risk of developing severe, life-threatening (although reversible) agranulocytosis, with an incidence of about 1 to 2 percent (Tschen et al., 1999). White blood cell counts and absolute neutrophil counts must be monitored weekly for the first 6 months of therapy, then every 2 weeks for the next 6 months, then monthly thereafter, with more frequent monitoring if the white blood cell count decreases. Other drugs that can reduce white blood cell count (most notably carbamazepine; see Chapter 6) should not be taken concomitantly. The etiology of clozapine-induced agranulocytosis appears to involve an unusual cellular-toxic mechanism. Eutrecht (1992) demonstrated that clozapine could be metabolized not only in the liver but also by the white blood cells themselves (an extremely unusual situation). An intermediate compound in this metabolic process is reactive and is toxic to the cell, possibly destroying the white cells that produced the metabolite.

Risperidone

Risperidone (Risperdal; see Figure 4.3), the second atypical antipsychotic drug, was introduced in 1994. It is a potent antagonist at both D_2 and $5\text{-}HT_2$ receptors, resulting in improved control of psychotic symptoms with a minimum of neuroleptic-induced EPS at low doses, less than 6 milligrams per day. However, the incidence of parkinsonism and other effects of dopaminergic blockade (such as prolactin release) increases at higher doses. In 2008, the FDA approved the first generic versions of risperidone tablets, again lowering the cost.

Pharmacokinetics. Risperidone is well absorbed when taken orally, is highly bound to plasma proteins, and is metabolized to an active intermediate, 9-hydroxy-risperidone. A long-acting injectable form of risperidone (Risperdal Consta) has now been approved. Using novel technology, the drug in this formulation is encapsulated in biodegradable polymer microspheres suspended in a water-based solution. A single intramuscular injection can last up to two weeks (Fleishhacker et al., 2003; Kane et al., 2003).

In 2009, Risperdal Consta (risperidone) long-acting injection was approved for a new indication, as either a monotherapy or as adjunctive therapy to lithium or valproate in the maintenance treatment of bipolar I disorder. One clinical trial showed that, over the course of 2 years, it was better than placebo, or monotherapy, at delaying time to relapse for any mood episode (depression, mania, hypomania, or mixed). A second study showed that over the course of 52 weeks, for patients already on lithium or valproate, it delayed the time to relapse compared with a combination of current treatment plus placebo.

The metabolic half-life of risperidone is about 3 hours; that of the metabolite, which accounts for much of risperidone's action, is about 23 hours. In fact, recognition of this characteristic led to the approval in 2006 of the active metabolite 9-hydroxy-risperidone (paliperidone), under the trade name Invega. This metabolite is a once-daily oral medication, available in 3-, 6-, or 9-milligram doses, that delivers the drug through the OROS[3] extended-release formulation, with a recommended dose of 6 milligrams and a range of 3 to 12 milligrams. Invega is not metabolized in the liver, so patients with liver failure can take it. Nussbaum and Stroup (2008) analyzed five studies comparing paliperidone with placebo, olanzapine, or Risperidal. Paliperidone was more effective than placebo, with a side

---

[3] OROS is a trademarked delivery system. It is a capsule-shaped tablet consisting of a multilayer core surrounded by a semipermeable membrane that allows slow release of the drug from the tablet. Concerta (methylphenidate; Chapter 18) is formulated in this OROS formulation.

effect profile similar to that of risperidone. But unlike risperidone, paliperidone cannot be crushed and administered in food.

An injectable, long-lasting form (1 month) of paliperidone was recently compared with placebo. The average time to first recurrence on placebo was 163 days (after being stable on a fixed dose for 12 weeks). So few paliperidone patients had relapsed that the corresponding number could not be calculated. In mid-2009, the FDA approved Invega Sustenna (paliperidone palmitate), an extended-release injectable suspension, for the acute and maintenance treatment of schizophrenia in adults. It is the first once-monthly, long-acting, injectable atypical antipsychotic approved in the United States for this use (Sedky et al., 2010). Unfortunately, its expense may limit its use.

Pharmacodynamics. Risperidone is as effective as haloperidol in reducing the positive symptomatology of schizophrenia at doses that do not produce a high incidence of EPS. Although this drug might not be quite as effective as clozapine, its safety profile can make it a first-line agent for treating schizophrenia.

Side Effects. Common side effects of risperidone include somnolence, agitation, anxiety, insomnia, headache, elevation of prolactin levels, EPS at high doses, and nausea. Weight gain is about 50 percent of that seen with either clozapine or olanzapine. Extrapyramidal symptoms are minimal at low doses (6 milligrams or less), although even low doses may elicit EPS in newly diagnosed patients with no previous exposure to antipsychotic drugs (Rosebush and Mazurek, 1999). Risperidone is considered to be safe in breast-fed infants; infant levels are only about 4 percent of the mother's (Ilett et al., 2004).

In 2004 the manufacturer reported an increased incidence of strokes and CNS ischemic attacks in elderly patients taking risperidone (see Chapter 19 for a more complete discussion).

Olanzapine

Introduced in 1996, olanzapine (Zyprexa; see Figure 4.3) structurally and pharmacologically resembles clozapine, without clozapine's toxicity on white blood cells.

Pharmacokinetics. Olanzapine is well absorbed orally. Peak plasma levels occur in about 5 to 8 hours. Metabolized in the liver, olanzapine has an elimination half-life in the range of 27 to 38 hours in both adults and children (Grothe et al., 2000). Gardiner and coworkers (2003) and Ambresin and coworkers (2004) studied olanzapine levels in infants of breast-feeding mothers who were taking the drug. They reported that infants received doses of only about 1 to 4 percent of that given to the mother, resulting in plasma levels of about 38 percent of those in the mother with no adverse effects.

Pharmacodynamics. Olanzapine is at least comparable to haloperidol in efficacy (Rosenheck et al., 2003), with minimal EPS, although it is much more expensive and produces much more weight gain. There is a complete block of 5-HT$_2$ receptors at low doses (5 milligrams/day), with increasing D$_2$ blockade as doses increase from 5 to 20 milligrams/day. Olanzapine has not been reported to cause agranulocytosis, which eliminates the need for white blood cell counts and may improve adherence.

Zyprexa IntraMuscular was as or more effective than either lorazepam or haloperidol in treating aggressive and agitated behaviors, usually in an emergency room scenario. In December 2009, a long-acting depot formulation of olanzapine was approved by the FDA, which had rejected it the previous year. Called Zyprexa Relprevv, it is given IM every 2 to 4 weeks, depending on the dose approved for treatment of schizophrenia in adults. Previous concerns were raised about a side effect called post-injection delirium/sedation syndrome (PDSS), which occurs in about 2 percent of patients. Patients have fallen asleep in public places or walked into walls. Labeling now includes a requirement that patients stay under observation at a health care facility for at least 3 hours after each injection and have an escort when leaving the facility. Dispensers must also register in a patient care education program to learn about the risks.

Sertindole

Sertindole (Serlect) was released in 1997 as the fourth atypical antipsychotic. It is primarily a 5-HT$_2$ receptor antagonist with lesser blockade of D$_2$ receptors. It therefore provides the requisite dual action of blocking 5-HT$_2$ and D$_2$ receptors thought to define SGAs. This dual action predicted therapeutic efficacy in treating schizophrenia, with a low incidence of EPS. Unlike risperidone and clozapine, sertindole has no affinity for histamine receptors and therefore is less sedative.

The drug can adversely affect the heart, an action that can lead to severe cardiac arrhythmias. For this reason, sertindole was removed from the market in 1998. However, it is undergoing postmarketing review to determine whether there might be an acceptably safe way to use it (Lewis et al., 2005). Sertindole may induce fewer movement disorders but more cardiac effects, weight change, and male sexual dysfunction than risperidone. However, these data are based on only two studies and are too limited to allow firm conclusions. Nothing can be said about the effects of sertindole compared with second-generation antipsychotics other than risperidone. There are several relevant trials under way or completed and about to be reported (Komossa et al., 2009a).

Quetiapine

Quetiapine (Seroquel; see Figure 4.3) is the fifth SGA with 5-HT$_2$/D$_2$ receptor-blocking action (Arvanitis and Miller, 1997). It is comparable to haloperidol in reducing positive symptoms, with little EPS. Quetiapine is currently approved for treatment of schizophrenia and acute bipolar depression and mania and for adjunctive maintenance therapy of bipolar disorder. The initial formulation has a relatively short biological half-life (about six hours); a long-acting version, quetiapine XR, was approved in June 2007 in 200-, 300-, and 400-milligram doses. In December 2008, tentative approval was given to market the generic tablet version. Consequently, efforts are under way to show that the drug is useful for a number of other disorders (Adityanjee, 2002). Seroquel is used a great deal to treat adolescent mania (Chapter 18). Unfortunately, its potent sedative/anxiolytic action has led to abuse, especially in prisons, where it is used to promote sleep and reduce anxiety and drug cravings.

Ziprasidone

Ziprasidone (Geodon; see Figure 4.3), approved in 2001, shows efficacy for treating schizophrenia with low liability for causing EPS (Arato et al., 2002; Goodnik, 2001; Gunasekara et al., 2002). Its half-life appears to be short, in the range of six hours. Perhaps its major clinical advantage is that it causes negligible weight gain. Ziprasidone has some unique receptor actions. In addition to blocking 5-HT$_2$ and D$_2$ receptors, it is a partial agonist at 5-HT$_{1A}$ receptors and a moderate inhibitor of serotonin and norepinephrine uptake. These receptor actions confer antidepressant and anxiolytic effects to the drug. Indeed, ziprasidone reduces both depressive and psychotic symptoms in people with schizoaffective disorder (Keck et al., 2001; Swainston and Scott, 2006). Ziprasidone was the first SGA to be approved for intramuscular use; an injectable formulation was approved in 2003 for rapid control of agitated behavior and psychotic symptoms. The limiting factor to the wide use of ziprasidone is its effect on the heart. The drug prolongs the QT interval, causing concern, but as yet no fatal reactions have occurred. However, QT prolongation may be a more serious problem in children and adolescents (Blair et al., 2005).

Aripiprazole

Aripiprazole (Abilify; see Figure 4.3) was approved in 2002 as perhaps the first of a new "third generation" (Potkin et al., 2003) because it has a different mechanism of action from those of the FGAs and SGAs. Aripiprazole is a partial agonist at D$_2$ and 5-HT$_{1A}$ receptors as well as an antagonist at 5-HT_2 receptors (Jordan et al., 2002). This "dopaminergic partial agonism" is meant to "stabilize" the system because, although the drug binds with high affinity to D_2 receptors, it has lower intrinsic activity (less efficacy). This means that under conditions of high dopamine levels, aripiprazole may replace dopamine at the receptor, but it will not produce as strong an effect as the natural transmitter. Conversely, when dopamine concentration is low, aripiprazole can produce a net increase in dopaminergic action (Lieberman, 2004; Stahl, 2002; Tamminga and Carlsson, 2002). Partial agonism at 5-HT_{1A} receptors confers anxiolytic or antidepressant actions, and this drug has been reported to augment the effect of SSRIs in patients with depression and anxiety disorders who were partial responders to the antidepressants (Schwartz et al., 2007). In 2007, the FDA approved aripiprazole as an adjunctive, or add-on, treatment to antidepressant therapy in adults with major depressive disorder. This was the first medication approved by the FDA as an add-on treatment for major depressive disorder. In addition, Abilify was approved in 2008 as an adjunct in patients whose manic episodes have not responded to lithium or valproate. This approval was based on a trial in 384 patients, with most receiving 15 milligrams during a 6-week period. The reduction in the Young Mania Rating Scale for aripiprazole was −13.3 versus −10.7 for placebo, with 19 percent of aripiprazole patients reporting akathisia (Vieta et al., 2008).

In late November 2009, the FDA approved an expanded indication for aripiprazole for the treatment of irritability associated with autism spectrum disorder in children aged 6 to 17 years. Oral aripiprazole had previously been approved for acute and maintenance treatment (with or without lithium or valproate) of manic and mixed episodes of bipolar disorder in patients aged 10 years and older as well as for acute and maintenance treatment of schizophrenia in patients aged 13 years and older (see Chapter 18).

To date, aripiprazole appears to be as effective as conventional and other second-generation agents. It does not cause QT prolongation or prolactin elevation, and it is not associated with weight gain or other glucose or lipid abnormalities. However, although rare, some cases of neuroleptic malignant syndrome have been reported after treatment with this drug, and some evidence for the development of movement disorders, like akathisia, has been noted.

Amisulpride

Amisulpride (Solian; see Figure 4.3) has a unique psychopharmacological profile. It selectively blocks D_2 and D_3 receptors in the limbic system but not in the basal ganglia, and it does not bind to D_1, D_4, or D_5 receptors, which may account for its lower incidence of EPS. Unlike all other SGAs, amisulpride does not block 5-HT_2 receptors, nor does it antagonize cholinergic, adrenergic, or histaminergic receptors. At low doses (50 to 300 milligrams per day) it preferentially blocks presynaptic dopamine receptors, which increases dopamine release. As a result, low doses increase dopaminergic activity in the mesolimbic system (Bressan et al., 2003). This may be the reason it has been reported to be effective in the treatment of dysthymia and depression as well as the negative symptoms of schizophrenia and to provide a better quality of life than haloperidol. In addition to its possible benefit for dysthymia and depression, this drug may be helpful in affective psychosis and chronic fatigue syndrome. In higher doses (up to 1200 milligrams per day), it was at least as effective as haloperidol, risperidone, and olanzapine in relieving psychosis, with EPS effects lower than those of haloperidol and comparable to those of risperidone and olanzapine. Although amisulpride has the benefit of producing less weight gain than risperidone and olanzapine and does not seem to be associated with diabetogenic effects, it may increase plasma prolactin levels. It has a half-life of about 12 hours—16 hours in the elderly (McKeage and Plosker, 2004). At this time, amisulpride has not been approved by the FDA for use in the United States.

Prominent Side Effects of Second-Generation Antipsychotics

Although the use of SGAs is generally associated with fewer parkinsonianlike symptoms than the use of FGAs, the SGAs are not without side effects, the most prominent of which are weight gain, a propensity to produce glucose intolerance (diabetes) along with elevation in blood lipids, and specific cardiac electrographic abnormalities that can be serious and even fatal. Collectively, these side effects have been termed the *metabolic syndrome*.

Weight Gain

As a group, SGAs have a propensity to induce weight gain, with clozapine and olanzapine inducing the most, ziprasidone and aripiprazole the least (amisulpride probably also shares this advantage) (Allison and Casey, 2001) (Figure 4.4). Weight gain occurs in 20 to 30 percent of people taking risperidone, olanzapine, and quetiapine, although the gain with risperidone is about half that brought on by the other two drugs. Weight gain in adolescents may be even greater than in adults (Ratzoni et al., 2002; Correll, 2007). This side effect may contribute to patient noncompliance with treatment and may adversely affect clinical outcome (Poyurovsky et al., 2003).

The mechanism responsible for this weight gain is still being elucidated (Newcomer, 2005); however, data suggest that this phenomenon is

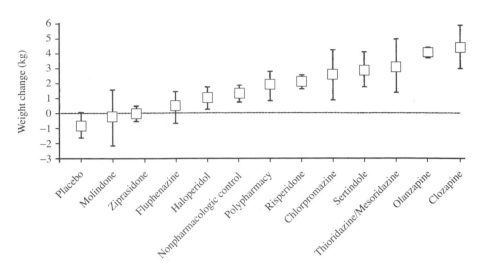

FIGURE 4.4 Estimated weight change after 10 weeks of treatment with standard drug doses. Shown are mean values and 95 percent confidence intervals. [From Allison and Casey (2001), p. 24.]

associated with the antihistaminergic aspects of the second-generation antipsychotics. Snyder and colleagues (discussed by Hampton, 2007) found a relationship between the SGAs that are most associated with this side effect and the stimulation of a hypothalamic AMP-activated protein kinase (AMPK). This enzyme, AMPK, is important for maintaining energy balance and has been linked to the regulation of food intake. The investigators found that histaminergic antagonism stimulated AMPK, and histamine decreased this stimulation. In mice given clozapine, AMPK activity quadrupled. This discovery may lead to the development of antipsychotics that retain their therapeutic benefit but do not produce weight gain and other metabolic problems.

Diabetes and Hyperglycemia

Patients who receive certain atypical antipsychotics are 9 to 14 percent more likely to develop adult-onset (type 2) diabetes than patients who receive traditional first-generation antipsychotic drugs (Lindenmayer et al., 2003; Newcomer, 2005; Sernyak et al., 2002). Increases in diabetes rates are seen in patients over 40 years of age who were taking clozapine, olanzapine, and quetiapine but not risperidone (Gianfrancesco et al., 2003). In patients under 40 years old, all agents increase the incidence of diabetes. These changes are independent of the weight gain induced by these drugs and seem to reflect a more rapid onset of diabetes. The American Diabetes Association and American Psychiatric Association have published suggested monitoring schedules for insulin resistance, recommending that blood levels be taken at 6 months and 1 year and then every 5 years thereafter. The long-term consequences of small elevations in blood glucose are unknown at this time but may include increased risk of cardiovascular disease (Wirshing et al., 2002). In one meta-analytic review, it was determined that the antidiabetic drug metformin significantly reduced body weight in nondiabetic patients who had gained weight on their antipsychotic medications. But there was a great deal of variability among the studies, and metformin is not approved for this indication (Björkhem-Bergman et al., 2010).

Electrocardiographic Abnormalities (Sudden Cardiac Death)

The "pacemaker" of the heart is the sinoatrial node, located in the right atrium of the heart. An electrical signal from the pacemaker flows over the atria and into the ventricles through the atrioventricular node. The ventricles then contract, propelling blood forward into the aorta and the arteries. Following depolarization and mechanical contraction, the ventricles repolarize to be ready for the next depolarization. Figure 4.5 illustrates the electrocardiogram (ECG) for one electrical cycle. The QT interval is the time from the start of spread of electricity to the ventricles to the end of ventricular repolarization. In essence, if this period is prolonged to about 500 milliseconds (0.5 second), the patient is at significant risk of developing the arrhythmia *torsades de pointes* (Figure 4.6), which can result in sudden death. The normal range for the QT interval for men below the age of 55 years is 350 to 430 milliseconds; for women, it is 350 to 450 milliseconds. Concern should arise when the QT interval is between 450 and 500 milliseconds; that is, the risk increases with a prolongation of 20 milliseconds or more. Besides drug-induced QT interval prolongation, *torsades de pointes* arrhythmias may at least partly be involved in sudden death in athletes and in infants (SIDS).

Many psychotropic medications, including neuroleptics, antidepressants, stimulants, and anxiolytics, may cause *torsades de pointes* (Glassman and Bigger, 2001; Khatib et al., 2003; Witchel et al., 2003). Even nonpsychotropic drugs have caused it, and some drugs, such as the antihistamine Seldane and the gastric stimulant Propulsid, have been removed from the market for this reason. Among the FGAs, thioridazine is most associated with this side effect and is rarely prescribed. Among the SGAs, this was one reason sertindole was removed from the market. In 2009 an FDA review found that patients taking sertindole had a significantly higher risk of sudden cardiac death (SCD) compared with those taking risperidone (13 versus 3). Approval of ziprasidone was delayed until additional safety data could be examined: it prolongs the interval about 10 or 15 milliseconds. Commonly used atypical drugs have electrophysiological effects that are similar to

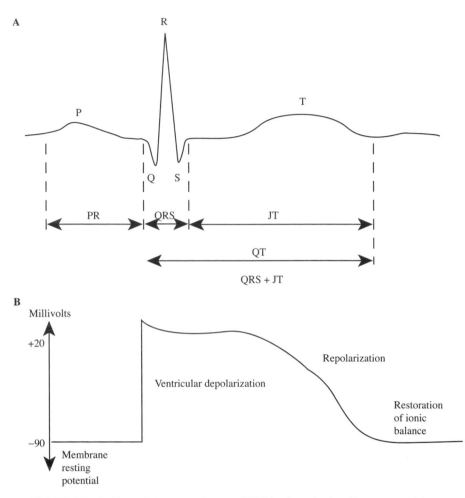

FIGURE 4.5   A. Normal electrocardiogram (ECG) in sinus rhythm. P wave = atrial electrical depolarization and leads to muscular contraction of the right and left ventricles. QRS complex = ventricular electrical depolarization and leads to muscular contraction of the right and left ventricles. JT = the time from the end of ventricular depolarization (QRS) to the end of ventricular repolarization. The QT interval includes both ventricular depolarization (QRS) and ventricular repolarization. **B.** Rapid ventricular depolarization and slower repolarization. Most of the QT interval represents ventricular repolarization.

those of the older drugs. There are now case reports that document the occurrence of *torsades de pointes* among users of several atypicals. In a large retrospective cohort of adults, current users of the atypicals had a dose-dependent increase in the risk of sudden cardiac death that was essentially identical to that among users of the typical agents. With regard to this side effect, the SGAs are no safer than the older drugs (Ray et al., 2009).

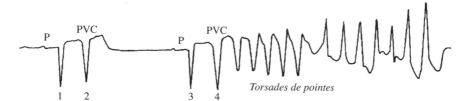

FIGURE 4.6 Characteristic development of *torsades de pointes* ventricular arrhythmia. Sinus beat with normal ventricular complex (1) followed by a premature ventricular contraction (PVC; 2) closely coupled to the sinus beat. After a long pause (2–3), this paired complex is repeated (3–4). The second PVC initiates a bizarre ventricular arrhythmia consistent with *torsades de pointes.* This ventricular arrhythmia is accompanied by poor contraction of ventricular muscle and therefore loss of contractility and output of blood from the heart, leading to a cardiac arrest.

New Agents and Updated Recommendations for the Treatment of Schizophrenia

In 2009 the FDA approved iloperidone (Fanapt) for the acute treatment of schizophrenia in adults. Two placebo and active control short-term trials (of 4 weeks and 6 weeks) showed efficacy, and safety data have been obtained from more than 2000 patients. Final doses are usually 12 to 24 mg/day, and titration to 12 mg should be gradually achieved over 4 days, because of the potent alpha antagonism. Like older SGAs, iloperidone is a D_2/5-HT_{2A} antagonist. It is also a 5-HT_{2C} and 5-HT_6 antagonist as well as a partial agonist at 5-HT_{1A} receptors (suggesting antidepressant benefit; Chapter 5), with relatively high alpha-1 blockade, which would be expected to produce orthostatic hypotension. But low histamine blockade should produce less sedation and weight gain, and little muscarinic antagonism might predict low anticholinergic side effects. This drug has had a long history of development, and early trials did not always show an impressive degree of efficacy relative to the comparator drug. It produced dose-dependent increases in QT interval, mild weight gain similar to risperidone, with mild glucose elevation. However, it elicited less akathisia than other compounds.

Asenapine (Saphris) was approved in 2009 for the treatment of schizophrenia (5 mg, 2 times a day) and manic or mixed episodes of bipolar disorder (10 mg, 2 times a day). Asenapine has a chemical structure related to the antidepressant mirtazepine. It is unique in that it must be dissolved under the tongue, with no eating or drinking for 10 minutes afterward; otherwise, it will not be adequately absorbed into the bloodstream. Bioavailability is less than 2 percent orally but 35 percent sublingually. It binds to more receptors than most other antipsychotics, with strong antagonism of D_1 through D_4,

5-HT$_{2A}$ and 5-HT$_{2C}$, 5-HT$_{1A}$, alpha-1 and H$_1$ receptors (Lincoln and Preskorn, 2009). As of December 2009, only a single study had been published regarding schizophrenia, a 6-week comparison of asenapine with risperidone and placebo in 174 patients. Notably, patients who had failed other drug treatments were excluded. Both drugs separated from placebo. A single paper has been published on a 3-week trial that assigned 488 patients with acute mania to Saphris, Zyprexa, or placebo. Adverse events were reported as 60.8 percent for Saphris, 52 percent for Zyprexa, and 36.2 percent for placebo. The most prominent side effects included weight gain, sleepiness, akathisia, dizziness, oral numbness, and, in some patients, a chalky sensation. However, the FDA advisory committee decision was based on efficacy data from more than 3000 patients and safety data from more than 45,000 patients. In addition, a long-term extension study (26 weeks, after 26 weeks of "acute" treatment) showed a favorable comparison with olanzapine. However, treatment-emergent adverse events were 85.1 percent for asenapine and 74.1 percent for olanzapine.

Lurasidone is an investigational atypical antipsychotic for the treatment of schizophrenia. Data have been obtained from 40 clinical studies and approximately 2500 patients. Lurasidone is also in late-stage clinical testing for acute and chronic schizophrenia, bipolar mania, and monotherapy and adjunctive treatment of bipolar depression. It is a potent antagonist of 5-HT$_{2A}$, D$_2$, 5-HT$_7$, and 5-HT$_{1A}$ receptors, with little affinity for most other receptors. It seems to produce minimal metabolic side effects, EPS, and akathisia, and it does not affect QTc prolongation. The dose range seems to be 20 to 40 mg/day for acute exacerbation of schizophrenia.

Cariprazine is another drug in clinical testing for schizophrenia, acute bipolar mania, bipolar depression, and treatment-resistant depression. It "prefers" D$_3$ over D$_2$, with both effects being partial agonism rather than antagonism. This selectivity would theoretically predict higher doses for mania and schizophrenia, for greater antagonist action, and lower doses for depression, for greater agonistic effect. Little weight gain or other metabolic problems have been reported so far. This agent has two long-acting active metabolites, which might offer the option of weekly to monthly depot administration.

The schizophrenia Patient Outcomes Research Team (PORT) recommendation summary has been updated. The review groups identified 41 treatment areas for review and conducted literature searches to identify all clinical studies published since the last review in 2002. Studies in areas not covered in 2002 were also reviewed. A total of 16 psychopharmacologic and 8 psychosocial treatments were recommended; another 13 psychopharmacologic and 4 psychosocial treatments had insufficient evidence for a recommendation (Kreyenbuhl et al., 2010).

Additional Applications for Second-Generation Antipsychotics

The use of SGAs in nonpsychotic disorders has rapidly increased in the last few years (Tables 4.3 and 4.4) (Trémeau and Citrome, 2006). With the exception of bipolar disorder, most of these applications have been "off-label," that is, they have not received FDA approval (Crystal et al., 2009). Although the FGAs were also known to be efficacious in some of these disorders, the improved neurological profile of the new agents and the inadequate response of many patients to their approved FGA medications for the respective illnesses have expanded the use of SGAs. While most information has been obtained from studies of risperidone and olanzapine, there are numerous case reports and open-label studies describing benefits of all the SGAs in a variety of conditions. At present, it should be kept in mind that most of the available evidence comes from evaluations of SGAs as adjuncts to other psychotropics, that few direct comparisons between FGAs and SGAs have been published, and that there is not yet a great deal of information on the long-term safety of the new agents. Current reports suggest that FDA-required warnings about risks concerning the use of atypical antipsychotics are not receiving sufficient attention (Kuehn, 2010).

As we will now see, atypical antipsychotic drugs are being used both on-label and off-label for multiple disorders, such as bipolar disorder, resistant depression, dysthymia, behavioral problems associated with dementia, autism spectrum disorders, severe resistant anxiety disorders, borderline personality disorder, and anger, aggression, and tantrums in various behavioral dyscontrol disorders. In these treatments the term "antipsychotic" seems inappropriate. Therefore, we introduce the term *thymic stabilizer* to encompass a variety of uses—comparable to use of the terms *mood stabilizer* or *neuromodulator* to refer to antiepileptic drugs used in nonepileptic disorders.

Bipolar Disorder

Except for clozapine, all the newer antipsychotics are approved by the FDA for treatment of some aspect of bipolar disorder. Olanzapine (in 2000), risperidone (in 2004), quetiapine (in 2004), ziprasidone (in 2004; Keck et al., 2003b), and aripiprazole (in 2004; Keck et al., 2003a) are approved for monotherapy of acute bipolar mania and (with the exception of quetiapine) for mixed episodes. Olanzapine, risperidone, and quetiapine are also approved as add-ons for treating bipolar mania in patients with a poor response to monotherapy.

A combination product containing olanzapine and fluoxetine (Symbyax) was approved (in 2003) for treating acute bipolar depression. However, in August 2009, the label for Symbyax was updated, and

TABLE 4.3 Nonpsychotic indications in Adults for second-generation antipsychotic agents

SGA[a]	Bipolar mania	Bipolar depression	Bipolar maintenance	Other
Aripiprazole	Acute mania or mixed episodes	Bipolar I disorder; most recent episode manic or mixed	Maintenance therapy	Resistant depression, irritability in autism
Asenapine	Acute mania or mixed episodes			
Clozapine				Risk of recurrent suicidal behavior in schizophrenia or schizoaffective disorders
Olanzapine	Acute mania or mixed episodes; monotherapy or with lithium or valproate for manic episodes		Bipolar disorder maintenance monotherapy	
Olanzapine/fluoxetine combination		Bipolar depressive episodes		Resistant depression
Quetiapine	Acute manic episodes; monotherapy or with lithium or valproate	Bipolar depressive episodes	Maintenance therapy	Resistant depression (XR formulation)
Risperidone	Acute mania or mixed episodes; monotherapy or with lithium or valproate			Irritability in autism
Ziprasidone	Acute mania or mixed episodes		Maintenance therapy	

[a]SGA = second-generation antipsychotic (oral form)
Safety issues. SGAs' safety profiles warrant caution. SGAs are less likely than first-generation antipsychotics (FGAs) to cause extrapyramidal symptoms (EPS) and tardive dyskinesia (TD) at therapeutic dosages, but they increase the risks of weight gain, diabetes, glucose intolerance, dyslipidemia, and hyperprolactinemia. Akathisia and hypotension also may occur.
Prescribing decisions. SGAs' potential adverse effects complicate clinical decision making. First it must be decided whether to use an SGA for the patient with a nonpsychotic disorder.
Adapted from Trémeau and Citrome (2006), p. 39.

TABLE 4.4 Second-generation antipsychotic uses in nonpsychotic disorders supported by evidence from published double-blind clinical trials[a]

SGA[b]	Unipolar depression	OCD[c]	Anxiety disorders	Dementia	Developmental disorders	Borderline personality disorder
Aripiprazole	Yes[d]				Yes	Yes[d]
Clozapine						
Olanzapine	Yes[d]	Yes	Yes	Yes		Yes
Quetiapine	Yes[d]	Yes				
Risperidone	Yes[d]	Yes	Yes	Yes	Yes	
Ziprasidone						

[a]Does not include studies of bipolar disorders, results from open trials, case reports, or studies not classified as double-blind with adequate numbers of subjects.
[b]SGA = second-generation antipsychotic
[c]OCD = obsessive-compulsive disorder
[d]Augmentation in treatment-resistant depression
Adapted from Trémeau and Citrome (2006), p. 39.

in October, labels were revised for olanzapine to warn of the possible development of leukopenia/neutropenia and agranulocytosis, that is, low white blood cells or neutrophils

Quetiapine is also approved for treating bipolar depressive episodes. For a series of articles that review the use of SGAs in bipolar disorder, see Volume 66, Supplement 3, of the *Journal of Clinical Psychiatry* (Hirschfeld, 2005).

Unipolar Depression

Only about one-third of patients with major depressive disorder (MDD) receiving initial antidepressant treatment achieve remission (see STAR*D study in Chapter 5). Among the many agents used for augmentation, the traditional antipsychotic drugs were known to be effective, but the risk of TD and EPS discouraged their use. The first report of an SGA for augmentation in MDD appeared in 1999, when eight patients with lack of response to selective serotonin reuptake inhibitors (SSRIs) showed rapid improvement with risperidone. This was followed by the first placebo-controlled study of the olanzapine-fluoxetine combination in fluoxetine-resistant depression (Shelton et al., 2005). Currently, the evidence for SGAs is greater than that for any other strategy, and they are becoming widely used for this purpose (Papakostas et al., 2004, 2005; Rapaport et al., 2006; Simon and Nemeroff, 2005; Yargic et al., 2004). As noted, in 2008 aripiprazole was the first atypical agent and first pharmacologic treatment of any type to be approved by the FDA for use as an augmentation agent in MDD. In December of 2009, quetiapine (extended release) was the second SGA approved for this indication.[4] One possible reason for quetiapine's antidepressant effects is the metabolite norquetiapine's potent inhibition of the NE transporter.

Nelson and Papakostas (2009) recently reviewed this area and reported no significant differences in efficacy among the different atypical agents. Efficacy did not appear to be affected by the duration of the trial or how treatment resistance was determined. However, the discontinuation rate due to adverse events was significantly higher for the atypicals, 9.1 percent compared to 2.3 percent for placebo. While rates of discontinuation did not differ among the SGAs, rates of specific side effects may be very different.

---

[4] Perhaps because the immediate-release formulation loses its patent in 2011, the manufacturer of quetiapine applied for approval of the drug as monotherapy for MDD and general anxiety disorder (GAD). The FDA advisory committee concluded that quetiapine was effective as an adjunctive therapy for MDD and monotherapy for MDD and GAD, but there was concern about safety. In the end, the panel voted that quetiapine was not safe to use as *monotherapy* for MDD or GAD. Increases in glucose and lipids were greater for quetiapine.

Dementia

Although not approved for this indication, antipsychotic drugs are widely used to treat delusions, aggression, and agitation in elderly patients (Carson et al., 2006; Jeste et al., 2005). Because FGAs may cause EPS, lower blood pressure, and increase the risk of falls, the use of SGAs for this population has become more common. The National Institute of Mental Health sponsored the CATIE-AD study to compare olanzapine, risperidone, and quetiapine with placebo in outpatients with symptoms of psychosis, agitation, and aggressiveness. Results showed no significant differences in effectiveness, measured as discontinuation for any cause, among the medications (Schneider et al., 2006). Other data suggest that olanzapine and quetiapine, perhaps because of their anticholinergic potency, may worsen cognition in older patients with dementia (Ballard et al., 2005).

However, an increased risk of stroke was noted in manufacturer-sponsored trials of risperidone and olanzapine (Wang et al., 2005), and in 2005 the FDA released an advisory stating that treatment with SGA medications of behavioral disorders in elderly patients with dementia is associated with a slight increase in mortality. This was extended to FGAs in 2008. Most of the deaths were due to heart-related events or infections (primarily pneumonia). Because the four SGAs that were studied belong to three different chemical classes, the FDA concluded that the effect was probably common across all atypical antipsychotics. The agency announced that it would require a "black box" warning describing this risk on the labels of the drugs and that it would also so designate the olanzapine-fluoxetine combination of Symbyax. To assess the impact of the warning, Dorsey and colleagues (2010) evaluated antipsychotic use in patients 65 and older with dementia, from 2003 to 2008. In the first year after the advisory, atypical antipsychotic prescriptions decreased by 2% overall, and by 19% for patients with dementia (discussed further in Chapter 19).

Autism Spectrum Disorders, Pervasive Developmental Disorder, Agitation, and Aggression

Antipsychotics represent one-third of all filled psychotropic prescriptions for patients with pervasive developmental disorders (PDD). Conventional antipsychotics are known to be effective in treating agitation, hyperactivity, aggression, stereotypic behaviors, tics, and affective lability in PDD (Lott et al., 2004) and autism spectrum disorders (McDougle et al., 1998, 2005; McCracken et al., 2002). Impairments of communication and social interaction are less affected. The undesirable neurologic side effects of FGAs, especially when used on a long-term basis, have shifted the focus toward SGAs. Indeed, in 2007 risperidone received FDA approval for the treatment of irritability associated with autistic behavior in children. Nevertheless, even in short-term studies, as many as 30 percent of children may fail to respond to risperidone, and after 6 months 33 percent of initial responders may fail to maintain their improvement. Concerns have also been raised about the long-term safety of this agent in children, particularly because of the increased release of prolactin. Chronic prolactin elevation may exert variable effects on puberty; may reduce bone mass; and is a risk factor in infertility, breast cancer, heart disease, and prostate abnormalities (Gagliano et al., 2004). Like other SGAs, risperidone, even in low doses, has been associated with weight gain and symptoms of the metabolic syndrome; in higher doses, it has been associated with EPS, tardive dyskinesia, and the neuroleptic malignant syndrome. As with risperidone, olanzapine has improved symptoms associated with PDD in children and adults. The use of antipsychotics in the management of agitation and aggression in youth has been reviewed and is covered in more detail in Chapter 18, where the use of antipsychotic drugs for aggression is compared with other agents.

Posttraumatic Stress Disorder

There is evidence for the effectiveness of SGAs in treating psychotic symptoms of posttraumatic stress disorder (PTSD). Most of the data come from studies of combat-related PTSD in patients either unresponsive or partially responsive to antidepressants. Clinical case reports support the use of risperidone (Bartzokis et al., 2005), olanzapine (Stein et al., 2002), quetiapine (Adityanjee, 2002), ziprasidone (Siddiqui et al., 2005), and aripiprazole (Lambert, 2006) in war veterans for reducing such symptoms as hyperarousal, reexperiencing, avoidance, nightmares, and flashbacks. Similarly, risperidone monotherapy was found useful for women with a current diagnosis of PTSD as a result of domestic violence or sexual abuse. A mean final risperidone dose of 2.6 milligrams per day significantly reduced avoidant and hyperarousal PTSD symptoms compared with the response of the placebo group, although there were no differences between the two groups on the Hamilton Rating Scales for Anxiety or Depression (Padala et al., 2006).

Obsessive-Compulsive Disorder

Risperidone (McDougle et al., 2000), olanzapine (Bystritsky et al., 2004), quetiapine (Atmaca et al., 2002; Denys et al., 2004; Mohr et al., 2002), and aripiprazole (Storch et al., 2008) have been reported to be effective in augmenting the clinical response of patients with obsessive-compulsive disorder who were treatment-refractory to antidepressants. Other anxiety disorders that have been responsive to SGAs, as either monotherapy or add-on, include social anxiety (Barnett et al., 2002), generalized anxiety (Brawman-Mintzer et al., 2005), and panic disorder (Khaldi et al., 2003). Gao and coworkers (2006) reviewed the use of SGAs in the management of anxiety disorders.

Borderline Personality Disorder

Borderline personality disorder (BPD) affects about 2 percent of the population: about 75 percent of patients with the diagnosis are female. The condition is characterized by brief, intense episodes of impulsiveness, hostility, and anger (including self-injurious behavior), as well as anxiety and depression.

Several reports had shown positive results with SGAs, including risperidone (Rocca et al., 2002), clozapine (Grootens and Verkes, 2005), quetiapine (Villeneuve and Lemelin, 2005), olanzapine (Bogenschutz and Nurnberg, 2004), and aripiprazole (Nickel et al., 2006). However, in two meta-analyses of pharmacotherapy for severe personality disorders, antipsychotics were found to have a very small effect (with aripiprazole being more effective than other antipsychotics; Mercer et al., 2009), whereas mood stabilizers were more efficacious (Ingenhoven et al., 2010; Mercer et al., 2009). Mood stabilizers were also found to be more effective for specific symptoms of BPD than antidepressants in a review by Lieb and colleagues (2010), although these authors concluded that aripiprazole and olanzapine were also beneficial.

Parkinson's Disease

It has long been appreciated that clozapine can reduce psychotic reactions in patients with Parkinson's disease who are receiving dopaminergic agents. Because of clozapine's undesirable side effect profile, quetiapine has become the preferred treatment (Comaty and Advokat, 2001; Reddy et al., 2002). The efficacy of these drugs may be due to their low affinity for the dopamine receptor, which prevents interference with the treatment of Parkinson's disease. This is supported by a report that aripiprazole was not very effective for medication-induced psychosis in "probable" parkinsonian patients (Fernandez et al., 2004).

Experimental Agents and Future Developmental Efforts

To determine whether *omega-3 polyunsaturated fatty acids* (omega-3-PUFA) reduce the rate of progression to first-episode psychotic disorder in adolescents and young adults aged 13 to 25 years with subthreshold psychosis, a randomized, double-blind, placebo-controlled trial was conducted between 2004 and 2007 in the "psychosis detection" unit of a large public hospital in Vienna, Austria. It included 81 patients at high risk of psychotic disorder. A 12-week intervention period of 1.2 grams/day of omega-3-PUFA or placebo was followed by a 40-week monitoring period, for a total study period of 12 months. Of the 81 participants, 76 completed the protocol (93.8%). At the end, 2 of 41 patients in the omega group and 11 of 40 in the placebo group had transitioned to psychotic disorder. Omega-3-PUFA may offer a safe and efficacious preventive strategy for young people with subthreshold psychotic states (Amminger et al., 2010).

The NIMH is launching a large-scale research project to explore whether using early and aggressive treatment, individually targeted and integrating a variety of different therapeutic approaches, will reduce the symptoms and prevent the gradual deterioration of functioning that is characteristic of chronic schizophrenia. The Recovery After an Initial Schizophrenia Episode (RAISE) project is being funded by the NIMH, with additional support from the American Recovery and Reinvestment Act (ARRA).

Efforts have been especially directed toward novel pharmacological approaches to treat cognitive deficits and negative symptoms. These efforts have focused on the cholinergic and glutamatergic systems, both of which may be involved in cognitive function. The two cholinergic receptor types are nicotinic and muscarinic. In 2008, a trial of one compound, a partial agonist of the alpha-7 nicotinic receptor subtype named anabaseine (DMXB-A), was conducted in 31 schizophrenic patients. DMXB-A was added to the patients' antipsychotic medications, mostly nonclozapine SGAs. Unfortunately, neither of the two DMXB-A doses differentiated from placebo on the battery of cognitive tests, although there was some evidence for effectiveness against negative symptoms. In the same year, a pilot clinical trial was conducted of the muscarinic agonist xanomeline in 20 schizophrenic patients. The xanomeline group showed significantly greater improvement in symptomatology and in some cognitive measures. But one drawback of this drug is that it also activates M_2, M_3, and M_5 receptors, which produces undesirable side effects. For this reason, Eli Lilly and Company and collaborators at several institutions developed a drug, LY2033298, that is an allosteric modulator of M_4 receptors. That is, it acts on a site that is different from the one at which acetylcholine binds, and it potentiates the action of the neurotransmitter. Preclinical laboratory studies were promising and research is ongoing (Leach et al., 2009).

Several observations implicate glutamate in the etiology of schizophrenia, although it is not clear what the most relevant mechanism might be. Antagonists of the ionotropic NMDA receptor, like PCP and ketamine, increase cortical excitability, which suggests that drugs that reduce such *hyperexcitation* might be antipsychotic.

Presynaptic metabotropic glutamate receptors, of the 2/3 subtype, modulate glutamate release. Agonists at this receptor decrease glutamate release, reducing neuronal excitation and possibly the pathological substrate of schizophrenia. In fact, mGlu2/3 receptor agonists block the effects of PCP and ketamine, as well as those of other neurotransmitter stimulants, on some behaviors and are under development as a new category of antipsychotic.

At the same time, PCP itself elicits some characteristic symptoms of schizophrenia. This led to the hypothesis that schizophrenia involves *hypofunction* of the NMDA receptor. The neuromodulator glycine is a required coagonist of the NMDA receptor, and administration of glycine has shown some modest improvement in schizophrenic patients. This suggests that increasing glycine levels and *enhancing* NMDA function might be therapeutic. For this reason, there is interest in the development of drugs that inhibit the transport system for glycine, specifically, the GlyT1 type, which has a similar distribution in the brain as the NMDA receptor. By blocking the glycine transporter, such drugs would increase NMDA activity and reverse the hypothesized deficit (Conn et al., 2008).

STUDY QUESTIONS

1. What are the positive and negative symptoms of schizophrenia? Why are these symptoms important in drug therapy?

2. Which neurotransmitters are most involved in the pathogenesis of schizophrenia?

3. What are the primary clinical differences between traditional and atypical antipsychotic drugs?

4. Discuss the mechanisms of action of traditional antipsychotics and atypical antipsychotics.

5. Discuss the side effects of first- and second-generation antipsychotics.

6. Name the currently available atypical antipsychotic drugs. How are they alike? How do they differ? What appears unique about ziprasidone, aripiprazole, and amisulpride?

7. Why might antipsychotic drugs induce weight gain and/or diabetes?

8. Compare and contrast the newer atypical antipsychotics in terms of their efficacy, diabetes potential, effect on weight gain, QT effects, and other side effects.

REFERENCES

Adityanjee, S. C. (2002). "Clinical Use of Quetiapine in Disease States Other Than Schizophrenia." *Journal of Clinical Psychiatry* 63, Supplement 13: 32–38.

Advokat, C. (2005). "Differential Effects of Clozapine, Compared with Other Antipsychotics, on Clinical Outcome and Dopamine Release in the Brain." *Essential Psychopharmacology* 6: 73–90.

Advokat, C. (2010). "A Brief Overview of Iatrogenic Akathisia." *Clinical Schizophrenia & Related Psychoses* 3: 226–236.

Allison, D. B., and Casey, D. E. (2001). "Antipsychotic-Induced Weight Gain: A Review of the Literature." *Journal of Clinical Psychiatry* 62, Supplement 7: 22–31.

Ambresin, G., et al. (2004). "Olanzapine Excretion into Breast Milk: A Case Report." *Journal of Clinical Psychopharmacology* 24: 93–95.

American Psychiatric Association. (2004). "Practice Guideline for the Treatment of Patients with Schizophrenia," 2nd ed. *American Journal of Psychiatry* 161 (February Supplement).

Amminger, G. P., et al., (2010). "Long-Chain Omega-3 Fatty Acids for Indicated Prevention of Psychotic Disorders: A Randomized Placebo-Controlled Trial." *Archives of General Psychiatry* 67: 146–154.

Arato, M., et al. (2002). "A 1-Year, Double-Blind, Placebo-Controlled Trial of Ziprasidone 40, 80 and 160 mg/day in Chronic Schizophrenia: The Ziprasidone Extended Use in Schizophrenia (ZEUS) Study." *International Clinical Psychopharmacology* 17: 207–215.

Arvanitis, L. A., and Miller, B. G. (1997). "Multiple Fixed Doses of 'Seroquel' (Quetiapine) in Patients with Acute Exacerbation of Schizophrenia: A Comparison with Haloperidol and Placebo. The Seroquel Trial 13 Study Group." *Biological Psychiatry* 42: 233–246.

Atmaca, M., et al. (2002). "Quetiapine Augmentation in Patients with Treatment Resistant Obsessive-Compulsive Disorder: A Single-Blind, Placebo-Controlled Study." *International Clinical Psychopharmacology* 17: 115–119.

Ballard, C., et al. (2005). "Quetiapine and Rivastigmine and Cognitive Decline in Alzheimer's Disease: Randomized Double Blind Placebo Controlled Trial." *British Medical Journal* 330: 874.

Barnett, S. D., et al. (2002). "Efficacy of Olanzapine in Social Anxiety Disorder: A Pilot Study." *Journal of Psychopharmacology* 16: 365–368.

Bartzokis, G., et al. (2005). "Adjunctive Risperidone in the Treatment of Combat-Related Posttraumatic Stress Disorder." *Biological Psychiatry* 57: 474–479.

Björkhem-Bergman, L., et al. (2010). "Metformin for Weight Reduction in Non-Diabetic Patients on Antipsychotic Drugs: A Systematic Review and Meta-Analysis." *Journal of Psychopharmacology*. In press.

Blair, J., et al. (2005). "Electrocardiographic Changes in Children and Adolescents Treated with Ziprasidone: A Prospective Study." *Journal of the American Academy of Child and Adolescent Psychiatry* 44: 73–79.

Bobes, J., et al. (2010). "Prevalence of Negative Symptoms in Outpatients with Schizophrenia Spectrum Disorders Treated with Antipsychotics in Routine Clinical Practice: Findings from the CLAMORS Study." *Journal of Clinical Psychiatry* 71; 280–286.

Bogenschutz, M. P., and Nurnberg, G. (2004). "Olanzapine versus Placebo in the Treatment of Borderline Personality Disorder." *Journal of Clinical Psychiatry* 65: 104–109.

Brawman-Mintzer, O., et al. (2005). "Adjunctive Risperidone in Generalized Anxiety Disorder: A Double-Blind, Placebo-Controlled Study." *Journal of Clinical Psychiatry* 66: 1321–1325.

Bressan, R. A., et al. (2003). "Is Regionally Selective D_2/D_3 Dopamine Occupancy Sufficient for Atypical Antipsychotic Effect? An In Vivo Quantitative [^{123}I] Epidepride SPET Study of Amisulpride-Treated Patients." *American Journal of Psychiatry* 160: 1413–1420.

Bystritsky, A., et al. (2004). "Augmentation of Serotonin Reuptake Inhibitors in Refractory Obsessive-Compulsive Disorder Using Adjunctive Olanzapine: A Placebo-Controlled Trial." *Journal of Clinical Psychiatry* 65: 565–568.

Carpenter, W. T., Jr., and Gold, J. M. (2002). "Another View of Therapy for Cognition in Schizophrenia." *Biological Psychiatry* 52: 969–971.

Carson, S., et al. (2006). "A Systematic Review of the Efficacy and Safety of Atypical Antipsychotics in Patients with Psychological and Behavioral Symptoms of Dementia." *Journal of the American Geriatric Society* 54: 354–361.

Ciranni, M. A., et al. (2009). "Comparing Acute Toxicity of First- and Second-Generation Antipsychotic Drugs: A 10-year, Retrospective Cohort Study." *Journal of Clinical Psychiatry* 70: 122–129.

Comaty, J. E., and Advokat, C. (2001). "Indications for the Use of Atypical Antipsychotics in the Elderly." *Journal of Clinical Geropsychology* 7: 285–309.

Conn, P. J., et al. (2008). "Schizophrenia: Moving Beyond Monoamine Antagonists." *Molecular Interventions* 8: 99–107.

Correll, C. U. (2007). "Weight Gain and Metabolic Effects of Mood Stabilizers and Antipsychotics in Pediatric Bipolar Disorder: A Systematic Review and Pooled Analysis of Short-Term Trials." *Journal of the American Academy of Child and Adolescent Psychiatry* 46: 687–700.

Correll, C. U., et al. (2004). "Lower Risk for Tardive Dyskinesia Associated with Second-Generation Antipsychotics: A Systematic Review of 1-Year Studies." *American Journal of Psychiatry* 161: 414–425.

Crystal, S., et al. (2009). "Broadened Use of Atypical Antipsychotics: Safety, Effectiveness, and Policy Challenges." *Health Affairs* 28: W770–W781.

Davis, J. M., and Chen, N. (2004). "Dose Response and Dose Equivalence of Antipsychotics." *Journal of Clinical Psychopharmacology* 24: 192–208.

Davis, J. M., et al. (2003). "A Meta-Analysis of the Efficacy of Second-Generation Antipsychotics." *Archives of General Psychiatry* 60: 553–564.

Denys, D., et al. (2004). "A Double-Blind, Randomized, Placebo-Controlled Trial of Quetiapine Addition in Patients with Obsessive-Compulsive Disorder Refractory to Serotonin Reuptake Inhibitors." *Journal of Clinical Psychiatry* 65: 1040–1048.

Dorsey, E. R., et al. (2010). "Impact of FDA Black Box Advisory on Antipsychotic Medication Use." *Archives of Internal Medicine* 170: 96–103.

Eutrecht, J. P. (1992). "Metabolism of Clozapine by Neutrophils: Possible Implications for Clozapine-Induced Agranulocytosis." *Drug Safety* 7, Supplement 1: 51–56.

Farber, N. B. (2003). "The NMDA Receptor Hypofunction Model of Psychosis." *Annals of the New York Academy of Sciences* 1003: 119–130.

Fazel, S., et al. (2009). "Schizophrenia, Substance Abuse and Violent Crime." *Journal of the American Medical Association* 301: 2016–2023.

Fernandez, H. H., et al. (2004). "Aripiprazole for Drug-Induced Psychosis in Parkinson Disease: Preliminary Experience." *Clinical Neuropharmacology* 27: 4–5.

Fleishhacker, W. W., et al. (2003). "Treatment of Schizophrenia with Long-Acting Injectable Risperidone: A 12-Month Open-Label Trial of the First Long-Acting, Second-Generation Antipsychotic." *Journal of Clinical Psychiatry* 64: 1250–1257.

Freedman, R. (2003). "Schizophrenia." *New England Journal of Medicine* 349: 1738–1749.

Freudenreich, O., et al. (2009). "Modafinil for Clozapine-Treated Schizophrenia Patients: A Double-Blind, Placebo-Controlled Pilot Trial." *Journal of Clinical Psychiatry* 70: 1674–1680.

Gagliano, A., et al. (2004). "Risperidone Treatment of Children with Autistic Disorder: Effectiveness, Tolerability, and Pharmacokinetic Implications." *Journal of Child and Adolescent Psychopharmacology* 14: 39–47.

Gao, K., et al. (2006). "Efficacy of Typical and Atypical Antipsychotics for Primary and Comorbid Anxiety Symptoms or Disorders: A Review." *Journal of Clinical Psychiatry* 67: 1327–1340.

Gardiner, S. J., et al. (2003). "Transfer of Olanzapine into Breast Milk, Calculation of Infant Drug Dose, and Effect on Breast-Fed Infants." *American Journal of Psychiatry* 160: 1428–1431.

Gianfrancesco, F., et al. (2003). "Antipsychotic-Induced Type 2 Diabetes: Evidence from a Large Health Plan Database." *Journal of Clinical Psychopharmacology* 23: 328–335.

Glassman, A. H., and Bigger, J. T. (2001). "Antipsychotic Drugs: Prolonged QTc Interval, Torsade de Pointes, and Sudden Death." *American Journal of Psychiatry* 158: 1774–1782.

Goodnik, P. J. (2001). "Ziprasidone: Profile on Safety." *Expert Opinions in Pharmacotherapy* 2: 1655–1662.

Grootens, K. P., and Verkes, R. J. (2005). "Emerging Evidence for the Use of Atypical Antipsychotics in Borderline Personality Disorder." *Pharmacopsychiatry* 38: 20–23.

Grothe, D. R., et al. (2000). "Olanzapine Pharmacokinetics in Pediatric and Adolescent Inpatients with Schizophrenia." *Journal of Clinical Psychopharmacology* 20: 220–225.

Grunder, G., et al. (2003). "Mechanism of New Antipsychotic Medications: Occupancy Is Not Just Antagonism." *Archives of General Psychiatry* 60: 974–977.

Gunasekara, N. S., et al. (2002). "Ziprasidone: A Review of Its Use in Schizophrenia and Schizoaffective Disorder." *Drugs* 62: 1217–1251.

Hampton, T. (2007). "Antipsychotic's Link to Weight Gain Found." *Journal of the American Medical Association* 297: 1305–1306.

Hirschfeld, R. M. A. (2005). "Introduction: The Role of Atypical Antipsychotics in the Treatment of Bipolar Disorder." *Journal of Clinical Psychiatry* 66, Supplement 3: 3–4.

Horacek, J., et al. (2006). "Mechanism of Action of Atypical Antipsychotic Drugs and the Neurobiology of Schizophrenia." *CNS Drugs* 20: 389–409.

Ilett, K., et al. (2004). "Transfer of Risperidone and 9-Hydroxyrisperidone into Human Milk." *Annals of Pharmacotherapy* 38: 273–276.

Ingenhoven, T., et al. (2010). "Effectiveness of Pharmacotherapy for Severe Personality Disorders: Meta-Analyses of Randomized Controlled Trials." *Journal of Clinical Psychiatry* 71: 14–25.

Janicak, P., et al. (2006). *Principles and Practice of Psychopharmacotherapy.* New York: Lippincott Williams & Wilkins.

Javitt, D. C., and Coyle, J. T. (2004). "Decoding Schizophrenia: A Fuller Understanding of Signaling in the Brain of People with This Disorder Offers a New Hope for Improved Therapy." *Scientific American* 290: 48–56.

Jeste, D. V., et al. (2005). "Atypical Antipsychotics in Elderly Patients with Dementia or Schizophrenia: Review of Recent Literature." *Harvard Review of Psychiatry* 13: 340–351.

Jones, P. B., et al. (2006). "Randomized Controlled Trial of the Effect on Quality of Life of Second- vs First-Generation Antipsychotic Drugs in Schizophrenia: Cost Utility of the Latest Antipsychotic Drugs in Schizophrenia Study (CUtLASS 1)." *Archives of General Psychiatry* 63: 1079–1087.

Jordan, S., et al. (2002). "The Antipsychotic Aripiprazole Is a Potent, Partial Agonist at the Human 5-HT1A Receptor." *European Journal of Pharmacology* 441: 137–140.

Kane, J. M., et al. (2003). "Long-Acting Injectable Risperidone: Efficacy and Safety of the First Long-Acting Atypical Antipsychotic." *American Journal of Psychiatry* 160: 1125–1132.

Kapur, S., and Remington, G. (2001). "Atypical Antipsychotics: New Directions and New Challenges in the Treatment of Schizophrenia." *Annual Reviews of Medicine* 52: 503–517.

Kapur, S., and Seeman, P. (2001). "Does Fast Dissociation from the Dopamine D2 Receptor Explain the Action of Atypical Antipsychotics? A New Hypothesis." *American Journal of Psychiatry* 158: 360–369.

Keck, P. E., et al. (2001). "Ziprasidone in the Short-Term Treatment of Patients with Schizoaffective Disorder: Results from Two Double-Blind, Placebo-Controlled, Multicenter Studies." *Journal of Clinical Psychopharmacology* 21: 27–35.

Keck, P. E., et al. (2003a). "A Placebo-Controlled, Double-Blind Study of the Efficacy and Safety of Aripiprazole in Patients with Acute Bipolar Disorder." *American Journal of Psychiatry* 160: 1651–1658.

Keck, P. E., et al. (2003b). "Ziprasidone in the Treatment of Acute Bipolar Mania: A Three-Week, Placebo-Controlled, Double-Blind, Randomized Trial." *American Journal of Psychiatry* 160: 741–748.

Kelly, D. L., et al. (2009). "Randomized Double-Blind Trial of Atomoxetine for Cognitive Impairments in 32 People with Schizophrenia." *Journal of Clinical Psychiatry* 70: 518–525.

Keltner, N. L., and Folks, D. G. (2005). *Psychotropic Drugs,* 4th ed. Philadelphia: Mosby.

Khaldi, S., et al. (2003). "Usefulness of Olanzapine in Refractory Panic Attacks." *Journal of Clinical Psychopharmacology* 23: 100–101.

Khatib, S. M. al-, et al. (2003). "What Clinicians Should Know About the QT Interval." *Journal of the American Medical Association* 289: 2120–2127.

Komossa, K., et al. (2009a). "Sertindole versus Other Atypical Antipsychotics for Schizophrenia." *Cochrane Database System Review.* Issue 4. Art. No. CD006752.

Komossa, K., et al. (2009b). "Ziprasidone versus Other Atypical Antipsychotics for Schizophrenia." *Cochrane Database System Review.* Issue 4. Art. No. CD006627.

Kreyenbuhl, J., et al. (2010). "The Schizophrenia Patient Outcomes Research Team (PORT): Updated Treatment Recommendations." *Schizophrenia Bulletin* 36: 94–103.

Kuehn, B. M. (2010). "Questionable Antipsychotic Prescribing Remains Common, Despite Serious Risks." *Journal of the American Medical Association* 303:1582–1584.

Lambert, M. T. (2006). "Aripiprazole in the Management of Post-Traumatic Stress Disorder Symptoms in Returning Global War on Terrorism Veterans." *International Clinical Psychopharmacology* 21: 185–187.

Laruelle, M., et al. (2003). "Glutamate, Dopamine and Schizophrenia from Pathophysiology to Treatment." *Annals of the New York Academy of Sciences* 1003: 138–158.

Leach, K., et al. (2009). "Molecular Mechanisms of Action and *In Vivo* Validation of an M_4 Muscarinic Acetylcholine Receptor Allosteric Modulator with Potential Antipsychotic Properties." *Neuropsychopharmacology* 35: 855–869.

Leucht, S., et al. (2003). "New Generation Antipsychotics versus Low-Potency Conventional Antipsychotics: A Systematic Review and Meta-Analysis." *Lancet* 361: 1581–1589.

Leucht, S., et al. (2009). "Second-Generation versus First-Generation Antipsychotic Drugs for Schizophrenia: A Meta-Analysis." *Lancet* 373: 31–41.

Lewis, R., et al. (2005). "Sertindole for Schizophrenia." *Cochrane Database System Review*. Issue 3. Art. No. CD001715.

Lieb, K., et al. (2010). "Pharmacotherapy for Borderline Personality Disorder: Cochrane Systematic Review of Randomised Trials." *British Journal of Psychiatry* 196: 4–12.

Lieberman, J. A. (2004). "Dopamine Partial Agonists: A New Class of Antipsychotic." *CNS Drugs* 18: 251–267.

Lieberman, J. A., et al. (2005). "Effectiveness of Antipsychotic Drugs in Patients with Chronic Schizophrenia." *New England Journal of Medicine* 353: 1209–1223.

Lincoln, J., and Preskorn, S. (2009). "Asenapine for Schizophrenia and Bipolar I Disorder." *Current Psychiatry* 8: 75–85.

Lindenmayer, J.-P., et al. (2003). "Changes in Glucose and Cholesterol in Patients with Schizophrenia Treated with Typical or Atypical Antipsychotics." *American Journal of Psychiatry* 160: 290–296.

López-Muñoz, F., et al. (2005). "History of the Discovery and Clinical Introduction of Chlorpromazine." *Annals of Clinical Psychiatry* 17: 113–135.

Lott, I. T., et al. (2004). "Longitudinal Prescribing Patterns for Psychoactive Medications in Community-Based Individuals with Developmental Disabilities: Utilization of Pharmacy Records." *Journal of Intellectual Disabilities Research* 48, Part 6: 563–571.

McCracken, J. T., et al. (2002). "Risperidone in Children with Autism and Serious Behavioral Problems." *New England Journal of Medicine* 347: 314–321.

McDougle, C. J. (1998). "A Double-Blind, Placebo-Controlled Study of Risperidone in Adults with Autistic Disorder and Other Pervasive Developmental Disorders." *Archives of General Psychiatry* 55: 633–641.

McDougle, C. J., et al. (2000). "A Double-Blind, Placebo-Controlled Study of Risperidone Addition in Serotonin Reuptake Inhibitor-Refractory Obsessive-Compulsive Disorder." *Archives of General Psychiatry* 57: 794–801.

McDougle, C. J., et al. (2005). "Risperidone for the Core Symptom Domains of Autism: Results from the Study by the Autism Network of the Research Units on Pediatric Psychopharmacology." *American Journal of Psychiatry* 162: 1142–1148.

McEvoy, J. P., et al. (2006). "Effectiveness of Clozapine versus Olanzapine, Quetiapine and Risperidone in Patients with Chronic Schizophrenia Who Did Not Respond to Prior Atypical Antipsychotic Treatment." *American Journal of Psychiatry* 163: 600–610.

McGowan, S., et al. (2004). "Presynaptic Dopaminergic Dysfunction in Schizophrenia: A Positron Emission Tomographic [^{18}F] Fluorodopa Study." *Archives of General Psychiatry* 61: 134–142.

McKeage, K., and Plosker, G. L. (2004). "Amisulpride: A Review of Its Use in the Management of Schizophrenia." *CNS Drugs* 18: 933–956.

Meltzer, H. Y. (2002). "Commentary on 'Clinical Studies on the Mechanism of Action of Clozapine: The Dopamine–Serotonin Hypothesis of Schizophrenia.'" *Psychopharmacology* 163: 1–3.

Meltzer, H. Y., et al. (2003). "Clozapine Treatment for Suicidality in Schizophrenia: International Suicide Prevention Trial (InterSePT)." *Archives of General Psychiatry* 60: 82–91.

Mercer, D., et al. (2009). "Meta-Analyses of Mood Stabilizers, Antidepressants and Antipsychotics in the Treatment of Borderline Personality Disorder: Effectiveness for Depression and Anger Symptoms." *Journal of Personality Disorders* 23: 156–174.

Mesholam-Gately, R. I. (2009). "Neurocognition in First-Episode Schizophrenia: A Meta-Analytic Review." *Neuropsychology* 23: 315–336.

Miyamoto, S., et al. (2003). "Recent Advances in the Neurobiology of Schizophrenia." *Molecular Interventions* 3: 27–39.

Moghaddam, B. (2003). "Bringing Order to the Glutamate Chaos in Schizophrenia." *Neuron* 40: 881–884.

Mohr, N., et al. (2002). "Quetiapine Augmentation of Serotonin Reuptake Inhibitors in Obsessive-Compulsive Disorder." *International Clinical Psychopharmacology* 17: 37–40.

Nelson, J. C., and Papakostas, G. I. (2009). "Atypical Antipsychotic Augmentation in Major Depressive Disorder: A Meta-Analysis of Placebo-Controlled Randomized Trials." *American Journal of Psychiatry* 166: 980–991.

Newcomer, J. W. (2005). "Second-Generation (Atypical) Antipsychotics and Metabolic Effects: A Comprehensive Literature Review." *CNS Drugs* 19, Supplement 1: 1–93.

Nickel, M. K., et al. (2006). "Aripiprazole in the Treatment of Patients with Borderline Personality Disorder: A Double-Blind, Placebo-Controlled Study." *American Journal of Psychiatry* 163: 833–838.

Nussbaum, A., and Stroup, S. (2008). "Paliperidone for Treatment of Schizophrenia." *Schizophrenia Bulletin* 34: 419–422.

Padala, P. R., et al. (2006). "Risperidone Monotherapy for Post-Traumatic Stress Disorder Related to Sexual Assault and Domestic Abuse in Women." *International Clinical Psychopharmacology* 21: 275–280.

Papakostas, G. I., et al. (2004). "Ziprasidone Augmentation of Selective Serotonin Reuptake Inhibitors (SSRIs) for SSRI-Resistant Major Depressive Disorder." *Journal of Clinical Psychiatry* 65: 217–221.

Papakostas, G. I., et al. (2005). "Aripiprazole Augmentation of Selective Serotonin Reuptake Inhibitors for Treatment-Resistant Major Depressive Disorder." *Journal of Clinical Psychiatry* 66: 1326–1330.

Parkinson Study Group (1999). "Low-Dose Clozapine for the Treatment of Drug-Induced Psychosis in Parkinson's Disease." *New England Journal of Medicine* 340: 757–763.

Peritogiannis, V., and Tsouli, S. (2009). "Can Atypical Antipsychotics Improve Tardive Dyskinesia Associated with Other Atypical Antipsychotics? Case Report and Brief Review of the Literature." *Journal of Psychopharmacology* 24: 1121–1125.

Potkin, S. G., et al. (2003). "Aripiprazole, an Antipsychotic with a Novel Mechanism of Action, and Risperidone vs. Placebo in Patients with Schizophrenia and Schizoaffective Disorder." *Archives of General Psychiatry* 60: 681–690.

Poyurovsky, M., et al. (2003). "Attenuation of Olanzapine-Induced Weight Gain with Reboxetine in Patients with Schizophrenia: A Double-Blind, Placebo-Controlled Study." *American Journal of Psychiatry* 160: 297–302.

Rapaport, M. H., et al. (2006). "Effects of Risperidone Augmentation in Patients with Treatment-Resistant Depression: Results of Open-Label Treatment Followed by Double-Blind Continuation." *Neuropsychopharmacology* 31: 2501–2513.

Ratzoni, G., et al. (2002). "Weight Gain Associated with Olanzapine and Risperidone in Adolescent Patients: A Comparative Prospective Study." *Journal of the American Academy of Child and Adolescent Psychiatry* 41: 337–343.

Ray, W. A., et al. (2009). "Atypical Antipsychotic Drugs and the Risk of Sudden Cardiac Death." *New England Journal of Medicine* 360: 225–235.

Reddy, S., et al. (2002). "The Effect of Quetiapine on Psychosis and Motor Function in Parkinsonian Patients with and Without Dementia." *Movement Disorders* 17: 676–681.

Rocca, P., et al. (2002). "Treatment of Borderline Personality Disorder with Risperidone." *Journal of Clinical Psychiatry* 63: 241–244.

Rosebush, P. I., and Mazurek, M. F. (1999). "Neurologic Side Effects in Neuroleptic-Naive Patients Treated with Haloperidol or Risperidone." *Neurology* 52: 782–785.

Rosenheck, R., and Sernyak, M. J. (2009). "Developing a Policy for Second-Generation Antipsychotic Drugs." *Health Affairs* 28: 782–793.

Rosenheck, R., et al. (2003). "Effectiveness and Cost of Olanzapine and Haloperidol in the Treatment of Schizophrenia: A Randomized Controlled Trial." *Journal of the American Medical Association* 290: 2693–2702.

Rujescu, D., et al. (2006). "A Pharmacological Model for Psychosis Based On N-Methyl-D-Aspartate Receptor Hypofunction: Molecular, Cellular, Functional and Behavioral Abnormalities." *Biological Psychiatry* 59: 721–729.

Sadock, B. J., and Sadock, V. A. (2007). *Kaplan and Sadock's Synopsis of Psychiatry.* New York: Lippincott Williams & Wilkins.

Schneider, L. S., et al. (2006). "Effectiveness of Atypical Antipsychotic Drugs in Patients with Alzheimer's Disease." *New England Journal of Medicine* 355: 1525–1538.

Schwartz, T. L., et al. (2007). "Aripiprazole Augmentation of Selective Serotonin or Serotonin Norepinephrine Reuptake Inhibitors in the Treatment of Major Depressive Disorder." *Primary Psychiatry* 14: 67–69.

Sedky, K., et al. (2010). "Paliperidone Palmitate: Once-Monthly Treatment Option for Schizophrenia." *Current Psychiatry* 9: 48–50.

Sernyak, M. J., et al. (2002). "Association of Diabetes Mellitus with Use of Atypical Neuroleptics in the Treatment of Schizophrenia." *American Journal of Psychiatry* 159: 561–566.

Shelton, R. C., et al. (2005). "Olanzapine/Fluoxetine Combination for Treatment-Resistant Depression: A Controlled Study of SSRI and Nortriptyline Resistance." *Journal of Clinical Psychiatry* 66: 1289–1297.

Siddiqui, Z., et al. (2005). "Ziprasidone Therapy for Post-Traumatic Stress Disorder." *Journal of Psychiatry & Neuroscience* 30: 430–431.

Simon, J. S., and Nemeroff, C. B. (2005). "Aripiprazole Augmentation of Antidepressants for the Treatment of Partially Responding and Nonresponding Patients with Major Depressive Disorder." *Journal of Clinical Psychiatry* 66: 1216–1220.

Stahl, S. M. (2002). "Dopamine System Stabilizers, Aripiprazole, and the Next Generation of Antipsychotics. Part 1: Goldilocks Actions at Dopamine Receptors; Part 2: Illustrating Their Mechanism of Action." *Journal of Clinical Psychiatry* 62: 841–842, 923–924.

Stein, M. B., et al. (2002). "Adjunctive Olanzapine for SSRI-Resistant Combat-Related PTSD: A Double-Blind, Placebo-Controlled Study." *American Journal of Psychiatry* 159: 1777–1779.

Storch, E. A., et al. (2008). "Aripiprazole Augmentation of Incomplete Treatment Response in an Adolescent Male with Obsessive-Compulsive Disorder." *Depression and Anxiety* 25: 172–174.

Stroup, T. S., et al. (2006). "Effectiveness of Olanzapine, Quetiapine, Risperidone, and Ziprasidone in Patients with Chronic Schizophrenia Following Discontinuation of a Previous Atypical Antipsychotic." *American Journal of Psychiatry* 163: 611–622.

Swainston, H. T., and Scott, L. J. (2006). "Ziprasidone: A Review of Its Use in Schizophrenia and Schizoaffective Disorder." *CNS Drugs* 20: 1027–1052.

Tamminga, C. A., and Carlsson, A. (2002). "Partial Dopamine Agonists and Dopaminergic Stabilizers, in the Treatment of Psychosis." *Current Drug Targets—CNS & Neurological Disorders* 1: 141–147.

Tenback, D. E., et al. (2009). "Incidence and Persistence of Tardive Dyskinesia and Extrapyramidal Symptoms in Schizophrenia." *Journal of Psychopharmacology* 24: 1031–1035.

Tollefson, G. D., et al. (1999). "Controlled, Double-Blind Investigation of the Clozapine Discontinuation Symptoms with Conversion to Either Olanzapine or Placebo." *Journal of Clinical Psychopharmacology* 19: 435–443.

Torrey, E. F. (2002). "Studies of Individuals with Schizophrenia Never Treated with Antipsychotic Medications: A Review." *Schizophrenia Research* 58: 101–115.

Trémeau, F., and Citrome, L. (2006). "Antipsychotics for Patients Without Psychoses?" *Current Psychiatry* 5: 33–44.

Tschen, A. C., et al. (1999). "The Cytotoxicity of Clozapine Metabolites: Implications for Predicting Clozapine-Induced Agranulocytosis." *Clinical Pharmacology and Therapeutics* 65: 526–532.

Vieta, E., et al. (2008). "Efficacy of Adjunctive Aripiprazole to Either Valproate or Lithium in Bipolar Mania Patients Partially Nonresponsive to Valproate/Lithium Monotherapy: A Placebo-Controlled Study." *American Journal of Psychiatry* 165: 1316–1325.

Villeneuve, E., and Lemelin, S. (2005). "Open-Label Study of Atypical Neuroleptic Quetiapine for Treatment of Borderline Personality Disorder: Impulsivity as Main Target." *Journal of Clinical Psychiatry* 66: 1298–1303.

Volavka, J., et al. (2002). "Clozapine, Olanzapine, Risperidone, and Haloperidol in the Treatment of Patients with Chronic Schizophrenia and Schizoaffective Disorder." *American Journal of Psychiatry* 159: 255–262.

Wang, P. S., et al. (2005). "Risk of Death in Elderly Users of Conventional vs. Atypical Antipsychotic Medications." *New England Journal of Medicine* 353: 2335–2341.

Weickert, T., et al. (2003). "Comparison of Cognitive Performance During a Placebo Period and an Atypical Antipsychotic Treatment Period in Schizophrenia: Critical Examination of Confounds." *Neuropsychopharmacology* 28: 1491–1500.

Weiss, E. M., et al. (2002). "The Effects of Second-Generation Atypical Antipsychotics on Cognitive Functioning and Psychosocial Outcomes in Schizophrenia." *Psychopharmacology* 162: 11–17.

Wheeler, A., et al. (2009). "Outcomes for Schizophrenia Patients with Clozapine Treatment: How Good Does It Get?" *Journal of Psychopharmacology* 23: 957–965.

Wirshing, D. A., et al. (2002). "The Effects of Novel Antipsychotics on Glucose and Lipid Levels." *Journal of Clinical Psychiatry* 63: 856–865.

Witchel, H. J., et al. (2003). "Psychotropic Drugs, Cardiac Arrhythmia, and Sudden Death." *Journal of Clinical Psychopharmacology* 23: 58–77.

Yargic, L. I., et al. (2004). "A Prospective Randomized Single-Blind, Multicenter Trial Comparing the Efficacy and Safety of Paroxetine with and Without Quetiapine Therapy in Depression Associated with Anxiety." *International Journal of Psychiatry in Clinical Practice* 8: 205–211.

Chapter 5

Antidepressant Drugs

Depression

Depression, or major depressive disorder (MDD), is a chronic, recurring, and potentially life-threatening illness. MDD is currently the fourth most disabling disease worldwide, and by the year 2020, it will be the second leading cause of disability across the globe. According to a May 2007 report of the World Health Organization, depression accounts for 4.5 percent of the total worldwide burden of disease in terms of disability-adjusted life years. Depression worsens the health of people with other chronic illnesses, has a tendency to recur, and is associated with increasing disability over time. About 10 percent of men and up to 25 percent of women experience depression in their lifetime, and each year about 9 to 10 percent of the U.S. population, or approximately 30 million Americans, suffer with this illness. Depression is responsible for up to 70 percent of psychiatric hospitalizations and about 40 percent of suicides. Unfortunately, it has been estimated that only about 21 percent of persons with depression are adequately treated (Kessler et al., 2003), and the personal and societal costs are enormous (World Health Organization, 2007).

Depression is an *affective disorder*, characterized by (sometimes profound) alterations of emotion or mood. The diagnosis of a "major depressive episode" is based on the following criteria, of which at least five must be evident daily or almost every day for at least two weeks (American Psychiatric Association, 1994):

- Depressed or irritable mood
- Decreased interest in pleasurable activities and in the ability to experience pleasure

- Significant weight gain or loss (> 5 percent change in a month)
- Insomnia or hypersomnia
- Psychomotor agitation or retardation
- Fatigue or loss of energy
- Feelings of worthlessness or excessive guilt
- Diminished ability to think or concentrate
- Recurrent thoughts of death or suicide (pp. 320–321)

Symptoms may be mild, moderate, or severe, depending on the extent of impairment in daily social and occupational functioning. Severe depression may be associated with symptoms of psychosis or loss of touch with reality. People with relatively mild but prolonged symptoms that persist for at least two years are considered to have "dysthymia." Other subtypes include *atypical depression* (Pae et al., 2009a) and depressive symptoms that occur after a significant trauma (for example, death of a loved one).

Symptoms of anxiety are also seen in many people with depression. Although many of the anxiety disorders have historically been treated with benzodiazepine anxiolytics (Chapter 7), today antidepressant treatment is also indicated for anxiety disorders. Not only are the antidepressant drugs efficacious for treating anxiety, they are less prone to compulsive use and less likely to impair learning, memory, and concentration than the benzodiazepines.[1]

Pathophysiology of Depression

Classically, depression was conceptualized as a deficiency involving neurotransmitters, particularly the "monoamines" serotonin, norepinephrine, and dopamine. Restoring these neurotransmitters, usually by prolonging their presence in the synaptic cleft, was responsible for recovering a normal mood state. One weakness of this model was that the neurotransmitter changes occurred soon after drug administration—but the clinical antidepressant effect develops more slowly, often during several weeks of continuous treatment. This delay was hypothesized to be due to changes in receptor sensitivity caused by the chronic increase in synaptic levels of neurotransmitter. However, in the last few years, this view has broadened, and attention has shifted to the study of the long-term actions of antidepressant treatments on intracellular processes, such as second messengers, and their functions in the neuron.

---

[1] According to current diagnostic criteria, anxiety disorders include panic disorder (PD), obsessive-compulsive disorder (OCD), posttraumatic stress disorder (PTSD), social phobia, and generalized anxiety disorder (GAD).

Two of these second-messenger functions are (1) to protect neu-rons from damage due to injury or trauma and (2) to promote and maintain the health and stability of newly formed neurons. Research into these processes has led to a new way of thinking about depression (and the effect of antidepressant treatment) called the *neurogenic theory of depression*.

The neurogenic theory is a result of the relatively recent discovery that, contrary to what we once believed, (1) existing neurons are able to "repair" or "remodel" themselves and (2) the brain is capable of making new neurons. In particular, it is now known that new neurons are pro-duced throughout life in the hippocampus and the frontal cortex of several species, including humans. The birth of new neurons is called *neurogenesis*. This finding is especially relevant to understanding depres-sive disorders because the hippocampus influences many functions that are impaired in a depressed person, such as attention, concentration, and memory. At the same time, we know that the hippocampus is also very vulnerable to the effects of trauma, such as hypoglycemia, lack of oxygen, toxins, infections, and especially stress, and to the hormones that are activated by stressful situations (such as corticosterone). In fact, stressful situations are known both to reduce hippocampal and frontal cortical neurogenesis and to damage existing neurons.

Among the stressful conditions that can damage the hippocampus is a state of depression—not surprising, as stress is believed to be one of the most significant causes of depression; about 50 percent of de-pressed patients have some abnormality in their physiological re-sponses to stress. Moreover, hippocampal nerve cells are among the most sensitive to stress-induced damage. In fact, it has been shown that the hippocampus physically shrinks in response to various stres-sors, including depression (Frodl et al., 2007), and that the longer an episode of depression goes untreated, the greater the amount of shrinkage (Figure 5.1). Consequently, depression is now viewed as a type of neurodegenerative disorder (Lucassen et al., 2010).

Just as a variety of stimuli can damage neurons and decrease neu-rogenesis, several factors are known to repair neurons and increase neurogenesis—among them, antidepressant drugs.[2] It has been pro-posed that the therapeutic delay in the clinical effect of antidepres-sants occurs because of the time required for new neurons to develop, mature, and become functional. This hypothesis is supported by the observation that the increase in neurogenesis requires chronic antide-pressant administration, which is consistent with the time course for the therapeutic action of these medications (Duman, 2004; Krishnan and Nestler, 2008).

---

[2] Other stimuli include electroconvulsive therapy, exercise, light therapy, and so on.

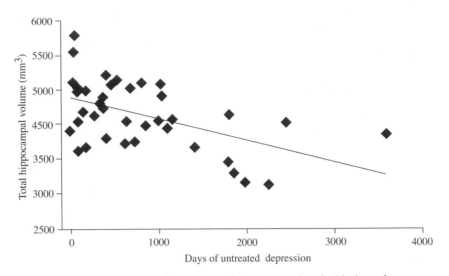

FIGURE 5.1 Reduction in total hippocampal volume correlated with days of untreated depression. The total time each patient had been in a depressive episode was divided into days during which the patient was receiving antidepressant medication versus days during which no antidepressant medication was given. The regression plot depicts the significant inverse relationship between total hippocampal volume and the length of time depression went untreated. [Adapted from Y. I. Sheline et al., "Untreated Depression and Hippocampal Volume Loss," *American Journal of Psychiatry* 160 (2003), p. 1517, Figure 1.]

A major focus of current research is to identify the cellular processes in the hippocampus and frontal cortex that are responsible for the protective effects of antidepressants. Most current studies are directed toward the second-messenger systems, which are activated by the synaptic action of neurotransmitters. This action in turn stimulates production of intracellular proteins that control the expression of certain genes.

One of the intracellular targets of second-messenger systems is called *cAMP response-element-binding protein* (CREB). The fact that the amount of CREB protein increases in the hippocampus during chronic antidepressant treatment provides additional evidence for the neurogenic hypothesis (Blendy, 2006; Malberg and Blendy, 2005). In turn, it is known that CREB activates genes that control the production of a protein called *brain-derived neurotrophic factor* (BDNF). BDNF is one of a group of substances called *neurotrophins*, produced by many brain structures, which are important for the normal development and health of the nervous system. For example, when injected into the brain of rats, BDNF not only prevents the spontaneous death of some neurons but also helps to protect neurons that have been poisoned with various toxins. Conversely, in animals, chronic stress decreases the production and amount of BDNF (and other neurotrophic substances) in the brain and increases cell death. As predicted by the neurogenic hypothesis, levels of BDNF (and some other neurotrophic substances) increase in the hippocampus of rats chronically exposed to a wide range of antidepressants (Saarelainen et al., 2003). Of particular significance, several reports have shown that blood levels of BDNF are decreased in depressed patients, and some studies have found that antidepressant treatment can reverse this effect (Angelucci et al., 2005; Duman and Monteggia, 2006; Jeanneteau and Chao, 2006; Kuipers and Bramham, 2006; Nair and Vaidya, 2006) (Figure 5.2).

In summary, several lines of evidence suggest that depression is a consequence of stress, which, like any injury, disease, or other type of

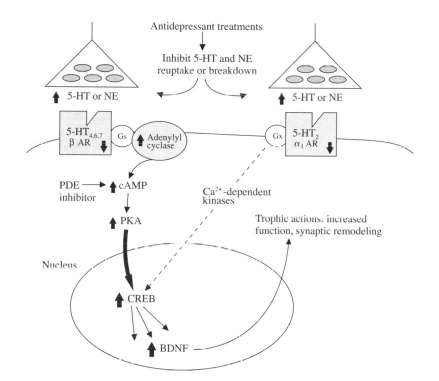

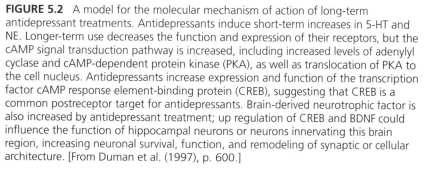

FIGURE 5.2   A model for the molecular mechanism of action of long-term antidepressant treatments. Antidepressants induce short-term increases in 5-HT and NE. Longer-term use decreases the function and expression of their receptors, but the cAMP signal transduction pathway is increased, including increased levels of adenylyl cyclase and cAMP-dependent protein kinase (PKA), as well as translocation of PKA to the cell nucleus. Antidepressants increase expression and function of the transcription factor cAMP response element-binding protein (CREB), suggesting that CREB is a common postreceptor target for antidepressants. Brain-derived neurotrophic factor is also increased by antidepressant treatment; up regulation of CREB and BDNF could influence the function of hippocampal neurons or neurons innervating this brain region, increasing neuronal survival, function, and remodeling of synaptic or cellular architecture. [From Duman et al. (1997), p. 600.]

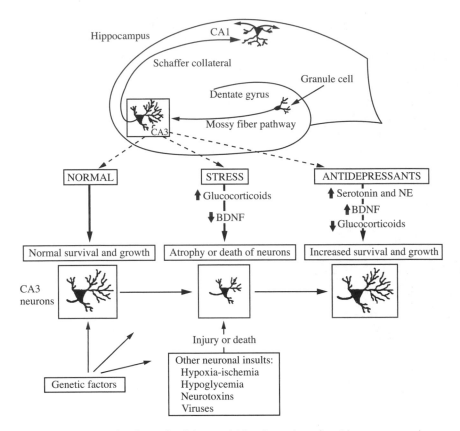

FIGURE 5.3 A molecular and cellular model for the action of antidepressants and the pathophysiology of stress-related disorders. Chronic stress decreases the expression of BDNF in the hippocampus, contributing to atrophy or death of neurons in the hippocampus. Elevated levels of glucocorticoids also decrease survival of these neurons, as do many other insults. Antidepressants increase the expression of BDNF and prevent the down regulation of BDNF elicited by stress, increasing neuronal survival or helping repair or protect neurons from further damage. [From Duman et al. (1997), p. 603.]

physical trauma, damages the brain and weakens its ability to recover. Antidepressants relieve depressed mood by acting at the cellular level to promote neuronal survival and reverse stress-induced neuronal damage (Figure 5.3). Although the immediate effect of antidepressants is to modulate synaptic levels of neurotransmitters, their ultimate targets are the intracellular molecules responsible for maintaining neuronal health and plasticity. This reconceptualization of depressive disorder has broadened the search for new drug treatments, including agents that block the effect of stress hormones or that directly stimulate neurotrophic processes, as described later in this chapter (Krishnan and Nestler, 2008; Marazziti et al., 2009).

Evolution of Antidepressant Drug Development

Over fifty years ago, the antidepressant properties of the drug *imipramine* were discovered accidentally. Since then, it has been learned that imipramine and similar drugs, called *tricyclic antidepressants* (TCAs; Table 5.1), block the presynaptic transporter protein receptors for the neurotransmitters norepinephrine and serotonin. Note that the term *tricyclic antidepressant* refers to a commonality in chemical *structure*, in contrast to newer antidepressants, which are defined by their mechanism of action. That is because, when the antidepressant effect of imipramine was discovered, its mechanism of action was unknown; thus, a structural classification had to suffice and persists today.

At about the same time the TCAs were discovered, another class of early antidepressant drugs, called the *monoamine oxidase inhibitors* (MAOIs), was identified. The MAOIs bind to and block the enzyme monoamine oxidase. This enzyme normally metabolizes and regulates the amount of the biogenic amine transmitters in the presynaptic nerve terminal. Thus, the levels of these neurotransmitters increase and more transmitter is available for release when stimulated by an action potential reaching the nerve terminal. Both the TCAs and the MAOIs are effective in the treatment of major depression, but both possess adverse side effects, discussed later in this chapter. Together, we refer to these two classes of drugs as *first-generation antidepressants*.

Many problems with the first-generation agents prompted the search for new antidepressants that were equally effective and better tolerated, but less toxic. First was the development of several drugs that were slight modifications of the basic tricyclic structure but that still exhibited antidepressant efficacy. These drugs were termed *second-generation*, or *atypical, antidepressants* (see Table 5.1).

During the late 1980s and continuing through the 1990s, the *selective serotonin reuptake inhibitors* (SSRIs) were developed, the first of which was fluoxetine (Prozac; see Table 5.1). Five more were eventually marketed. Today, because of the limitations and side effects of the SSRIs, antidepressant drug research is progressing to identify compounds that act by different mechanisms. These drugs are not necessarily more clinically efficacious than the older TCAs, but they may have a more favorable profile of toxicity or side effects (Richelson, 2003). The availability of the newer drugs has not yet reduced the number of treatment-resistant patients with major depression; the new drugs have only altered the profile of side effects. Three main therapeutic improvements have still to be met: (1) superior efficacy, especially in the treatment of therapy-resistant depression, (2) faster onset of action, and (3) improved side effect profile. The following discussion of specific antidepressant drugs is subdivided into categories according to the chronology of their introduction into medicine and the neurotransmitters on which each group is thought to act.

TABLE 5.1 Drugs used to treat depression

Drug name: Generic (trade)	Sedative activity	Anticholinergic activity[a]	Elimination half-life (h)	Reuptake inhibition		
				Norepinephrine	Serotonin	Dopamine
TRICYCLIC COMPOUNDS						
Imipramine (Tofranil)	Moderate	Moderate	10–20	++	++	0
Desipramine (Norpramin)	Low	Low	12–75	+++	+	0
Trimipramine (Surmontil)	High	Moderate	8–20	+	+	0
Protriptyline (Vivactil)	Low	Moderate	55–125	+++	+	0
Nortriptyline (Pamelor, Aventil)	Low	Low	15–35	++	++	0
Amitriptyline (Elavil)	High	High	20–35	++	++	0
Doxepin (Adapin, Sinequan)	High	High	8–24	++	++	0
Clomipramine (Anafranil)	Low	Low	19–37	++	++++	0
SECOND-GENERATION (ATYPICAL) COMPOUNDS						
Amoxapine (Asendin)[b]	Moderate	Moderate	8–10	++	+	0
Maprotiline (Ludiomil)	Moderate	Moderate	27–58	+++	0	0
Trazodone (Desyrel)	High	Low	6–13	0	++	0
Bupropion (Wellbutrin)	Low	Low	8–14	0/+	0/+	++
Venlafaxine (Effexor)	Moderate	None	3–11	++	++++	0
Desvenlafaxine (Pristiq)	Moderate	None	3–11	++	++++	0

[a]Anticholinergic side effects include dry mouth, blurred vision, tachycardia, urinary retention, and constipation.
[b]Also has antipsychotic effects due to blockage of dopamine receptors (Chapter 4).
0 = no effect; + = mild effect; ++ = moderate effect; +++ = strong effect; ++++ = maximal effect.

TABLE 5.1 Drugs used to treat depression (continued)

Drug name: Generic (trade)	Sedative activity	Anticholinergic activity[a]	Elimination half-life (h)	Reuptake inhibition		
				Norepinephrine	Serotonin	Dopamine
SELECTIVE SEROTONIN REUPTAKE INHIBITORS						
Fluoxetine (Prozac)	Moderate	None	24–96	0	++++	0
Sertraline (Zoloft)	Moderate	None	26	0	++++	0
Paroxetine (Paxil)	Moderate	None	24	+	++++	0
Citalopram (Celexa)	Moderate	None	33	0	++++	0
Fluvoxamine (Luvox)	Moderate	None	15	0	++++	0
Escitalopram (Lexapro)	Low	None	2–5	0	++++	0
DUAL-ACTION ANTIDEPRESSANTS						
Nefazodone (Serzone)	High	None	3–4	0	++++	0
Mirtazapine (Remeron)	High	Low	20–40	++	++++	0
Duloxetine (Cymbalta)	Moderate	Low	11–16	+++	+++	0
MAO INHIBITORS: IRREVERSIBLE						
Phenelzine (Nardil)	Moderate	None	2–4[c]	0	0	0
Isocarboxazid (Marplan)	Low	None	1–3[c]	0	0	0
Tranylcypromine (Parnate)	Moderate	None	1–3[c]	0	0	0
SELECTIVE NOREPINEPHRINE REUPTAKE INHIBITORS						
Reboxetine (Edronax)[d]	None	Low	13	+++	0	0
Atomoxetine (Strattera)	None	Low	5	+++	0	0

[a]Half-life does not correlate with clinical effect (see text).
[d]Not available in United States.
0 = no effect; + = mild effect; ++ = moderate effect; +++ = strong effect; ++++ = maximal effect.

First-Generation Antidepressants

The first two classes of antidepressants (TCAs and MAOIs) were introduced into medicine in the late 1950s and early 1960s. Drugs of both
classes increased the levels of norepinephrine and serotonin in the
brain, leading to the concept that depression resulted from a relative
deficiency of these neurotransmitters. Conversely, excesses in the
amounts of these transmitters were thought to lead to a state of mania.
This was called the *monoamine (receptor) hypothesis of mania and
depression.* Although this interpretation is much too simplistic, until
recently the concept has been extremely useful for guiding the development of new antidepressants.

Tricyclic Antidepressants

The term *tricyclic antidepressant* describes a class of drugs that all have
a characteristic three-ring molecular core (Figure 5.4). TCAs not only
effectively relieve symptoms of depression; they also possess significant anxiolytic and analgesic actions. Historically, the TCAs were
drugs of first choice for the treatment of major depression. The SSRIs,
which today are widely prescribed, are no more effective and may be
considerably more expensive; they are, however, less toxic, and their
use is associated with a higher rate of patient comfort and compliance.

Imipramine (Tofranil) is the prototype TCA, but another clinically
available TCA, *desipramine* (Norpramin), is the pharmacologically active

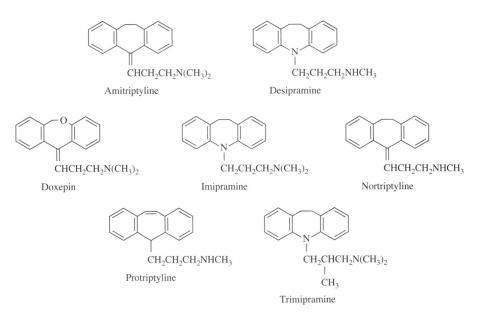

FIGURE 5.4 Chemical structures of seven tricyclic antidepressants.

intermediate metabolite of imipramine. Likewise, *amitriptyline* (Elavil) has an active intermediate metabolite, *nortriptyline* (Pamelor, Aventil). In fact, these two active intermediates may actually be responsible for much of the antidepressant effect of both imipramine and amitriptyline.

Mechanism of Action. TCAs exert two significant pharmacologic actions that are presumed to account for both the therapeutic effects and most side effects of these drugs:

1. They block the *presynaptic reuptake transporter* for norepinephrine and/or serotonin.
2. They block *postsynaptic receptors* for histamine, acetylcholine, and norepinephrine.

The therapeutic effects of the TCAs result from blockade of presynaptic serotonin and norepinephrine reuptake transporters. Blockade of histamine receptors results in drowsiness and sedation, an effect similar to the sedation seen after administration of the classic antihistamine diphenhydramine (Benadryl). Blockade of acetylcholine receptors results in confusion, memory and cognitive impairments, dry mouth, blurred vision, increased heart rate, and urinary retention. Blockade of norepinephrine receptors affects blood pressure; one result may be a "dizzy" feeling when standing up too quickly from a sitting or reclining position. In general, nortriptyline and desipramine are reasonable choices for initial treatment of depression when therapy with a TCA is chosen. These two TCAs cause less sedation and exert fewer anticholinergic side effects, such as cognitive impairment, than most other TCAs. Moreover, nortriptyline is known to have a therapeutic range, or window: the maximum response is most likely at blood levels of the drug between 0.05 and 0.15 micrograms per milliliter.

Pharmacokinetics. The TCAs are well absorbed when administered orally. Because most of them have relatively long half-lives (see Table 5.1), taking them at bedtime can reduce the impact of unwanted side effects, especially persistent sedation. These drugs are metabolized in the liver, and, as discussed earlier, two TCAs are converted into pharmacologically active intermediates that are detoxified later (Figure 5.5). This combination of a pharmacologically active drug and active metabolite results in a clinical effect lasting up to four days, even longer in elderly patients (who can be adversely affected by the detrimental cognitive effects of these drugs; Chapter 19).

TCAs readily cross the placental barrier. However, in utero exposure does not affect global IQ, language development, or behavioral development in preschool children. No fetal abnormalities from these drugs have yet been reported.

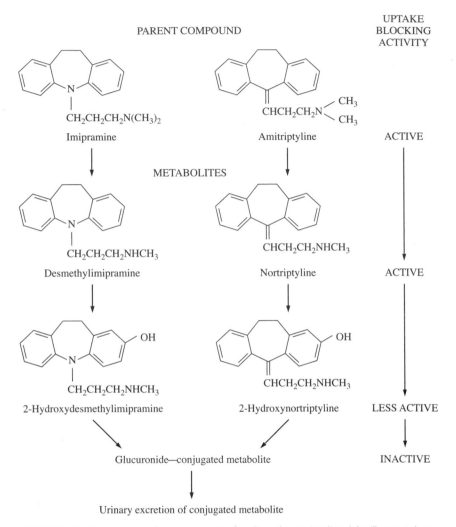

FIGURE 5.5 Metabolism of imipramine (Tofranil) and amitriptyline (Elavil). Note that the two active intermediates (desmethylimipramine and nortriptyline) are marketed commercially as Norpramin and Pamelor or Aventil, respectively.

Pharmacological Effects. All the TCAs attach to and inhibit (to varying degrees) the presynaptic transporter proteins for both norepinephrine and serotonin, which is thought to account for their therapeutic efficacy. The TCAs, however, have three clinical limitations. First, they are claimed to have a slow onset of action, although overall, TCAs seem to start acting as fast as any other antidepressant drug, provided that comparable dosage strategies can be tolerated. Second, the TCAs exert a wide variety of effects on the CNS, causing numerous adverse side effects that the SSRIs do not cause. Third, in overdosage (as in suicide attempts), TCAs are cardiotoxic and potentially fatal because they can cause cardiac arrhythmias.

Because TCAs do not produce euphoria in normal people, they have no recreational or addictive liability. Therefore, abuse and psychological dependence are not concerns. The clinical choice of TCA is determined by effectiveness, tolerance of side effects, prior good response, family history of good response, and duration of action of the particular agent.

In depressed patients, TCAs elevate mood, increase physical activity, improve appetite and sleep patterns, and reduce morbid preoccupation. They are useful in treating acute episodes of major depression as well as in preventing relapses. Some patients resistant to other antidepressants respond favorably to a TCA. In addition, TCAs are clinically effective in the long-term therapy of dysthymia and in treating bipolar depression (as an adjunct to a mood stabilizer), although the SSRIs are equally efficacious and better tolerated.

TCAs are effective analgesics in a variety of clinical pain syndromes; they are consistently superior to placebo in the treatment of chronic pain. Uses include diabetes-associated peripheral neuropathies, postherpetic neuralgia, migraine headache, fibromyalgia, chronic back pain, myofascial pain, and chronic fatigue. The antidepressant action may not only provide analgesic relief but promote well-being and improve affect as it reduces physical discomfort. One review compared the analgesic effect of three types of antidepressants, and it concluded that the TCAs were slightly more efficacious than the selective norepinephrine reuptake inhibitors (SNRIs), which were more analgesic than the selective serotonin reuptake inhibitors (Sindrup et al., 2005).

Side Effects. Side effects follow from the anticholinergic, antihistaminic, and antiadrenergic actions. In the patient on long-term TCA therapy, tolerance may develop to many of these side effects, but some will persist. Often, choosing a particular TCA with an awareness of its side effects can turn a disadvantage into a therapeutic advantage. For example, amitriptyline and doxepin are the most sedating of the TCAs, making them useful in treating people with comorbid depression and insomnia. Administering one of these drugs at bedtime would provide both the antidepressant effect and the needed sedation.

The effects of TCAs on memory and cognitive function are significant. The direct adverse effects on cognition are related to the anticholinergic and antihistaminic properties of the drugs, which may be partly compensated for by the improvement in mood. Relatively nonsedating compounds with minimal anticholinergic side effects cause less impairment of psychomotor or memory functions. Therefore, because the young and the elderly may be more susceptible to the anticholinergic-induced impairment of memory, patients at the extremes of age, if treated with TCAs, should probably receive a drug with low potency at blocking histaminic and cholinergic receptors.

As already noted, cardiac effects can be life-threatening when an overdose is taken, as in suicide attempts. The patient commonly exhibits excitement, delirium, and convulsions, followed by respiratory depression and coma, which can persist for several days. Cardiac arrhythmias can lead to ventricular fibrillation, cardiac arrest, and death. Thus, all TCAs can be lethal in doses that are commonly available to depressed patients. For this reason, it is unwise to dispense more than a week's supply of an antidepressant to an acutely depressed patient.

There have been reports of about 12 cases of sudden death in children receiving desipramine for the treatment of attention deficit/hyperactivity disorder (ADHD) or depression. These deaths are certainly cause for concern when using TCAs to treat depression in children, and the therapeutic efficacy of TCAs in treating major depression in children is questionable anyway (Chapter 18). In cases where efficacy is more demonstrable—enuresis (bed-wetting), obsessive-compulsive disorder (OCD), and ADHD—use may be appropriate, but caution is warranted.

Monoamine Oxidase Inhibitors

Monoamine oxidase (MAO) is one of two enzymes that regulate the amount of monoamine neurotransmitters (as well as other substances) in the body, including norepinephrine, dopamine, and serotonin. There are two forms of the enzyme: MAO-A metabolizes dopamine, norepinephrine, and serotonin, as well as some other substances, such as tyramine; MAO-B also metabolizes dopamine, tyramine, and other substances. It is generally presumed that drug-induced inhibition of MAO-A is responsible for the antidepressant activity. The blockade of metabolism causes transmitter molecules to build up in the terminal, which means that more transmitter than usual is released into the synaptic cleft when the neuron fires an action potential.

Three monoamine oxidase inhibitors have been available since the late 1950s for treating major depressive illnesses (see Table 5.1). Their use is limited by serious side effects involving potentially fatal interactions when taken with certain foods and medicines, such as adrenalinelike drugs found in nasal sprays, antiasthma medications, and cold medicines. The foods include those that contain tyramine, a by-product of fermentation, such as many cheeses, wines, beers, liver, and some beans. Because MAO is also found in the gastrointestinal tract, inhibition of the enzyme blocks the metabolism of dietary tyramine. This substance increases blood pressure, and in the absence of MAO, the blood pressure increase may occasionally cause heart attacks or strokes. Nevertheless, although they are potentially dangerous, MAOIs can be used safely with strict dietary restrictions. A review of drug interactions supports the conclusion that caution is warranted when combining antidepressants with other CNS drugs, particularly MAOIs (Nieuwstraten et al., 2006).

Interest in MAOIs has remained strong because (1) they can be as safe as SSRIs, (2) they can work in many patients who respond poorly to both TCAs and SSRIs, and (3) they are particularly effective drugs for the treatment of atypical depression, masked depression (such as hypochondriasis), anorexia nervosa, bulimia, bipolar depression, dysthymia, depression in the elderly, panic disorder, and phobias.

All three orally administered MAOIs are irreversible in their effect, since they form a chemical bond with the MAO enzyme that cannot be broken; enzyme function returns only as new enzyme is biosynthesized. For this reason, patients who need to switch from an MAOI to another type of antidepressant must still observe the dietary restrictions and other precautions for approximately 10 to 14 days, until new enzyme is produced. A few years ago, a specific MAO-A inhibitor (moclobemide) was developed that was reversible. That is, moclobemide did not bond as tightly to the enzyme as the classic MAOIs. Therefore, when levels of tyramine or similar substances increased sufficiently, moclobemide was eventually forced to detach from MAO. When detachment occurred, MAO was again able to metabolize the tyramine and the cardiotoxic risk was minimized. Unfortunately, although this was a logical approach for developing a better MAOI, moclobemide was not a very efficacious antidepressant. The drug was marketed in Canada and European countries, but it was not released in the United States.

Although the reversible MAO-A inhibitor, moclobemide, was not as efficacious as hoped, a reversible MAO-B inhibitor may prove more useful, because MAO-B is the predominant form of the enzyme in the brain. At least one reversible MAO-B agent is currently under development and was shown to bind to MAO-B in the human brain (Hirvonen et al., 2009).

Interest in the MAOIs has undergone resurgence because of the availability of a new formulation. In 2006, the MAOI *selegiline* (Eldapril; Chapter 19) became commercially available as a transdermal patch that allows for slow, continuous absorption (in this form, it was marketed under the new trade name Emsam). At the low doses absorbed across the skin, food and drug interactions were not a concern because transdermal administration bypasses the gastrointestinal tract and because at doses less than 10 milligrams, selegiline does not inhibit MAO-A.[3] As initially reported by Amsterdam (2003), selegiline (as a 6-milligram patch applied daily) was robustly effective in reducing moderate to severe depression, with onset of effect in only a few days. Sexual functioning was not impaired, and compliance was excellent. Skin irritation was the only significant side effect. These initial positive results were confirmed in a long-term study in which patients with MDD who responded to selegiline during acute treatment (10 weeks) were either maintained on the drug or switched to placebo. After 52 weeks, significantly fewer patients taking selegiline relapsed (16.8 percent) compared with the placebo group (30.7 percent), and they did so after a significantly longer time on the drug than those given the placebo (Amsterdam and Bodkin, 2006). This new formulation promises to be a very useful option for situations in which MAOIs are preferred (Goodnick, 2007).

Second-Generation (Atypical) Antidepressants

Efforts from the late 1970s to the mid-1980s to find structurally different agents that might overcome some of the disadvantages of the TCAs (slow onset of action, limited efficacy, and significant side effects) produced the so-called second-generation, or atypical, antidepressants (Figure 5.6; see Table 5.1).

Maprotiline (Ludiomil) was one of the first clinically available antidepressants (other than the MAOIs) that modified the basic tricyclic structure (see Figure 5.6). It has a long half-life, blocks norepinephrine reuptake, and is as efficacious as imipramine (the gold standard of TCAs). However, it offers few, if any, therapeutic advantages. A major limitation of maprotiline is that it can cause seizures (although it rarely does), presumably because of the accumulation of active metabolites that excite the CNS. It is generally not an antidepressant of first choice.

Amoxapine (Ascendin) (see Figure 5.6) is the second atypical antidepressant, structurally different from the TCAs (see Figure 5.4). It is primarily a norepinephrine reuptake inhibitor, clinically as effective as imipramine, although it may be slightly better at relieving accompanying anxiety and agitation. Amoxapine may produce parkinsonianlike side effects as a result of postsynaptic dopamine receptor blockade.

---

[3] There is some evidence, however, that with the 9- and 12-milligram patches, the effect may be no different than with any other oral MAOI and dietary restrictions may again be needed.

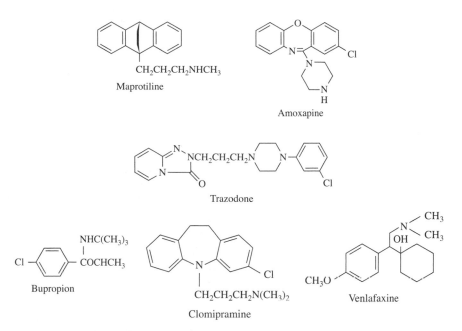

FIGURE 5.6 Chemical structures of six second-generation "atypical" antidepressants.

The drug is metabolized to an active intermediate, 8-hydroxy-amoxapine, which may be responsible for the dopamine receptor blockade. As with TCAs, overdosage can result in fatality. Amoxapine is not generally an antidepressant of first choice.

Trazodone (Desyrel) is the third atypical antidepressant (see Figure 5.6), therapeutically as efficacious as the TCAs. However, it is not a potent reuptake blocker of either norepinephrine or serotonin, although its active metabolite, m-chlorophenylpiperazine, is a serotonin agonist. Drowsiness is the most common side effect, and, until recently, the drug's main use was as an antidepressant sleeping pill. Taken at bedtime, in the 25–100-mg range, trazodone essentially blocks all $5HT_{2A}$ receptors (at 10 milligrams), and about half of the alpha-1 adrenergic receptors and histamine receptors, producing a good night's sleep. While about 50 percent of the serotonin transporters are also blocked at these doses, that is not enough for an antidepressant action. Therefore, traditional trazodone, available as a short-acting immediate-release (IR) formulation, has often been used as a hypnotic (even though the Food and Drug Administration has not approved it for this indication). Its peak effect is reached and then declines relatively rapidly, and this "pulsatile" action is less likely to produce tolerance.

However, a new formulation of trazodone—an extended-release, once-daily preparation with the trade name Oleptro—was approved in February 2010 for the treatment of MDD in adults. This formulation, in a dose of 300 milligrams, apparently provides sufficient constant blood levels for an antidepressant effect; tolerance gradually develops to the sedation over several days. With this pharmacokinetic modification, it may be possible to regain the antidepressant benefit of trazodone.

Trazodone's main side effect can be serious: in rare instances, priapism (prolonged and painful penile erection) occurs. This side effect requires prompt attention because it can lead to permanent impotence and infertility. Any detrimental effects of an overdose of trazodone on cognitive functioning appear modest.

Clomipramine (Anafranil) (see Figure 5.6) is structurally a TCA (see Figure 5.4), but it has a greater effect on serotonin reuptake than the classic TCAs (Suhara et al., 2003). In addition, it and its active metabolite, desmethylclomipramine, also inhibit norepinephrine reuptake. Thus, it is classified as a *mixed serotonin-norepinephrine reuptake inhibitor*, similar to venlafaxine. Clomipramine is approximately equal to the TCAs in both its efficacy and its profile of side effects.

Clomipramine has long been used to treat obsessive-compulsive disorder (OCD); about 40 to 75 percent of patients with OCD respond favorably. The drug has also been used in the treatment of panic disorder and phobic disorders. Historically, it was the first antidepressant medication to be appreciated as having efficacy in the treatment of anxiety disorders, an observation later applied to the SSRI-type antidepressants. The remaining two second-generation atypical antidepressants, venlafaxine and bupropion, will be discussed later in this chapter.

Selective Serotonin Reuptake Inhibitors

Six SSRIs are currently available: fluoxetine (Prozac), paroxetine (Paxil), sertraline (Zoloft), fluvoxamine (Luvox), citalopram (Celexa), and escitalopram (Lexapro). All except escitalopram are shown in Figure 5.7. These drugs are all potent blockers of the presynaptic transporter for serotonin reuptake. The degree to which they block reuptake of other neurotransmitters, primarily norepinephrine, varies greatly, with more than a twelvefold difference between citalopram (the most selective for serotonin) and fluoxetine (the least selective for serotonin). They do not block postsynaptic serotonin receptors of any subtype. Therefore, the primary acute neuronal effect of SSRIs is to make more serotonin available in the synaptic cleft, which activates all of the many postsynaptic receptors for serotonin. The action of serotonin at all its postsynaptic receptors is believed to be responsible for all the actions of the six serotonin antidepressants—both their therapeutic actions and their serotonergic side effects.

The current view is that increased serotonin availability at 5-HT_1-type receptors is associated with antidepressant and anxiolytic effects, whereas increased serotonin availability at 5-HT_2-type and 5-HT_3-type

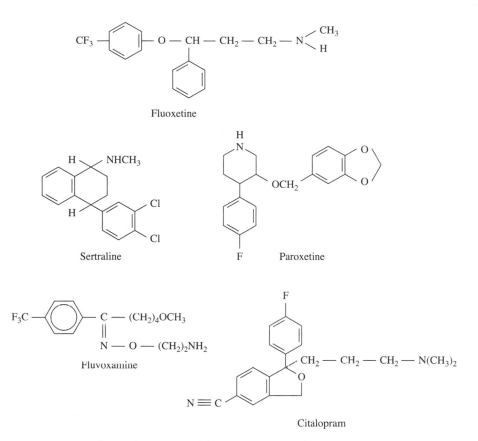

FIGURE 5.7 Chemical structures of five selective serotonin reuptake inhibitor (SSRI) antidepressants. The sixth SSRI, escitalopram, is the active isomer of citalopram and is therefore not shown.

receptors produces adverse effects. Increased 5-HT$_2$ receptor activity is associated with insomnia, anxiety, agitation, sexual dysfunction, and the production of a *serotonin syndrome* at higher doses (see below). Increased 5-HT$_3$ receptor activity is responsible for the nausea that these drugs can cause (which has led to the development of 5-HT$_3$ antagonists as antiemetics). Because of their receptor selectivity, SSRIs demonstrate few anticholinergic or antihistaminic side effects. Nevertheless, some of them, especially fluoxetine, are sedating. Wadsworth and coworkers (2005) demonstrated that long-term treatment with SSRIs may produce some cognitive impairment. Most important, these drugs are not fatal in overdose because they are devoid of the cardiac toxicity produced by TCAs.

As a general statement, the clinical differences among individual SSRIs are minimal; all are equally effective (Kroenke et al., 2001). As noted in one review (Ruhé et al., 2006), after a first SSRI, any switch,

TABLE 5.2 Ability of SSRIs to inhibit various subtypes of CYP liver enzymes

Drug	CYP-450 1A2	CYP-450 2C9	CYP-450 2C19	CYP-450 2D6	CYP-450 3A4
Citalopram (Celexa)	0	0	0	+	0
Escitalopram (Lexapro)	0	0	0	+	0
Fluoxetine (Prozac)	+	++	+/++	+++	+/++
Paroxetine (Paxil)	+	+	+	+++	+
Sertraline (Zoloft)	+	+	+	+/++	+
Fluvoxamine (Luvox)	+	++	++	+++	++

either within or between all classes of antidepressants, appears legitimate. For an excellent table summarizing the procedure for switching from each antidepressant category to any of the others, see Bezchlibnyk-Butler and Jeffries (2005, pp. 59–60). No unequivocal evidence is available to prove an advantage of a between-class switch. Hansen and coworkers (2005) arrived at the same conclusion. However, the six SSRIs are not necessarily interchangeable: patients who discontinue one SSRI for lack of tolerability or response can sometimes be treated effectively with another. Differences lie in individual pharmacokinetics and in effects that inhibit cytochrome P (CYP) drug-metabolizing enzymes in the liver (Table 5.2), thus adversely and possibly dangerously interacting with other medicines that the patient may be taking. Genetic testing (Chapter 1) is commercially available to identify people with altered ability to metabolize SSRIs.

Approved therapeutic indications for SSRI therapy include major depression, dysthymia, and all the anxiety disorders (panic disorder, OCD, GAD, PTSD, phobias), although SSRIs also have benefit in other clinical situations. The conditions for which each of the newer drugs is currently FDA-approved are summarized in Table 5.3.

Before discussing individual SSRIs, we address several concerns associated with SSRI therapy: (1) the serotonin syndrome, (2) the SSRI withdrawal syndrome, (3) SSRI-induced sexual dysfunction, and (4) problems with long-term treatment. A fifth issue, the possible fetal effects if the mother takes the SSRI during pregnancy or while breast-feeding, is discussed in Chapter 18.

Serotonin Syndrome

High doses of an SSRI or the combination of an SSRI plus another serotonergic drug can induce the disturbing reaction termed the *serotonin syndrome* (Birmes et al., 2003). Accumulation of serotonin leads to

TABLE 5.3 FDA-approved indications for antidepressant medications

	ADHD	MDD	GAD	OCD	Panic	PTSD	Social anxiety	Bulimia	Premenstrual dysphoria	Smoking cessation	Diabetic neuropathy	Fibromyalgia
SSRI												
Fluoxetine		✓		✓	✓			✓	✓			
Sertraline		✓		✓	✓	✓	✓		✓			
Fluvoxamine				✓		✓	✓(CR)					
Paroxetine		✓	✓	✓	✓	✓	✓		✓(CR)			
Citalopram		✓										
Escitalopram		✓	✓									
SSNRI												
Duloxetine		✓	✓								✓	✓
Venlafaxine		✓	✓(XR)		✓(XR)		✓(XR)					
Mirtazepine		✓										
Desvenlafaxine		✓										
Milnacepran												✓
SNRI												
Atomoxetine	✓											
NDRI												
Bupropion		✓								✓		

SSRI = selective serotonin reuptake inhibitor
SSNRI = selective serotonin norepinephrine reuptake inhibitor
SNRI = selective norepinephrine reuptake inhibitor
NDRI = norepinephrine dopamine reuptake inhibitor
CR = controlled-release formulation
XR = extended-release formulation

a cluster of responses, characterized by cognitive disturbances (disorientation, confusion, hypomania), behavioral agitation and restlessness, autonomic nervous system dysfunctions (fever, shivering, chills, sweating, diarrhea, hypertension, tachycardia), and neuromuscular impairment (ataxia, increased reflexes, myoclonus). Visual hallucinations have even been reported. Some of these symptoms might result from excess serotonin at 5-HT$_2$ receptors, the site of action of the psychedelic drug LSD (Chapter 15). There is a positive relationship between the specificity of the SSRI for blocking the 5-HT transporter and the likelihood of producing the syndrome. For example, paroxetine (Paxil) is one of the most specific SSRIs, and it is perhaps the SSRI most implicated in causing the serotonin syndrome.

In theory, any drug that has the net effect of increasing serotonin function can produce the syndrome; usually, however, it results from the combination of an SSRI and other serotonergic drugs, especially since these drugs can inhibit each other's metabolic detoxification and potentiate each other's effects. The syndrome can even occur when SSRIs are combined with herbal substances such as St. John's wort or valerian (Chapter 8). Once the drugs are discontinued, the syndrome usually resolves within 24 to 48 hours; during this time, support is the primary treatment.

SSRI Withdrawal Syndrome

A discontinuation syndrome occurs in perhaps 60 percent of SSRI-treated patients following abrupt cessation of drug intake. This SSRI withdrawal syndrome was originally associated with discontinuation from paroxetine, but it can occur following discontinuation of any SSRI, although it is least likely with fluoxetine because of the drug's long half-life. Onset of withdrawal is usually within a few days and persists perhaps three to four weeks. There are six core sets of somatic symptoms, usually including these "FINISH" effects (Muzina, 2010):

- Flulike symptoms (fatigue, lethargy, myalgias, chills, headache)
- Insomnia (sleep disturbances, vivid dreams)
- Nausea (gastrointestinal symptoms, vomiting, diarrhea)
- Imbalance (dizziness, vertigo, ataxia)
- Sensory disturbances (paresthesia sensation of electric shocks in the arms, legs, or head)
- Hyperarousal (anxiety, agitation)

Other, less frequently reported symptoms of SSRI withdrawal include hyperactivity, depersonalization, depressed mood, and memory problems (confusion, decreased concentration, and slowed thinking). The tricyclic antidepressants, venlafaxine (Effexor), and duloxetine (Cymbalta), because of their serotoninergic action, also produce this discontinuation syndrome (Warner et al., 2006). Venlafaxine and duloxetine are discussed later.

Withdrawal from other antidepressants (MAOIs, bupropion, mirtazepine and nefazodone) may present a little differently. For example, rapid termination from MAOIs may be associated with severe anxiety, agitation, pressured speech, sleeplessness or drowsiness, hallucinations, delirium, and even paranoid psychosis.

Risk factors for antidepressant withdrawal symptoms include abrupt termination of the antidepressant (or noncompliance or drug holidays), short half-life of the drug, long treatment duration, female gender, pregnancy, younger age, newborn infants of mothers who have been on antidepressants (Chapter 18), and vulnerability to depressive relapse.

All the somatic and psychological phenomena abate over time and obviously disappear when the SSRI is restarted. It is believed that the syndrome results from a relative deficiency of serotonin when the SSRI is stopped; however, the exact mechanism may be more complex. Therefore, tapering of all antidepressants that are being discontinued is recommended.

SSRI-Induced Sexual Dysfunction

Sexual dysfunction is often associated with major depressive disorder, and SSRI medications can further compound it (Schweitzer et al., 2009). Up to 80 percent of depressed patients treated with SSRIs exhibit sexual dysfunction, including problems with orgasm, erection, sexual interest, desire, and psychological arousal (Stimmel and Gutierrez, 2006). In males, ejaculatory dysfunction seems most prominent. Loss of desire and sexual dysfunction can affect medication compliance and impair interpersonal relationships. Treatment of sexual dysfunction may involve discontinuation of the SSRI and switching to an antidepressant in another class (for example, bupropion), although. sildenafil (Viagra) has been found useful for some patients (Nurnberg et al., 2001; Seidman et al., 2001).

Additional Side Effects of SSRIs

In addition to the specific issues described above, there are several other notable consequences of long-term antidepressant use (Moret et al., 2009):

- *Suicidality*. A review of FDA trials in pediatric and adolescent patients indicated that antidepressants increased the risk of suicidal ideation/behavior. In 2005, the FDA required that manufacturers include a warning in product labeling, recommending that young patients be monitored for the occurrence of suicidality. After that, the number of prescriptions for youth fell dramatically, followed by an *increase* in adolescent suicide. In 2007, the FDA extended the suicidality warning to young adults aged 18 to 24, with the emphasis that depression itself may lead to suicide and that anyone started on antidepressants should be monitored for worsening symptoms. This warning is supported by a study showing that the risk of suicide or hospitalization due to self-harm is equal across all antidepressant agents (Schneeweiss et al., 2010). The use of antidepressants in children and adolescents is discussed further in Chapter 18.

- *Sleep Disturbance.* SSRIs interfere with sleep function, although these difficulties vary among the agents. They may produce insomnia with sleep fragmentation (episodes of awakening).

- *Apathy.* Although rare, lack of motivation and apathy have been reported in children and adults treated with SSRIs.

- *Physiological Symptoms.* A variety of physiological symptoms have been reported with these drugs. Hyponatremia (serum sodium concentration below 130 mEq/L) may occur within the first few weeks of treatment but will resolve after discontinuation. Symptoms include nausea, headache, lethargy, muscle cramps, seizures, coma, and possibly respiratory arrest. In adults over 50 years of age, SSRI use may increase the risk of sustaining fractures in a fall and of osteoporosis. SSRIs increase the risk of gastrointestinal bleeding, although this is usually not common unless other drugs with this risk are also taken, such as nonsteroidal anti-inflammatory agents. Rare cases of cardiovascular problems, such as arrhythmias, prolonged QTc intervals, and cardiovascular depressant effects, have been reported. In patients 65 years of age and older, the risk of extrapyramidal symptoms appears to be increased. Weight gain is not as prominent with these drugs as with other antidepressants.

The wide use of SSRI antidepressants has perhaps increased awareness of these symptoms. Suicidality, sexual dysfunction, and pregnancy problems might be more easily recognized, while sleep disturbances, apathy, weight changes, and other physiological effects might be associated with depression itself and less likely to be differentiated from the disorder.

Specific SSRIs

Fluoxetine. Fluoxetine (Prozac; see Figure 5.7) became clinically available in the United States in 1988 as the first SSRI-type antidepressant and the first non-TCA that could be considered a first-line antidepressant (not just for patients who have failed therapy with TCAs). Fluoxetine's efficacy is comparable to that of the TCAs, with few or no anticholinergic or antihistaminic side effects.

Besides major depression, fluoxetine has been used in the treatment of dysthymia, bulimia (an eating disorder), alcohol withdrawal, and virtually all the various subtypes of anxiety disorders. Specific formulations of fluoxetine, sertraline, and paroxetine have been shown to be effective in relieving the symptoms of a controversial syndrome termed *premenstrual dysphoric disorder.* Pearlson and coworkers (2003) further demonstrated that symptoms of premenstrual dysphoric disorder recur when fluoxetine administration is stopped. For this use, the manufacturer of Prozac marketed fluoxetine under the trade name Sarafem.

Fluoxetine has a half-life of about 2 to 3 days, but its active metabolite *(norfluoxetine,* which is an even stronger reuptake inhibitor than fluoxetine) has a half-life of about 6 to 10 days. This prolonged action distinguishes fluoxetine from other SSRIs, which have half-lives of about 1 day and no active intermediates. Also because of its long half-life, fluoxetine need not be administered every day; it can be taken as infrequently as once a week, and a once-weekly oral formulation of fluoxetine is commercially available under the trade name Prozac Weekly.

As with all SSRIs, fluoxetine's antidepressant action is of slow onset (about 4 to 6 weeks), and the drug and its metabolite thus tend to accumulate with repeated doses over about 2 months, presumably because levels of both compounds continue to increase. This action can explain not only the slow onset of peak therapeutic effect but also the late onset of side effects and the prolonged duration of action following drug discontinuation. Therapeutic trials with fluoxetine should continue for at least 8 weeks before the drug is determined to be ineffective (Quitkin et al., 2003).

Significant and important side effects of fluoxetine include anxiety, agitation, and insomnia, which at the extreme can result in the serotonin syndrome. As discussed, sexual dysfunction is common.

Fluoxetine, sertraline, paroxetine, and fluvoxamine inhibit certain of the drug-metabolizing enzymes in the liver (see Table 5.2). Therefore, coadministration of any of these four drugs can increase the level of other drugs that the patient might be taking.

In 2004, the FDA approved a novel combination of fluoxetine and olanzapine (discussed in Chapter 4) for the treatment of depressive episodes associated with bipolar disorder (Chapter 6). The trade name of the combination product is Symbyax. One review supports the benefit of this combination in treatment-resistant depression (Bobo and Shelton, 2009), although it produced greater increases in body weight, prolactin, and total cholesterol than either of the two agents independently or a combination of fluoxetine plus an atypical antipsychotic with less potential for weight gain (Chapter 4).

Sertraline. Sertraline (Zoloft; see Figure 5.7) was the second **SSRI** approved for clinical use in the United States. Clinically, like all

SSRIs, it is as effective as TCAs in the treatment of major depression and dysthymia, and it has fewer side effects and improved patient compliance (Ravindran et al., 2000).

Sertraline is four to five times more potent than fluoxetine in blocking serotonin reuptake and is more selective. Because of increased selectivity, serotonin-associated side effects (serotonin syndrome and serotonin discontinuation syndrome) may be more intense than with fluoxetine. Steady-state levels of the drug in plasma are achieved within 4 to 7 days, and its metabolites are less cumulative and less pharmacologically active. Like all SSRIs, sertraline has few anticholinergic, antihistaminic, and adverse cardiovascular effects, as well as a low risk of toxicity in overdose.

Paroxetine. Paroxetine (Paxil; see Figure 5.7) was the third SSRI to become available in the United States for clinical use in treating major depression, dysthymia, various anxiety disorders, and premenstrual dysphoric disorder. Paroxetine is also approved by the FDA for treating generalized anxiety disorder (GAD), although this capability is probably shared by all SSRIs.

Like sertraline, paroxetine is more selective than fluoxetine in blocking serotonin reuptake. The drug's metabolic half-life is about 24 hours, and steady state is achieved in about 7 days; its metabolites are relatively inactive.

Paroxetine is perhaps the SSRI most associated with serotonin syndrome, serotonin discontinuation syndrome, new onset or precipitation of psychosis, paranoid ideations, temper dyscontrol, delusions, and even visual hallucinations. In 2006, it was reported that the use of paroxetine was associated with a small but statistically significant increase in the risk of cleft lip/palate deformities in newborns of women who took the drug during their pregnancy. In December 2006, the American College of Obstetricians and Gynecologists published a position statement that paroxetine probably should not be used during pregnancy (Chapter 18).

In February 2010, it was reported that among women who were being treated for breast cancer with the drug tamoxifen, paroxetine was associated with significantly greater mortality than other SSRIs. This increased cancer mortality was presumed to be due to the fact that paroxetine inhibited the enzyme that converted tamoxifen to its active metabolite. As a result, the benefits of tamoxifen were blocked by paroxetine. Clinicians were advised to avoid prescribing paroxetine to women with breast cancer who are receiving tamoxifen (Kelly et al., 2010). In their review, Desmarais and Looper (2009) describe interactions between tamoxifen and other antidepressants as well.

Fluvoxamine. Fluvoxamine (Luvox) is a structural derivative of fluoxetine (see Figure 5.7). Like all SSRIs, fluvoxamine has well-described antidepressant properties, comparable in efficacy to the

TCA imipramine, but fewer serious side effects and superior patient compliance. It has been shown effective in the treatment of all anxiety disorders. A new, once-a-day extended-release formulation of this drug (Luvox CR) was approved by the FDA in 2008 for the treatment of social anxiety disorder and OCD in adult patients.

Citalopram. Citalopram (Celexa; see Figure 5.7) is an SSRI available in Europe since 1989 and introduced into the United States in 1998 as the fifth SSRI. Citalopram is claimed to have a more rapid onset of action than fluoxetine, but this observation is probably related to differences in half-life and therefore to different times to peak plasma levels with continued dosing. Extremely large doses of citalopram have been associated with ECG irregularities, seizures, and rare fatalities. It has a lower incidence of inhibition of drug-metabolizing hepatic enzymes, so it might be better for patients who are taking multiple medications (Brosen and Naranjo, 2001).

Citalopram is well absorbed orally; peak plasma levels are reached in about 4 hours. Steady state is achieved in about 1 week, and maximal effects are seen in about 5 to 6 weeks. The elimination half-life is about 33 hours, enabling once-per-day dosing. The elderly have a reduced ability to metabolize citalopram; for older people, a 33 to 50 percent reduction in dose is necessary.

Citalopram has been reported to moderately reduce alcohol consumption in problem alcoholics. Citalopram might be expected to exert anxiolytic effects similar to those exerted by other SSRIs. Adverse effects of citalopram resemble those of other SSRIs.

Escitalopram. Escitalopram (Lexapro) was released in the United States in 2002 for the treatment of major depression. It is also approved for the treatment of GAD. The drug is the therapeutically active isomer (mirror-image molecule; Figure 5.8) of citalopram.

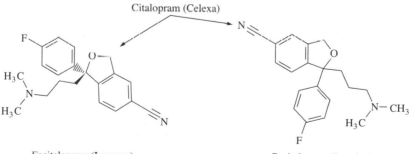

Citalopram (Celexa)

Escitalopram (Lexapro)   R-citalopram (inactive)

FIGURE 5.8 The SSRI citalopram (Celexa) is a racemic mixture of two enantiomers. The R-enantiomer is inactive; the S-enantiomer (Escitalopram) is active and is marketed as Lexapro. Citalopram is composed of both structures (one active and one inactive) present in equal amounts; escitalopram is the active half.

As an active isomer, the major difference is potency: escitalopram is twice as potent as citalopram, so the prescribed dose is 50 percent of the dose of citalopram. In other words, 10 milligrams of escitalopram is equivalent to 20 milligrams of citalopram. Otherwise the two drugs are identical.

Dual-Action Antidepressants

Historically, the TCAs were the first dual-action antidepressants: they block the presynaptic reuptake of both norepinephrine and serotonin, but side effects limited their widespread use. The unitary action of the SSRIs, while associated with efficacy against a wide variety of anxiety and depressive disorders, is limited by side effects common to serotonin overactivity. Therefore, attempts have been made to expand on the concept that actions at two different synaptic sites may improve or maintain efficacy while limiting side effects. Most attempts to develop a dual-action antidepressant have resulted in medicines that inhibit the active presynaptic reuptake of both serotonin and norepinephrine.

Nefazodone

Nefazodone (Serzone; Figure 5.9) is a dual-action antidepressant chemically related to trazodone (see Figure 5.6) but with some important pharmacological distinctions. Nefazodone's strongest pharmacological action is 5-HT$_2$ receptor blockade, which distinguishes it from the SSRIs; however, it also inhibits both serotonin and norepinephrine

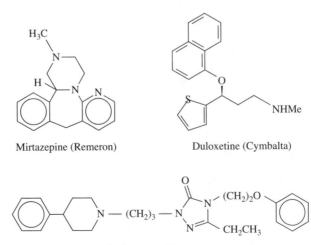

Mirtazepine (Remeron)

Duloxetine (Cymbalta)

Nefazodone (Serzone)

FIGURE 5.9   Chemical structures of three dual-action antidepressants.

reuptake at its therapeutic dose. In 2003, a new warning was added to the information about this drug, stating that it produced liver failure at a rate about three to four times greater than that in the general population, resulting in death or necessitating liver transplantation. The drug was removed from the market in Canada in 2004, and although it is still available in the United States, only some generic formulations will still be marketed once present supplies are exhausted.

Milnacipran

Milnacipran (Savella) is another drug that blocks norepinephrine and serotonin reuptake (Tran et al., 2003), but it has not been approved by the FDA as an antidepressant. Although it is not significantly different from other antidepressants, it is claimed to produce fewer adverse effects (Nakagawa et al., 2009).

Interest in milnacipran has centered on efficacy in the treatment of fibromyalgia (Pae et al., 2009b), a disorder for the treatment of which pregabalin (Lyrica) and duloxetine (discussed later) have received FDA approval. Milnacipran reduces the chronic pain associated with fibromyalgia with concomitant improvements in global well-being, fatigue, and other domains of the disorder (Gendreau et al., 2005; Rooks, 2007). In 2009 the FDA approved this indication for milnacipran, under the brand name Savella.

Venlafaxine

Venlafaxine (Effexor) (see Figure 5.6) is classified as a mixed *serotonin-norepinephrine reuptake inhibitor.* The serotonin blockade occurs at lower doses than does the norepinephrine blockade, and at higher doses venlafaxine also inhibits the reuptake of dopamine. Venlafaxine lacks anticholinergic or antihistaminic effects, a distinct advantage. On the other hand, it was reported that, while the response and remission rates to venlafaxine XR were the same as to bupropion XL, venlafaxine produced significantly more sexual side effects (Thase et al., 2006). Some evidence also suggests that venlafaxine may be more likely than other antidepressants to trigger a manic state in people who are taking the drug as treatment for bipolar depression. This suggests a possibility that venlafaxine might precipitate agitated or aggressive behavior in some patients.

Concern was raised about venlafaxine's known association with blood pressure elevation in some 3 to 4 percent of patients using the sustained-release formulation and 2 to 13 percent of those taking the immediate-release preparation. Essentially, higher overdose fatality rates were seen according to studies using population datasets. In December 2006, the U.S. manufacturer issued a warning stating that prescriptions for Effexor should be written for the smallest quantity of capsules consistent with good patient management, in order to reduce the risk of overdose. However, in 2010, a large population study from the United Kingdom looked at the sudden cardiac death, or near death, rate of new users (18 to 89 years old) of several antidepressants. The results of this large study found no association of venlafaxine, used for either depression or anxiety, with increased cardiac risk, compared with other antidepressants, over a period of 3.3 years (Martinez et al., 2010).

In an extended-release formulation (Effexor XR), venlafaxine is FDA-approved for the treatment of GAD as well as panic and social anxiety. Venlafaxine appears to have only minimal effects on drug-metabolizing enzymes, and drug interactions are few. Venlafaxine's primary metabolite, desvenlafaxine, is pharmacologically active; the half-lives of the parent compound and the primary metabolite are 5 hours and 11 hours, respectively. Desvenlafaxine has antidepressant efficacy, safety, and tolerability, it requires only once-daily dosing, and it has minimal impact on metabolic enzymes (Perry and Cassagnol, 2009). In 2008 desvenlafaxine was approved for the treatment of MDD under the brand name Pristiq (Pae et al., 2009c). This drug has also been shown to reduce the frequency and severity of hot flashes in postmenopausal women, which may lead eventually to FDA approval for this indication (Archer et al., 2009).

Duloxetine

Duloxetine (Cymbalta; see Figure 5.9) is another dual-action antidepressant that binds to and blocks the reuptake transporters for norepinephrine and serotonin (Karpa et al., 2002). The blockade seems to be more complete than that of venlafaxine (Bymaster et al., 2005). The manufacturer that markets Prozac developed duloxetine, and now that fluoxetine is available in less expensive generic form, Cymbalta is being promoted as a replacement.

Studies have shown duloxetine to be clinically effective in the treatment of both depression (Gartlehner et al., 2009) and anxiety (Dunner et al., 2003). Duloxetine was reported to significantly reduce physical symptoms of pain (such as backaches, headache, muscle and joint pain, and back and shoulder pain), to reduce interference with daily activities, and to reduce time in pain while awake. This drug has been approved for the management of neuropathic pain associated with diabetic peripheral neuropathy and fibromyalgia (Arnold et al., 2009; Mease, 2009). There is also evidence that this agent may induce a manic or hypomanic episode in patients with bipolar disorder (Peritogiannis et al., 2009). Duloxetine has been shown to be effective for the treatment of urinary stress incontinence (Norton et al., 2002). The mechanism underlying this action is unclear. In 2007, duloxetine was FDA-approved for the treatment of generalized anxiety disorder (Endicott et al., 2007; Rynn et al., 2008).

The half-life of duloxetine is about 12 hours, allowing once-daily dosing. Nausea is the most common side effect. Weight gain and sexual dysfunction have not yet been problems with the drug. Elevations in blood pressure (hypertension), thought to be possible with duloxetine, have not yet been a major problem in clinical studies.

Mirtazepine

Mirtazepine (Remeron; see Figure 5.9) was introduced into clinical use in the United States in 1997. Overall, mirtazepine is a dual-action anti-depressant that increases the presynaptic release of both norepinephrine and serotonin through several actions:

1. It blocks central alpha$_2$ autoreceptors. By blocking adrenergic autoreceptors, it causes an increase in the release of norepinephrine.

2. It blocks adrenergic heteroreceptors located on the terminals of serotonin-releasing neurons, where they normally inhibit the release of serotonin. When these adrenergic heteroreceptors are blocked, 5-HT neurons release more serotonin.

3. The increased release of serotonin stimulates only 5-HT$_1$ receptors because 5-HT$_2$- and 5-HT$_3$-type receptors are specifically blocked by mirtazepine.

Although complicated, this mechanism explains how mirtazepine enhances both norepinephrine and serotonin neurotransmission. Because mirtazepine is a potent antagonist of postsynaptic 5-HT$_2$ and 5-HT$_3$ receptors, it does not produce the side effects of SSRIs (especially anxiety, insomnia, agitation, nausea, and sexual dysfunction). Mirtazepine is also a potent blocker of histamine receptors, and drowsiness is a prominent and often therapeutically limiting side effect. Sedation may be advantageous in depressed patients with symptoms of anxiety and insomnia, a common occurrence. Because of the drowsiness, the drug is best taken at bedtime and probably should not be combined with alcohol or other CNS depressants.

Other side effects of mirtazepine include increased appetite and weight gain. The drug may therefore be advantageous in certain situations, such as in the treatment of patients with anorexia, in patients with wasting diseases (for example, cancers and AIDS), and in the elderly where bedtime sedation and maintenance of body weight are a goal. Nelson and colleagues (2006) studied mirtazepine in elderly nursing home patients (average dose 20 milligrams at bedtime) and found it safe and effective; the depression scores of 50 percent of elderly patients were markedly reduced. An average weight gain of 1.3 pounds was considered to be beneficial in this population.

Mirtazepine is rapidly absorbed orally; peak blood levels occur 2 hours after administration. The elimination half-life is 20 to 40 hours, allowing once-a-day administration, usually at bedtime to maximize sleep and minimize daytime sedation.

Dopamine-Norepinephrine Reuptake Inhibitor: Bupropion

Bupropion (Wellbutrin, Zyban; see Figure 5.6) is a dopamine-norepinephrine reuptake inhibitor (DNRI). It is mechanistically unique as an antidepressant because it is the only available antidepressant that selectively inhibits the reuptake transporter for these two transmitters. It is without effect on serotonin neurons, and therefore it does not have the side effects associated with the use of SSRIs. Because of its potentiation of dopamine, it has been used to treat children with ADHD (Chapter 18), although efficacy is not very robust. Although bupropion is not commonly used as an anxiolytic, Zisook and coworkers (2001) reported that the drug was effective in treating grief following the death of a loved one. Bupropion is also useful as add-on, or augmenting, therapy in patients only partially responsive or nonresponsive to SSRIs (DeBattista et al., 2003) and in patients with difficult-to-treat bipolar depression (Erfurth et al., 2002). Unlike SSRIs, bupropion exhibits evidence of inducing enhanced sexual functioning or minimal sexual dysfunction and can be combined with SSRIs to counteract that side effect (Clayton et al., 2004). It may also reduce the fatigue associated with depression (Schonfeldt-Lecuona et al., 2006). Short-term treatment with long-acting bupropion (Wellbutrin SR) may result in weight loss, an advantage in patients for whom weight gain is a problem, although tolerance to this action appears to develop.

As an anticraving drug (Zyban), bupropion is widely used as part of nicotine replacement therapies for smoking cessation. Treatment of nicotine dependence is discussed further in Chapter 11.

Side effects of bupropion include anxiety, restlessness, tremor, and insomnia. More serious side effects include the induction of psychosis de novo and generalized seizures at higher doses. Bupropion is not effective in the treatment of panic disorder, and it may even exacerbate or precipitate panic in susceptible people. Higher-than-recommended doses of bupropion may cause a manic switch in patients with bipolar depression (Foley et al., 2006).

Because bupropion and cocaine share similar mechanisms of action (blockade of dopamine reuptake), it's possible that bupropion exerts a reinforcing or dependency-inducing action. One study has shown that rats will self-administer bupropion. Although there are a couple of reports of youth snorting this drug, it does not seem to have

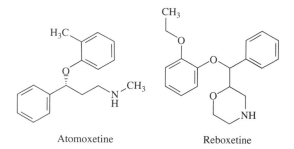

FIGURE 5.10 Chemical structures of two adrenergic (primarily norepinephrine) reuptake inhibitor antidepressants.

a high abuse potential in humans, perhaps because of the occurrence of seizures, but this conclusion remains unproven and the reason for the lack of abuse-liability is unclear (Tella et al., 1997).

Selective Norepinephrine Reuptake Inhibitors

Until recently, no antidepressant exhibited specific norepinephrine reuptake blockade in the absence of dopamine or serotonin reuptake blockade. Then two agents, *reboxetine* (Vestra, Edronax; Figure 5.10) and *atomoxetine* (Strattera; Figure 5.10), were developed as selective norepinephrine reuptake inhibitors (SNRIs). Unfortunately, in two separate clinical trials, reboxetine was not found to have any more effect than placebo, and it was not found to be very effective in a meta-analysis (Cipriani et al., 2009); it has since been withdrawn from the market. Atomoxetine became commercially available in 2003 as the first nonstimulant drug to be approved by the FDA for the treatment of ADHD in children, adolescents, and adults. It is claimed to be as effective as methylphenidate, probably without abuse potential. The use of atomoxetine in children and adolescents is discussed in Chapter 18. Simpson and Plosker (2004) and Spencer and coworkers (2004) reviewed the use of atomoxetine in adult ADHD.

STAR*D Study

While basic research continues to improve our understanding of the pathophysiology of depressive disorders and the mechanisms of action of antidepressants, progress is also being made in the clinical management of depression. A nationwide clinical trial, the Sequenced Treatment Alternatives to Relieve Depression (STAR*D) study, was conducted to determine the effectiveness of antidepressants as normally used in standard clinical practice, particularly for patients who had not responded to their initial antidepressant. The aim was to identify specific treatment strategies that would improve the long-term outcome of people with MDD.

Procedure

There were four study levels; each tested different medications or medication combinations. At each step, those who did not become symptom-free or could not tolerate the treatment's side effects could enter the next level of treatment. The study was designed to mimic clinical practice by using psychiatrists and primary care physicians in both private practice and public clinics and by allowing participants, who were already seeking care at these facilities, to choose which of the available treatments were acceptable to them. This was the first study to provide solid scientific evidence regarding which next steps were best for treatment-resistant depression.

Over a 7-year period, a total of 4041 outpatients, ages 18 to 75 years, were enrolled from 41 clinical sites around the country. Of these, 1165 were excluded because they either did not meet the study requirements of having "at least moderate" depression (based on rating scales used in the study) or they chose not to participate. Thus, 2876 "evaluable" people were included in Level 1 results. Level 2 results included 1439 people who did not become symptom-free (did not achieve remission) in Level 1 and chose to continue. Level 3 results included 377 people, and Level 4 results included 142 people.

All Level 1 participants were treated with citalopram for 12 to 14 weeks. Citalopram was chosen for the first treatment because it is easy to administer (once a day), it does not interact with other medications, and it is safe for older and medically fragile patients. Participants who became symptom-free moved on to a 12-month follow-up period during which citalopram was continued and patients were monitored.

In Level 2, patients had the option of switching to a different medication or adding to the existing citalopram. For those who wanted to switch, the choices were sertraline (Zoloft), bupropion-SR (Wellbutrin SR), or venlafaxine-XR (Effexor XR); add-on choices were either bupropion-SR or buspirone (Chapter 7). Participants who became symptom-free in Level 2 continued with the treatment in a follow-up period; participants who did not or who experienced intolerable side effects could continue on to Level 3. In Level 3, participants who chose to switch were randomly assigned to either mirtazepine (Remeron) or nortriptyline (Aventyl or Pamelor, a TCA) for up to 14 weeks. Both drugs work differently than the medications of Levels 1 and 2. In the Level 3 add-on group, participants were randomly prescribed either lithium (a mood stabilizer commonly used to treat bipolar disorder; Chapter 6) or triiodothyronine (T3) (a medication commonly used to treat thyroid conditions).

In Level 4, participants who had not become symptom-free in any of the preceding levels were taken off all other medications and randomly switched to one of two treatments, the MAOI tranylcypromine (Parnate) or the combination of extended-release venlafaxine (Effexor XR) with mirtazepine.

Results

Only about 30 percent of the participants in the Level 1 portion reached "remission," and about 10 to 15 percent more were "responders," who did not achieve remission but whose symptoms decreased to at least half of what they had been at the start of the trial. On average, it took nearly 6 weeks for a participant to respond and nearly 7 weeks to achieve remission. The average number of visits with the respective physician was between 5 and 6. Overall, about 9 percent of the participants in Level 1 stopped citalopram because of side effects. Considering that the historical response to placebo is usually around 20 to 25 percent, these results were very discouraging because they documented the poor efficacy of the chosen SSRI to achieve significant therapeutic benefits.

In Level 2, only 21 of the 1439 participants said that all the choices were equally acceptable and allowed themselves to be randomized to a switch or an augmentation treatment. For all the other participants at least one option was unacceptable, and they chose to limit the range of treatments to which they would be randomized. Of those, 727 (51 percent) agreed to switch their medication (Rush et al., 2006) and 565 (39 percent) agreed to receive "medication augmentation" (Trivedi et al., 2006); the rest received cognitive therapy. About 25 percent of the participants who switched became symptom-free. This result was the same for each of the three medication groups: no one drug was best, none worked more quickly than another, and there was no difference in side effects or serious problems. About one-third of the participants in the augmentation group achieved remission.

Subsequent results describe comparisons between cognitive-behavioral therapy (CBT) and the various medications (Thase et al., 2007). Among patients who did not respond adequately to citalopram, CBT produced outcomes comparable to those of medications; antidepressant therapy was more rapidly effective than CBT, but CBT was better tolerated than were the antidepressants.

In the Level 3 switch group, 10 to 20 percent of participants achieved remission, with no significant overall difference between the two medications, although there were more troublesome side effects with lithium. In Level 4, 7 to 10 percent of participants became symptom-free. Although there were no significant differences between the two treatments, patients taking the venlafaxine-XR/mirtazapine combination reported more symptom reduction and were less likely to stop taking the medication because of side effects than the patients taking the MAOI tranylcypromine.

Conclusions

Over the course of all four treatment levels (12 weeks each, with the option of adding 2 more weeks), about two-thirds of participants were able to achieve remission if they did not withdraw from the study. However, a substantial number of participants did withdraw: 21 percent after Level 1, 30 percent after Level 2, and 42 percent after Level 3. The data show that, overall, many patients with treatment-resistant depression can get better, but the odds of remission diminish with every additional treatment strategy needed. Furthermore, relapse rates were higher for those who entered the 12-month follow-up phase after more treatment steps. This was the case regardless of whether the participants had or had not reached remission. Interestingly, the time to relapse for those who did relapse was similar across all levels, ranging from 2.5 to 4.5 months. Nevertheless, relapse rates were much lower for those who achieved remission, confirming that remission is associated with a better prognosis even if it is achieved after several treatments. For a review of the STAR*D, study see Rush and colleagues (2009).

Enhancing Responsiveness to Antidepressant Treatment

In spite of the overall disappointing outcomes, the STAR*D study led to some important conclusions. First, it was appreciated that initial medication may need to be continued for a longer period of time than was typically assumed before improvement occurs. Second, if, after a sufficient duration, the response is still not sufficient, the two available options are to increase the dose or to augment the subthreshold effect with another treatment. As a result, the therapeutic benefit of augmentation is gaining more acceptances (Blier et al., 2010; Rush et al., 2009). Third, the number of people who respond sufficiently is much smaller than the population needing treatment, and the dropout rate is great. One reason for this might be the adverse side effects of the medications. Fourth, there is increasing interest in determining whether antidepressant response or side effects might be predicted by a person's genetic makeup (Kato and Serretti, 2010).

Since the STAR*D study, there have been additional efforts to determine whether any of the current, newer antidepressants show a clinical advantage over the others, in regard to either effectiveness or tolerability (such as Ciprianai et al., 2009). Sertraline and escitalopram were found to be slightly better in effectiveness and tolerability than several other agents, with mirtazapine and venlafaxine the next in line. However, it was acknowledged that even these conclusions were not definitive because (1) many of the studies were funded by the manufacturer of sertraline, (2) for some drugs the data were scarce, and (3) the differences among the drugs were rarely statistically significant. Overall, there appears to be no antidepressant that is superior to all the

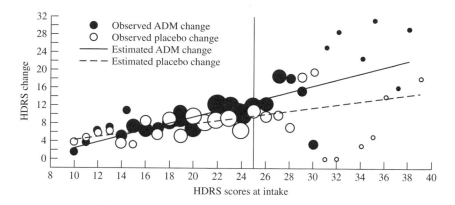

FIGURE 5.11 Efficacy of antidepressant medication and depression severity. Shown are the positive changes in the Hamilton Depression Rating Scale (HDRS, ordinate) after treatment versus the HDRS at the beginning of treatment (abscissa) in patients taking antidepressant medication (ADM, solid circles) or placebo (open circles). As illustrated, higher levels of depression at the start of treatment predicted greater medication response. The size of each circle is proportional to the number of patients at each HDRS score at intake. As illustrated, the few patients with very severe depression (i.e., HDRS scores > 30) taking placebo pills exhibited wide variability in response. [From Fournier et al. (2010), p. 51, Figure 2.]

others, and clinical decisions need to be based not only on effectiveness but also on side effects, cost, and patient preference.

Another important variable that appears to be relevant to the effectiveness of antidepressant treatment is the severity of the symptoms. In most clinical trials, that measure is represented by the score on the Hamilton Depression Rating Scale (HDRS). Although the benefit of antidepressants is well established when the HDRS is very high (28 or greater), the difference between antidepressant and placebo treatment is not always evident in clinical trials when baseline symptomatology is lower, even at values that indicate "very severe depression" (around 23; Fournier et al., 2010). Fournier and colleagues determined the relationship between baseline severity of depressive symptoms and response to antidepressants compared with placebo by analyzing numerous databases from 1980 to March 2009. They found that, compared with placebo, antidepressant drugs seemed to be effective mainly in people with severe depression, with HDRS scores of about 25 and above, than in patients with lower baseline severity (Figure 5.11).

Antidepressants of the Future

The history of antidepressant drugs now encompasses almost 50 years. As is apparent in the descriptions of current drugs, we are still seeking the "perfect" antidepressant, one that is widely effective in bringing about the remission of acute episodes and preventing future relapses in the absence of significant side effects (Schechter et al., 2005). In this section, potential agents of the future are briefly examined. Because they come from numerous and diverse neurochemical categories, it is useful to organize these potential antidepressant medications into several groups.

Augmenting Agents

Modafinil (Provigil) is a nonstimulant wakefulness-promoting drug used to combat daytime fatigue in patients with narcolepsy. It does not produce typical psychostimulant-induced side effects, and, in narcoleptic patients, modafinil may also improve subjective well-being, reduce fatigue, and enhance concentration. One open-label study (Konuk et al., 2006) was consistent with previous reports demonstrating the efficacy and safety of modafinil as an augmenting agent for patients with only partial response to traditional antidepressant drugs.

Modafinil has two isomers, each of which is active. One is eliminated from the body much more quickly than the other, so essentially the activity really comes from one isomer. Nuvigil is the longer-acting isomer formulation of Provigil; in 2009 it was marketed and being tested as an augmenting agent for bipolar depression. Given that the Provigil version becomes generic (and less expensive) in 2012, the manufacturer's interest in promoting Nuvigil is understandable.

The possible significance of *folate* in depression has also been appreciated (Fava and Mischoulon, 2009). Folate is a water-soluble B vitamin that occurs naturally in food. Folic acid is the synthetic form of folate that is found in supplements and added to fortified foods. The relationship between folate and antidepressants is that folate enhances the production of all three monoamines, dopamine, norepinephrine, and serotonin. Therefore, a deficiency of folate may increase the risk of depression. Some people have a genetic defect that reduces folate formation and increases the risk of folate deficiency, and perhaps depression. There is evidence that in depressed patients with folate deficiency who have not responded to antidepressants, augmentation with any one of several folate formulations may be helpful.

Other drugs that may well serve as augmenting agents to supplement antidepressant medications in partially responsive patients include mood stabilizers/anticonvulsants (Vigo and Baldessarini, 2009) (Chapter 6); the newer atypical antipsychotic drugs (Papakostas et al., 2007; Nelson and Papakostas, 2009), such as *quetiapine, aripiprazole,* and *amisulpride* (Chapter 4); and certain of the omega-3 fatty acids (discussed later in this chapter). Indeed, quetiapine and aripiprazole are approved by the FDA for the treatment of resistant depression. The superiority of the olanzapine/fluoxetine combination (Symbyax) to either of the two drugs alone was also reported in a pooled analysis of five trials (Tohen et al., 2010).

Serotonin 5-HT₁ Agonists and Antagonists

Chapter 7 discusses *buspirone* (BuSpar) as an anxiolytic agent and notes that it exerts its effects secondary to weak stimulation of serotonin 5-HT_{1A} receptors. Its poor absorption remains a clinical limitation. Antidepressive effects should be produced by either antagonizing presynaptic 5-HT_{1A} autoreceptors (which would increase serotonin release) or by directly stimulating postsynaptic 5-HT_{1A} receptors (which is believed to be responsible for the antidepressive/anxiolytic action). Feiger and coworkers (2003) reported efficacy of another serotonin 5-HT_1 partial agonist, *gepirone-ER*, as monotherapy for depression.

One experimental agent, vilazodone, combines the characteristic of serotonergic reuptake inhibition with partial 5-HT_{1A} agonism, and positive results have been reported in two controlled trials by the manufacturer (Khan, 2009).[5]

New Drugs Affecting Serotonin, Norepinephrine, and/or Dopamine

Because many side effects of the SSRIs are due to the stimulation of 5-HT_2 receptors, combinations of 5-HT_2 blocking drugs and SSRIs may be more tolerable. Some new compounds with this action are under study, and older drugs with this property are being reassessed. [In fact, the current drug mirtazepine (Remeron) has this characteristic.] Similar logic has led to additional combinations, such as a drug that stimulates postsynaptic 5-HT_{1A} receptors and blocks alpha₂ receptors.

One new class of compounds is much more potent at blocking both 5-HT/NE reuptake (Mahaney et al., 2006). Other experimental agents block the reuptake of both 5-HT and dopamine (minaprine, bazinaprine), and one drug in this class, called serdaxin, is currently undergoing preclinical investigation. There is particular interest in exploring the potential of triple reuptake blockers, which would block the transporters for dopamine, norepinephrine, and serotonin (Guiard

---

[5] It has been suggested that some people are nonresponsive to antidepressants because they have a specific genetic variant that produces too many 5-HT_{1A} serotonin autoreceptors. Normally, when serotonin is released, some of the transmitter molecules bind to the autoreceptors, which shut down and turn off further serotonin release from that neuron. Therefore, if some people have too many of these receptors, then the increase in serotonin produced by SSRIs may actually counteract the effect of the drug (because of the increased autoreceptor activation) and prevent any therapeutic benefit. Evidence for this theory has been shown by researchers who were able to develop a genetic mouse that had more autoreceptors than the normal mouse. On animal models of depression, the drug fluoxetine had no effect. But when levels of their autoreceptors were lowered, they responded to the drug (Richardson-Jones et al., 2010). These researchers are now trying to find out if depressed patients who don't respond to serotonergic antidepressants also have elevated 5-HT_{1A} autoreceptors.

et al., 2009; Marks et al., 2008). One such drug is DOV 216,303 (azabi-cyclohexane; Skolnick et al., 2006).

Tianeptine (Stablon) increases the presynaptic neuronal uptake of serotonin in the brain and thus decreases serotonin neurotransmission. However, tianeptine appears to reduce stress-induced atrophy of neuronal dendrites, exerting a neuronal protective effect against stress (Czeh et al., 2001; Nickel et al., 2003) and restoring intracellular mechanisms adversely affected by stress and other insults (Shakesby et al., 2002). Its efficacy against major depression is well documented (Dalery et al., 2001; Loo et al., 2001). It does not appear to produce adverse cognitive, psychomotor, sleep, cardiovascular, body weight, or sexual side effects. Tianeptine is also effective in bipolar depression, dysthymia, and anxiety. It seems quite useful in the elderly and in patients with chronic alcoholism. This unusual compound offers both an alternative medication to standard antidepressants and new insights into the pathophysiology of depression and anxiety.

Drugs Affecting Glutamate and GABA

There are several reasons for studying the possible role of excitatory (glutamate) and inhibitory transmitters (GABA) in depression. First, stressful stimulation increases levels of glutamate in the brain. Second, the receptors for glutamate and GABA are found in the brain structures associated with emotional regulation. Third, chronic antidepressant treatment (in laboratory animals) affects the major glutamate receptors. This approach benefits from the fact that we already have drugs that act on the glutamatergic neurotransmitter system. They are usually developed as anticonvulsants, as neuroprotective agents (to prevent neuronal death after stroke or brain damage), or to treat dementia. Because there are so many important therapeutic possibilities for such drugs, many are being evaluated as treatments for a variety of disorders, including depression and anxiety (Machado-Vieira et al., 2008; Moskal and Burgdor, 2009; Skolnick et al., 2009).

The possibility that the GABAergic system is dysfunctional in MDD was suggested by a study that found deficits in inhibitory control in people who were depressed, especially in those resistant to current treatment (Levinson et al., 2010).

Drugs Affecting Peptide Systems

All the antidepressant drugs discussed so far have therapeutic short-comings such as limited efficacy and significant side effects. The neurogenic hypothesis of depression suggests novel therapeutic approaches involving neuroactive proteins (neuropeptides) that affect synaptic and intracellular metabolic processes (Madaan and Wilson, 2009; Paschos et al., 2009).

Tachykinins. The endogenous neurochemicals known as tachykinins were discovered 70 years ago, but compounds that antagonize their action are just now being developed. The tachykinins are products of two genes that produce substance P (SP) and the various neurokinins. The tachykinin peptides share a common chemical structure and act through three types of neurokinin receptors—termed neurokinin$_1$ (NK$_1$), neurokinin$_2$ (NK$_2$), and neurokinin$_3$ (NK$_3$)—to regulate a variety of physiological processes, especially processes related to inflammatory reactions, such as asthma, inflammatory bowel disorder, and migraine. SP is the most abundant tachykinin in the CNS and reacts with the NK$_1$ receptor. Neurons containing SP occur in many regions of the brain implicated in the pathogenesis of depression (midbrain, hypothalamus, amygdala, and hippocampus), and the protein is sometimes found with 5-HT and NE or their receptors. SP is released in response to stress and pain, and depressed patients have increased levels of SP in plasma and cerebrospinal fluid. Because chronic antidepressant treatment reduces SP, SP antagonists (also called NK$_1$ antagonists) might be expected to reduce stress, pain, and depression. Recent studies demonstrate that two experimental NK$_2$ antagonists, saredutant and osanetant, have antidepressant effects in animals (Salome et al., 2006). For an update on this class of drugs, see Quartara (2009).

Hypothalamic Peptides. During the past decade, there has been a dramatic increase in research involving peptides, located in the hypothalamus, that regulate feeding behavior. Recent observations have linked a couple of these "feeding peptides" to depression. One group of neurons in the hypothalamus produces melanin-concentrating hormone (MCH), which promotes appetite. Consequently, antagonists of the MCH$_1$ receptor are usually studied as possible diet drugs. In a battery of tests using laboratory animals, MCH$_1$ antagonists produced "antidepressant effects" (Borowsky et al., 2002). Interest in this application continues (Shimazaki et al., 2006).

A second peptide, called alpha-melanocyte stimulating hormone (αMSH) produces the opposite effect—it acts to suppress appetite. The release of αMSH is controlled by two other hormones called melanocyte-stimulating hormone release-stimulating factor and melanocyte-stimulating hormone release-inhibiting factor (MIF). Older literature suggested that MIF had antidepressantlike effects in animals, which led to the development of an analog of this peptide hormone, called *nemifitide,* which also looked like an antidepressant in laboratory animal tests and in clinical trials. Nemifitide interacts with several different types of peptide receptors, and serotonin receptors. It was reported to have minimal side effects, and there were no dropouts due to adverse reactions (Montgomery et al., 2006). Unfortunately, nemifitide must be administered by subcutaneous injection, so further development may depend on the ability to produce an oral formulation or a transdermal patch.

Corticotropin-Releasing Factor and Glucocorticoid Peptides.

Because stress is associated with depression, it is not surprising that a great deal of effort has been directed toward understanding the physiological regulation of stress and its possible role in the etiology of major depressive disorder. A person's ability to cope with stress is primarily regulated by the physiological system known as the hypothalamic-pituitary-adrenal (HPA) axis. *Corticotropin-releasing* factor (CRF) is the driving force of this circuit. CRF is produced in the hypothalamus. Once synthesized, CRF is transported to the anterior lobe of the pituitary gland, where it stimulates the release of adrenocorticotropic hormone (ACTH). ACTH is then carried by the circulation to the adrenal cortex, where it promotes release of the glucocorticoid hormone cortisol. Cortisol is an essential response to stressful situations; it activates functions that are necessary for coping with stress, such as the release of glucose for energy, an increase in alertness and concentration, and a sharpening of cognitive processes. Cortisol levels are sensed by cells in the hypothalamus, reducing CRF release (a negative feedback inhibition). This feedback inhibition is important because too much cortisol is toxic to neurons in the hippocampus and inhibits neurogenesis.

In a depressed person, the HPA axis is hyperactive, and increased cortisol has been proposed as the reason the hippocampus of a depressed person may be smaller than normal. Moreover, hyperactivity of the HPA axis in a depressed patient may be normalized after successful antidepressant treatment. Accordingly, there has been intense effort to develop drugs that can intervene at some point in this system and restore balance to the HPA (Surget et al., 2008).

One glucocorticoid antagonist is already available—the drug mifepristone (which is a progesterone receptor antagonist and is used clinically to induce chemical abortion of early pregnancy). Although preclinical research is ongoing (Wulsin et al., 2010), results of clinical trials for psychotic major depression were not impressive (Blaseyab et al., 2009).

Other neurochemical mediators of stress include substances that promote inflammation and trigger immune responses. One such substance, which is activated by stress and reduces hippocampal neurogenesis and produces depressivelike behaviors in rats, is called nuclear factor-κB (NF-κB). In one study, various stressors administered to rats decreased neurogenesis, and inhibition of NF-κB reversed this effect (Koo et al., 2010).

Drugs Affecting Second Messengers and Neurotropins

As discussed at the beginning of this chapter, attention has recently been directed to studying the intracellular effects of antidepressants, that is, the processes that take place after receptors have been activated. This has led to renewed interest in second-messenger systems, such as the cAMP pathway, and the beneficial effects of these biochemical events on neuronal health and survival. Many second-messenger pathways, whether activated by transmitters, hormones, or neurotrophins, converge on the cAMP response element, or CREB, protein, and it has been shown that various antidepressants—SSRIs, TCAs, and MAOIs—activate CREB (see Figure 5.2). Furthermore, there is some evidence for decreased CREB levels and less responsiveness to CREB activation in depressed people. These observations suggest that manipulations that increase second-messenger levels may have antidepressant potential.

One method of doing so is to block the degradation of cAMP by inhibiting the enzymes, called phosphodiesterases (PDEs), that break it down. Moreover, PDE4 inhibitors have been reported to induce the expression of brain-derived neurotrophic factor (BDNF) in the hippocampus. Unfortunately, although such inhibitors have been developed, their side effects so far have precluded clinical usefulness.

Substances with Miscellaneous Mechanisms of Action

Dehydroepiandrosterone.   Dehydroepiandrosterone (DHEA) is a glucocorticoid hormone secreted by the adrenal glands, but its physiological role is unclear. It is a weakly active adrenal androgen that serves as a precursor to testosterone and estradiol, hormones that can have a positive effect on mood when administered exogenously. It may increase the amount of available neurotrophins, which may also affect mood. Secretion of the hormone peaks at 20 to 25 years of age and declines by about 90 percent by age 70.

DHEA has been promoted to prevent a variety of disorders; perhaps the most enduring claims have been that DHEA may delay the aging process, improve mood, and delay the cognitive decline that occurs with age. A randomized, double-blind, crossover trial of DHEA in two dosages (low dose for three weeks followed by high dose for three weeks) showed antidepressive effects in middle-aged men and women during the six weeks of treatment, relative to baseline and to placebo treatment (Schmidt et al., 2005). DHEA treatment was also effective, relative to placebo, in reducing symptoms of mild depression or dysthymia in a group of HIV-positive adults with few adverse effects and no worsening of their HIV status (Rabkin et al., 2006). In spite of these positive results, a review of the literature found "equivocal" support across all types of clinical reports for the long-term antidepressant benefits of DHEA in older men (Shamlian and Cole, 2006).

Because DHEA is usually classified as an androgen, it would not be surprising to see its use accompanied by the characteristic side effects of acne, male-pattern baldness, hirsutism, voice changes, and so on. In fact, the most common adverse effects in the 2005 study were acne and oily skin. More serious effects include the theoretical potential for causing breast or prostate cancer and liver damage. Ebinger and colleagues (2009) provide a critical overview on the current literature regarding testosterone and depression.

Agomelatine. Abnormal circadian rhythms are common in depression and other mood disorders. For many patients symptoms are worse in the morning, with some improvement during the day. One major component in the regulation of diurnal rhythm is the hormone melatonin, which is derived from serotonin and has connections with serotonergic and noradrenergic structures. These considerations led to the development of a novel antidepressant, agomelatin (or agomelatine), which is an agonist at melatonin 1 and melatonin 2 receptors and an antagonist at 5-HT$_2$ receptors, with no detectable affinity for any other receptors.

In late-phase trials for the treatment of major depressive disorder, symptoms of depression significantly improved with agomelatine compared with placebo, and the drug appeared to be as efficacious as other SSRI/SNRI antidepressants but with fewer adverse effects. Agomelatine is being developed under the brand name Valdoxan as a once-daily treatment for MDD and its symptoms, particularly anxiety, and for sleep and circadian disturbances. According to one review, agomelatine does not have any significant advantages over other antidepressants, but it has a different mode of action and might be more tolerable for patients who do not respond to or cannot tolerate current options (Howland, 2009) or who have prominent anxiety (Dubovsky and Warren, 2009).

S-Adenosyl-Methionine. S-adenosyl-methionine (SAM; SAMe) itself is not abundant in the diet but is normally produced in the liver from the amino acid methionine, which is plentiful in most diets. SAMe functions by donating its methyl group to any of a wide range of molecules that are subsequently transformed to homocysteine. The homocysteine is transformed to methionine and the process repeats. Folic acid and vitamin B$_{12}$ are necessary for its synthesis, and deficiencies of these vitamins result in low concentrations of SAMe in the central nervous system. Low blood or central nervous system levels of SAMe have been detected in people with cirrhosis of the liver, coronary heart disease, Alzheimer's disease, and depression.

Although SAMe is widely marketed for the treatment of depression, evidence remains inconclusive (Papakostas, 2009). Part of this difficulty may be due to the fact that oral absorption is poor, and less than 1 percent of the ingested drug reaches the bloodstream; oral doses have ranged from 200 to 1600 milligrams. Although several studies have found SAMe effective, most were small and poorly conducted. One of the best-designed studies, a double-blind, placebo-controlled study of 133 depressed people, actually failed to find intravenous SAMe more effective than placebo (Delle Chiaie and Pancheri, 1999).

No formulation of SAMe is regulated by the FDA; some formulations were found to contain no SAMe at all. Because oral absorption is low, side effects are minimal and include mild insomnia, lack of appetite, constipation, nausea, dry mouth, sweating, dizziness, and nervousness; there is little information on drug interactions. Because SAMe is metabolized to homocysteine and because elevated homocysteine levels have been associated with early onset of atherosclerosis and coronary artery disease, there is concern that overuse of SAMe may predispose to these diseases. No reports of safety in pregnancy or breast-feeding are available.

Omega-3 Fatty Acids. Two types of omega-3 fatty acids are found in fatty fish like salmon, sardines, and mackerel: eicosapentaenoic acid, or EPA, and docosahexaenoic acid, or DHA. A third omega-3, alpha-linolenic acid, is found in plant foods such as flaxseed, soybean oil, walnuts, and canola oil. The American Heart Association recommends eating at least two servings of fatty fish each week, based on strong evidence that the omega-3 fats found in the fish help protect against cardiovascular disease.

Several lines of evidence also indicate an association between omega-3 polyunsaturated fatty acids and mood disorders. In his book *The Omega-3 Connection*, Stoll (2001) theorized a link between depression and heart disease: People with depression are more likely to develop heart problems than people without depression. When they do, they suffer more and are more likely to die than people who are not depressed. Low omega-3 fatty acid status is often present in heart disease and depression, and when people with heart disease or depression increase their intake of the long-chain omega-3 fatty acids EPA and DHA, their condition often improves.

Infrequent fish consumption is also associated with depression in epidemiological studies (Parker et al., 2006). In addition, some case reports and cohort studies show that lower omega-3 concentrations are associated with unipolar and postpartum depression (Sontrop and Campbell, 2006), an increased risk for depression in adolescents (Mamalakis et al., 2006), or the likelihood of reporting symptoms of mild to moderate depression (Conklin et al., 2007).

However, in spite of the evidence linking low levels of omega-3 to mood disorders, there is less evidence that EPA and DHA are effective antidepressants. One review concluded that four of seven double-blind randomized controlled trials showed significant improvement of depression with treatment of at least 1 gram per day of an omega-3 fatty acid; that is, this treatment was effective only about half the time. In patients with coronary heart disease, augmentation with omega-3 plus sertraline treatment for depression was ineffective (Carney et al., 2009), yet there is some evidence for a positive relationship between omega-3 fatty acid levels and depression in adults with coronary heart disease (see Chapter 8). And, although one study concluded that omega-3 fatty acids were effective in the treatment of postpartum depression, this interpretation is weakened because there was no placebo treatment (Freeman et al., 2006). It therefore remains unclear whether omega-3 supplementation is effective independent of antidepressant treatment for depressed patients in general or only for those with abnormally low concentrations of these substances (Freeman, 2009; Sontrop and Campbell, 2006).

In addition to these more well-recognized agents, many other substances have been proposed as putative antidepressants. Arguments have been made for the endocannabinoids (Hill et al., 2009), for the herb curcumin (turmeric) (Kulkarni et al., 2009), and for ceramide, a natural lipid substance in the body (Kornhuber et al., 2009).

Moreover, although beyond the scope of this book, there are a variety of other somatic treatments for depression, particularly various forms of brain stimulation. In addition to the long-standing and well-established procedure of electroconvulsive shock therapy, newer approaches include transcranial magnetic stimulation, vagus nerve stimulation, deep brain stimulation, magnetic seizure therapy, and cortical stimulation. Such concerted effort in developing better antidepressant treatments attests to the serious nature of the depressive disorders and the continuing lack of sufficient benefit from current therapies.

STUDY QUESTIONS

1. What is the relationship between depression and the biological amine transmitters in the brain?

2. Describe the probable mechanism of both acute and ultimate effects of antidepressant drugs. What might account for the delay in clinical effect?

3. List and differentiate the major classes of antidepressants.

4. Compare and contrast imipramine and fluoxetine.

5. Discuss what happens when a patient overdoses on a tricyclic antidepressant.

6. Discuss the side effects of SSRIs. What is the serotonin syndrome? What is the SSRI withdrawal syndrome? Discuss the effects of these drugs on sexual function.

7. Which drug or class of drugs do you think is the "best" antidepressant? Why?

8. Which antidepressants are used in the treatment of anxiety disorders? Why? How do these drugs differ from the benzodiazepine-type anxiolytics?

9. Discuss the strategies being used to discover the next generation of antidepressant drugs and the types of drugs that are being developed from those approaches.

REFERENCES

American College of Obstetricians and Gynecologists. (2006). "Position Statement on Paroxetine." *Obstetrics and Gynecology* 108: 1601–1603.

American Psychiatric Association. (1994). *Diagnostic and Statistical Manual of Mental Disorders,* 4th ed. (DSM-IV). Washington, DC: American Psychological Association.

Amsterdam, J. D. (2003). "A Double-Blind, Placebo-Controlled Trial of the Safety and Efficacy of Selegiline Transdermal System Without Dietary Restrictions in Patients with Major Depressive Disorder." *Journal of Clinical Psychiatry* 64: 208–214.

Amsterdam, J. D., and Bodkin, A. (2006). "Selegiline Transdermal System in the Prevention of Relapse of Major Depressive Disorder: A 52-Week, Double-Blind, Placebo-Substitution, Parallel-Group C Clinical Trial." *Journal of Clinical Psychopharmacology* 26: 579–586.

Angelucci, F., et al. (2005). "BDNF in Schizophrenia, Depression and Corresponding Animal Models." *Molecular Psychiatry* 10: 345–352.

Archer, D. F., et al. (2009). "Desvenlafaxine for the Treatment of Vasomotor Symptoms Associated with Menopause: A Double-Blind, Randomized, Placebo-Controlled Trial of Efficacy and Safety." *American Journal of Obstetrics and Gynecology* 200: 238.c1–238.c10.

Arnold, L. M., et al. (2009). "Efficacy of Duloxetine in Patients with Fibromyalgia: Pooled Analyses of 4 Placebo-Controlled Clinical Trials." *Primary Care Companion Journal of Clinical Psychiatry* 11: 237–244.

Bezchlibnyk-Butler, K. Z., and Jeffries, J. J., eds. (2005) *Clinical Handbook of Psychotropic Drugs*, 15th ed. Toronto: Hogrefe & Huber.

Birmes, P., et al. (2003). "Serotonin Syndrome: A Brief Review." *Journal of the Canadian Medical Association* 168: 1439–1442.

Blaseyab, C. M., et al. (2009). "A Multisite Trial of Mifepristone for the Treatment of Psychotic Depression: A Site-By-Treatment Interaction." *Contemporary Clinical Trials* 30: 284–288.

Blendy, J. A. (2006). "The Role of CREB in Depression and Antidepressant Treatment." *Biological Psychiatry* 59: 1144–1150.

Blier, P., et al. (2010). "Combination of Antidepressant Medications from Treatment Initiation for Major Depressive Disorder: A Double-Blind Randomized Study." *American Journal of Psychiatry* 167: 281–288.

Bobo, W.V., and Shelton, R. C. (2009). "Fluoxetine and Olanzapine Combination Therapy in Treatment-Resistant Major Depression: Review of Efficacy and Safety Data." *Expert Opinion in Pharmacotherapy* 10: 2145–2159.

Borowsky, B., et al. (2002). "Antidepressant, Anxiolytic and Anorectic Effects of a Melanin-Concentrating Hormone-1 Receptor Antagonist." *Nature Medicine* 8: 825–830.

Brosen, K., and Naranjo, C. A. (2001). "Review of Pharmacokinetic and Pharmacodynamic Interaction Studies with Citalopram." *European Neuropsychopharmacology* 11: 275–283.

Bymaster, F. P., et al. (2005). "The Dual Transporter Inhibitor Duloxetine: A Review of Its Preclinical Pharmacology, Pharmacokinetic Profile, and Clinical Results in Depression." *Current Pharmaceutical Design* 11: 1475–1493.

Carney, R.M., et al. (2009). "Omega-3 Augmentation of Sertraline in Treatment of Depression in Patients with Coronary Heart Disease. A Randomized Controlled Trial." *Journal of the American Medical Association* 302: 1651–1657.

Ciprianai, A., et al. (2009). "Comparative Efficacy and Acceptability of 12 New-Generation Antidepressants: A Multiple-Treatments Meta-Analysis." *Lancet* 373: 746–758.

Clayton, A. H., et al. (2004). "A Placebo-Controlled Trial of Bupropion SR as an Antidote for Selective Serotonin Reuptake Inhibitor-Induced Sexual Dysfunction." *Journal of Clinical Psychiatry* 65: 62–67.

Conklin, S. M., et al. (2007)."Serum Omega-3 Fatty Acids Are Associated with Variation in Mood, Personality and Behavior in Hypercholesterolemic Community Volunteers." *Psychiatry Research* 152: 1–10.

Czeh, B., et al. (2001). "Stress-Induced Changes in Cerebral Metabolites, Hippocampal Volume, and Cell Proliferation Are Prevented by Antidepressant Treatment with Tianeptine." *Proceedings of the National Academy of Sciences* 22: 12796–12801.

Dalery, J., et al. (2001). "Efficacy of Tianeptine vs Placebo in the Long-Term Treatment (16 Months) of Unipolar Major Recurrent Depression." *Human Psychopharmacology* 16: S39–S47.

DeBattista, C., et al. (2003). "A Prospective Trial of Bupropion-SR Augmentation of Partial and Non-Responders to Serotonergic Antidepressants." *Journal of Clinical Psychopharmacology* 23: 27–30.

Delle Chiaie, R., and Pancheri, P. (1999). "Combined Analysis of Two Controlled, Multicentric, Double Blind Studies to Assess Efficacy and Safety of Sulfo-Adenosyl-Methionine (SAMe) vs. Placebo (MC1) and SAMe vs. Clomipramine (MC2) in the Treatment of Major Depression [in Italian; English Abstract]. *Giornale Italiano di Psicopatologia* 5: 1–16.

Desmarais, J. E., and Looper, K.J. (2009). "Interactions Between Tamoxifen and Antidepressants via Cytochrome P450 2D6." *Journal of Clinical Psychiatry* 70: 1688–1697.

Dubovsky, S. L., and Warren, C. (2009). "Agomelatine, a Melatonin Agonist with Antidepressant Properties." *Expert Opinion on Investigational Drugs* 18: 1533–1540.

Duman, R. S. (2004). "Depression: A Case of Neuronal Life and Death?" *Biological Psychiatry* 56: 140–145.

Duman, R. S., and Monteggia, L. M. (2006). "A Neurotrophic Model for Stress-Related Mood Disorders." *Biological Psychiatry* 59: 1116–1127.

Duman, R. S., et al. (1997). "A Molecular and Cellular Theory of Depression." *Archives of General Psychiatry* 54: 597–606.

Dunner, D., et al. (2003). "Duloxetine in Treatment of Anxiety Symptoms Associated with Depression." *Depression and Anxiety* 18: 53–61.

Ebinger, M., et al. (2009). "Is There a Neuroendocrinological Rationale for Testosterone as a Therapeutic Option in Depression?" *Journal of Psychopharmacology* 23: 841–853.

Endicott, J., et al. (2007). "Duloxetine Treatment for Role Functioning Improvement in Generalized Anxiety Disorder: Three Independent Studies." *Journal of Clinical Psychiatry* 68: 518–524.

Erfurth, A., et al. (2002). "Bupropion as Add-On Strategy in Difficult-to-Treat Bipolar Depressive Patients." *Neuropsychobiology* 45, Supplement 1: 33–36.

Fava, M., and Mischoulon, D. (2009). "Evidence for Folate in Combination with Antidepressants at Initiation of Therapy." *Journal of Clinical Psychlopedia*. Retrieved December 2009 from www.cmeinstitute.com/psychlopedia/depression/9cam/default.asp

Feiger, A. D., et al. (2003). "Gepirone Extended Release: New Evidence for Efficacy in the Treatment of Major Depressive Disorder." *Journal of Clinical Psychiatry* 64: 243–249.

Foley, K. F., et al. (2006). "Bupropion. Pharmacology and Therapeutic Applications." *Expert Review of Neurotherapeutics* 6: 1249–1265.

Fournier, J. C., et al. (2010). "Antidepressant Drug Effects and Depression Severity. A Patient-Level Meta-Analysis." *Journal of the American Medical Association* 303: 47–53.

Freeman, M. P. (2009). "Omega-3 Fatty Acids in Major Depressive Disorder." *Journal of Clinical Psychiatry* 70, Supplement 5: 7–11.

Freeman, M. P., et al. (2006). "Randomized Dose-Ranging Pilot Trial of Omega-3 Fatty Acids for Postpartum Depression." *Acta Psychiatrica Scandinavia* 113: 31–35.

Frodl, T., et al. (2007). "Association of the Brain-Derived Neurotrophic Factor Val66Met Polymorphism with Reduced Hippocampal Volumes in Major Depression." *Archives of General Psychiatry* 64: 410–416.

Gartlehner, G., et al. (2009). "The General and Comparative Efficacy and Safety of Duloxetine in Major Depressive Disorder: A Systematic Review and Meta-Analysis." *Drug Safety* 32: 1159–1173.

Gendreau, R. M., et al. (2005). "Efficacy of Milnacipran in Patients with Fibromyalgia." *Journal of Rheumatology* 32: 1975–1985.

Goodnick, P. J. (2007). "Seligiline Transdermal System in Depression." *Expert Opinion in Pharmacotherapy* 8: 59–64.

Guiard, B. P., et al. (2009). "Prospect of a Dopamine Contribution in the Next Generation of Antidepressant Drugs." *Current Drug Targets* 10: 1069–1084.

Hansen, R. A., et al. (2005). "Efficacy and Safety of Second-Generation Antidepressants in the Treatment of Major Depressive Disorder." *Annals of Internal Medicine* 143: 415–426.

Hill, M. N., et al. (2009). "The Therapeutic Potential of the Endocannabinoid System for the Development of a Novel Class of Antidepressants." *Trends in Pharmacological Sciences* 30: 484–493.

Hirvonen, J., et al. (2009). "Assessment of MAO-B Occupancy in the Brain With PET and [^{11}C]-L-Deprenyl-D$_2$: A Dose-Finding Study with a Novel MAO-B Inhibitor, EVT 301. *Clinical Pharmacology and Therapeutics* 85: 506.

Howland, R. H. (2009). "Critical Appraisal and Update on the Clinical Utility of Agomelatine, a Melatonergic Agonist, for the Treatment of Major Depressive Disease in Adults." *Neuropsychiatric Disease and Treatment* 5: 563–576.

Jeanneteau, F., and Chao, M. V. (2006). "Promoting Neurotrophic Effects by GCPR Ligands." *Novartis Foundation Symposium* 276: 181–189.

Karpa, K. D., et al. (2002). "Duloxetine Pharmacology: Profile of a Dual Mono-Amine Modulator." *CNS Drug Reviews* 8: 361–376.

Kato, M., and Serretti, A. (2010). "Review and Meta-Analysis of Antidepressant Pharmacogenetic Findings in Major Depressive Disorder." *Molecular Psychiatry* 15: 473–500.

Kelly, C. M., et al. (2010). "Selective Serotonin Reuptake Inhibitors and Breast Cancer Mortality in Women Receiving Tamoxifen: A Population Based Cohort Study." *British Medical Journal* 340: c693.

Kessler, R. C., et al. (2003). "The Epidemiology of Major Depressive Disorder: Results from the National Comorbidity Survey Replication (NCS-R)." *Journal of the American Medical Association* 289: 3095–3105.

Khan, A. (2009). "Vilazodone, a Novel Dual-Acting Serotonergic Antidepressant for Managing Major Depression." *Expert Opinion on Investigational Drugs* 18: 1753–1764.

Konuk, N., et al. (2006). "Open-Label Study of Adjunct Modafinil for the Treatment of Patients with Fatigue, Sleepiness, and Major Depression Treated with Selective Serotonin Uptake Inhibitors." *Advances in Therapy* 23: 646–654.

Koo, J. W., et al. (2010). "Nuclear Factor-κB Is a Critical Mediator of Stress-Impaired Neurogenesis and Depressive Behavior." *Proceedings of the National Academy of Sciences* 107: 2669–2674.

Kornhuber, J., et al. (2009). "The Role of Ceramide in Major Depressive Disorder." *European Archives of Psychiatry and Clinical Neurosciences* 259, Supplement 2: S199–S204.

Krishnan, V., and Nestler, E. J. (2008). "The Molecular Neurobiology of Depression." *Nature* 455: 894–902.

Kroenke, K., et al. (2001). "Similar Effectiveness of Paroxetine, Fluoxetine, and Sertraline in Primary Care: A Randomized Trial." *Journal of the American Medical Association* 286: 2947–2955.

Kuipers, S. D., and Bramham, C. R. (2006). "Brain-Derived Neurotrophic Factor Mechanisms and Function in Adult Synaptic Plasticity: New Insights and Implications for Therapy." *Current Opinion in Drug Discovery Development* 9: 580–586.

Kulkarni, S., et al. (2009). "Potentials of Curcumin as an Antidepressant." *Scientific World Journal* 9: 1233–1241.

Levinson, A. J., et al. (2010). "Evidence of Cortical Inhibitory Deficits in Major Depressive Disorder." *Biological Psychiatry* 67: 458–464.

Loo, H., et al. (2001). "Efficacy and Safety of Tianeptine in the Treatment of Depressive Disorders in Comparison with Fluoxetine." *Human Psychopharmacology* 16: S31–S38.

Lucassen, P. J., et al. (2010). "Regulation of Adult Neurogenesis by Stress, Sleep Disruption, Exercise and Inflammation: Implications for Depression and Antidepressant Action." *European Neuropsychopharmacology* 20: 1–17.

Machado-Vieira, R., et al. (2008). "Rapid Onset of Antidepressant Action: A New Paradigm in the Research and Treatment of Major Depressive Disorder." *Journal of Clinical Psychiatry* 69: 946–958.

Madaan, V., and Wilson, D. R. (2009). " Neuropeptides: Relevance in Treatment of Depression and Anxiety Disorders." *Drug News Perspective* 22: 319–324.

Mahaney, P. E., et al. (2006). "Synthesis and Activity of a New Class of Dual Acting Norepinephrine and Serotonin Reuptake Inhibitors: 3-(1H-Indol-1-yl)-3-Arylpropan-1-Amines." *Bioorganic and Medicinal Chemistry* 14: 8455–8466.

Malberg, J. E., and Blendy, J. A. (2005). "Antidepressant Action: To the Nucleus and Beyond." *Trends in Pharmacological Sciences* 26: 631–638.

Mamalakis, G., et al. (2006). "Depression and Serum Adiponectin and Adipose Omega-3 and Omega-6 Fatty Acids in Adolescents." *Pharmacology, Biochemistry and Behavior* 85: 474–479.

Marazziti, D., et al. (2009). "Second Messenger Modulation: A Novel Target of Future Antidepressants?" *Current Medicinal Chemistry* 16: 4679–4690.

Marks, D. M., et al. (2008). "Triple Reuptake Inhibitors: The Next Generation of Antidepressants." *Current Neuropharmacology* 6: 338–343.

Martinez, C., et al. (2010). "Use of Venlafaxine Compared with Other Antidepressants and the Risk of Sudden Cardiac Death or Near Death: A Nested Case-Control Study." *British Medical Journal* 340: c249.

Mease, P. J. (2009). "Further Strategies for Treating Fibromyalgia: The Role of Serotonin and Norepinephrine Reuptake Inhibitors." *American Journal of Medicine* 122, Supplement 12: S44–S55.

Montgomery, S. A., et al. (2006). "Efficacy and Safety of 30 mg/d and 45 mg/d Nemifitide Compared to Placebo in Major Depressive Disorder." *International Journal of Neuropsychopharmacology* 9: 517–528.

Moret, C., et al. (2009). "Problems Associated With Long-Term Treatment with Selective Serotonin Reuptake Inhibitors." *Journal of Psychopharmacology* 23: 967–974.

Moskal, J., and Burgdor, J. (2009). "The Anti-Depressant and Anxiolytic Properties of GLYX-13: A Glycine-Site Functional Partial Agonist (GFPA), a Novel Mechanism for Modulating NMDA Receptors." Paper presented at the 2009 Annual Meeting of the American College of Neuropsychopharmacology, Hollywood, FL.

Muzina, D. J. (2010). "Discontinuing an Antidepressant? Tapering Tips to Ease Distressing Symptoms." *Current Psychiatry* 9: 51–61.

Nair, A., and Vaidya, V. A. (2006). "CyclicAMP Response Element Binding Protein and Brain-Derived Neurotrophic Factor: Molecules That Modulate Our Mood?" *Journal of Bioscience* 31: 423–434.

Nakagawa, A., et al. (2009). "Milnacipran versus Other Antidepressive Agents for Depression." *Cochrane Database of Systematic Reviews* CD006529.

Nelson, J. C., and Papakostas, G. I. (2009). "Atypical Antipsychotic Augmentation in Major Depressive Disorder: A Meta-Analysis of Placebo-Controlled Randomized Trials." *American Journal of Psychiatry* 166: 980–991.

Nelson, J. C., et al. (2006). "Mirtazepine Orally Disintegrating Tablets in Depressed Nursing Home Residents 85 Years of Age and Older." *International Journal of Geriatric Psychiatry* 21: 898–901.

Nickel, T., et al. (2003). "Clinical and Neurobiological Effects of Tianeptine and Paroxetine in Major Depression." *Journal of Clinical Psychopharmacology* 23: 155–168.

Nieuwstraten, C., et al. (2006). "Systematic Overview of Drug Interactions with Antidepressant Medications." *Canadian Journal of Psychiatry* 51: 300–316.

Norton, P. A., et al. (2002). "Duloxetine versus Placebo in the Treatment of Stress Urinary Incontinence." *American Journal of Obstetrics and Gynecology* 187:40–48.

Nurnberg, H. G., et al. (2001). "Efficacy of Sildenafil Citrate for the Treatment of Erectile Dysfunction in Men Taking Serotonin Reuptake Inhibitors." *American Journal of Psychiatry* 158: 1926–1928.

Pae, C. U., et al. (2009a). "Atypical Depression: A Comprehensive Review." *CNS Drugs* 23: 1023–1037.

Pae, C. U., et al. (2009b). "Milnacipran: Beyond a Role of Antidepressant." *Clinical Neuropharmacology* 32: 355–363.

Pae, C. U., et al. (2009c). "Desvenlafaxine: A New Antidepressant or Just Another One?" *Expert Opinion on Pharmacotherapy* 10: 875–887.

Papakostas, G. I. (2009). "Evidence for S-Adenosyl-L-Methionine (SAM-e) for the Treatment of Major Depressive Disorder." *Journal of Clinical Psychiatry* 70: 18–22.

Papakostas, G. I., et al. (2007). "Augmentation of Antidepressants with Atypical Antipsychotic Medications for Treatment-Resistant Major Depressive Disorder: A Meta-Analysis." *Journal of Clinical Psychiatry* 68: 826–831.

Parker, G. P., et al. (2006). "Omega-3 Fatty Acids and Mood Disorders." *American Journal of Psychiatry* 163: 969–978.

Paschos, K. A., et al. (2009). "Neuropeptide and Sigma Receptors as Novel Therapeutic Targets for the Pharmacotherapy of Depression." *CNS Drugs* 23: 755–772.

Pearlson, T., et al. (2003). "Recurrence of Symptoms of Premenstrual Dysphoric Disorder After the Cessation of Luteal-Phase Fluoxetine Treatment." *Journal of Obstetrics and Gynecology* 188: 887–895.

Peritogiannis, V., et al. (2009). "Duloxetine-Induced Hypomania: Case Report and Brief Review of the Literature on SNRIs-Induced Mood Switching." *Journal of Psychopharmacology* 23: 592–596.

Perry, R., and Cassagnol, M. (2009). "Desvenlafaxine: A New Serotonin-Norepinephrine Reuptake Inhibitor for the Treatment of Adults with Major Depressive Disorder." *Clinical Therapeutics* 31(Pt. 1): 1374–1404.

Quartara, L. (2009). "Tachykinin Receptor Antagonists in Clinical Trials." *Expert Opinion on Investigational Drugs* 18: 1843–1864.

Quitkin, F. M., et al. (2003). "When Should a Trial of Fluoxetine for Major Depression Be Declared Failed?" *American Journal of Psychiatry* 160: 734–740.

Rabkin, J. G., et al. (2006). "Placebo-Controlled Trial of Dehydroepiandrosterone (DHEA) for Treatment of Nonmajor Depression in Patients with HIV/AIDS." *American Journal of Psychiatry* 163: 59–66.

Ravindran, A. V., et al. (2000). "Treatment of Dysthymia with Sertraline: A Double-Blind, Placebo-Controlled Trial in Dysthymic Patients Without Major Depression." *Journal of Clinical Psychiatry* 61: 821–827.

Richardson-Jones, J. W., et al. (2010). "5-HT$_{1A}$ Autoreceptor Levels Determine Vulnerability to Stress and Response to Antidepressants." *Neuron* 65: 40–52.

Richelson, E. (2003). "Interactions of Antidepressants with Neurotransmitter Transporters and Receptors and Their Clinical Relevance." *Journal of Clinical Psychiatry* 64, Supplement 13: 5–12.

Rooks, D. S. (2007). "Fibromyalgia Treatment Update." *Current Opinions in Rheumatology* 19: 111–117.

Ruhé, H. G., et al. (2006). "Switching Antidepressants After a First Selective Serotonin Reuptake Inhibitor in Major Depressive Disorder." *Journal of Clinical Psychiatry* 67: 1836–1855.

Rush, A. J., et al. (2006). "Bupropion-SR, Sertraline, or Venlafaxine-XR After Failure of SSRIs for Depression." *New England Journal of Medicine* 354: 1231–1242.

Rush, A. J., et al. (2009). "STAR*D: Revising Conventional Wisdom." *CNS Drugs* 23: 627–647.

Rynn, M. et al. (2008). "Efficacy and Safety of Duloxetine in the Treatment of Generalized Anxiety Disorder: A Flexible-Dose, Progressive-Titration, Placebo-Controlled Trial." *Depression and Anxiety* 25: 182–189.

Saarelainen, T., et al. (2003). "Activation of the TrkB Neurotrophin Receptor Is Induced by Antidepressant Drugs and Is Required for Antidepressant-Induced Behavioral Effects." *Journal of Neuroscience* 23: 349–357.

Salome, N., et al. (2006). "Selective Blockade of NK2 or NK3 Receptors Produces Anxiolytic- and Antidepressant-like Effects in Gerbils." *Pharmacology, Biochemistry, and Behavior* 83: 533–539.

Schechter, L. E., et al. (2005). "Innovative Approaches for the Development of Antidepressant Drugs: Current and Future Strategies." *NeuroRx: Journal of the American Society for Experimental NeuroTherapeutics* 2: 590–611.

Schmidt, P. J., et al. (2005). "Dehydroepiandrosterone Monotherapy in Mid-Life Onset Major and Minor Depression." *Archives of General Psychiatry* 62: 154–162.

Schneeweiss, S., et al. (2010). "Variation in the Risk of Suicide Attempts and Completed Suicides by Antidepressant Agent in Adults: A Propensity Score-Adjusted Analysis of 9 Years' Data." *Archives of General Psychiatry* 67: 497–506.

Schonfeldt-Lecuona, C., et al. (2006). "Bupropion Augmentation in the Treatment of Chronic Fatigue Syndrome with Coexistent Major Depression Episode." *Pharmacopsychiatry* 39: 152–154.

Schweitzer, I., et al. (2009). "Sexual Side-Effects of Contemporary Antidepressants: Review." *Australian and New Zealand Journal of Psychiatry* 43: 795–808.

Seidman, S. N., et al. (2001). "Treatment of Erectile Dysfunction in Men with Depressive Symptoms: Results of a Placebo-Controlled Trial with Sildenafil Citrate." *American Journal of Psychiatry* 158: 1623–1630.

Shakesby, A. C., et al. (2002). "Overcoming the Effects of Stress on Synaptic Plasticity in the Rat Hippocampus: Rapid Actions of Serotoninergic and Antidepressant Agents." *Journal of Neuroscience* 22: 3638–3644.

Shamlian, N., and Cole, M. G. (2006). "Androgen Treatment of Depressive Symptoms in Older Men: A Systematic Review of Feasibility and Effectiveness." *Canadian Journal of Psychiatry* 51: 295–299.

Shimazaki, T., et al. (2006). "Melanin-Concentrating Hormone MCH1 Receptor Antagonists: A Potential New Approach to the Treatment of Depression and Anxiety Disorders." *CNS Drugs* 20: 801–811.

Simpson, D., and Plosker, G. L. (2004). "Atomoxetine: A Review of Its Use in Adults with Attention Deficit Hyperactivity Disorder." *Drugs* 64: 205–222.

Sindrup, S. H., et al. (2005). "Antidepressants in the Treatment of Neuropathic Pain." *Basic and Clinical Pharmacology and Toxicology* 96: 399–409.

Skolnick, P., et al. (2006). "Preclinical and Clinical Pharmacology of DOV 216,303, a 'Triple' Reuptake Inhibitor." *CNS Drug Review* 12: 123–134.

Skolnick, P., et al. (2009). "Glutamate-Based Antidepressants: 20 Years On." *Trends in Pharmacological Sciences* 30: 563–569.

Sontrop, J., and Campbell, M. K. (2006). "Omega-3 Polyunsaturated Fatty Acids and Depression: A Review of the Evidence and a Methodological Critique." *Preventive Medicine* 42: 4–13.

Spencer, T., et al. (2004). "Nonstimulant Treatment of Adult Attention-Deficit/Hyperactivity Disorder." *Psychiatric Clinics of North America* 27: 373–383.

Stimmel, G. L., and Gutierrez, M. A. (2006). "Sexual Dysfunction and Psychotropic Medications." *CNS Spectrum* 8, Supplement 9: 24–30.

Stoll, A. (2001). *The Omega-3 Connection.* New York: Simon & Schuster.

Suhara, T., et al. (2003). "High Levels of Serotonin Transporter Occupancy with Low-Dose Clomipramine in Comparative Occupancy Study with Fluvoxamine Using Positron Emission Tomography." *Archives of General Psychiatry* 60: 386–391.

Surget, A., et al. (2008). "Drug-Dependent Requirement of Hippocampal Neurogenesis in a Model of Depression and of Antidepressant Reversal." *Biological Psychiatry* 64: 293–301.

Tella, S. R., et al. (1997). "Differential Regulation of Dopamine Transporter After Chronic Self-Administration of Bupropion and Nomifensine." *Journal of Pharmacology and Experimental Therapeutics* 281: 508–518.

Thase, M. E., et al. (2006). "A Double-Blind Comparison Between Bupropion XL and Venlafaxine XR: Sexual Functioning, Antidepressant Efficacy, and Tolerability." *Journal of Clinical Psychopharmacology* 26: 482–488.

Thase, M. E., et al. (2007). "Cognitive Therapy versus Medication in Augmentation and Switch Strategies as Second-Step Treatments: A STAR*D Report." *American Journal of Psychiatry* 164: 739–752.

Tohen, M. et al. (2010). "Olanzapine/Fluoxetine Combination in Patients with Treatment-Resistant Depression: Rapid Onset of Therapeutic Response and Its Predictive Value for Subsequent Overall Response in a Pooled Analysis of 5 Studies." *Journal of Clinical Psychiatry* 71: 451–462.

Tran, P. V., et al. (2003). "Dual Monoamine Modulation for Improved Treatment of Major Depressive Disorder." *Journal of Clinical Psychopharmacology* 23: 78–86.

Trivedi, M. H., et al. (2006). Medication Augmentation After the Failure of SSRIs for Depression." *New England Journal of Medicine* 354: 1243–1252.

Vigo, D. V., and Baldessarini, R. J. (2009). "Anticonvulsants in the Treatment of Major Depressive Disorder: An Overview." *Harvard Review of Psychiatry* 17: 231–241.

Wadsworth, E. J., et al. (2005). "SSRIs and Cognitive Performance in a Working Sample." *Human Psychopharmacology* 8: 561–572.

Warner, C. H., et al. (2006). "Antidepressant Discontinuation Syndrome." *American Family Physician* 74: 449–456.

World Health Organization. (2007). *World Health Statistics 2007*, p. 16. Geneva: WHO Press.

Wulsin, A. C., et al. (2010). "Mifepristone Decreases Depression-Like Behavior and Modulates Neuroendocrine and Central Hypothalamic-Pituitary-Adrenocortical Axis Responsiveness to Stress." *Psychoneuroendocrinology.* In press.

Zisook, S., et al. (2001). "Bupropion Sustained Release for Bereavement: Results of an Open Trial." *Journal of Clinical Psychiatry* 62: 227–230.

Chapter 6

Drugs Used to Treat Bipolar Disorder

Bipolar Disorder

Bipolar disorder (manic-depressive disorder) is one of the ten most disabling conditions in the world, with a prevalence of about 1 percent across all populations, regardless of nationality, race, or socioeconomic status. People who have the disorder lose many years of healthy functioning, in which their livelihood, marriage, social relationships, and even life may be destroyed. The course of the illness is episodic, with alternating periods of mania and/or depression nearly half the time and intervening periods of at least some degree of remission. Although it may appear in childhood or adolescence, the diagnosis is difficult and it is still being debated (Chapter 18). The main problems in diagnosis are that mania or hypomania may be underreported, that symptoms of unipolar and bipolar depression overlap, and that there is a high degree of comorbidity with many other psychiatric conditions (Hirschfeld, 2009). Generally, onset occurs in the third decade or later, often with a significant delay between the appearance of symptoms and a correct diagnosis and treatment. Most patients experience several episodes during the course of their lives. The risk of recurrence has recently been reported to be 24 percent by six months, 36 percent by one year, and 61 percent by four years (Baldassano, 2009).

A patient with bipolar disorder (BD) may be diagnosed with any of several subtypes of the disorder. The traditional subtype, bipolar disorder I (BP-I), includes at least one episode of full-blown mania with or without an episode of major depression. The disorder is classified as bipolar II (BP-II) if the manic episode is less severe, or "hypomanic," and episodes of major depression also occur. A patient is said to be a "rapid cycler" if at least four illness episodes occur in a 12-month period. Several other bipolar subtypes have been described, exhibiting varying degrees of severity in recurrent mood swings. Together, the variants bring the prevalence of all bipolar disorders to 4.4 percent of U.S. residents (Merikangas et al., 2007).

Despite intensive care and treatment, outpatients with bipolar disorder have a considerable degree of illness-related morbidity, including a threefold greater amount of time spent depressed than time spent manic (Post et al., 2005). Moreover, there is a high rate of mortality (Kupfer, 2005); one of every four or five untreated or inadequately treated patients commits suicide during the course of the illness, a rate ten times that of the general population. Other predictors of mortality in bipolar patients include male gender, history of alcoholism, and poor occupational status before the index episode, as well as a history of previous episodes, psychotic features, symptoms of depression during the index manic episode (termed "mixed mania"), and residual affective symptoms between episodes.

Diagnostic and Treatment Issues

Similar to unipolar depression, the symptoms of bipolar depression, as described by patients, include (in decreasing order of prevalence) sadness, insomnia, feelings of worthlessness, loss of energy and ability to concentrate, inability to enjoy everyday activities, thoughts of death and suicide, and an inability to function. Manic symptoms include various aspects of behavioral and physiological hyperactivity, such as erratic sleep, increased sexual interest, emotional elation and racing thoughts, increased physical activity, impulsiveness, poor judgment, and reckless and aggressive behavior.

Comorbid substance abuse affects at least 60 percent of bipolar I and 50 percent of bipolar II patients, with reported rates for alcohol (82 percent), cocaine (30 percent), marijuana (29 percent), sedatives or amphetamines (21 percent), and opioids (13 percent). It may, at least initially, represent an attempt at self-medication for the symptoms accompanying the affective disorder. Unfortunately, substance abuse is associated with a greater risk of switching from a depressive episode to one of mania, hypomania, or a mixed mood state (Ostacher et al., 2010), sometimes referred to as a "flip."

Although a patient with bipolar disorder may present initially with either mania or depression, most patients seek treatment for depression. As a result, many are incorrectly diagnosed with unipolar depression and consequently receive inappropriate treatment with antidepressants alone. Unfortunately, while antidepressants can be effective against depressive symptomatology, they may induce or trigger a manic episode, that is, produce a "switch," or "flip," resulting in serious adverse consequences for the patient. As stated in a review of the neurobiology of the switch phenomenon: "[T]he process of switching from depression to a state of mania or hypomania is a unique and core feature of bipolar disorder" (Salvadore et al., 2010, p. e1). The risk of such an event is apparently greater if patients have more severe manic symptoms at baseline, before addition of the antidepressant (Frye et al., 2009). Interestingly, it has been reported that electroconvulsive shock treatment (ECT) is also effective for bipolar depression (Bailine et al., 2010). Goldberg (2010) provides an excellent review of the role of antidepressants in treating patients with bipolar disorder.

Because of the risk that antidepressants may trigger a manic switch, administration or addition of a *mood stabilizer* (MS) is the most recommended pharmacological treatment for bipolar depression (Bauer and Mitchner, 2004; Mundo et al., 2006). Unfortunately, even combinations may still increase the risk of a manic flip, and the risk varies among the different antidepressants (Leverich et al., 2006). Long-term treatment with antidepressant/mood stabilizer combinations may even worsen manic symptom severity (Goldberg et al., 2007) or increase the likelihood of a switch in patients who are rapid cyclers (Schneck et al., 2008). Given that maintenance treatment with antidepressants may not prevent depressive relapses, weaning patients off antidepressants 6 to 12 months after remission has been advised. Yet, considering the scarcity of definitive data, even this advice may change in the future (Amsterdam and Shults, 2010).

Obviously, because of these significant differences in recommended pharmacological treatment, it is important to be able to differentiate between unipolar and bipolar depression. Although the distinction is not always easy to make, some clinical features have been proposed to help (Perlis et al., 2006b). Unipolar depression usually develops after the age of 25 years and may be preceded by an extended period of gradually worsening symptoms. Unipolar patients usually have no history of mania or hypomania. In contrast, bipolar depression typically occurs before the age of 25 years, with a more abrupt onset of hours or days, and may be periodic or seasonal. Bipolar disorder is highly heritable and may run in families, which makes a thorough family history a crucial component of the diagnosis. Similarly, a personal history of disruptive behavioral patterns or evidence of mania, hypomania, increased energy, or decreased need for sleep may suggest a bipolar diagnosis, as would treatment-emergent mania or hypomania during antidepressant monotherapy. It has recently been proposed that postpartum depression may also be misdiagnosed as major depressive disorder, when, in fact, more than half of patients who received a referral diagnosis of postpartum depression were later found to have bipolar disorder (Sharma et al., 2009, and references therein).

Medications are currently available to treat acute manic/mixed states and acute bipolar depression and for the prophylactic prevention of recurrent episodes. However, the quality of evidence for efficacy in each of these phases differs among the putative mood stabilizers. Table 6.1 summarizes the relative effectiveness of the available agents for each phase (see also Bauer, 2005). These drugs include the lithium ion, several anticonvulsant "neuromodulators," second-generation antipsychotics (SGAs), and a dietary supplement of the omega-3 fatty acids (Parker et al., 2006a).

The classic mood stabilizer is *lithium*. Although lithium may effectively control manic symptoms and reduce the recurrence of both manic and depressive episodes, its bothersome and serious side effects

---

TABLE 6.1 Quality of Evidence for the Use of Mood Stabilizers in Bipolar Disorder

A Double-blind placebo-controlled trials with adequate samples
B Double-blind comparator studies with adequate samples
C Open trials with adequate samples
D Uncontrolled observation or controlled study with ambiguous result
E No published evidence
F Available evidence negative

	Acute mania/Mixed	Mood stabilizer prophylaxis	Acute bipolar depression
Lithium	A+	A+	A
Valproic acid	A+	A−	D
Carbamazepine	A	B−	D
Lamotrigine	F	A+	A
Gabapentin	F	E	D
Topiramate	D	E	D
Aripiprazole	A	E	E
Haloperidol	A	E	E
Olanzapine	A+	E	A
Risperidone	A	E	D
Quetiapine	A	E	E
Ziprasidone	A	E	E
Omega-3	E	D	E

A+ is reserved for those instances when fewer than 40 studies have been reported and more than one double-blind placebo-controlled study supports the same finding. A− indicates positive outcomes on some but not all relevant measures. From G. S. Sachs, "Decision Tree for the Treatment of Bipolar Disorder," *Journal of Clinical Psychiatry* 64, Supplement 8 (2003), p. 37.

have necessitated a search for equally effective, safer, and more tolerable agents. Today, it is recognized that combination treatment with two or more medications is often required, preferably with adjunctive psychosocial interventions.

In 1996, the American Psychiatric Association published its first clinical practice guideline for the treatment of patients with bipolar disorder. A revision was published in 2002, emphasizing that the major objectives of intervention are to treat acute manic episodes and to reduce their frequency of recurrence. The most recent update was the result of a consensus conference in May 2004, which reinforced the general treatment goals of (1) symptomatic remission, (2) full return of psychosocial functioning, and (3) prevention of relapses and recurrences (Suppes et al., 2005). A recent guideline for monitoring the safety of drug treatment in bipolar disorder recognizes the challenging side effect burden of many of these drugs, as described below (Ng et al., 2009).

Drug therapy is the cornerstone of bipolar disorder treatment. For less severe acute manic episodes, first-line treatment is monotherapy with lithium, valproate (divalproex), or a second-generation antipsychotic (Suppes et al., 2005). The same guidelines apply for mixed episodes, except that lithium is less efficacious for that condition. For more severe situations, the combination of either lithium or valproate (or another neuromodulator anticonvulsant) and an antipsychotic is recommended.

First-line treatment of less severe acute bipolar depression is monotherapy with the "third-generation" neuromodulator/anticonvulsant lamotrigine, with the addition of an antimanic agent if there is a history of severe mania. For maintenance treatment, regardless of whether the most recent episode was manic, depressed, or mixed, it is acceptable to stay on the acute-phase medication if it is well tolerated. However, if additional options are necessary, antipsychotics are recommended when the most recent episode is manic or mixed; if the most recent episode is depressed, either lithium or the combination of an antimanic and an antidepressant may be helpful. In 2004 a new combination product was approved for treating bipolar depression. Trade-named Symbyax, it contains the antipsychotic olanzapine (for mania; Chapter 4) and the antidepressant fluoxetine (for depression; Chapter 5). The treatment of bipolar disorder in children and adolescents is discussed in Chapter 18.

Pathophysiology and Mechanisms of Drug Action

Identifying the therapeutic action of mood stabilizers in the treatment of bipolar disorder has been particularly challenging, and as yet there is no unifying hypothesis. It is difficult to understand how any single drug class can reduce symptoms of both mania and depression, and it has proven difficult to find a mechanism among the relevant drug classes that would account for this dual therapeutic efficacy. Such a mechanism might also need to be linked to common genes. However, a recent study looking at the possible genetic basis of a clinical response to lithium did not find any specific associations (Perlis et al., 2009).

Mood stabilizers may have some neurobiological actions in common with antidepressants. This conclusion comes from growing evidence of similarities between the damaging effects of depression and bipolar disorder on the brain. As discussed in Chapter 5, severe depression is associated with an increase in neuronal vulnerability to injury or trauma, including stress, which may damage neural structures and produce functional impairment. Imaging and postmortem studies have shown similar types of structural changes in the brains of patients diagnosed with bipolar disorder. As in major depressive disorder, reductions in the volume of the prefrontal cortex and hippocampus are significant (Bertolino et al., 2003); the number of neurons and glial cells in the prefrontal cortex is decreased; and levels of the neurochemical N-acetyl-aspartate, which is considered a marker of neuronal "health," are lower (Zarate et al., 2005).

Like antidepressants, mood stabilizers may reverse some of the impairments in brain structure and levels of brain-derived neurotrophic factor (BDNF; Figure 6.1), reversals that could be relevant to the therapeutic benefit of mood stabilizers in bipolar disorder (Yasuda et al., 2009). In laboratory models, lithium was found to protect neurons against a variety of toxic agents and to promote the growth of neuronal processes; in the human brain, lithium increases levels of N-acetyl-aspartate and gray matter volume. However, in spite of their common neuroprotective effects, no universal mechanism has

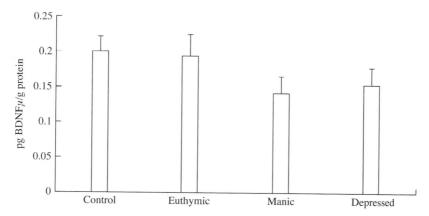

FIGURE 6.1 Serum BDNF levels in BD patients and healthy controls. Measurement is picograms of BDNF protein per microgram of total serum protein. [From A. B. M. Cunha et al., "Serum Brain-Derived Neurotrophic Factor Is Decreased in Bipolar Disorder During Depressive and Manic Episodes," *Neuroscience Letters* 398 (2006), p. 216.].

yet been identified to account for the therapeutic and neurobiological similarities between antidepressants and mood stabilizers. While antidepressants and antipsychotics have some common effects on neurotransmitter receptors in the brain (which could be relevant to their common antidepressant efficacy; Yatham et al., 2005), neither lithium nor the "neuromodulatory" anticonvulsants share these mechanisms of action. That is, unlike antidepressants and antipsychotics, lithium and many of the anticonvulsants do not exert their primary effect at neuronal synapses. Rather, these drugs seem to act intracellularly to produce changes that "stabilize" neuronal membranes.

Currently, the most extensively studied putative mechanisms of mood stabilizers are the second- and third-messenger systems, that is, the intracellular biochemical processes produced by activation of G-protein-coupled receptors (see Figure 2.7). It has already been established that lithium, valproate, and carbamazepine interact with various enzymes involved in these intracellular signaling pathways. Although individual drugs may interact at different sites within the neurochemical systems, they may all ultimately produce some final common effect that is responsible for their clinical efficacy in bipolar disorder (Gould et al., 2004; Rapoport et al, 2009).[1] "Thus, the mood stabilizers may act to restore the balance among aberrant signaling pathways in specific areas of the brain and prevent degeneration" (Brunello, 2004).

STEP-BD Study

As with the antidepressants for major depression, progress is also being made in determining the best approach for the clinical management of bipolar illness. To provide therapeutic guidelines for practitioners, a large-scale, federally funded trial, called the STEP-BD study, compared pharmacological treatments for bipolar disorder. The study was recently completed.

STEP-BD stands for Systematic Treatment Enhancement Program for Bipolar Disorder; it was one of the first of several studies funded by the National Institute of Mental Health (NIMH)

---

[1] One possibility is suggested by the fact that lithium and valproate, like antidepressants (as discussed in Chapter 5), increase the levels of proteins, such as cAMP response element-binding protein (CREB), which, in turn, activates genes that produce additional proteins (in particular, one called bcl-2) and a neurotrophic factor (BDNF) that are known to protect neurons from the toxic effects of injury or trauma. Because of this, the two drugs are sometimes referred to as "neuroprotective" agents. Such a broad, general effect on neuronal health may be the reason these drugs are also useful in the management of other clinical conditions, such as aggressive disorders, pain, and so on, discussed later in this chapter.

designed to determine the real-world effectiveness of the major psychiatric drug classes. Like the companion studies for depression (the STAR*D trial, discussed in Chapter 5) and schizophrenia (the CATIE trial, discussed in Chapter 4), this investigation involved large numbers of typical patients and used few exclusion criteria in an effort to make the results more generalizable for treatment in standard clinical practice.

To be enrolled at one of the 20 sites in the United States, patients had to meet the criteria for any type or subtype of bipolar disorder. After study entry, patients were assigned a "STEP-BD-certified" psychiatrist, who received 20 hours of training in standard care procedures in the treatment of bipolar disorder. The guidelines for the procedures were written by a group of experts who identified nine separate decision points, corresponding to nine typical clinical situations. At each point there is a specified "menu of reasonable choices" that provides recommendations rather than rigid algorithms for appropriate, standard care. For the most part, participants were managed with an optimized mood stabilizer regimen (lithium, valproate, combined lithium and valproate, or carbamazepine) plus either one or two antidepressants. Additionally, patients were systematically monitored for suicidal symptoms. Patients were seen every three months for the first year, then every six months thereafter, and were encouraged to stay in the trial for five years.

The study began in 1998, and data collection from the final total of 4360 patients was completed in September 2005. Results are gradually being analyzed, and several major findings have been published. One of the first papers (Perlis et al., 2006c) described the results in a subset of 1469 patients who had participated for at least two years (Figure 6.2). The researchers found that only 58.4 percent (858 patients) of this group achieved recovery (defined as having only two symptoms of the disorder for at least eight weeks). During the two-year follow-up period, almost half of this group, 48.5 percent, or 416 patients, had a recurrence at some point, more commonly to a depressive episode (72 percent) than to a manic, hypomanic, or mixed episode (28 percent). Recurrence was most likely in those who had residual symptoms at recovery or had an additional psychiatric illness (for example, anxiety, an eating disorder, or substance abuse).

In March 2007, Sachs and coworkers published results of another STEP-BD trial. In this trial, patients received a mood stabilizer (lithium, valproate, carbamazepine, or another FDA-approved agent) combined with either an antidepressant (bupropion or paroxetine) ($n = 179$) or placebo ($n = 187$). Subjects with bipolar I or bipolar II disorder were treated for up to 26 weeks to evaluate the effectiveness, safety, and tolerability of the adjunctive use of antidepressant medication. Unfortunately, the results showed no difference between the

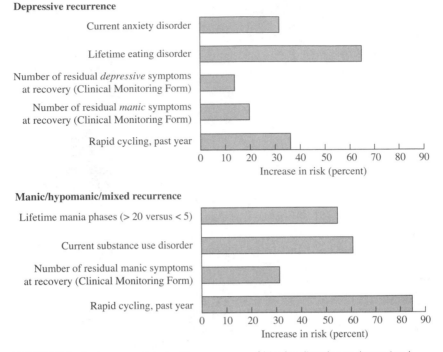

FIGURE 6.2 Factors associated with recurrence of bipolar disorder as determined from the STEP-BD study. [From R. H. Perlis et al. (2006c).].

groups that received adjunct antidepressants and the groups that received placebo. At each criterion of response, the percent of patients in the respective groups was the same: only 23.5 percent of patients on the antidepressants and 27.3 percent of patients on placebo achieved recovery, which was defined as 8 consecutive weeks of euthymia (a normal mood). Only 17.9 percent on the antidepressant and 21.4 percent on the placebo experienced a transient remission (1 to 7 consecutive weeks of euthymia), while only 32.4 percent on antidepressant and 38 percent on placebo showed a 50 percent improvement in symptoms. The groups also did not differ in the percentage of patients who showed symptoms of switching into an episode of mood elevation (hypomania or mania): 10.1 percent on the antidepressant and 10.7 percent on placebo showed symptoms of switching. In summary, for the treatment of bipolar depression, mood-stabilizing monotherapy provided as much benefit and a comparable risk of switching as treatment with mood stabilizers combined with a standard antidepressant. Clearly, these results are disappointing and illustrate how much we have yet to achieve in the pharmacological treatment of bipolar disorder.

Patients who were treatment-resistant to the combination of a mood stabilizer and at least one antidepressant could choose to enter the last portion of the program. Each of the 66 participants who agreed was randomly assigned one of three additional agents: the anticonvulsant lamotrigine (Lamictal), the antipsychotic risperidone (Risperdal), or inositol (a sugar, which is an isomer of glucose and is normally a component of one of the second-messenger pathways). Recovery rates were 23.8 percent, 4.6 percent, and 17.4 percent, respectively, and were not statistically different from one another (perhaps because of the small number of subjects), although the relatively poor effect of the antipsychotic was unexpected (Nierenberg et al., 2006).

One particularly important finding of the STEP-BD study was the confirmation of the notion that valproic acid may increase the risk of polycystic ovarian syndrome (PCOS). The large sample of 230 women (ages 18 to 44) made it possible to test this concern. They found PCOS symptoms (menstrual irregularities, acne, male-pattern hair loss, elevated testosterone, and excessive body hair) in 9 of 86 women (10.5 percent) on valproate compared to only 2 of 144 women on another agent (1.4 percent). These results show a clear increase in the risk of developing PCOS for women on valproic acid (Joffe et al., 2006). Valproate also increases the risk of certain birth defects and is not recommended for women who are pregnant (Chapter 18).

Lithium

Lithium has historically been the drug of first choice for treating bipolar disorder and reducing its rate of relapse.[2] Unfortunately, its clinical effectiveness is less than that predicted by clinical trials; relapse often occurs because of patient nonadherence to therapy. Therefore, the pharmacology of lithium and the reasons for patient noncompliance with this drug therapy need to be recognized and alternative agents considered.

Lithium (Li^+) is the lightest of the alkali metals (Figure 6.3) and shares some characteristics with sodium (Na^+). In nature, lithium is abundant in some alkaline mineral spring waters. Devoid of psychotropic effects in normal people, lithium is effective in treating 60 to 80 percent of acute manic and hypomanic episodes, although in the last few years its use has declined because of limitations with regard to toxicities, side effects, compliance, and relapse as well as the prospect of more alternatives.

---

[2] For a historical overview of lithium therapy and commentaries on lithium, see four related letters in *Archives of General Psychiatry* 54 (1997): 9–23.

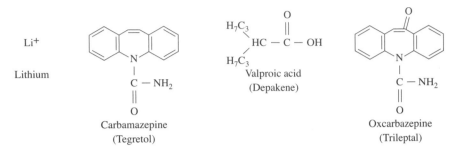

FIGURE 6.3   Drugs classically used in the treatment of bipolar disorder. Structures of newer anticonvulsants used in bipolar disorder are shown in Figure 7.7.

History

During the late 1940s, lithium chloride was recommended as a salt substitute for patients with heart disease. Wide use for this purpose resulted in cases of severe toxicity and death, causing it to be abandoned as a medicine. In 1949, however, an Australian physician, John Cade, noted that when lithium was administered to guinea pigs, the animals became lethargic. Taking an intuitive leap, Cade administered lithium to patients with acute mania and noted remarkable improvement. However, because of the earlier problems with lithium as a salt substitute, the medical community took more than 20 years to accept this agent as an effective treatment for mania. Fortunately, research in the 1970s found lithium to be clearly superior to placebo in the prophylaxis of bipolar disorder; less than a third of lithium-treated patients relapsed, compared with 80 percent of placebo-treated patients.

Many controlled studies demonstrate lithium's efficacy for acute mania, acute depressive episodes, and maintenance treatment for relapse prevention (Geddes et al., 2010). Baldessarini and Tondo (2000) recommended lithium as a drug of first choice for both the treatment of acute manic attacks and the long-term management of bipolar disorder:

> We suggest that the growing American urge to abandon lithium maintenance therapy as ineffective, excessively toxic, or complicated is unwarranted. No other proposed mood-stabilizing treatment has such substantial research evidence of long-term efficacy in both type I and type II bipolar disorders, as well as yielding a substantial reduction of mortality risk. (p.190)

Lithium has been referred to as the "gold standard" of bipolar treatment. Nevertheless, real-world evidence may show poorer outcomes than expected. An early study (Maj et al., 1998) reported that 28 percent of patients discontinued the drug, 38 percent experienced recurrence of the disorder even while they were taking the drug, and only 23 percent did not have recurrent episodes. Perhaps such results have led to the present situation, in which fewer clinicians are prescribing lithium in favor of neuromodulator anticonvulsants and second-generation antipsychotics. Yet lithium can be effective over long periods of time. One recent study compared clinical outcome to lithium in patients with and without atypical features. In this case, atypical features included mixed states, incomplete remissions, poor cognitive functioning in between episodes, comorbid psychiatric disorders, and poor social functioning. Data were presented from 20 years of lithium treatment across five centers. In each case, the response to lithium was stable. The drug was not better in one group compared to the other, showing that atypical features do not predict poor maintenance control (Berghöfer et al., 2008).

Pharmacokinetics

Peak blood levels of lithium are reached within 3 hours of oral administration, complete absorption by 8 hours. The drug crosses the blood-brain barrier slowly and incompletely, and, although the clinical significance of the observation is unclear, there can be a twofold variation in the concentration of lithium in the brain compared with its concentration in plasma. However, the therapeutic efficacy of lithium is directly correlated with its blood level.

Lithium is not metabolized and is excreted unchanged by the kidneys, with only small amounts excreted through the skin. About half an oral dose is eliminated within 18 to 24 hours and the rest, which is taken up by the cells of the body, is excreted over the next 1 to 2 weeks. Thus, when therapy is initiated, lithium slowly accumulates over about 2 weeks until a steady state is reached, making once-daily dosing appropriate for many patients.

Lithium has a very narrow therapeutic range below which the drug is ineffective and above which side effects and toxicity are prevalent. Usually guidelines recommend about 0.8 to 1.2 milliequivalents per liter of blood (mEq/l) for acute treatment and 0.6 to 0.8 for maintenance. More adverse effects, increasing the likelihood of noncompliance, occur at levels above 1.5 mEq/l, and levels above 2.0 mEq/l are potentially lethal. Because lithium closely resembles table salt, when a patient lowers his or her salt intake or loses excessive amounts of salt, such as through sweating, lithium blood levels may rise, inadvertently producing intoxication. Consequently, patients taking lithium should avoid marked changes in sodium intake or excretion and replenish salts after excessive exercise or illness-induced dehydration.

Pharmacodynamics

In therapeutic concentrations, lithium has almost no discernible psychotropic effect in normal persons and, unlike many psychoactive drugs, does not produce sedation, depression, or euphoria. In general, a consensus is developing that the mood-stabilizing actions of lithium and other effective antibipolar agents (Li et al., 2002) may be due to effects on intracellular second-messenger signaling systems, particularly protein kinase enzyme pathways (Hashimoto et al., 2002; Kopnisky et al., 2003). Lithium, valproate, and lamotrigine are all known to inhibit the intracellular enzyme glycogen synthase kinase-3 (GSK-3). One consequence is an increase in the level of a protein, β-catenin, that promotes cell survival and stimulates axonal growth. GSK-3 is also involved in producing amyloid-β, which is a major component of the plaques that are found in Alzheimer's disease, suggesting that GSK-3 inhibitors might someday be treatments for that disorder. In that regard, a nationwide study of lithium prescription registry data from Denmark found a decreased risk of dementia in patients who continued lithium use over a 10-year period (Kessing et al., 2008). This result supports a neuroprotective effect of lithium.

As another example, Cui and coworkers (2007) found that lithium and valproate also protected neurons in the brains of rats (in culture) from damage due to oxidative stress. Oxidative stress occurs when intracellular enzymes cannot sufficiently reduce the levels of toxic substances produced by metabolic activity. In this environment, lithium and valproate increased the amount of the antioxidant enzyme glutathione, which plays an important role in reducing oxidative damage. Furthermore, chronic treatment with lamotrigine and carbamazepine had similar effects. Valproate also influences DNA to alter genetic processes that could protect cells from injury or toxic agents. These interactions are believed to increase levels of cellular protective proteins, such as CREB and *bcl-2* and other neurotrophic substances such as BDNF (Einat and Manji, 2006; Zarate et al., 2006).

Clinical evidence shows that the laboratory results may be relevant to the therapeutic effect of these drugs. It has been reported that levels of BDNF were significantly decreased in the blood serum of patients with bipolar disorder who were either manic or depressed compared to patients who were euthymic or to healthy controls (see Figure 6.2). Another study found that the volume of gray matter in the brains of patients on lithium was as much as 15 percent larger in areas that are critical for paying attention and controlling emotions, compared to the brain volume of people without the disorder and of bipolar patients not on lithium (Bearden et al., 2007). The possibility that lithium may affect how genes are controlled means that it might also be helpful for treating genetic disorders. Evidence for this possibility was reported by researchers working with a mouse model of a lethal neurodegenerative disease called spinocerebellar ataxia type 1. Mice with this disease that were fed lithium showed improvement in coordination and memory, although lithium did not increase their life span (Watase et al., 2007). Reviews by Beaulieu and Caron (2008) and Marmol (2008) provide thorough discussions of the history, clinical application, and neurochemistry of lithium, including evidence for its neuroprotective effects in brain injury, Parkinson's disease, Huntington's chorea, and Alzheimer's disease, Unfortunately, early reports of benefit in ALS (amyotrophic lateral sclerosis) were not confirmed (Aggarwal et al., 2010).

Side Effects and Toxicity

Because of lithium's extremely narrow therapeutic range, lithium blood levels must be closely monitored. The occurrence and intensity of side effects and toxic reactions are usually related to plasma drug concentrations and involve the nervous system, the gastrointestinal (GI) tract, the kidneys, the thyroid, the cardiovascular system, and the skin.

At plasma levels of 1.5 to 2.0 mEq/l and sometimes lower, most reactions involve the GI tract, resulting in nausea, vomiting, diarrhea, and abdominal pain. Nevertheless, weight gain may be substantial during long-term therapy—up to 30 percent of patients become obese, a prevalence three times greater than in the general population that can profoundly affect compliance (Keck and McElroy, 2003).

Lithium may elicit a variety of dermatological reactions. These include rashes, acne, psoriasis, hair and nail disorders, lesions of the mucosal tissue, and other conditions (Jafferany, 2008). Chronic lithium treatment may enlarge the thyroid. As many as 60 percent of patients on lithium may experience increased thirst, water intake, and urine output (due to an impairment of renal concentrating ability). Although kidney function should be assessed periodically, permanent damage is rare.

Neurological side effects include a slight tremor, lethargy, impaired concentration, dizziness, slurred speech, ataxia, muscle weakness, and nystagmus (uncontrollable, jerky eye movements in any direction). Lithium-induced tremor is very common, and more than 30 percent of patients report this reaction even at therapeutic doses of 0.6 to 1.2 mEq/l. A hypothyroid condition may develop, and enlargement of the gland can occur at normal doses. Adverse effects on memory and cognition are common, and patients often complain of memory problems. Consistent with these effects, some researchers found improvements in motor performance, cognition, and creative ability after lithium withdrawal. Severe cognitive deficits are seen with lithium intoxication.

At plasma lithium levels above 2.0 mEq/l, more severe side effects include fatigue, muscle weakness, slurred speech, and worsening tremors. Thyroid gland function becomes more depressed and the gland may enlarge further, resulting in goiter. Muscle fasciculations, abnormal motor movements, psychosis, and stupor may occur. Above

2.5 mEq/l, toxic symptoms include muscle rigidity, coma, renal failure, cardiac arrhythmias, and death.

Treatment of poisoning or overdose is nonspecific; there is no antidote to lithium. Usually drug administration is stopped and sodium-containing fluids are infused immediately. If toxic signs are serious, hemodialysis, gastric lavage, diuretic therapy, antiepileptic medication, and other supports may be needed. Complete recovery may be prolonged, with full return of renal and neurological function taking weeks or months.

Effects in Pregnancy

In general, lithium is not advised during pregnancy, particularly in the first trimester, as the risk of fetal malformation of the cardiovascular system—in particular, the tricuspid valve—is increased (Ernst and Goldberg, 2002). If mood stabilization is necessary during pregnancy, other agents (such as lamotrigine) are preferred, if possible. When a pregnant woman is on lithium therapy, the drug should be discontinued several days before delivery because (1) when the water breaks, acute dehydration will quickly increase lithium to toxic levels and (2) the newborn will have difficulty excreting the drug. On the other hand, it is important for the mother to restart her lithium within 24 hours of delivery to reduce the risk of relapse. Breast-feeding is also contraindicated during lithium therapy because lithium passes easily into breast milk. The use of lithium and alternatives for bipolar patients in pregnancy is discussed further in Chapter 18.

Noncompliance

Noncompliance is associated with significant morbidity, recurrent manic episodes, and greatly increased suicide risk. Nevertheless, up to 50 percent of patients on lithium stop taking the drug against medical advice. Some years ago it was felt that discontinuation of lithium treatment would result in treatment resistance when therapy was resumed, but this does not appear to be the case.

Noncompliance seems to result primarily from intolerance of side effects, particularly memory impairment and cognitive slowing, weight gain, and the subjective feeling of reduced energy and productivity. Other reasons include missing the manic "highs," belief that the disorder has resolved and the drug is unnecessary, and feelings of stigmatism in having a psychiatric illness.

Lithium therapy reduces suicidal behaviors in bipolar patients. Unfortunately, when patients stopped taking the drug, the rate of suicide attempts increased fourteenfold and the rate of completed suicides thirteenfold. The prophylactic effect of lithium was confirmed by Cipriani and coworkers (2005), who reported that lithium was effective in the prevention of suicide, deliberate self-harm, and death from all causes in patients with mood disorders. It should be appreciated that reduction of suicidal behavior occurs independently of lithium's effect on mood. There is growing evidence for the effectiveness of lithium as an antisuicide agent, even when used as an adjunct medication, in any situation in which suicide is a concern (Baldessarini et al., 2006).

Combination Therapy

Combination therapy—often lithium plus an antiepileptic or antipsychotic drug—can provide both greater therapeutic efficacy and better protection against relapse than lithium therapy alone. In fact, combination therapy has become the rule rather than the exception (Geddes et al., 2004), with lithium most effective for mania, for augmenting antidepressant efficacy in refractory patients, and for maintenance; and an anticonvulsant such as lamotrigine often helpful against bipolar depression as well as mania (Goodwin et al., 2004). Moreover, there is some evidence that such combinations may also exert greater neuroprotective effects on the brain (Leng et al., 2008).

"Neuromodulator" Anticonvulsant Mood Stabilizers

Only about 60 to 70 percent of patients with bipolar disorder can be adequately controlled by lithium alone, both for maintenance and for relapse prevention; and lithium is even less effective in controlling episodes of rapid-cycling mania. Therefore, there is a need for alternative agents effective in patients who are treatment-refractory, noncompliant with therapy, or intolerant of lithium's side effects. One alternative is anticonvulsants (Chapter 7, Appendix). The variety of disorders for which these drugs are now used is much broader than their original indication for epilepsy. Their use in alcohol detoxification and relapse prevention is described in Chapter 13; Chapter 7 describes their use in the treatment of anxiety disorders and the control of emotional outbursts in such disorders as posttraumatic stress disorder (PTSD); Chapter 18 describes their use in treating aggressive and explosive behavioral disorders in children and adolescents. Treating people afflicted with this variety of disorders with an antiepileptic drug may give the wrong impression that somehow they are "epileptic." To avoid this misconception, we introduce the broader term *neuromodulator* (to be used interchangeably with *anticonvulsant*), reflecting the diverse clinical applications of these agents.

First-generation anticonvulsants included phenobarbital, other barbiturates, and phenytoin and its derivatives, none of which were useful in treating bipolar illness.[3] Second-generation anticonvulsants included valproic acid (Divalproex, Depakote), and carbamazepine (Tegretol), which have significant side effects that limit their use.

In particular, many of the antiepileptic drugs (AEDs) produce birth defects. However, there is great variability among reports. This variability may be because the baseline rate of all major congenital anomalies in newborns in the U.S. population is between 2 and 4 percent (Montouris, 2005) and because epilepsy per se is associated with an increased risk of such anomalies (Perucca, 2005). There is also agreement that the magnitude of the risk increases in offspring exposed to polypharmacy (Perucca, 2005). The most common congenital malformations from anticonvulsants are the same as the malformations in the general population, for example, heart defects, club foot, and cleft palate. This topic is discussed more extensively in Chapter 18.

In addition to these concerns, the FDA notified health care professionals in January 2008 that the agency had analyzed the reports of suicidality (suicidal behavior or ideation) from anticonvulsant studies and found a significantly greater risk (0.43 percent) compared to patients receiving placebo (0.22 percent). Nearly a year later, a study (Gibbons et al., 2009) stated that patients with bipolar disorder treated with anticonvulsants attempted suicide at the same rate as patients who received either lithium or no medication. In this population, the suicide attempt rate was higher *before* the patients received the medications than afterwards. Nevertheless, the FDA warning has been supported by an analysis of individual medications based on a large dataset of more than 250,000 patients who started taking an anticonvulsant for any indication from July 2001 to December 2006 (Patorno et al., 2010). Although not all anticonvulsants were associated with an increased risk, the results showed that the classwide warning was warranted.

Carbamazepine

Studies conducted in the early 1990s indicated that carbamazepine (Tegretol; see Figure 6.3) might be as effective as lithium in preventing the recurrence of mania. However, in bipolar patients not previously treated with mood stabilizers, lithium is superior to carbamazepine in prophylactic efficacy (Hartong et al., 2003). Nevertheless, some patients who do not respond adequately to either agent alone are helped by the combination of the two drugs (Keck and McElroy, 2002). Because of the correlation between therapeutic effectiveness and plasma level, one reason patients may fail to respond to carba-

---

[3] Phenytoin was never widely used as a mood stabilizer, although there are some positive reports from one group of investigators (Mishory et al., 2000; Bersudsky, 2005).

mazepine is inadequate blood levels. The therapeutic level for epilepsy and for bipolar disorder is estimated to be the same, between 8 and 12 µg/ml.

Several possible mechanisms have been proposed to explain carbamazepine's action in treating epilepsy and bipolar disorder. Its anticonvulsant effects may occur because it reduces neuronal excitation by blocking sodium channels and thus the ability of sodium to initiate action potentials. Its benefit for bipolar disorder may be related to the fact that carbamazepine, like lithium, inhibits enzyme activity in intracellular second-messenger systems. In the treatment of bipolar disorder, carbamazepine is useful for prophylaxis—that is, reducing the frequency of episodes—and it may be the better choice for episodes of mixed mania and rapid cycling.

Adverse effects of carbamazepine include GI upset, sedation, ataxia, visual disturbances, and rare but life-threatening dermatological reactions, many of which may be caused by a metabolite, carbamazepine-epoxide. While the risk of the skin reactions is 1 to 6 per 10,000 new users of the drug in countries with mainly Caucasian populations, the risk is estimated to be about 10 times higher in some Asian countries. Consequently, the FDA announced, in late 2007, that manufacturers must add a recommendation to the labeling that patients of Asian ancestry get a genetic blood test that would indicate whether they were in the population at risk. Although impairment of higher-order cognitive functioning is modest, some patients may be particularly sensitive to this side effect. More serious reactions involve the blood and range from a relatively benign reduction in white blood cell count (leucopenia) to, on rare occasions, a severe reduction, called agranulocytosis. For this reason it received a "black box" warning and a recommendation for periodic blood analyses.[4]

Drug interactions involving carbamazepine are common and result from drug-induced stimulation of drug-metabolizing enzymes, especially CYP-3A4 in the liver. As a result, acute blood levels may decrease, which may require increasing the dose by up to 100 percent to maintain a therapeutic blood level. This effect also extends to other drugs metabolized by the same enzyme family when combined with carbamazepine.

As stated, because carbamazepine is potentially teratogenic, it should not be administered during pregnancy if at all possible.

It was approved by the FDA in 2005 for the treatment of manic and mixed episodes in an extended-release form (Equetro).

---

[4] A black box warning is an FDA-mandated list of adverse effects placed in a large black box just below the drug name on the package insert that accompanies every container of prescription medication received by a pharmacy.

Oxcarbazepine

Oxcarbazepine (Trileptal) can be considered a safer carbamazepine, capable of replacing carbamazepine for all its uses with comparable efficacy and greatly improved safety. The difference is the result of a small structural variation between the two drugs (see Figure 6.3). Oxcarbazepine is essentially carbamazepine with an oxygen molecule attached to one of the rings. The liver can thus easily metabolize the drug by a process called hydroxylation. In fact, this process occurs within 5 minutes after drug absorption, and the monohydroxy derivative is the active form of the drug; oxcarbazepine is therefore an inactive "prodrug." Because of this easy metabolic process, there is no enzyme induction, no alteration in liver enzymes, no white blood cell problems, no required blood monitoring, and few drug interactions.

Oxcarbazepine is approved for use in epilepsy, and it is becoming widely used to treat bipolar disorder and other disorders treatable with carbamazepine (Ghaemi et al., 2003). It has been shown to be superior to placebo in the treatment of acute mania in adults and comparable to lithium, valproate, and the antipsychotic haloperidol. However, Wagner and coworkers (2006) found no difference between oxcarbazepine and placebo in children and adolescents. There is less information about its use in pregnant women (Chapter 18).

Valproic Acid

Valproate (valproic acid, divalproex, Depakene, Depacon, Depakote; see Figure 6.3) is the second anticonvulsant that was systematically studied for treatment of bipolar illness, and it has been used for this disorder since its introduction in 1994. In 2008 the FDA approved a delayed-release valproate therapy in soft gel capsule (Stavzor), for BD, epilepsy, and migraine headache. In 2009 the FDA approved a generic version of Depakote extended-release (ER) tablets.

Several actions of valproic acid have been identified. First, it binds to and inhibits GABA transaminase, the enzyme that breaks down GABA. Therefore, the drug's anticonvulsant activity may be related to increased brain concentrations of GABA, as a result of its metabolic inhibition. Second, valproic acid may increase GABA by blocking its reuptake into glia and nerve endings. Third, valproic acid may also work by suppressing repetitive neuronal firing through inhibition of voltage-sensitive sodium channels. A fourth mechanism was proposed by Chen and coworkers (1999), who observed an effect of valproate on enzymes associated with the cellular organization of DNA. By influencing these enzymes and altering DNA function, valproate may be involved in gene transcription.

Valproate is particularly effective in the treatment of acute mania, mixed states, schizoaffective disorder, and rapid-cycling bipolar disorder. It may be more effective than other agents in treating lithium-resistant patients, producing a positive response in up to 71 percent of patients. The combination of valproate and lithium may be more efficacious than either agent alone. A recent, randomized, open-label, multisite, international, two-year trial compared the effectiveness of lithium, valproate, and their combination in preventing relapse. Relapse, defined as intervention for a new mood episode, occurred in 54 percent of the combination subgroup, 59 percent of those on lithium alone, and 69 percent of those on valproate alone. The first two treatments were not different from each other and were statistically better than the third. The combination seemed best at preventing manic episodes and lithium alone in preventing depressive episodes. Results were not affected by the baseline severity, the polarity of the most recent episode, drug doses, or blood levels. Although the study had no placebo group, it was a real-world design and argues for greater use of lithium (Geddes et al., 2010). Valproate is not more effective than lithium for rapid-cycling BD (Calabrese et al., 2005a) or for rapid-cycling BD with comorbid substance abuse (Kemp et al., 2009).

Valproic acid has traditionally been administered in divided doses through the day. An extended-release preparation allows once-daily dosing, usually at bedtime, to improve compliance and help alleviate daytime sedation and memory impairment. There is no consistent evidence to show that giving this drug intravenously would speed the onset of action, which normally takes 3 to 10 days (Phrolov et al., 2004). Depakene comes in capsules and as a syrup, while Depacon is the intravenous solution and Depakote is the formulation of tablets or delayed-release tablets.

Side effects associated with valproate include GI upset, sedation, lethargy, hand tremor, alopecia (hair loss), and some metabolic changes in the liver. In females starting valproate before the age of 20, the drug has been associated with an 8 percent prevalence of marked obesity, polycystic ovaries, and markedly increased levels of serum androgens (increased testosterone levels). Valproate may be slightly more detrimental to cognitive function than carbamazepine.

Like lithium and carbamazepine, valproate can be teratogenic, increasing the risk of spina bifida, neural tube defects, and developmental deficits in the infant. In fact, it has been suggested that this property may be related to its interaction with DNA. Withdrawal symptoms, including irritability, jitteriness, abnormal tone, feeding difficulties, and seizures, have been described in infants whose mothers took valproate during pregnancy. Consequently, caution must be exercised in using valproate in women who may become pregnant during drug therapy (see Chapter 18).

Other serious side effects of valproate, which have resulted in black box warnings, include hepatotoxicity (liver damage) and pancreatitis (inflammation of the pancreas).

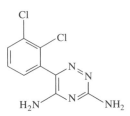

Lamotrigine
(Lamictal)

FIGURE 6.4 Chemical structure of lamotrigine (Lamictal); also shown in Figure 7.7.

Lamotrigine

The third-generation anticonvulsant neuromodulator lamotrigine (Lamictal; Figure 6.4) has rapidly been accepted as an important monotherapeutic drug for treatment of acute bipolar depression and rapid-cycling bipolar II disorder as well as the prevention of recurrent bipolar depressive episodes. It was as effective as lithium in preventing relapse to any manic episode and better than lithium in preventing relapse to a depressive episode (Bowden et al., 2003). Conversely, it is not useful for acute mania. It is now a first-line therapy for patients with rapid-cycling bipolar II as well as bipolar depression, and it is less likely to cause a manic shift compared with the conventional antidepressants (Goldberg et al., 2009; Keck et al., 2003).

In 2003 lamotrigine was approved for the long-term maintenance of adults with bipolar I disorder, that is, for delaying the time to relapse to depressive and manic symptoms in BP-I disorder. This benefit is most evident if patients respond acutely to lamotrigine. Although this clinical effect suggests that lamotrigine might be effective for acute bipolar depression, this was not the case in five different studies; that is, lamotrigine performed no better than placebo. Although most of these data were not published, the manufacturer, GlaxoSmithKline, has posted results of all its studies on its Web site (http://ctr.gsk.co.uk/Summary/lamotrigine/studylist.asp).

Generic lamotrigine tablets were approved in 2008 and the chewable tablet formulation in 2009. In 2009 the FDA also approved Lamictal (lamotrigine) orally disintegrating tablets for long-term treatment of BP I to lengthen the time between mood episodes in people 18 years or older who have been treated with other medicine for mood episodes. The doses will match the current tablets.

The major mechanism of action of lamotrigine is blockade of voltage-dependent sodium channel conductance. It has been found to inhibit depolarization of the glutaminergic presynaptic membrane, thus reducing release of glutamate, particularly in the cortex and hippocampus. This decrease in neuronal excitability may account for its antiepileptic, mood-stabilizing, and analgesic effects (Ketter et al., 2003), and it may also have some neuroprotective effects in people who suffer traumatic brain injuries (Pachet et al., 2003).

After oral administration, lamotrigine is rapidly and completely absorbed, reaching peak plasma concentrations in 1 to 5 hours. It is metabolized before excretion, with a half-life of 26 hours, which can decrease to about 7.4 hours when used with phenytoin or carbamazepine (requiring increased doses of lamotrigine) or increase to 60 hours when used with valproate (requiring decreased doses of lamotrigine) (Hurley, 2002). Therapeutic blood concentrations of lamotrigine used to treat epilepsy are in the range of about 1.5 to 5 μg/ml (mg/L), with adverse effects increasing with higher doses (Hirsch et al, 2004). It is presumed that the same concentration range applies to treatment of bipolar disorder.

Side effects associated with lamotrigine include dizziness, tremor, somnolence, headache, nausea, and rash. The most serious side effect is rash, which conceivably may be severe enough to require hospitalization and prove fatal. Adolescents are believed to be more prone to this reaction, so the drug is not indicated for patients younger than 16 years of age. The incidence of rash is currently about 1 in 500, which has not recently been a problem; a slow titration of dose over about 6 weeks is thought to reduce the incidence (Calabrese et al., 2002).

In marked contrast to other antiepileptic agents, lamotrigine can improve cognitive functioning. In one study (Khan et al., 2004), after discontinuation of other drugs, separate groups of patients, diagnosed with either mania (349) or depression (966), were maintained for 8 to 16 weeks on lamotrigine monotherapy. Both groups showed cognitive improvements, manic patients more than depressed patients. Even after correcting for improvements in mood, there were significant improvements in cognition when switching from other medications.

Data are still inadequate to determine the risks of developmental effects of fetal exposure to lamotrigine; however, current evidence indicates that the risk is much lower than for valproate or carbamazepine. Today, lamotrigine appears to be the drug of choice for pregnant women with bipolar disorder (Ornoy, 2006; see Chapter 18 for further discussion).

Gabapentin and Pregabalin

Introduced in the United States in 1993 as an anticonvulsant for the treatment of partial complex seizures, *gabapentin* (Neurontin) is also used for the treatment of anxiety, neuropathic pain, substance dependency, and behavioral dyscontrol, as well as bipolar disorder. Mechanistically, it is a GABA analogue, but it has little or no action on the GABA receptor. Although it increases GABA levels, it is not clear how much the increase contributes to the efficacy of the drug. A derivative of gabapentin, *pregabalin* (Lyrica), was approved for use in the United States in 2005 for the treatment of pain states, such as diabetic peripheral neuropathy and postherpetic neuralgia, and as adjunctive therapy in the treatment of partial seizures in adults (Beydoun et al., 2005). In June 2007 the FDA approved Lyrica for the treatment of fibromyalgia.

The most recent hypothesis for the mechanism of action of these two drugs is that they interact with a component of the calcium channels in presynaptic neuronal membranes to decrease the influx of calcium ions. As a result, less neurotransmitter is released, which translates into antiepileptic, analgesic, and anxiolytic effects (Chiu et al., 2005).

Gabapentin has an excellent pharmacokinetic profile: it is not bound to plasma proteins; it is not metabolized; it is excreted unchanged through the kidneys, with an elimination half-life of 5 to 7 hours; and it has few pharmacokinetic drug interactions. Gabapentin is absorbed by a saturable active transport mechanism from intestine to plasma, so doses up to 1500 milligrams can be given at any one time. Like gabapentin, pregabalin is excreted unchanged, and therefore it has no effect on the liver. Because it is excreted unchanged, it can be safely used in the treatment of alcoholism (Chapter 13). It is two to three times as potent as gabapentin and has a slightly longer half-life of 6 to 8 hours. It is clear that gabapentin (and presumably pregabalin) is not effective as monotherapy for bipolar disorder. However, there is evidence that these drugs may be very beneficial for neuropathic pain and at least some types of anxiety disorders, as described below.

Topiramate

Topiramate (Topamax), discussed in Chapter 13 as an antiepileptic drug used to prevent relapse to detrimental drinking patterns in people with alcoholism, is a very potent anticonvulsant and has been approved by the FDA for the treatment of migraine headaches. Structurally different from other agents in this group, it is derived from the sugar D-fructose and was initially developed as an antidiabetic drug. Topiramate has multiple mechanisms of action. It exerts an inhibitory effect on sodium conductance, decreasing the duration of spontaneous bursts and the frequency of generated action potentials; it enhances GABA by unknown mechanisms; and it blocks the AMPA subtype glutamate receptor.

The initial positive results of open-label studies of the drug used to treat bipolar disorder were not supported by four recent clinical trials showing topiramate monotherapy to be ineffective in acute mania (Kushner et al., 2006). In addition, topiramate was no different than placebo when combined with either valproate or lithium for the treatment of bipolar I disorder (Chengappa et al., 2006). The main advantage of topiramate is that it is associated with weight loss rather than weight gain. This characteristic may make the drug useful as an adjunctive agent to offset the weight gain associated with other antimanic drugs. Preliminary evidence indicates positive effects in comorbid bipolar disorder and bulimia and bipolar disorder and binge eating (McElroy et al., 2004), and it may be preferred in obese patients with either unipolar or bipolar disorder who want to lose weight.

Unfortunately, the cognitive impairment (especially problems in word-finding) induced by topiramate is greater than that produced by other anticonvulsants, although impairment may occur more frequently at higher doses and with rapid dose increases. Other side effects include tingling in the extremities, irritability, anxiety, and depression. However, these effects may subside within a few weeks.

Topiramate is excreted unchanged and has a reduced likelihood of being involved in drug interactions mediated by the liver. However, this drug has the potential to increase plasma levels of other drugs excreted by the kidneys, such as lithium. It may also increase the incidence of kidney stones. In 2009 the FDA approved generic Topamax, as topiramate tablets, and a generic version of Topamax (Sprinkle) as topiramate capsules (Sprinkle).

Zonisamide

Zonisamide (Zonegran) is an antiepileptic drug long available in Japan, which became available in the United States in mid-2000 for the treatment of epilepsy. Its major mechanism of action is reduction of neuronal repetitive firing by blocking sodium channels and preventing neurotransmitter release. It also acts on calcium channels, preventing the influx of calcium ions, and it may exert neuroprotective effects.

Preliminary studies showing positive effects in small numbers of patients with bipolar disorder were not supported by subsequent research. Overall, zonisamide has inconsistent effects against mania or bipolar depression and a high dropout rate, mostly due to side effects such as worsening of mood and sedation or lack of efficacy (Goodnick, 2007; Wilson and Findling, 2007). Other side effects include reduced white blood cell counts, elevated liver enzymes, and several drug interactions. Like topiramate, this drug may be of use in treating binge eating.

Tiagabine and Retigabine

The mechanism of action of tiagabine as an anticonvulsant involves inhibition of the active reuptake of GABA by inhibiting the GABA transporter in the hippocampus and cerebral cortex. In spite of some initial positive reports, this drug has not been found efficacious in the treatment of bipolar disorder.

Retigabine is a newer antiepileptic drug, expected to become commercially available for the treatment of seizure disorders (Porter et al., 2007). Early evidence indicates that the drug may be effective in mania (Amann et al., 2006), as a neuroprotective agent (Boscia et al., 2006), and as an anxiolytic (Korsgaard et al., 2005).

Other Uses for Anticonvulsant Mood Stabilizers

Neuropathic Pain

The overlap between the underlying pathophysiologic mechanisms of some epilepsy models and neuropathic pain models supports the rationale for using certain anticonvulsant drugs in the treatment of neuropathic pain. Patients with trigeminal neuralgia have been treated with carbamazepine for decades, and topiramate is the second antiepileptic drug, after valproate, to be approved for the prevention of migraine (in 2004). Because recommended doses are much lower than those for other indications, the cognitive side effects may not be as troublesome for migraine. Gabapentin has proven effective against neuropathic pain induced by diabetic neuropathy, postherpetic neuralgia, and spinal cord injury. Data from clinical studies show that pregabalin (Lyrica) shares this analgesic effectiveness. Efficacy has been demonstrated in a number of clinical studies, including those in patients with diabetic neuropathy and fibromyalgia. Treatment of neuropathic pain is seen as the drug's leading indication. McDonald and Portenoy (2006) provide an excellent review of the use of anticonvulsants in neuropathic pain states.

Anxiety Disorders

Pregabalin has shown early onset of action and short-term and long-term efficacy in patients with generalized anxiety disorder (Feltner et al., 2003; Pande et al., 2003). A ten-week, randomized, open-label trial of tiagabine and paroxetine found that both agents significantly reduced anxiety and depressive symptoms and improved sleep quality and overall functioning (Rosenthal, 2003). In addition, topiramate has been found useful for the treatment of posttraumatic stress disorder (Berlant and van Kammen, 2002) in decreasing nightmares and flashbacks in the majority of patients. In social phobia, gabapentin was found to be superior to placebo (Pande et al., 1999), and one randomized placebo-controlled study found that gabapentin reduced panic symptoms in severe panic disorder (Pande et al., 2000).

Borderline Personality Disorder

Borderline personality disorder is characterized by emotional instability, impulsivity, and aggression and is associated with considerable morbidity and mortality. It is a common comorbid condition with bipolar disorder. All the medications routinely used in treating bipolar disorder have been shown in published studies to have some value in treating borderline personality disorder: antidepressants, mood stabilizers, and antipsychotics ameliorate the irritability and anger and reduce the tempestuousness of the relationships and the impulsive aggressiveness of these patients. However, numerous studies indicated that the neuromodulator anticonvulsants had a particular benefit in this regard, and this has recently been supported in two reviews (Lieb et al., 2010; Mercer et al., 2009) and a meta-analysis of randomized controlled trials (Ingenhoven et al., 2010). Mood stabilizers had a pronounced effect on impulsive behavioral dyscontrol, anger and anxiety; antipsychotics had a moderate effect on the various symptoms; and antidepressants were the least effective in this situation.

Aggression and Behavioral Dyscontrol

Impulsive aggressive behavior is common in psychiatric disorders and accounts for significant morbidity and mortality. In a multicenter, randomized placebo-controlled study, Hollander and colleagues (2003) evaluated the effect of valproic acid in outpatients diagnosed with intermittent explosive disorder, posttraumatic stress disorder, or Cluster B personality disorders (borderline, antisocial, histrionic, and narcissistic disorders). They found statistically significant treatment effects only for the Cluster B group on measures such as verbal assault and assault against objects: valproate was superior to placebo in the treatment of impulsive aggression, irritability, and global severity. In a comparison study, carbamazepine and valproate were reported to produce a significant reduction in "impulsive aggression" compared with placebo (Stanford et al., 2005). As an adjunct medication, oxcarbazepine has reduced aggressive behavior in developmentally disabled adults (Jankowsky et al., 2003).

Atypical Antipsychotics for Bipolar Disorder

For decades, traditional antipsychotic drugs have been used to help control the symptoms and behaviors associated with acute mania. In fact, the use of traditional antipsychotic drugs predated the use of lithium by 20 years. Recently, the antimanic potency of the typical antipsychotics was found to be positively associated with their affinity for D_2 receptors, which supported a "dopamine-blockade" hypothesis of antimanic drug action (Harrison-Read, 2009). These observations are consistent with the possibility that schizophrenia and BD share some common genetic origin (Lichtenstein et al., 2009).

All the second-generation antipsychotics have also shown efficacy either as monotherapy or as adjunctive agents for acute mania, and they have all been approved for this indication. Recent comparisons show that there is no difference among them compared with placebo (Perlis et al., 2006a). Furthermore, the first-generation antipsychotic haloperidol was also shown to be as good as risperidone, olanzapine, carbamazepine, or valproate when used alone or as an add-on medication—although it was less efficacious than aripiprazole (Vieta et al., 2005). Not surprisingly, haloperidol also produced less weight gain but more movement disorders than the other agents (Cipriani et al., 2006).

In their meta-analysis, Scherk and coworkers (2007) concluded:

> SGAs as add-on medication to mood stabilizers are superior to mood stabilizers alone for acute manic symptoms, as indicated by greater reductions in mania scores, higher response rates, and fewer dropouts due to inefficacy. . . . Combination treatment with a second-generation atypical antipsychotic and a mood stabilizer should be the treatment of choice, in particular for severe manic episodes. (p. 442)

A consensus guideline on the use of aripiprazole for the treatment of mania was recently published in the United Kingdom (Aitchison et al., 2009).

Subsequent trials have examined the efficacy of the SGAs for bipolar depression and maintenance of remission. Risperidone has been found effective in extension trials as monotherapy or adjunctive treatment in sustaining remission from mania while not inducing depression (Hirschfield et al., 2006; Rendell et al., 2006). Olanzapine (Tohen et al., 2006), quetiapine (Calabrese et al., 2005b), aripiprazole (Keck et al., 2006, 2007), and ziprasidone (Bowden et al., 2010) have all been found more effective than placebo for maintenance treatment, and olanzapine was reported comparable to lithium (Tohen et al., 2005).

Olanzapine alone has been reported to be as effective for bipolar depression as the antidepressant fluoxetine alone or in combination as the recently approved drug Symbyax (Amsterdam and Shults, 2005; Corya et al., 2006). Symbyax was also found to be as effective as lamotrigine for the treatment of bipolar depression (Brown et al., 2006). Both Symbyax and lamotrigine had an equally low risk of inducing mania, which is a serious concern with antidepressant treatment for bipolar disorder. To determine whether there is a difference among the newer antidepressants in inducing mania, studies have examined the relative risk of three other antidepressants—sertraline, bupropion, and venlafaxine—producing a "switch" when used as adjuncts to mood stabilizers. Overall, the rate was higher for bipolar I (30.8 percent) than bipolar II (18.6 percent), although eventually only 23.3 percent of patients did not switch. However, venlafaxine was reported to be more likely than the other two antidepressants to produce a switch (Leverich et al., 2006; Post et al.,

2006). These results suggest that people with bipolar II might be less vulnerable to an antidepressant-induced switch. This suggestion is supported by Altshuler and coworkers (2006), who found less switching with adjunctive selective serotonergic reuptake inhibitors in bipolar II than in bipolar I patients, and by Parker and coworkers (2006b), who successfully treated depressed bipolar II patients for nine months with SSRIs, without any worsening of symptoms.

Several recent studies have supported the use of quetiapine in treating bipolar depression. In a retrospective chart review, 69 percent of depressed bipolar patients showed improvement with quetiapine (Shajahan and Taylor, 2010). Two clinical trials reported that quetiapine was statistically better than placebo in treating bipolar depression, whereas neither lithium (Young et al., 2010) nor paroxetine (McElroy et al., 2010) differed from the respective placebo control groups. In 2009, Seroquel XR (quetiapine fumarate) extended-release tablets were approved by the FDA for acute treatment for depressive, manic, and mixed bipolar disorder episodes and for maintenance therapy as adjunctive treatment to lithium or divalproex. The new formulation was not approved for patients with dementia-related psychosis or for patients younger than 18 years.

Although the SGAs may be less likely to elicit movement disorders than the older drugs in schizophrenic patients, there is evidence that patients with bipolar disorder may be more susceptible to these side effects (Ghaemi et al., 2006). One meta-analysis (Gao et al., 2008) concluded that bipolar patients were approximately twice as likely as schizophrenia patients to suffer movement disorders (extrapyramidal symptoms, akathisia) and an increase in anticholinergic drug treatment of these symptoms. Only olanzapine was not different from placebo, in either bipolar or schizophrenia patients, while aripiprazole was more likely to cause akathisia in bipolar patients but not schizophrenic patients.

Omega-3 Fatty Acids for Bipolar Disorder

In countries where the diet is rich in fish oils, the incidence of bipolar disorder is quite low (Noaghiul and Hibbeln, 2003). Therefore, it is possible that fish oils may prevent BD, perhaps by protecting the brain from the neuronal injuries now being identified in this disorder. Omega-3 fatty acids, obtained from marine or plant sources, are known to damp these signal transduction pathways in a variety of cell systems (Parker et al., 2006a).

Stoll and coworkers (1999) found that augmentation of antimanic treatment with omega-3 fatty acids compared to placebo greatly increased the time before recurrence of a bipolar episode, even in patients who were not taking any other medication. Two reviews (Parker et al., 2006a; Marengell et al., 2006) summarized the subsequent research regarding the association of omega-3 fatty acid consumption with rates of mood disorders, the relationship between physiological markers of omega-3 fatty acids and mood disorders, and results of omega-3 fatty acid treatment of mood disorders. But although there is some support for the role of omega-3 fatty acids in slowing the recurrence of episodes of bipolar and other mood disorders, the results of clinical trials have been inconsistent. Similarly, a subsequent review (Montgomery and Richardson, 2008) also concluded that, despite "intriguing" findings, there is still not enough evidence to say whether this treatment is useful for bipolar disorder. Results of a small study of children with bipolar disorder are consistent with this conclusion. Over an eight-week period, only about 35 percent of the patients (6 to 17 years of age) had even a modest response of a 50 percent decrease in manic symptoms (Wozniak et al., 2007).

Miscellaneous Agents

Many patients are unresponsive to or intolerant of present medications, and alternative agents are much needed. Several different types of drugs have been tried.

The anticholinergic drug *scopolamine* produces some effects resembling manic symptoms, such as flight of ideas, talkativeness, and difficulties in concentration. Therefore, agents that potentiate the effect of acetylcholine might have some antimanic action. *Donepezil* inhibits the enzyme acetylcholinesterase and therefore might help patients with bipolar disorder. However, a double-blind placebo-controlled trial found no effect of adjunctive donepezil in patients with refractory mania (Evins et al., 2006).

Because lithium interferes with membrane ion function, *calcium channel blockers,* such as *verapamil,* have been tried, but their effectiveness remains questionable. *Clonidine,* an antihypertensive drug, has been tried in treatment-refractory patients with bipolar disorder. It was hypothesized that the action of clonidine in decreasing the release of norepinephrine might reduce manic episodes. Despite initial positive results, effectiveness remains unproved.

Kulkarni and colleagues (2006) reported that the hormonal agents *tamoxifen* and *medroxyprogesterone acetate* were more effective than placebo in improving the symptoms of mania in 13 women with acute bipolar affective disorder. Although most commonly used for its anti-estrogenic property in the treatment of breast cancer, tamoxifen is a potent inhibitor of the enzyme protein kinase C, which is involved in intracellular signal transduction. It is this mechanism that may be the route by which it affects bipolar disorder.

Although not considered a mood stabilizer, the wakefulness-promoting agent *modafinil* has been useful for alleviating fatigue accompanying many medical conditions, including depression.[5] A retrospective chart review study found modafinil effective in relieving fatigue and sleepiness in adults with unipolar or bipolar depression (Nasr et al., 2006). The authors report that no patient demonstrated a switch into mania or hypomania while on modafinil. A small prospective study (which excluded patients with a history of stimulant-induced mania) also found a significantly greater improvement in depression symptoms, and in remission, in adults with bipolar depression (Frye et al., 2007).

Psychotherapeutic and Psychosocial Treatments

Increasing focus on the pharmacologic treatment of bipolar disorders has sometimes led clinicians to forgo psychological interventions as an adjunctive treatment (Colom et al., 2003, p. 402). Patients with bipolar disorder suffer from the psychosocial consequences of past episodes, the ongoing vulnerability to future episodes, and the burdens of adhering to a long-term treatment plan that may involve some unpleasant side effects. In addition, many patients have clinically significant mood instability between episodes.

Successful treatment involves a social network primed to recognize the early symptoms of an episode, to seek help for patients who lack insight into their condition, and to assist with recognition of side effects and toxicities, thus aiding in compliance with therapy. Issues of importance include the following:

* Emotional consequences of periods of major mood disorder and diagnosis of a chronic mental illness
* Developmental deviations and delays caused by past episodes
* Problems associated with stigmatization
* Problems regulating self-esteem
* Fears of recurrence and consequent inhibition of normal psychosocial functioning
* Interpersonal difficulties
* Marriage, family, childbearing, and parenting issues
* Academic and occupational problems
* Other legal, social, and emotional problems that arise from reckless, violent, withdrawn, or bizarre behavior that may occur during episodes

---

[5] Modafinil (as Provigil) is approved by the FDA for helping persons with the disease *narcolepsy* stay awake during the day, maintaining daytime wakefulness, and promoting more tiredness at bedtime.

It is also important to ensure that the manic state is not being caused by medications, such as antidepressants, caffeine, herbals containing ephedrine, behavioral stimulants (including illegal drugs, such as cocaine), corticosteroids (cortisone), anabolic steroids, antiparkinsonian drugs, over-the-counter cough and cold preparations, and diet aids. One must also rule out thyroid disease because mania secondary to thyroid hyperactivity is common.

Among psychotherapeutic interventions used concomitantly with pharmacotherapy are group psychoeducation (Colom et al., 2003), cognitive-behavioral therapy (Lam et al., 2003; Otto et al., 2003), psychodynamically oriented therapy, family therapy, couples therapy, interpersonal psychotherapy, and self-help groups. As part of the STEP-BD study, Miklowitz and coworkers (2007) studied the efficacy of four disorder-specific psychotherapies in conjunction with pharmacotherapy in treating bipolar depression. Intensive psychotherapy given weekly or biweekly was superior to less intensive interventions in shortening the time to recovery and increasing the likelihood of remaining well (see also Geller and Goldberg, 2007). Chapter 20 provides a general discussion concerning the integration of psychopharmacological and psychological treatments for mental illness.

STUDY QUESTIONS

1. What are the major pharmacological drug categories useful in the treatment of bipolar disorder and the major drugs in each category?

2. List the clinical uses of lithium.

3. Describe the correlations between plasma levels of lithium and the therapeutic and side effects of lithium.

4. What are the major organ systems affected by lithium and the drug's major side effects on each system?

5. Discuss the effects of the various mood stabilizers on memory and cognitive behaviors.

6. Discuss the comorbidity of bipolar disorder with other psychological disorders.

7. List the advantages and disadvantages of the antiepileptic drugs used to treat BD.

8. What medications, drugs, or diseases might precipitate or worsen bipolar illness?

9. Describe the possible role of omega-3 fatty acids in bipolar illness.

10. How can a health care professional who is not the prescribing physician contribute to the well-being of the bipolar patient?

REFERENCES

Aggarwal, S. P., et al. (2010). "Safety and Efficacy of Lithium in Combination with Riluzole for Treatment of Amyotrophic Lateral Sclerosis: A Randomized, Double-Blind, Placebo-Controlled Trial." *Lancet Neurology* 9: 481–488.

Aitchison. K. J., et al. (2009). "A UK Consensus on the Administration of Aripirazole for the Treatment of Mania." *Journal of Psychopharmacology* 23: 231–240.

Altshuler, L. L., et al. (2006). "Lower Switch Rate in Depressed Patients with Bipolar II than Bipolar I Disorder Treated Adjunctively with Second-Generation Antidepressants." *American Journal of Psychiatry* 163: 313–315.

Amann, B., et al. (2006). "An Exploratory Open Trial on Safety and Efficacy of the Anticonvulsant Retigabine in Acute Manic Patients." *Journal of Clinical Psychopharmacology* 26: 534–536.

American Psychiatric Association. (2002). "Practice Guideline for the Treatment of Patients with Bipolar Disorder (Revision)." *American Journal of Psychiatry* 159, Supplement (April).

Amsterdam, J. D., and Shults, J. (2005). "Comparison of Fluoxetine, Olanzapine, and Combined Fluoxetine plus Olanzapine Initial Therapy of Bipolar Type I and Type II Major Depression—Lack of Manic Induction." *Journal of Affective Disorders* 87: 121–130.

Amsterdam, J. D., and Shults, J. (2010). "Efficacy and Safety of Long-Term Fluoxetine versus Lithium Monotherapy of Bipolar II Disorder: A Randomized, Double-Blind, Placebo-Substitution Study." *American Journal of Psychiatry* 167: 792–800.

Bailine, S., et al. (2010). "Electroconvulsive Therapy Is Equally Effective in Unipolar and Bipolar Depression." *Acta Psychiatrica Scandinavica* 121: 431–436,.

Baldassano, C. F. (2009). "Promoting Wellness in Patients with Bipolar Disorder: Strategies to Move Beyond Maintaining Stability and Minimizing Adverse Events in Effective Long-Term Management." *Current Psychiatry,* Supplement *Maintaining Wellness in Patients with Bipolar Disorder: Moving Beyond Efficacy to Effectiveness* (October 2009): S12–S18.

Baldessarini, R. J., and Tondo, L. (2000). "Does Lithium Treatment Still Work? Evidence of Stable Responses over Three Decades." *Archives of General Psychiatry* 57: 187–190.

Baldessarini, R. J., et al. (2006). "Decreased Risk of Suicides and Attempts During Long-Term Lithium Treatment: A Meta-Analytic Review." *Bipolar Disorders* 8: 625–639.

Bauer, M. S. (2005) "How Solid Is the Evidence for the Efficacy of Mood Stabilizers in Bipolar Disorder?" *Essential Psychopharmacology* 6: 301–318.

Bauer, M. S., and Mitchner, L. (2004). "What Is a 'Mood Stabilizer'? An Evidence-Based Response." *American Journal of Psychiatry* 161: 3–18.

Bearden, C. E., et al. (2007). "Greater Cortical Gray Matter Density in Lithium-Treated Patients with Bipolar Disorder." *Biological Psychiatry* 62: 7–16.

Beaulieu, J.-M., and Caron, M. G. (2008). "Looking at Lithium: Molecular Moods and Complex Behavior." *Molecular Interventions* 8: 230–241.

Berghöfer, A., et al. (2008). "Long-Term Effectiveness of Lithium in Bipolar Disorder: A Multicenter Investigation of Patients with Typical and Atypical Features." *Journal of Clinical Psychiatry* 69: 1860–1868.

Berlant, J., and van Kammen, D. P. (2002). "Open-Label Topiramate as Primary or Adjunctive Therapy in Chronic Civilian Posttraumatic Stress Disorder: A Preliminary Report." *Journal of Clinical Psychiatry* 63: 15–20.

Bersudsky, Y. (2005). "Phenytoin: An Anti-Bipolar Anticonvulsant?" *International Journal of Neuropsychopharmacology* 9(4): 479–484.

Bertolino, A., et al. (2003). "Neuronal Pathology in the Hippocampal Area of Patients with Bipolar Disorder: A Study with Proton Magnetic Resonance Spectroscopic Imaging." *Biological Psychiatry* 53: 906–913.

Beydoun, A., et al. (2005). "Safety and Efficacy of Two Pregabalin Regimens for Add-On Treatment of Partial Epilepsy." *Neurology* 64: 475–480.

Boscia, F., et al. (2006). "Retigabine and Flupirtine Exert Neuroprotective Actions in Organotypic Hippocampal Cultures." *Neuropharmacology* 51: 283–294.

Bowden, C. L., et al. (2003). "A Placebo-Controlled 18-Month Trial of Lamotrigine and Lithium Maintenance Treatment in Recently Manic or Hypomanic Patients with Bipolar I Disorder." *Archives of General Psychiatry* 60: 392–400.

Bowden, C. L., et al. (2010). "Ziprasidone plus a Mood Stabilizer in Subjects with Bipolar I Disorder: A 6-Month, Randomized, Placebo-Controlled, Double-Blind Trial." *Journal of Clinical Psychiatry* 71: 130–137.

Brown, E. B., et al. (2006). "A 7-Week, Randomized Double-Blind Trial of Olanzapine/Fluoxetine Combination versus Lamotrigine in the Treatment of Bipolar I Depression." *Journal of Clinical Psychiatry* 67: 1025–1033.

Brunello, N. (2004). "Mood Stabilizers: Protecting the Mood . . . Protecting the Brain." *Journal of Affective Disorders* 79: 15–20.

Calabrese, J. R., et al. (2002). "Rash in Multicenter Trials of Lamotrigine in Mood Disorders: Clinical Relevance and Management." *Journal of Clinical Psychiatry* 63: 1012–1019.

Calabrese, J. R., et al. (2005a). "A 20-Month, Double-Blind, Maintenance Trial of Lithium versus Divalproex in Rapid-Cycling Bipolar Disorder." *American Journal of Psychiatry* 162: 2152–2161.

Calabrese, J. R., et al. (2005b). "A Randomized, Double-Blind, Placebo-Controlled Trial of Quetiapine in the Treatment of Bipolar I or II Depression." *American Journal of Psychiatry* 162: 1351–1360.

Chen, G., et al. (1999). "Valproate Robustly Enhances AP-1 Mediated Gene Expression." *Brain Research: Molecular Brain Research* 64: 52–58.

Chengappa, R., et al. (2006). "Adjunctive Topiramate Therapy in Patients Receiving a Mood Stabilizer for Bipolar I Disorder: A Randomized, Placebo-Controlled Trial." *Journal of Clinical Psychiatry* 67: 1698–1706.

Chiu, S. (2005). "GABApentin Treatment Response in Selective Serotonin Reuptake Inhibitor (SSRI)-Refractory Panic Disorder." *Psychiatry-Online.* http://www.priory.com/psych/gabapentin.htm.

Cipriani, A., et al. (2005). "Lithium in the Prevention of Suicidal Behavior and All-Cause Mortality in Patients with Mood Disorders: A Systematic Review of Randomized Trials." *American Journal of Psychiatry* 162: 1805–1819.

Cipriani, A., et al. (2006). "Haloperidol Alone or in Combination for Acute Mania." *Cochrane Database of Systematic Reviews* 3CD004362.

Colom, F., et al. (2003). "A Randomized Trial on the Efficacy of Group Psycho-Education in the Prophylaxis of Recurrences in Bipolar Patients Whose Disease Is in Remission." *Archives of General Psychiatry* 60: 402–407.

Corya, S. A., et al. (2006). "A 24-Week Open-Label Extension Study of Olanzapine-Fluoxetine Combination and Olanzapine Monotherapy in the Treatment of Bipolar Depression." *Journal of Clinical Psychiatry* 67: 798–806.

Cui, J., et al. (2007). "Role of Glutathione in Neuroprotective Effects of Mood Stabilizing Drugs Lithium and Valproate." *Neuroscience* 144: 1447–1453.

Einat, H., and Manji, H. K. (2006). "Cellular Plasticity Cascades: Genes-to-Behavior Pathways in Animal Models of Bipolar Disorder." *Biological Psychiatry* 59: 1160–1171.

Ernst, C. L., and Goldberg, J. F. (2002). "The Reproductive Safety Profile of Mood Stabilizers, Atypical Antipsychotics, and Broad-Spectrum Psychotropics." *Journal of Clinical Psychiatry* 63, Supplement 4: 42–55.

Evins, A. E., et al. (2006). "A Double-Blind, Placebo-Controlled Trial of Adjunctive Donepezil in Treatment-Resistant Mania." *Bipolar Disorders* 8: 75–80.

Feltner, D. E., et al. (2003). "High Dose Pregabalin Is Effective for the Treatment of Generalized Anxiety Disorder." *Journal of Clinical Psychopharmacology* 23: 240–249.

Frye, M., et al. (2007). "A Placebo-Controlled Evaluation of Adjunctive Modafinil in the Treatment of Bipolar Depression." *American Journal of Psychiatry* 164: 1242–1249.

Frye, M., et al. (2009). "Correlates of Treatment-Emergent Mania Associated with Antidepressant Treatment in Bipolar Depression." *American Journal of Psychiatry* 166: 164–172.

Gao, K., et al. (2008). "Antipsychotic-Induced Extrapyramidal Side Effects in Bipolar Disorder and Schizophrenia: A Systematic Review." *Journal of Clinical Psychopharmacology* 28: 203–209.

Geddes, J. R., et al. (2004). "Long-Term Lithium Therapy for Bipolar Disorder: Systematic Review and Meta-Analysis of Randomized Controlled Trials." *American Journal of Psychiatry* 161: 217–222.

Geddes, J. R., et al. for the BALANCE Investigators and Collaborators. (2010). "Lithium plus Valproate Combination Therapy versus Monotherapy for Relapse Prevention in Bipolar 1 Disorder (BALANCE): A Randomized Open-Label Trial." *Lancet* 375: 385–395.

Geller, R. E., and Goldberg, J. F. (2007). "A Review of Evidence-Based Psychotherapies for Bipolar Disorder." *Primary Psychiatry* 14: 59–69. Available online at www.primarypsychiatry.com.

Ghaemi, S. N., et al. (2003). "Oxcarbazepine Treatment of Bipolar Disorder." *Journal of Clinical Psychiatry* 64: 943–945.

Ghaemi, S. N., et al. (2006). "Extrapyramidal Side Effects with Atypical Neuroleptics in Bipolar Disorder." *Progress in Neuro-Psychopharmacology & Biological Psychiatry* 30: 209–213.

Gibbons, R., et al. (2009). "Relationship Between Antiepileptic Drugs and Suicide Attempts in Patients with Bipolar Disorder." *Archives of General Psychiatry* 66: 1354–1360.

Goldberg, J. F. (2010). "Antidepressants in Bipolar Disorder. 7 Myths and Realities." *Current Psychiatry* 9: 41–48.

Goldberg, J. F., et al. (2007). "Adjunctive Antidepressant Use and Symptomatic Recovery Among Bipolar Depressed Patients with Concomitant Manic Symptoms: Findings From the STEP-BD." *American Journal of Psychiatry* 164: 1348–1355.

Goldberg, J. F., et al. (2009). "Mood Stabilization and Destabilization During Acute and Continuation Phase Treatment for Bipolar I Disorder with Lamotrigine or Placebo." *Journal of Clinical Psychiatry* 70: 1273–1280.

Goodnick, P. J. (2007). "Bipolar Depression: A Review of Randomized Clinical Trials." *Expert Opinion in Pharmacotherapy* 8: 13–21.

Goodwin, G. M., et al. (2004). "A Pooled Analysis of Two Placebo-Controlled 18-Month Trials of Lamotrigine and Lithium Maintenance in Bipolar I Disorder." *Journal of Clinical Psychiatry* 64: 432–441.

Gould, T. D., et al. (2004). "Emerging Experimental Therapeutics for Bipolar Disorder: Insights from the Molecular and Cellular Actions of Current Mood Stabilizers." *Molecular Psychiatry* 9: 734–755.

Harrison-Read, P. E. (2009). "Antimanic Potency of Typical Neuroleptic Drugs and Affinity for Dopamine D2 and Serotonin 5-HT2A Receptors—A New Analysis of Data from the Archives and Implications for Improved Antimanic Treatments." *Journal of Psychopharmacology* 23: 899–907.

Hartong, E. G., et al. (2003). "Prophylactic Efficacy of Lithium versus Carbamazepine in Treatment-Naïve Bipolar Patients." *Journal of Clinical Psychiatry* 64: 144–151.

Hashimoto, R., et al. (2002). "Lithium Induces Brain-Derived Neurotrophic Factor and Activates TrkB in Rodent Cortical Neurons: An Essential Step for Neuroprotection Against Glutamate Excitotoxicity." *Neuropharmacology* 43: 1173–1179.

Hirsch, L. J., et al. (2004). "Correlating Lamotrigine Serum Concentrations with Tolerability in Patients with Epilepsy." *Neurology* 28: 1022–1026.

Hirschfield, R. M., et al. (2006). "An Open-Label Extension Trial of Risperidone Monotherapy in the Treatment of Bipolar I Disorder." *International Journal of Clinical Psychopharmacology* 21: 11–20.

Hirschfeld, R. M. A. (2009). "Making Efficacious Choices: The Integration of Pharmacotherapy and Nonpharmacologic Approaches to the Treatment of Patients with Bipolar Disorder." *Current Psychiatry*, Supplement *Maintaining Wellness in Patients with Bipolar Disorder: Moving Beyond Efficacy to Effectiveness* (October 2009): S6–S11.

Hollander, E., et al. (2003). "Divalproex in the Treatment of Impulsive Aggression: Efficacy in Cluster B Personality Disorders." *Neuropsychopharmacology* 28: 1186–1197.

Hurley, S. C. (2002). "Lamotrigine Update and Its Use in Bipolar Disorders." *Annals of Pharmacotherapy* 36: 860–873.

Ingenhoven, T., et al. (2010). "Effectiveness of Pharmacotherapy for Severe Personality Disorders: Meta-Analyses of Randomized Controlled Trials." *Journal of Clinical Psychiatry* 71: 14–25.

Jafferany, M. (2008). "Lithium and Skin: Dermatologic Manifestations of Lithium Therapy." *International Journal of Dermatology* 47: 1101–1111.

Janowsky, D. S., et al. (2003). "Effects of Topiramate on Aggressive, Self-Injurious, and Disruptive/Destructive Behaviors in the Intellectually Disabled: An Open-Label Retrospective Study." *Journal of Clinical Psychopharmacology* 23: 500–504.

Joffe, H., et al. (2006). "Valproate Is Associated with New-Onset Oligoamenorrhea with Hyperandrogenism in Women with Bipolar Disorder." *Biological Psychiatry* 59: 1078–1086.

Keck, P. E., and McElroy, S. L. (2002). "Carbamazepine and Valproate in the Maintenance Treatment of Bipolar Disorder." *Journal of Clinical Psychiatry* 63, Supplement 10: 13–17.

Keck, P. E., and McElroy, S. L. (2003). "Bipolar Disorder, Obesity, and Pharmacotherapy-Associated Weight Gain." *Journal of Clinical Psychiatry* 64: 1426–1435.

Keck, P. E., et al. (2003). "Advances in the Pharmacological Treatment of Bipolar Depression." *Biological Psychiatry* 53: 671–679.

Keck, P. E., et al. (2006). "A Randomized, Double-Blind, Placebo-Controlled 26-Week Trial of Aripiprazole in Recently Manic Patients with Bipolar I Disorder." *Journal of Clinical Psychiatry* 67: 626–637.

Keck, P. E., et al. (2007) "Aripirazole Monotherapy for Maintenance Therapy in Bipolar I Disorder: A 100 Week, Double-Blind Study versus Placebo." *Journal of Clinical Psychiatry* 68: 1480–1491.

Kemp, D. E., et al. (2009) "A 6-Month, Double-Blind, Maintenance Trial of Lithium Monotherapy versus the Combination of Lithium and Divalproex for Rapid-Cycling Bipolar Disorder and Co-Occurring Substance Abuse or Dependence." *Journal of Clinical Psychiatry* 70: 113–121.

Kessing, L., et al. (2008). "Lithium Treatment and Risk of Dementia." *Archives of General Psychiatry* 65: 1331–1335.

Ketter, T. A., et al. (2003). "Potential Mechanisms of Action of Lamotrigine in the Treatment of Bipolar Disorders." *Journal of Clinical Psychopharmacology* 23: 484 495.

Khan, A., et al. (2004). "Effect of Lamotrigine on Cognitive Complaints in Patients with Bipolar I Disorder." *Journal of Clinical Psychiatry* 65: 1483–1490.

Kopnisky, K. L., et al. (2003). "Chronic Lithium Treatment Antagonizes Glutamate-Induced Decrease of Phosphorylated CREB in Neurons via Reducing Protein Phosphorylase 1 and Increasing MEK Activities." *Neuroscience* 116: 425 435.

Korsgaard, M. P., et al. (2005). "Anxiolytic Effects of Maxipost (BMS-204352) and Retigabine via Activation of Neuronal Kv7 Channels." *Journal of Pharmacology & Experimental Therapeutics* 314: 282–292.

Kulkarni, J., et al. (2006). "A Pilot Study of Hormone Modulation as a New Treatment for Mania in Women with Bipolar Affective Disorder." *Psychoneuroendocrinology* 31: 543–547.

Kupfer, D. J. (2005). "The Increasing Medical Burden in Bipolar Disorder." *Journal of the American Medical Association* 293: 2528–2530.

Kushner, S. F., et al. (2006). "Topiramate Monotherapy in the Management of Acute Mania: Results of Four Double-Blind Placebo-Controlled Trials." *Bipolar Disorders* 8: 15–27.

Lam, D. H., et al. (2003). "A Randomized Controlled Study of Cognitive Therapy for Relapse Prevention for Bipolar Affective Disorder: Outcome of the First Year." *Archives of General Psychiatry* 60: 145–152.

Leng, Y., et al. (2008). "Synergistic Neuroprotective Effects of Lithium and Valproic Acid or Other Histone Deacetylase Inhibitors in Neurons: Roles of Glycogen Synthase Kinase-3 Inhibition." *Journal of Neuroscience* 28: 2576–2588.

Leverich, G. S., et al. (2006) "Risk of Switch in Mood Polarity to Hypomania or Mania in Patients with Bipolar Depression During Acute and Continuation Trials of Venlafaxine, Sertraline, and Bupropion as Adjuncts to Mood Stabilizers." *American Journal of Psychiatry* 163: 232–239.

Li, X., et al. (2002). "Synaptic, Intracellular, and Neuroprotective Mechanisms of Anticonvulsants: Are They Relevant for the Treatment and Course of Bipolar Disorders?" *Journal of Affective Disorders* 69: 1–14.

Lichtenstein, P., et al. (2009). "Common Genetic Determinants of Schizophrenia and Bipolar Disorder in Swedish Families: A Population-Based Study. *Lancet* 373: 234–239.

Lieb, K., et al. (2010). "Pharmacotherapy for Borderline Personality Disorder: Cochrane Systematic Review of Randomised Trials." *British Journal of Psychiatry* 196: 4–12.

Maj, M., et al. (1998). "Long-Term Outcome of Lithium Prophylaxis in Bipolar Disorder: A Five-Year Prospective Study of 402 Patients at a Lithium Clinic." *American Journal of Psychiatry* 155: 30–35.

Marengell, L. B., et al. (2006). "Omega-3 Fatty Acids in Bipolar Disorder: Clinical and Research Considerations." *Prostaglandins Leuokotrienes and Essential Fatty Acids* 75: 315–321.

Marmol, F. (2008). "Lithium: Bipolar Disorder and Neurodegenerative Diseases Possible Cellular Mechanisms of the Therapeutic Effects of Lithium." *Progress in Neuro-Psychopharmacology & Biological Psychiatry* 32: 1761–1771.

McDonald, A. A., and Portenoy, R. K. (2006). "How to Use Antidepressants and Anticonvulsants as Adjuvant Analgesics in the Treatment of Neuropathic Cancer Pain." *Journal of Supportive Oncology* 4: 43–52.

McElroy, S. L., et al. (2004). "Topiramate in the Long-Term Treatment of Binge-Eating Disorder Associated with Obesity." *Journal of Clinical Psychiatry* 65: 1463–1469.

McElroy, S. L., et al. (2010). "A Double-Blind Placebo-Controlled Study of Quetiapine and Paroxetine as Monotherapy in Adults with Bipolar Depression (EMBOLDEN II)." *Journal of Clinical Psychiatry* 71: 163–174.

Mercer, D., et al. (2009). "Meta-Analyses of Mood Stabilizers, Antidepressants and Antipsychotics in the Treatment of Borderline Personality Disorder: Effectiveness for Depression and Anger Symptoms." *Journal of Personality Disorders* 23: 156–174.

Merikangas, K. R., et al. (2007). "Lifetime and 12-Month Prevalence of Bipolar Spectrum Disorder in the National Comorbidity Survey Replication." *Archives of General Psychiatry* 64: 543–552.

Miklowitz, D. J., et al. (2007). "Psychosocial Treatments for Bipolar Depression." *Archives of General Psychiatry* 64: 419–426.

Mishory, A., et al. (2000). "Phenytoin as an Antimanic Anticonvulsant: A Controlled Study." *American Journal of Psychiatry* 157: 463–465.

Montgomery, P., and Richardson, A. J. (2008). "Omega-3 Fatty Acids for Bipolar Disorder." *Cochrane Database of Systematic Reviews* CD005169.

Montouris, G. (2005). "Safety of the Newer Antiepileptic Drug Oxcarbazepine During Pregnancy." *Current Medical Research Opinion* 21: 693–701.

Mundo, E., et al. (2006). "Clinical Variables Related to Antidepressant-Induced Mania in Bipolar Disorder." *Journal of Affective Disorders* 92: 227–230.

Nasr, S., et al. (2006). "Absence of Mood Switch with and Tolerance to Modafinil: A Replication Study from a Large Private Practice." *Journal of Affective Disorders* 95: 111–114.

Ng, F., et al. (2009). "The International Society for Bipolar Disorders (ISBD) Consensus Guidelines for the Safety Monitoring of Bipolar Disorder Treatments." *Bipolar Disorders* 11: 559–595.

Nierenberg, A. A., et al. (2006). "Treatment-Resistant Bipolar Depression: A STEP-BD Equipoise Randomized Effectiveness Trial of Antidepressant Augmentation with Lamotrigine, Inositol, or Risperidone." *American Journal of Psychiatry* 163: 210–216.

Noaghiul, S., and Hibbeln, J. R. (2003). "Cross-National Comparisons of Seafood Consumption and Rates of Bipolar Disorder." *American Journal of Psychiatry* 160: 2222–2227.

Ornoy, A. (2006). "Neuroteratogens in Man: An Overview with Special Emphasis on the Teratogenicity of Antiepileptic Drugs in Pregnancy." *Reproductive Toxicology* 22: 214–226.

Ostacher, M. J., et al. (2010). "Impact of Substance Use Disorders on Recovery from Episodes of Depression in Bipolar Disorder Patients: Prospective Data from the Systematic Treatment Enhancement Program for Bipolar Disorder (STEP-BD)." *American Journal of Psychiatry* 167: 289–297.

Otto, M. W., et al. (2003). "Psychoeducational and Cognitive-Behavioral Strategies in the Management of Bipolar Disorder." *Journal of Affective Disorders* 73: 171–181.

Pachet, A., et al. (2003). "Beneficial Behavioural Effects of Lamotrigine in Traumatic Brain Injury." *Brain Injury* 17: 715–722.

Pande, A. C., et al. (1999). "Treatment of Social Phobia with Gabapentin: A Placebo-Controlled Study." *Journal of Clinical Psychopharmacology* 19: 341–348.

Pande, A., et al. (2000). "Placebo-Controlled Study of GABApentin Treatment of Panic Disorder." *Journal of Clinical Psychopharmacology* 20: 467–471.

Pande, A., et al. (2003). "Pregabalin in Generalized Anxiety Disorder: A Placebo-Controlled Trial." *American Journal of Psychiatry* 160: 533–540.

Parker, G., et al. (2006a). "Omega-3 Fatty Acids and Mood Disorders." *American Journal of Psychiatry* 163: 969–978.

Parker, G., et al. (2006b) "SSRIs as Mood Stabilizers for Bipolar II Disorder? A Proof of Concept Study." *Journal of Affective Disorders* 92: 205–214.

Patorno, E., et al. (2010). "Anticonvulsant Medications and the Risk of Suicide, Attempted Suicide, or Violent Death." *Journal of the American Medical Association* 303: 1401–1409.

Perlis, R. H., et al. (2006a). "Atypical Antipsychotics in the Treatment of Mania: A Meta-Analysis of Randomized, Placebo-Controlled Trials." *Journal of Clinical Psychiatry* 67: 509–516.

Perlis, R. H., et al. (2006b). "Clinical Features of Bipolar Depression versus Major Depressive Disorder in Large Multicenter Trials." *American Journal of Psychiatry* 163: 225–231.

Perlis, R. H., et al. (2006c). "Predictors of Recurrence in Bipolar Disorder: Primary Outcomes from the Systematic Treatment Enhancement Program for Bipolar Disorder (STEP-BD)." *American Journal of Psychiatry* 163: 217–224.

Perlis, R. H., et al. (2009). "A Genomewide Association Study of Response to Lithium for Prevention of Recurrence in Bipolar Disorder." *American Journal of Psychiatry* 166: 718–725.

Perucca, E. (2005). "Birth Defects After Prenatal Exposure to Antiepileptic Drugs." *Lancet Neurology* 4: 781–786.

Phrolov, K., et al. (2004). "Single-Dose Intravenous Valproate in Acute Mania." *Journal of Clinical Psychiatry* 65: 68–70.

Porter, R. J., et al. (2007). "Randomized, Multicenter, Dose-Ranging Trial of Retigabine for Partial-Onset Seizures." *Neurology* 68: 1197–1204.

Post, R. M., et al. (2005). "The Impact of Bipolar Depression." *Journal of Clinical Psychiatry* 66, Supplement 5: 5–10.

Post, R. M., et al. (2006). "Mood Switch in Bipolar Depression: Comparison of Adjunctive Venlafaxine, Bupropion and Sertraline." *British Journal of Psychiatry* 189: 124–131.

Rapoport, S. I., et al. (2009). "Bipolar Disorder and Mechanisms of Action of Mood Stabilizers." *Brain Research Reviews* 61: 185–209.

Rendell, J. M., et al. (2006) "Risperidone Alone or in Combination for Acute Mania." *Cochrane Database of Systematic Reviews* CD004043.

Rosenthal, M. (2003). "Tiagabine for the Treatment of Generalized Anxiety Disorder: A Randomized, Open-Label, Clinical Trial with Paroxetine as a Positive Control." *Journal of Clinical Psychiatry* 64: 1245–1249.

Sachs, G. S., et al. (2007). "Effectiveness of Adjunctive Antidepressant Treatment for Bipolar Depression." *New England Journal of Medicine* 356: 1711–1722.

Salvadore, G., et al. (2010)."The Neurobiology of the Switch Process in Bipolar Disorder: A Review." *Journal of Clinical Psychiatry.* In press.

Scherk, H., et al. (2007). "Second-Generation Antipsychotic Agents in the Treatment of Acute Mania." *Archives of General Psychiatry* 64: 442–455.

Schneck, C. D., et al. (2008). "The Prospective Course of Rapid-Cycling Bipolar Disorder: Findings from the STEP-BD." *American Journal of Psychiatry* 165: 370–377.

Shajahan, P., and M. Taylor (2010). "The Uses and Outcomes of Quetiapine in Depressive and Bipolar Mood Disorders in Clinical Practice." *Journal of Psychopharmacology* 24: 565–572.

Sharma V., et al. (2009). "Bipolar II Postpartum Depression: Detection, Diagnosis, and Treatment." *American Journal of Psychiatry* 166: 1217–1221.

Stanford, M. S., et al. (2005). "A Comparison of Anticonvulsants in the Treatment of Impulsive Aggression." *Experimental and Clinical Psychopharmacology* 13: 72–77.

Stoll, A. L., et al. (1999). "Omega-3 Fatty Acids in Bipolar Disorder: A Preliminary Double-Blind, Placebo-Controlled Trial." *Archives of General Psychiatry* 56: 407–412.

Suppes, T., et al. (2005). "The Texas Implementation of Medication Algorithms: Update to the Algorithms for Treatment of Bipolar I Disorder." *Journal of Clinical Psychiatry* 66: 870–886.

Tohen, M., et al. (2005). "Olanzapine versus Lithium in the Maintenance Treatment of Bipolar Disorder: A 12-Month, Randomized, Double-Blind, Controlled Clinical Trial." *American Journal of Psychiatry* 162: 1281–1290.

Tohen, M., et al. (2006). "Randomized, Placebo-Controlled Trial of Olanzapine as Maintenance Therapy in Patients with Bipolar I Disorder Responding to Acute Treatment with Olanzapine." *American Journal of Psychiatry* 163: 247–256.

Vieta, E., et al. (2005). "Effectiveness of Aripiprazole v. Haloperidol in Acute Bipolar Mania: Double-Blind, Randomized, Comparative 12-Week Trial." *British Journal of Psychiatry* 187: 235–242.

Wagner, K. D., et al. (2006). "A Double-Blind, Randomized, Placebo-Controlled Trial of Oxcarbazepine in the Treatment of Bipolar Disorder in Children and Adolescents." *American Journal of Psychiatry* 163: 1179–1186.

Watase, K., et al. (2007) "Lithium Therapy Improves Neurological Function and Hippocampal Dendritic Arborization in a Spinocerebellar Ataxia Type 1 Mouse Model." *PLoS Med* 4(5): e182. doi:10.1371/journal.pmed.0040182.

Wilson, M. S., and Findling, R. L. (2007). "Zonisamide for Bipolar Depression." *Expert Opinion on Pharmacotherapy* 8: 111–113.

Wozniak, J., et al. (2007). "Omega-3 Fatty Acid Monotherapy for Pediatric Bipolar Disorder: A Prospective Open-Label Trial." *European Neuropsychopharmacology* 17: 440–447.

Yasuda, S., et al. (2009). "The Mood Stabilizers Lithium and Valproate Selectively Activate the Promoter IV of Brain-Derived Neurotrophic Factor in Neurons." *Molecular Psychiatry* 14: 51–59.

Yatham, L. N., et al. (2005). "Atypical Antipsychotics in Bipolar Depression: Potential Mechanisms of Action." *Journal of Clinical Psychiatry* 66, Supplement 5: 40–48.

Young, A. H., et al. (2010). "A Double-Blind, Placebo-Controlled Study of Quetiapine and Lithium Monotherapy in Adults in the Acute Phase of Bipolar Depression (EMBOLDEN I)." *Journal of Clinical Psychiatry* 71: 150–162.

Zarate, C. A., et al. (2005). "Molecular Mechanisms of Bipolar Disorder." *Drug Discovery Today: Disease Mechanisms* 2: 435–445.

Zarate, C. A., et al. (2006). "Cellular Plasticity Cascades: Targets for the Development of Novel Therapeutics for Bipolar Disorder." *Biological Psychiatry* 59: 1006–1020.

Chapter 7

Sedative-Hypnotic and Anxiolytic Medications

Anxiety and insomnia have long plagued mankind. Both have been the object of drug therapy, probably since the discovery of alcohol as a product of fermentation. We discuss the pharmacological treatment of anxiety and insomnia by introducing the historically significant and still widely used medicines that were used as sedatives, hypnotics, and antianxiety medications. Earlier chapters have discussed more modern medications that are not classified as sedative/hypnotics but nevertheless exert anxiolytic efficacy (atypical antipsychotic medications and certain antidepressants; Chapters 4 and 5). Indeed, in the modern-day treatment of severe anxiety and insomnia, these medications can be used in place of older sedative-hypnotic agents.

Prior to the appearance of the third edition of the *Diagnostic and Statistical Manual of Mental Disorders* (DSM-III) in 1980, all anxiety disorder subtypes (as we know them today) were lumped under the single diagnostic entity "anxiety neurosis." To treat anxiety neurosis, barbiturates and several older nonbarbiturate sedatives, as well as the benzodiazepines (introduced in about 1960), were considered appropriate. The barbiturates were also early drugs used to treat epilepsy and to induce a state of general anesthesia for surgical procedures. These uses are discussed later in this chapter. Today, the most widely used sedative/anxiolytics are the benzodiazepines and their variants.

Historical Background

In the mid-nineteenth century, *bromide* and *chloral hydrate* became available as early sleep-inducing agents, as alternatives to alcohol and opium. In 1912, *phenobarbital* was introduced into medicine as a sedative drug, the first of the structurally classified group of drugs called *barbiturates* (Figure 7.1). Between 1912 and 1950, about 50 different barbiturates were marketed commercially. In the early 1950s, several other sedatives, including meprobamate (Equanil) and carisoprodol (Soma), were marketed as potentially safer alternatives, but their safety was not significantly better than that of the barbiturates. In 1960, *chlordiazepoxide* (Librium) was marketed as the first sedative/anxiolytic

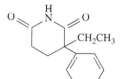

Barbiturate nucleus

Phenobarbital (a barbiturate)

Nonbarbiturate Sedatives

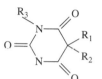

Glutethimide (Doriden)

Ethchlorvynol (Placidyl)

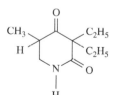

Methyprylon (Noludar)

Methaqualone (Quaalude)

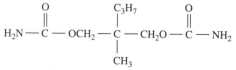

Meprobamate (Equanil, Miltown)

FIGURE 7.1 Chemical structures of classical sedatives. Barbiturates are defined by containing the barbiturate nucleus. Nonbarbiturate sedatives do not have this basic structure.

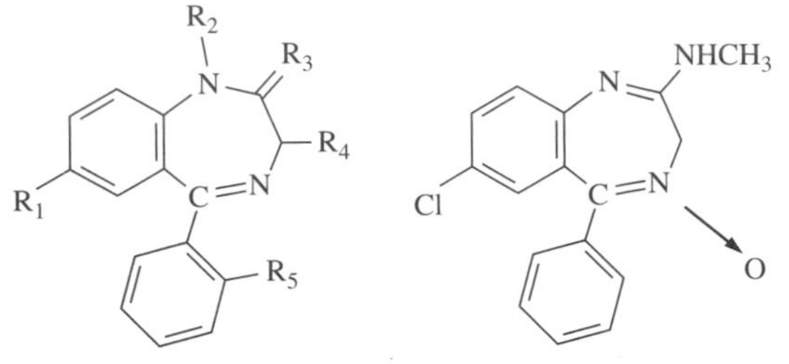

FIGURE 7.2 Structures of some benzodiazepines. The basic "benzodiazepine" nucleus, which structurally defines this class of drugs, is shown on the left; chlordiazepoxide (the first marketed benzodiazepine) is shown on the right. Variations in the basic structure are located at the R1–R5 positions on the basic structure.

of a new structural class of drugs called *benzodiazepines*. Diazepam (Valium), alprazolam (Xanax), clonazepam (Klonopin), and lorazepam (Ativan) are other commonly prescribed benzodiazepines. Several others are also available (Figure 7.2). The benzodiazepines had one major advantage over the barbiturates: they were rarely if ever fatal in overdosage, unless they were combined with alcohol. Because of improved safety, the benzodiazepine tranquilizers became incredibly popular (by physician prescription) for the treatment of anxiety and and insomnia.

Sites and Mechanisms of Action

Historically, the sedative-hypnotic, anxiolytic, anticonvulsant, and general anesthetic actions of the barbiturates were perceived to result from a nonselective neuronal depression throughout the brain. These compounds were presumed to depress diffuse neuronal pathways both in the brain stem and in the cerebral cortex. Brain-stem depression would continue as dosage was increased, accounting for the deep coma, cessation of respiration, and death that can follow drug overdosage. Today, we have much greater understanding of specific

Drug	R_1	R_2	R_3	R_4	R_5
Diazepam	Cl	CH_3	$=O$	H_2	H
Nitrazepam	NO_2	H	$=O$	H_2	H
Flurazepam	Cl	$(CH_2)_2N(C_2H_5)_2$	$=O$	H_2	H
Flunitrazepam	NO_2	H	$=O$	H_2	F
Oxazepam	Cl	H	$=O$	OH	H
Temazepam	Cl	CH_3	$=O$	H_2	H
Clonazepam	NO_2	H	$=O$	H_2	Cl
Lorazepam	Cl	H	$=O$	OH	Cl
Clorazepate	Cl	H	$=O$	COOH	H
Nordiazepam	Cl	H	$=O$	H_2	H

receptor-drug interactions that characterize the actions of these sedative/anxiolytic tranquilizers.

In our current era of drug development, we name new drugs not so much by their structure (as we did with barbiturates and benzodiazepines) as by the receptors that they they bind to or that underlie their major clinical action (for example, a selective serotonin reuptake inhibitor (SSRI), a serotonin 1_A agonist, a dopamine$_2$ blocker, and so on). If discovered today, a barbiturate or a benzodiazepine would be called a *GABA receptor agonist*. Because of what is now known of GABA receptors and because specific binding sites for both barbiturates and benzodiazepines on the GABA receptor have been identified, these and related drugs are called *benzodiazepine receptor agonists* (BZRAs). This term encompasses both the benzodiazepines and several newer non-benzodiazepines that are agonists at the same receptor and that are widely prescribed to improve the quality of sleep in the clinical management of insomnia (e.g., zolpidem, or Ambien). Note that the terms *GABA receptor agonist* and *BZRA* are not synonymous.

Benzodiazepines facilitate the binding of GABA to its receptor. They do not directly stimulate the GABA receptor; rather, they bind to a site adjacent to the GABA receptor, producing a three-dimensional conformational change in the receptor structure that, in turn, increases the affinity of GABA for the receptor. That action, in turn, increases the inhibitory synaptic action of GABA, facilitating the influx of chloride ions, causing hyperpolarization of the postsynaptic neuron, and depressing its excitability (Chapter 2).

Benzodiazepines exert their anxiolytic properties by acting on GABA neurons at limbic centers. Their actions at other regions (for example, the cerebral cortex and brain stem) produce side effects such as sedation, increased seizure threshold, cognitive impairment, amnesia, and muscle relaxation. Neuroanatomically, the *amygdala, orbitofrontal cortex*, and *insula* are associated with the production of behavioral responses to fearful stimuli and the central mediation of anxiety and panic. Electrical stimulation of these structures evokes behavioral and physiological responses that are associated with fear and anxiety. Electrical lesions of the amygdala in animals result in an anxiolytic effect. PET scanning of the brain demonstrates increased amygdala blood flow concomitant with anxiety responses; MRI scanning of the brain demonstrates amygdala abnormalities in panic disorder patients.

Artificially blocking GABAergic function can elicit anxiogeniclike effects, with both behavioral and physiologic alterations similar to symptoms of human anxiety states. Increasing the activity of amygdala function (with lowered GABAergic inhibition of function) produces anxiogenic responses. Thus, hypofunctional GABA$_A$ receptor activity may sensitize the amygdala to anxiogenic responses to what might otherwise be considered nondistressing stimuli. This mechanism might underlie pathological emotional responses, such as chronically high levels of anxiety. The benzodiazepines may reset the threshold of the amygdala to a more normal level of responsiveness. Sigel (2002) detailed the molecular biology of the interaction between benzodiazepines and GABA$_A$ receptor function.

Sedative-Induced Brain Dysfunction

High levels of alcohol (Chapter 13) can induce a "blackout" following attainment of extreme levels of alcohol in the blood (e.g., a blood alcohol level of about 0.25 to 0.30 grams% or higher) (Hartzler and Fromme, 2003; White, et al., 2004). A blackout is a state of *anterograde amnesia,* resulting in loss of memory for events or actions at a certain blood level of alcohol that persists until the level of alcohol drops again below the amnestic level. More correctly, alcohol-induced blackout is a manifestation of a *drug-induced, reversible, organic brain syndrome* (or state of dementia) that can follow use of any sedative, including barbiturates, benzodiazepines, or other BZRAs. Therefore, any sedative, in high enough doses, can produce amnesia. This amnestic effect is clearly distinct from higher dose effects that produce loss of consciousness (John and Prichap, 2005; Lee et al., 2009). Therefore, a person can be in blackout yet awake and capable of performing behavioral activities (as would be a patient with organic dementia).

This state of dementia (whether drug-induced or organic) produces characteristic behavioral, intellectual, and cognitive deficits. One way to diagnose drug-induced dementia is to perform a *mental status examination* while the patient is under the influence of the drug. The examination evaluates 12 areas of mental functioning (Table 7.1). When a person is in an amnestic state, 5 of the 12 components of the mental status examination are particularly altered (sensorium, affect, mental content, intellectual function, and insight and judgment). The sensorium becomes clouded, which causes disorientation in time and place; memory becomes impaired, which is manifested by loss of ability to form short-term memory (the blackout); the intellect becomes depressed; judgment is altered. Affect becomes shallow and labile; that is, the person becomes extremely vulnerable to external stimuli and may be sullen and moody one moment and exhibit mock anger or rage the next. This kind of mental status is diagnosed as a "brain syndrome" caused by depressed nerve cell function. This state of *anterograde amnesia* is reached when one achieves a certain blood level of drug or alcohol and terminates when these levels fall to lower levels. The reason these sedative drugs are called "date rape" drugs is that the person who takes the drug does not remember what happened during the period of intoxication. This occurs despite being in a state of wakefulness. In medicine, this is seen when medical professionals induce a state of

TABLE 7.1	Mental status examination: Twelve areas of mental functioning

1. General appearance
* 2. Sensorium
  a. Orientation to time, place, and person
  b. Clear vs. clouded thinking
3. Behavior and mannerisms
4. Stream of talk
5. Cooperativeness
6. Mood (inner feelings)
* 7. Affect (surface expression of feelings)
8. Perception
  a. Illusions (misperception of reality)
  b. Hallucinations (not present in reality)
9. Thought processes: logical vs. strange or bizarre
* 10. Mental content (fund of knowledge)
* 11. Intellectual function (ability to reason and interpret)
* 12. Insight and judgment

* Characteristically altered in both organic dementia and reversible, drug-induced dementia.

"conscious sedation," where the patient is awake and cooperative yet does not remember the medical procedure. One example is the administration of a short-acting benzodiazepine (midazolam, or Versed) so the patient does not remember a colonoscopy, despite having been awake during the procedure.

Certain people (such as the elderly) who already have some natural loss of nerve cell function are adversely affected by these drugs; they experience increased disorientation and further clouding of consciousness. Frequently these people exhibit a state of drug-induced paradoxical excitement, which is characterized by a labile personality with marked anger, delusions, hallucinations, and confabulations (unconscious fabrications of memory gaps). Treating drug-induced memory loss requires that administration of the sedative drug be stopped.

Barbiturates

In their decades of use, barbiturates were associated with thousands of suicides, deaths from accidental ingestion, widespread dependency and abuse, and many serious interactions with other drugs and alcohol. They are now rarely used; however, they remain the classic prototype of sedative-hypnotic drugs.

Pharmacokinetics

Barbiturates are all of similar structure, and classification of individual drugs is by their individual pharmacokinetics. As shown in Table 7.2, their half-lives can be quite short (3-minute redistribution half-life for thiopental) or as long as several days. The hypnotic action of ultrashort-acting barbiturates (such as thiopental) is terminated by redistribution, while the action of other barbiturates is determined by their rate of metabolism by enzymes in the liver.

Barbiturates are well absorbed orally and well distributed to most body tissues. The ultrashort-acting barbiturates are exceedingly lipid soluble, cross the blood-brain barrier rapidly, and induce sleep within seconds following their intravenous injection. Because the longer-acting barbiturates are more water soluble, they are slower to penetrate the central nervous system (CNS). Sleep induction with these compounds, therefore, is delayed for 20 to 30 minutes, and residual hangover is prominent (since the plasma half-lives of most barbiturates are longer than that needed for 8 hours of sleep).

Pharmacological Effects

Barbiturates have a low degree of selectivity, and it is not possible to achieve anxiolysis without evidence of sedation. Barbiturates are not analgesic; they cannot be relied on to produce sedation or sleep in the presence of even moderate pain. Sleep patterns are decidedly affected by barbiturates; rapid eye movement (REM) sleep is markedly suppressed. Because dreaming occurs during REM sleep, barbiturates suppress dreaming. During drug withdrawal, dreaming becomes vivid and excessive. Such rebound increase in dreaming during withdrawal (termed "REM rebound") is one example of a withdrawal effect following prolonged periods of barbiturate ingestion. The vivid nature of the dreams can lead to insomnia, which can be clinically relieved by restarting the drug, negating the attempt at withdrawal.

Since barbiturates depress memory functioning, they are *cognitive inhibitors.* Drowsiness and more subtle alterations of judgment, cognitive functioning, motor skills, physical coordination, and behavior may persist for hours or days until the barbiturate is completely metabolized and eliminated. Sedative doses of barbiturates have minimal effect on respiration, but overdoses (or combinations of barbiturates and alcohol) can result in death.

Barbiturates exert few significant effects on the cardiovascular system, the gastrointestinal tract, the kidneys, or other organs until toxic doses are reached. In the liver, barbiturates stimulate the synthesis of enzymes that metabolize barbiturates as well as other drugs, an effect that produces significant tolerance to the drugs.

TABLE 7.2 Half-lives and uses of some barbiturates

Drug name		R₁[a]	R₂[a]	R₃[a]	Distribution (min)	Elimination (h)	Uses		
Trade	Generic						Insomnia	Anesthesia	Epilepsy
Amytal	Amobarbital	Ethyl	Isopentyl	H		10–40	X		
Alurate	Aprobarbital	Allyl	Isopentyl	H		12–34	X		
Butisol	Butabarbital	Athyl	sec-Butyl	H		34–42	X		
Mebaral	Mephobarbital	Ethyl	Phenyl	CH₃		50–120			X
Brevital	Methohexital	Allyl	1-Methyl, 2-Pentynyl	CH₃		1–2		X	
Nembutal	Pentobarbital	Ethyl	Methyl butyl	H		15–50	X		
Luminal	Phenobarbital	Ethyl	Phenyl	H		24–120	X		X
Seconal	Secobarbital	Allyl	Methyl butyl	H		15–40	X		
Lotusate	Talbutal	Allyl	sec-Butyl	H			X		
Surital	Thiamylal	Allyl	Methyl butyl	H				X	
Pentothal	Thiopental	Ethyl	Methyl butyl	H	3	3–6		X	

[a] Symbols R₁, R₂, and R₃ refer to chemical substitution at these positions on the barbiturate nucleus shown in Figure 7.1.

Psychological Effects

The behavioral, motor, and cognitive inhibitions caused by barbiturates are similar to those caused by alcohol. A person may respond to low doses either with relief from anxiety (the expected effect) or with withdrawal, emotional depression, or aggressive and violent behavior. Higher doses lead to more general behavioral depression and sleep. Mental set and physical or social setting can determine whether relief from anxiety, mental depression, aggression, or another unexpected or unpredictable response is experienced. Driving skills, judgment, insight, and memory all become severely impaired during the period of intoxication.

Clinical Uses

Use of barbiturates has declined rapidly for several reasons: (1) they are lethal in overdose, (2) they have a narrow therapeutic-to-toxic range, (3) they have a high potential for inducing tolerance, dependence, and abuse, and (4) they interact dangerously with many other drugs. Because of these disadvantages, they have largely been replaced by benzodiazepines.

Adverse Reactions

Drowsiness is an inescapable accompaniment to the anxiolytic effect and is often the effect sought if the drug is intended to produce either daytime sedation or nighttime sleep. Barbiturates significantly impair motor and intellectual performance and judgment. It should be emphasized that all sedatives are equivalent to alcohol in their effects, that all are additive in their effects with alcohol, and that their effects persist longer than might be predicted. There are no specific antidotes with which one can treat barbiturate overdosage. Treatment is aimed at supporting the respiratory and cardiovascular system until the drug is metabolized and eliminated.

Tolerance

The barbiturates can induce tolerance by either of two mechanisms: (1) the induction of drug-metabolizing enzymes in the liver or (2) the adaptation of neurons in the brain to the presence of the drug. With the latter mechanism, tolerance develops primarily to the sedative effects, much less to the brain-stem depressant effects on respiration. Thus, the margin of safety for the person who uses the drug decreases.

Physical Dependence

Normal clinical doses of barbiturates can induce a degree of physical dependence, usually manifested by sleep difficulties during attempts at withdrawal. Withdrawal from high doses of barbiturates may result in hallucinations, restlessness, disorientation, and even life-threatening convulsions.

Effects in Pregnancy

Barbiturates, like all psychoactive drugs, are freely distributed to the fetus. Data are limited on whether deleterious fetal abnormalities occur as a result of a pregnant woman taking barbiturates, although it has been suggested that developmental abnormalities occur. This possibility can be a concern for pregnant women who are epileptic and must take a barbiturate to prevent seizures. At a minimum, there is uncertainly concerning the risk of fetal problems associated with the ingestion of barbiturates by pregnant women (Eadie, 2008); nevertheless, barbiturates are considered to be relatively safe during pregnancy (Timmermann et al., 2008, 2009).

Nonbarbiturate Sedative-Hypnotic Drugs

In the early 1950s, several "nonbarbiturate" sedatives—*glutethimide* (Doriden), *ethchlorvynol* (Placidyl), and *methyprylon* (Noludar), for example—were introduced as anxiolytics, daytime sedatives, and hypnotics. They somewhat resembled the barbiturates (see Figure 7.1), but they did not have the exact barbiturate nucleus and could not legally be called barbiturates, despite being pharmacologically interchangeable. These drugs offered no advantages over the barbiturates. Now considered obsolete for use in medicine, they are occasionally encountered as drugs of abuse.

Meprobamate (Equanil, Miltown) was marketed in 1955 as an alternative to the barbiturates for daytime sedation and anxiolysis. Around it developed the term *tranquilizer* in a marketing attempt to distinguish it from the barbiturates, a distinction that was not borne out in reality. Like barbiturates, meprobamate produces long-lasting daytime sedation, mild euphoria, and relief from anxiety. Meprobamate is not as potent a respiratory depressant as are the barbiturates; attempted suicides from overdosage are seldom successful unless the drug is mixed with opioid narcotics such as morphine or oxycodone. Despite a continuing reduction in clinical use, abuse and dependency continue and are difficult to treat. There is a possibility that use of meprobamate during pregnancy may be associated with an increased frequency of congenital malformations.

Carisoprodol (Soma) is a precursor compound to meprobamate; after it is absorbed, it is rapidly metabolized to meprobamate, which is the active form of the drug. Currently, carisoprodol, as an intoxicant, is increasingly encountered as a drug of abuse.

Methaqualone (Quaalude) was another nonbarbiturate sedative that had little to justify its widespread use. During the late 1970s, its popularity rivaled that of marijuana and alcohol in its level of abuse. The attention was due to an undeserved reputation as an aphrodisiac (as a sedative, it was actually an *anaphrodisiac*, much like alcohol). It was, however, a "date rape" drug since, as with all these drugs, the amnestic effect occurred at doses lower than the dose required to produce incapacitation or unconsciousness. Extensive illicit use and numerous deaths led to its being banned in the United States in 1984, although illicit supplies occasionally emerge as a drug of abuse.

Chloral hydrate (Noctec) is yet another drug of historical interest, having been available clinically since the late 1800s. It is rapidly metabolized to *trichlorethanol* (a derivative of ethyl alcohol), which is a nonselective CNS depressant and the active form of chloral hydrate. The drug is an effective sedative-hypnotic, with a plasma half-life of about 4 to 8 hours. Next-day hangover is less likely to occur than with compounds having longer half-lives. Withdrawal of the drug may be associated with disrupted sleep and intense nightmares. One interesting aside is that the combination of chloral hydrate with alcohol can produce increased intoxication, stupor, and amnesia. This mixture, called a *Mickey Finn*, was an early example of a "date rape" drug combination.

Paraldehyde, introduced into medicine before the barbiturates, is a polymer of acetaldehyde, an intermediate by-product in the body's metabolism of ethyl alcohol. Administered either rectally or orally, paraldehyde was historically used to treat delirium tremens (DTs) in alcoholics undergoing detoxification. Paraldehyde is rapidly absorbed (from both rectal and oral routes), sleep ensues within 10 to 15 minutes after hypnotic doses, and the drug is metabolized in the liver to acetaldehyde. Some paraldehyde is eliminated through the lungs, producing a characteristic breath odor.

Gamma hydroxybutyric acid (gamma hydroxybutyrate, GHB, Xyrem) is a potent CNS depressant used outside the United States as an intravenous general anesthetic. It is also a popular drug of abuse (Nicholson and Balster, 2001). As a sedative, GHB has disinhibition effects and has been abused as an aphrodisiac and a euphoriant. It has been sold illicitly under such names as RenewTrient, Revivarant, Blue Nitro, Remiforce, GH Revitalize, and Gamma G. It has been called "nature's Quaalude," among a variety of other names.

GHB has been implicated as an illicit "date rape" drug; it produces amnesia, although the victim is not necessarily asleep or unconscious. Often GHB is added to alcohol to produce this state. There is no evidence that GHB aids sexual performance: it is a potent sedative and depressant. Like any depressant, it can produce a state of disinhibition, excitement, drunkenness, and amnesia.

Because of GHB's notorious reputation and abuse, the U.S. Food and Drug Administration (FDA) classified it as a Schedule I controlled substance, implying high propensity for abuse and no therapeutic use. (The FDA also classifies heroin and marijuana as Schedule I drugs.) In

2003, although the drug was still scheduled in this manner, it was secondarily classified by the FDA as a Schedule III drug because of its new clinical indication for the treatment of narcolepsy. This was the first (and to date only) time that one drug has been scheduled under two FDA categories of control, depending on the intent of its use and the manner in which it is used or abused (Fuller et al., 2004).[1]

GHB has a rapid onset (about 30 minutes) and a short half-life (about 30 minutes). The drug is rapidly metabolized to inactive metabolites and ultimately to carbon dioxide and water. It is detectable in urine for only very brief periods of time. Overdoses are characterized by stupor, delirium, unconsciousness, coma, and death. Combined with alcohol, the drug's toxic potential is greatly magnified. Acute withdrawal in a GHB-dependent person results in rapid onset of a withdrawal syndrome that includes insomnia, anxiety, and tremors. Withdrawal symptoms usually resolve in about 3 to 10 days.

As stated earlier, GHB has beeen used intraveneously for the induction of general anesthesia. This use has been supplanted by superior anesthetics. However, GHB remains useful in treating narcolepsy, a life-long disorder characterized by fragmented sleep during the night, altered sleep patterns, and excessive sleepiness during the day. GHB is taken at bedtime and then 2.5 to 4 hours later, even if the patient has to be wakened to take the medicine. Taken in this fashion, the drug improves sleep and markedly reduces the number of daytime narcoleptic attacks.

Benzodiazepines

In the 1960s, the benzodiazepines replaced the barbiturates and quickly became the most widely used class of psychotherapeutic drugs; the terms *tranquilizer* and *anxiolytic* rapidly became synonymous with the *benzodiazepines*. These medications remain in wide use today (by prescription) and are widely abused or otherwise used inappropriately.

Pharmacokinetics

Fifteen benzodiazepine derivatives remain available (Table 7.3). They differ from one another mainly in their pharmacokinetic parameters and the routes through which they are administered. Pharmacokinetic differences include rates of metabolism to pharmacologically active intermediates and plasma half-lives of both the parent drug and any active metabolites. Twelve of the benzodiazepines are commercially available in the United States; all 12 are available in dosage forms intended

---

[1]A Schedule I classification means that to the FDA a drug has a high potential for abuse with no therapeutic use. Schedules II through V allow for therapeutic use under varying degrees of prescription regulation.

TABLE 7.3 Benzodiazepines

Drug name		Dosage form		Active metab- olite	Active compounds in blood	Mean elimination half-life in hours (range)
Generic	Trade	Oral	Paren- teral			
LONG-ACTING AGENTS						
Diazepam	Valium	X	X	Yes	Diazepam	24 (20–50)
					Nordiazepam	60 (50–100)
Chlordiazepoxide	Librium	X		Yes	Chlordiaze- poxide	10 (8–24)
					Nordiazepam	60 (50–100)
Flurazepam	Dalmane	X		Yes	Desalkylfluraz- epam	80 (70–160)
Halazepam	Paxipam	X		Yes	Halazepam Nordiazepam	14 (10–20)
Prazepam	Centrax	X		Yes	Nordiazepam	
Chlorazepate	Tranxene	X		Yes	Nordiazepam	
INTERMEDIATE-ACTING AGENTS						
Lorazepam	Ativan	X	X	No	Lorazepam	15 (10–24)
Clonazepam	Klonopin	X		No	Clonazepam	30 (18–50)
Quazepam	Dormalin	X		Yes	Quazepam	35 (25–50)
					Desalkylfluraz- epam	80 (70–160)
Estazolam	ProSom	X		Yes	Hydroxyestaz- olam	18 (13–35)
SHORT-ACTING AGENTS						
Midazolam	Versed		X	No	Midazolam	2.5 (1.5–4.5)
Oxazepam	Serax	X		No	Oxazepam	8 (5–15)
Temazepam	Restoril	X		No	Temazepam	12 (8–35)
Triazolam	Halcion	X		No	Triazolam	2.5 (1.5–5)
Alprazolam	Xanax	X		No	Alprazolam	12 (11–18)

only for oral ingestion, 2 (diazepam and lorazepam) are available for both oral use and use by injection, and 1 (midazolam) is available only in injectable formulation.

Absorption and Distribution. Benzodiazepines are well absorbed when they are taken orally; peak plasma concentrations are achieved in about 1 hour. Some (for example, oxazepam and lorazepam) are absorbed more slowly, while others (for example, triazolam) are absorbed more rapidly. Clorazepate is metabolized in gastric juice to an active metabolite (nordiazepam) that is completely absorbed.

Metabolism and Excretion. Psychoactive drugs are usually metabolized to pharmacologically inactive products, which are then excreted in urine (Chapter 1). Although some benzodiazepines behave this way, several are first metabolized to intermediate, pharmacologically active products; these products, in turn, are detoxified by further metabolism before they are excreted (Figure 7.3). As can be seen from Table 7.3 and Figure 7.3, several benzodiazepines are metabolized into long-lasting, pharmacologically active metabolites; the primary one is nordiazepam, the half-life of which is about 60 hours, much longer (perhaps 1 to 2 weeks) in the elderly. Thus, the long-acting benzodiazepines are long acting primarily because of the long half-life of a pharmacologically active metabolite. In contrast, the short-acting benzodiazepines are short acting because they are metabolized directly into inactive products.

Benzodiazepines in the Elderly. The elderly have a reduced ability to metabolize long-acting benzodiazepines and their active metabolites. In this population, the elimination half-life for diazepam and its active metabolite is about 7 to 10 days. Since it takes about six half-lives to rid the body completely of a drug (Chapter 1), it may take an elderly patient 6 to 10 weeks to become drug-free after stopping the drug. With short-acting benzodiazepines, such as midazolam, pharmacokinetics are not so drastically altered, but the dose necessary to achieve effect is reduced by about 50 percent.

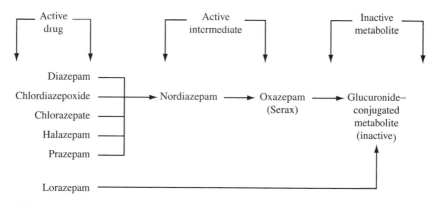

FIGURE 7.3 Metabolism of benzodiazepines. The intermediate metabolite nordiazepam is formed from many agents. Oxazepam (Serax) is commercially available and is also an active metabolite in the metabolism of nordiazepam to its inactive products.

Because all benzodiazepines can produce cognitive dysfunction, elderly patients can become clinically demented as a result. In general, benzodiazepines should be used only with great caution (if at all) in the elderly (Weston et al., 2010). Rang and Dale (1991) stated some twenty years ago:

> At the age of 91, the grandmother of one of the authors was growing increasingly forgetful and mildly dotty, having been taking nitrazepam for insomnia regularly for years. To the author's lasting shame, it took a canny general practitioner to diagnose the problem. Cancellation of the nitrazepam prescription produced a dramatic improvement. (p. 637)

Paterniti and coworkers (2002) followed over 130 benzodiazepine-using elderly people for up to four years. Even periodic use was associated with prolonged decreases in cognitive performance, compared with non-drug-taking elderly. Recently, Wu and coworkers (2009) reported that long-term benzodiazepine use was associated with a more than twofold increased risk of dementia. They concluded that bezodiazepines should be avoided in the elderly. They postulate that this dementing action in the elderly may follow from hyperpolarization of neuronal cell membranes, possibly reducing synaptic plasticity and hindering the individual's ability to form new memories.

Another significant problem with benzodiazepines in the elderly is a widely reported increase in the incidence of falls and bone fractures (Nurmi-Luthje et al., 2006; Allain et al., 2005). Atypical antipsychotic drugs, such as quetiapine (Chapter 4), are replacing the use of benzodiazepines for sedation and behavioral control in the elderly (Chapter 19).

Pharmacological Effects

All benzodiazepines are termed *pure GABA agonists* because they faithfully facilitate GABA binding at GABA receptors. Low doses moderate anxiety, agitation, and fear by their actions on receptors located in the amygdala, orbitofrontal cortex, and insula. Mental confusion and amnesia follow action on GABA neurons located in the cerebral cortex and the hippocampus. The mild muscle relaxant effects of the benzodiazepines are probably caused both by their anxiolytic actions and by effects on GABA receptors located in the spinal cord, cerebellum, and brain stem. The antiepileptic actions seem to follow from actions on GABA receptors located in the cerebellum and the hippocampus. The behavioral rewarding effects, drug abuse potential, and psychological dependency probably result from actions on GABA receptors that modulate the discharge of neurons located in the ventral tegmentum and the nucleus accumbens.

Clinical Uses and Limitations

From 1960 to the late 1990s, the benzodiazepines were the drugs of choice for the short-term pharmacological treatment of stress-related anxiety and insomnia. They are easy to use, have relatively low toxicity, and are effective in producing a "tranquil" state with reductions in anxiety. The benzodiazepines, however, are not antidepressant; in fact, they can intensify depression in much the same way that alcohol intensifies depression. The cognitive impairments and potential for producing dependency are generally conceded to limit their therapeutic use to relatively short periods of time and to conditions in which short-term therapy is beneficial. For longer-term treatment of such disorders as insomnia, generalized anxiety, phobias, panic disorder, and posttraumatic stress disorder, behavioral treatments and both antidepressant and atypical antipsychotic drugs are now preferred over benzodiazepine therapy. In instances where a combination of cognitive-behavioral therapies and benzodiazepines are used to treat anxiety, the benzodiazepines have the potential to interfere with the cognitive therapy, perhaps significantly reducing its efficacy. A cognitive inhibitor could certainly be predicted to block cognitive-based psychological therapies.[2]

Benzodiazepines are generally not utilized for chronic use or for treating depression. They should be avoided in situations requiring fine motor or cognitive skills or mental alertness, or in situations where alcohol or other CNS depressants are used. They should be used only with great caution in the elderly, in children or adolescents, and in anyone with a history of drug misuse or ongoing abuse.

One possible indication for benzodiazepine therapy is for the short-term treatment of anxiety that is so debilitating that the patient's life-style, work, and interpersonal relationships are severely hampered. A benzodiazepine may alleviate the symptoms of nervousness, dysphoria, and psychological distress without necessarily blocking the physiological correlates accompanying the state of anxiety.

Because they are sedating, benzodiazepines are used as hypnotics for the treatment of insomnia. Agents with rapid onset, a 2- to 3-hour half-life, and no active metabolites may be preferred to minimize daytime sedation (note that few benzodiazepines fit this profile; see Table 7.3). Use in treating insomnia is also limited by the development of dependence, as reflected by rebound increases in insomnia upon drug discontinuation.

The benzodiazepines have been used as muscle relaxants, both to directly reduce states associated with increased muscle tension and

---

[2] A patient is often unaware of this interaction since the long half-lives of benzodiazepines imply that a patient is seldom, if ever, free of drug. Neither the patient nor the therapist knows the patient's cognitive ability in the absence of drug.

to reduce the psychological distress that can predispose to muscle tension. However, they do not directly relax muscles. They relieve only the distress associated with muscle tension (much like alcohol).

Benzodiazepines are exceedingly effective in producing antero-grade amnesia (amnesia that starts at the time of drug administration and ends when the blood level of drug has decreased to a point where memory function is regained). For this use, two injectable benzodi-azepines are available—lorazepam, when long-lasting amnesia is desir-able, and midazolam, when shorter periods of amnesia are desirable.

Often, however, an amnestic effect is undesirable. For example, con-cern has been expressed about an illegally imported "date rape" drug, which turned out to be a benzodiazepine that is commercially marketed outside the United States. This drug, *flunitrazepam* (Rohypnol), is very similar to *triazolam* (Halcion; see Table 7.3); it produces anxiolysis, seda-tion, and amnesia, especially when taken with alcohol. When the drug and alcohol are ingested by an unknowing victim, the effect closely re-sembles the effect of a Mickey Finn (chloral hydrate in alcohol), and am-nesia is achieved without loss of unconsciousness.[3]

Panic attacks and phobias can be treated with benzodiazepines such as *alprazolam* (Xanax), although the efficacy of benzodiazepines may be less than that of the serotonin-type antidepressants, which are actually more specific anxiolytics (Stocchi et al., 2003). Moreover, un-like with the benzodiazepines, SSRI use is not accompanied by im-paired psychomotor performance, impaired learning and cognition, reduced alertness, and the potential for dependence and abuse (Arkowitz and Lilienfeld, 2007).

Because benzodiazepines can substitute for alcohol, they are used both in treating acute alcohol withdrawal and in long-term therapy to reduce the rate of relapse to previous drinking habits. Today, however, certain of the antiepileptic mood stabilizers (Chapter 6) are viable alternatives. Finally, all benzodiazepines exert antiepileptic actions be-cause they raise the threshold for generating seizures. In general, how-ever, benzodiazepines are used as secondary drugs or as adjuvants to other, more specific anticonvulsants.

In summary, perhaps the only well-accepted situation in which ben-zodiazepines cannot readily be replaced by other drugs is the intentional production of anterograde amnesia, for example, in hospital situations where it is desirable to block the memory for certain unpleasant or painful procedures. The newer antidepressant/anxiolytic agents continue

---

[3] Rohypnol intoxication (and the amnesia it causes) can begin within about 30 minutes, peak within 2 hours, and persist for up to 8 hours. With a combina-tion of Rohypnol and alcohol, the amnestic and intoxicating effects can last 8 to 18 hours. Disinhibition is another widely reported effect of Rohypnol when it is ingested alone or in combination with alcohol.

to reduce benzodiazepine use for the treatment of most anxiety disorders, although the benzodiazepines may have a faster onset of effect.

Side Effects and Toxicity

Common acute side effects associated with benzodiazepine therapy are usually dose-related extensions of the intended actions, including sedation, drowsiness, ataxia, lethargy, mental confusion, motor and cognitive impairments, disorientation, slurred speech, amnesia, and induction or extension of the symptoms of dementia. At higher doses, mental and psychomotor dysfunction progress to hypnosis. Used for the treatment of insomnia, benzodiazepines are especially controversial; drugs can cause the expected sedation, or they can induce paradoxical agitation (anxiety, aggression, hostility, and behavioral disinhibition). In addition, cessation of use results in rebound increases in insomnia (*REM rebound*) and anxiety.

Impairment of motor abilities—especially a person's ability to drive an automobile—is common. Verster and coworkers (2002a) demonstrated that low doses of alprazolam (Xanax), equivalent to a 0.15 gram% blood level of alcohol, markedly impaired driving ability. The ability to divide attention was especially impaired. This impairment is compounded by the drug-induced suppression of a person's ability to assess his or her own level of physical and mental impairment.

The cognitive deficits associated with benzodiazepine use are significant. In both children and adults, benzodiazepines can significantly interfere with learning behaviors, academic performance, and psychomotor functioning. Cognitive and generalized intellectual impairments can persist even long after the benzodiazepine is discontinued, although cognitive improvements after discontinuation are the norm. Stewart (2005) stated:

> Meta-analyses found that cognitive dysfunction did in fact occur in patients treated long-term with benzodiazepines, and although cognitive dysfunction improved after benzodiazepines were withdrawn, patients did not return to levels of functioning that matched benzodiazepine-free controls. (p. 9)

This statement is certainly cause for concern!

Tolerance and Dependence

When benzodiazepines are taken for prolonged periods of time, a pattern of dependence can develop. Early withdrawal signs include a return (and possible intensification) of the anxiety state for which the drug was originally given. Rebound increases in insomnia, restlessness, agitation, irritability, and unpleasant dreams gradually appear. In rare instances, hallucinations, psychoses, and seizures have been reported. Most of these withdrawal symptoms subside within one to four weeks.

Zitman and Couvee (2001) studied a large group of patients for whom benzodiazepines had been inappropriately prescribed for the treatment of depression. They were withdrawn from their benzodiazepine either with or without administration of concomitant paroxetine. Although two-thirds of the patients were successfully withdrawn, by two or three years after original discontinuation only 13 percent remained benzodiazepine-free. This illustration shows the attractiveness of the benzodiazepines and explains the inability of certain people to refrain from their use. Patients who have histories of drug or alcohol abuse are most apt to use these agents inappropriately, and abuse of benzodiazepines usually occurs as part of a pattern of abuse of more than one drug.

Effects in Pregnancy

During pregnancy, benzodiazepines and their metabolites freely cross the placenta and accumulate in the fetal circulation. Benzodiazepines administered during the first trimester of pregnancy have been reported to cause fetal abnormalities, although the risk is probably very small. Howland (2009) stated that "benzodiazepine drugs, used for anxiety or insomnia, have a small but significant risk of birth defects."

Near the time of delivery, if a mother is on high doses of benzodiazepines, a fetus can develop benzodiazepine dependence or even a "floppy-infant syndrome," followed after delivery by signs of withdrawal. Because benzodiazepines are excreted in breast milk and because they can accumulate in nursing infants, taking benzodiazepines while breast-feeding is not recommended.

Flumazenil: A Benzodiazepine Receptor Antagonist

Flumazenil (Romazicon) is a benzodiazepine that binds with high affinity to benzodiazepine receptors on the GABA$_A$ complex, but after binding, it exhibits no intrinsic activity. As a consequence, it competitively blocks the access of pharmacologically active benzodiazepines to the receptor, effectively reversing the antianxiety and sedative effects of any benzodiazepines administered before flumazenil.

Flumazenil is metabolized quite rapidly in the liver and has a short half-life (about 1 hour). Because this half-life is much shorter than that of most benzodiazepines, the benzodiazepine effects can reappear as flumazenil is lost, thus necessitating reinjection. Flumazenil is utilized as an antidote (administered by intravenous injection) when benzodiazepine overdosage is suspected.

Benzodiazepine Receptor Agonist Hypnotics

Any drug that activates the benzodiazepine receptor is termed a *benzodiazepine receptor agonist* (BZRA). The benzodiazepines are obviously in this category, since they all work by binding to the benzodiazepine receptor and exert a stimulant (or agonist) action to increase GABA activity. Benzodiazepines in lower doses exert anxiolytic effects, but at higher doses they exert hypnotic effects and are used for the treatment of insomnia.

Three other drugs that are currently available are structurally not classified as benzodiazepines but nevertheless are agonists at the benzodiazepine receptor. These *nonbenzodiazepine BZRAs* are prescribed as hypnotic drugs intended for the treatment of insomnia. They are not prescribed as anxiolytics, primarily because of their short half-lives. These three drugs, as well as the benzodiazepines, have been implicated in behavioral activities that occur while one is amnestic (for example, driving, eating, cooking a meal, or engaging in sexual activity and not remembering having done so).

Chronic insomnia can manifest itself as difficulty falling asleep, difficulty staying asleep, waking up too early, or waking in the morning without feeling "refreshed." About 10 percent of people experience chronic insomnia. Roughly 50 percent of people with other medical or psychological conditions complain of insomnia. Consequences of insomnia include daytime fatigue, lack of energy, poor concentration and memory, moodiness and irritability, and difficulty completing tasks. Treatments can be either psychological or pharmacological. Of the psychological therapies, cognitive-behavioral therapies have been shown to be at least as effective as pharmacotherapies (Sivertsen et al., 2006; Morin et al., 2006). Practice parameters for the psychological and behavioral treatment of insomnia are available (Morgenthaler et al., 2006). Pharmacotherapies include two types of FDA-approved insomnia medications: agonists of the benzodiazepine receptor (BZRAs) and a melatonin receptor agonist (ramelteon).

Benzodiazepine BZRAs

As discussed earlier, all benzodiazepines exhibit hypnotic properties. Five of them (flurazepam, estazolam, quazepam, temazepam, and triazolam) are formally indicated for the treatment of insomnia. Triazolam has the shortest half-life, 2 to 4 hours, and is associated with the least daytime sedation. It may not provide adequate sedation through the night. Conversely, the others have longer half-lives and increase sleep maintenance, but they have adverse cognitive consequences the next day (see Table 7.3). Dependence and tolerance are potentially harmful.

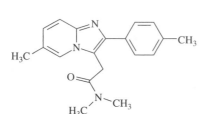

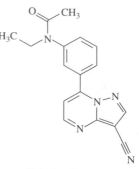

Zolpidem (Ambien)   Zaleplon (Sonata)

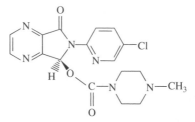

Eszopiclone (Lunesta)

FIGURE 7.4 Structural formulas of zolpidem (Ambien), zaleplon (Sonata), and eszopiclone (Lunesta). Note the close (but dissimilar) relationship of their basic three-ring structures to the benzodiazepine nucleus (see Figure 7.2). Thus, these three compounds are nonbenzodiazepines despite similar GABAergic actions and clinical effects.

Nonbenzodiazepine BZRAS

Three drugs that are structurally not benzodiazepines nevertheless bind to the same receptors to which benzodiazepines bind and exert the same agonist effects as the benzodiazepines (Figure 7.4). These three drugs are referred to as *nonbenzodiazepine BZRAs*.

Zolpidem. Zolpidem (Ambien, Edluar) is marketed for the treatment of insomnia. Binding to a specific subgroup, the $GABA_{1A}$ receptor, it exhibits primarily a hypnotic rather than an anxiolytic effect. It displays primarily sedative effects rather than anxiolytic effects; it seems that its sedative actions overwhelm any anxiolytic effects. With a half-life of about 2 to 2.5 hours, zolpidem is often compared to triazolam (Halcion), a benzodiazepine with similar pharmacokinetics; at comparable doses, there appears to be little to differentiate the two drugs. A controlled-release formulation of zolpidem (Ambien CR) is available. Due to slower dissolution in the gastrointestinal tract, it is absorbed at a slower rate. Thus, its half-life is a bit longer, perhaps about 3 hours.

Zolpidem is rapidly absorbed from the gastrointestinal tract after oral administration, with about 75 percent of the administered drug reaching the plasma and the remainder being rapidly metabolized as it is being absorbed. Peak plasma levels are reached in about 1 hour. Following metabolism in the liver, the kidneys excrete the inactive metabolites. At doses of 5 to 10 milligrams, zolpidem produces sedation and promotes a physiological pattern of sleep in the absence of anxiolytic, anticonvulsant, or muscle relaxant effects. Memory is adversely affected as it is by benzodiazepines, and drug-induced blackouts are common.

Dose-related adverse effects of zolpidem include drowsiness, dizziness, and nausea. In doses of 10 milligrams, zolpidem exhibits minimal next-day effects on memory or psychomotor performance, such as driving; however, doses of 10 to 20 milligrams significantly impair performance and memory even 4 hours after taking the drug (Verster et al., 2002b). Overdoses to 400 milligrams (40 times the therapeutic dose) have not been fatal.

In the elderly, confusion, falls, memory loss, and psychotic reactions have been reported. The calculated half-life is prolonged in the elderly and, here, the extended-release preparation may increase the risk of next-day sedation and cognitive impairment.

Zaleplon. Zaleplon (Sonata) is a second nonbenzodiazepine agonist that binds to the $GABA_{1A}$ receptor. In general, it exerts actions similar to those of zolpidem as a hypnotic agent. The half-life of zaleplon is very short (less than 1 hour), and only about 30 percent of the dose reaches the bloodstream; most undergoes first-pass metabolism in the liver. Because Zaleplon is so short acting, it does not require predicting that insomnia will occur on a particular night. Instead, if unable to fall asleep and stay asleep without pharmacological assistance, the person has the option of taking this very short-acting agent without fear of detrimental effects the next morning.

Sleep is quite rapidly induced with zaleplon at doses of 5 to 10 milligrams, and sleep quality is improved without rebound insomnia. Zaleplon appears particularly noteworthy in its lack of deleterious effects on psychomotor function and driving ability the morning following use (Verster et al., 2002b). Allowing at least 4 hours from drug intake to driving results in few adverse effects (Patat et al., 2001). In fact, at 4 hours after oral administration, most of the drug is eliminated from the body. Dependence is unlikely to develop because of the short half-life: by morning, the drug is metabolized. In essence, a person taking the drug withdraws daily, and drug does not persist in the body. At extremely high doses (25 to 75 milligrams), an abuse potential comparable to that seen for triazolam (Halcion) is seen.

Eszopiclone. Eszopiclone (Lunesta) is the third BZRA approved for the treatment of insomnia. It is the active isomer of zopiclone (Immovane), which has been used outside the United States for many years. Eszopiclone shares all the actions of zolpidem and traditional benzodiazepines. Because of a half-life of 5 to 7 hours, eszopiclone has the most prolonged action of the nonbenzodiazepine BZRAs. Therefore, it might be preferable to the others for improving both sleep latency and sleep maintenance. However, this benefit is offset by increased risk of next-day sedation. It was the first of these agents to have data reported from long-term trials, and thus it has been approved by the FDA for longer-term use. At its highest dose level (3 milligrams), next-day memory impairments and poor performance on measures of psychomotor performance have been reported.

Partial Agonists at GABA$_A$ Receptors

"Full" BZRA agonists are effective anxiolytics and/or sedatives; however, their use is limited by rebound anxiety (on discontinuation), physical dependence, abuse potential, and side effects that include ataxia, sedation, memory impairments, and cognitive disturbances. Therefore, attempts have been made to identify "partial" agonists of GABA receptors (*partial BZRAs*) in the hope of providing anxiolytics that may be equally as effective without the side effects that limit the use of the benzodiazepines. To date, several have been examined, although none are currently available in the United States. The best studied of these agents are alpidem (marketed in Europe), etizolam, imidazenil, abecarnil, and bretazenil. Each of these partial agonists is in various stages of experimentation or trial for various clinical uses, including use as anticonvulsants.

Sleep Driving and Sleep-Related Activities

In March 2007, the FDA released an advisory requesting that all manufacturers of sedative-hypnotic products that are used to induce and/or maintain sleep strengthen their product labeling to include risks of "sleep driving" and "sleep-related activities." Sleep driving is defined as driving while not fully awake after ingestion of a sedative-hypnotic product and having no memory of the event—in other words, driving while still in a drug-induced amnestic state. Sleep-related activities that can occur include making telephone calls, preparing and eating food and then having no later memory of having done so, and engaging in sexual activity and then having no later memory of having done so (Zammit, 2009). Thirteen products were listed on the FDA advisory. These included the three nonbenzodiazepine BZRAs (Ambien, Sonata, and Lunesta); the benzodiazepines Dalmane, Halcion, ProSom, and

Restoril; the barbiturates Butisol, Carbrital, and Seconal; the melatonin agonist Rozerem; and two miscellaneous agents (Doral and Placidyl). This advisory is probably not all-inclusive.

General Anesthetics

All sedatives in sufficient doses can produce amnesia and loss of consciousness. General anesthetics are drugs that are used to intentionally produce these effects for the performance of surgical procedures. The agents that are used as general anesthetics are of two types: (1) those that are administered by inhalation through the lungs and (2) those that are injected directly into a vein.

The inhalation anesthetics in current use include one gas (nitrous oxide) and five volatile liquids (isoflurane, halothane, desflurane, enflurane, and sevoflurane). These drugs produce a dose-related depression of all functions of the CNS—an initial period of sedation followed by the onset of sleep. As anesthesia deepens, both amnesia and unconsciousness are induced. Adding an opioid narcotic (such as morphine) to a volatile anesthetic adds analgesic action to this state of unconsciousness.

Occasionally, the inhaled anesthetic agents are subject to misuse. *Nitrous oxide,* a gas of low anesthetic potency, is an example. Currently used not only in anesthesia but also as a carrier gas in whipped cream charger cans (for example, Whippets), nitrous oxide induces a state of behavioral disinhibition, analgesia, and mild euphoria. Since the inhalation of nitrous oxide dilutes the air that a person is breathing, extreme caution must be exercised to prevent hypoxia. If the nitrous oxide is mixed only with room air, hypoxia results, which could produce irreversible brain damage. Other forms of inhalant abuse are discussed in Chapter 13.

Several *injectable anesthetics* are available. *Thiopental* (Pentothal) and *methohexital* (Brevital) are ultrashort-acting barbiturates. *Propofol* (Diprovan) and *etomidate* (Amidate) are structurally unique; propofol structurally resembles the neurotransmitter GABA. Because propofol and etomidate are now generically available (and inexpensive), more expensive preparations have been marketed. Fospropofol (Lusedra) is a prodrug to propofol; fospropofol is rapidly converted to propofol, its active form. Desmedetomidine (Precedex) is structurally related to etomidate and likely works with identical efficacy (Paris et al., 2007; Mizrak et al., 2010). The injectable anesthetic *ketamine* is discussed as a psychedelic anesthetic in Chapter 15.

Ramelteon: A Selective Melatonin Receptor Agonist

Melatonin, available for many years as an over-the-counter drug for the treatment of insomnia, has repeatedly failed to demonstrate significant effects, except perhaps on people with disrupted sleep-wake

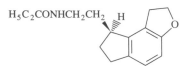

Ramelteon (Rozerem)

FIGURE 7.5 Structural formula of ramelteon (Rozerem).

cycles, such as shift workers and people with jet lag (Srinivasan et al., 2008). The sleep-wake cycle is controlled by homeostatic and circadian processes that regulate the drive for sleep that accumulates during waking. Neurons in the anterior hypothalamus coordinate the timing of this circadian system and maintain 24-hour periodicity, controlling the pineal gland in producing melatonin, with melatonin levels increasing as bedtime approaches, plateauing during the night, and decreasing as sleep ends in the morning. These anterior hypothalamic neurons contain a high concentration of melatonin receptors.

Ramelteon (Rozerem; Figure 7.5) is a melatonin receptor agonist that has been approved by the FDA for the treatment of insomnia characterized by difficulty with sleep onset. The drug is thought to be non-addicting and therefore devoid of abuse potential. Rebound insomnia following a period of nightly drug use has not been reported. In an available 8-milligram dose, it is taken 30 minutes before going to bed. A half-life of about 3 hours is thought to leave little morning drowsiness. In controlled trials, efficacy was quite modest, with sleep onset occurring only about 10 or 15 minutes earlier than after taking placebo and with total sleep time little affected (Simpson and Curran, 2008). Controlled trials against established anti-insomnia drugs, including the nonbenzodiazepine BZRAs, have not been reported. Therefore, its efficacy relative to other therapeutic options cannot be estimated at this time. Several reviews of the pharmacology of ramelteon are available (Sateia et al., 2008; Reynoldson et al., 2008; Pandi-Perumal et al., 2009).

Serotonin Receptor Agonists as Anxiolytics

Anxiety may, at least in part, result from defects in serotonin neurotransmission, and drugs that augment serotonin activity are useful in the treatment of anxiety disorders. Perhaps the most widely used class of serotonin agonists are the SSRI-type antidepressants (Chapter 5). The six clinically available SSRI antidepressants are widely used in the treatment of all anxiety disorders and are, in fact, considered to be drugs of first choice for such use. We focus here on several other agents that act through direct stimulation of the postsynaptic serotonin 5-HT$_{1A}$ receptor.

Serotonin 5-HT$_{1A}$ receptors are found in high density in the hippocampus, the septum, parts of the amygdala, and the dorsal raphe nucleus, areas all presumed to be involved in fear and anxiety responses. Activation of the 5-HT$_{1A}$ receptor is thought to diminish neuronal activity. Mice selectively bred without 5-HT$_{1A}$ receptors display increased fear responses, suggesting that reductions in 5-HT$_{1A}$ receptor activity or density (presumably due to genetic deficits or environmental stressors) result in heightened anxiety (Rambos et al., 1998).

Buspirone. Clinical interest in serotonin anxiolytics began 20 years ago with demonstration of the anxiolytic action of *buspirone*, a selective serotonin 5-HT$_{1A}$ agonist. In 1986 the drug was approved for clinical use, and it is marketed under the trade name BuSpar. Thereafter, other related agents were identified, but they have not yet been marketed. Gepirone, ipsapirone, and alnespirone are three examples of such drugs.

Buspirone (BuSpar) is a 5-HT$_{1A}$ agonist with demonstrable anxiolytic properties. It relieves anxiety in a unique fashion:

- Its anxiolysis occurs without significant sedation or hypnotic action, even in overdosage.
- Amnesia, mental confusion, and psychomotor impairment are minimal or absent.
- It does not potentiate the CNS depressant effects of alcohol, benzodiazepines, or other CNS sedatives (synergism does not occur).
- It does not substitute for benzodiazepines in treating anxiety or benzodiazepine withdrawal.
- It does not exhibit cross-tolerance or cross-dependence with benzodiazepines.
- It exhibits little potential for addiction or abuse.
- It exhibits an antidepressant effect in addition to its anxiolytic effect, making it potentially useful in depressive disorders with accompanying anxiety.
- Its effect has a gradual onset rather than the immediate onset of the action of the benzodiazepines.

Buspirone is a weak agonist at 5-HT$_{1A}$ receptors. As a result, it exerts both an anxiolytic action and an antidepressant action (the antidepressant role of 5-HT$_{1A}$ receptors is discussed in Chapter 7). Buspirone has some efficacy in the treatment of generalized anxiety disorder (Pollack, 2009). It has also been recommended for patients who suffer from mixed symptoms of anxiety and depression, as well as for elderly people with agitated dementia.

Buspirone is most helpful in anxious patients who do not demand the immediate symptom relief they associate with the benzodiazepine response. Slower and more gradual onset of anxiety relief is balanced by the increased safety and lack of dependency-producing aspects of

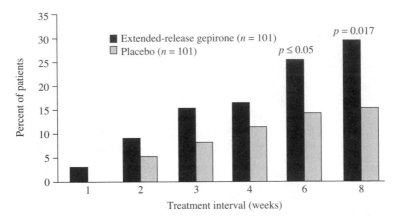

FIGURE 7.6 Percentage of patients achieving remission on a 17-item Hamilton Rating Scale for Depression. [Adapted from A. D. Feiger et al., "Gepirone Extended Release: New Evidence for Efficacy in the Treatment of Major Depressive Disorder," *Journal of Clinical Psychiatry* 4 (2003), p. 247, Figure 5.]

buspirone. It takes several weeks of continuous treatment to see clinical effects. Patients who have previously been taking benzodiazepines do poorly on buspirone.

Chapter 1 presents a likely reason that the effects of buspirone are so subtle: most of the drug is detoxified by first-pass metabolism; only about 5 percent of orally administered drug reaches the bloodstream. Inhibition of metabolism (for example, by concurrent drinking of grapefruit juice) improves its efficacy by increasing its intestinal absorption (Paine et al., 2006; Uno and Yasui-Furukori, 2006).

Gepirone. *Gepirone* (Arisa, Variza) is another 5-HT_{1A} agonist currently in clinical trial in the United States for use as both an antidepressant and an anxiolytic. In extended-release formulation, gepirone-ER (Figure 7.6) efficacy is comparable to standard agents, and side effects (for example, lightheadedness, nausea, dizziness) have been tolerable (Bielski et al., 2008). The drug is currently under FDA review in an extended-release formulation for use in treating anxiety and depression.

Antiepileptic Drugs

Sedative-hypnotic drugs used for the treatment of epilepsy have been called anticonvulsants or antiepileptic drugs. In recent years, their uses have been expanded to treatment of bipolar disorder (Chapter 6); treatment of *explosive behavioral disorders* in children, adolescents, and adults (Chapter 18); management of alcohol withdrawal and cravings (Chapter 13); treatment of chronic *pain*; and management of certain anxiety disorders such as posttraumatic stress disorder, generalized anxiety disorder, and even certain components of borderline personality disorder (Chapter 6). These nonepileptic uses necessitate the terms *mood stabilizer* or *neuromodulator* to cover this multitude of actions. In this section, these drugs are introduced for their original indication: antiepileptic agents or anticonvulsants. The plasma half-lives and therapeutic blood levels of available antiepileptic drugs are listed in Table 7.4.

TABLE 7.4 Antiepileptic drugs available in the United States

Year introduced	Generic name	Trade name	Half-life (hours)	Therapeutic blood level (mcg/ml) [a]
1912	Phenobarbital	Luminal	50+	15–40
1935	Mephobarbital	Mebaral	—[b]	—
1938	Phenytoin	Dilantin	18+	5–20
1946	Trimethadione	Tridione	6–13	>700
1947	Mephenytoin	Mesantoin	95	—
1949	Paramethadione	Paradione	—	—
1951	Phenacemide	Phenurone	—	—
1952	Metharbital	Gemonil	—	—
1953	Phensuximide	Milontin	8	—
1954	Primidone	Mysoline	5–20	5–40
1957	Methsuximide	Celontin	2–40	—
1957	Ethotoin	Peganone	4–9	15–50
1960	Ethosuximide	Zarontin	30+	40–400
1968	Diazepam	Valium	20–50	—
1974	Carbamazepine	Tegretol	18–50	4–12
1975	Clonazepam	Klonopin	18–60	20–80
1978	Valproic acid	Depakene	5–20	50–150
1981	Clorazepate	Tranxene	30–100	—
1981	Lorazepam	Ativan	14	—
1993	Felbamate	Felbatol	22	—
1994	Gabapentin	Neurontin	5–7	—
1995	Lamotrigine	Lamictal	33	1–5
1998	Topiramate	Topamax	19–23	—
1998	Tiagabine	Gabatril	6–9	—
1999	Levetiracetam	Keppra	7	10
2000	Zonisamide	Zonegran	60	—
2009	Lacosamide	Vimpat	13	4–10

[a] mcg/ml = micrograms of drug per milliliter of blood
[b] — = data not available

The chemical structures of the major antiepileptic drugs are presented in Figure 7.7. Phenobarbital (a barbiturate) was the first widely effective antiepileptic drug. This and other barbiturates, because of their sedative and adverse cognitive depressant effects, are today rarely used; equally effective, more specific, and less sedating antiepileptic agents are now available.

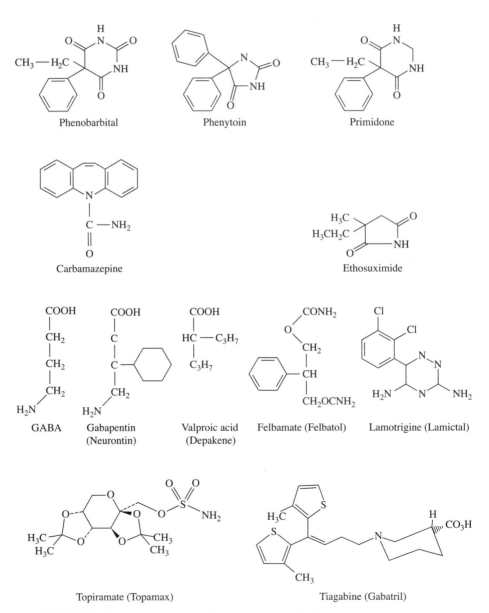

FIGURE 7.7 Chemical structures of antiepileptic medications.

Phenytoin (Dilantin) remains a commonly used *hydantoin* anticonvulsant, producing less sedation than do the barbiturates. Phenytoin has a half-life of about 24 hours; thus, daytime sedation can be minimized if the patient takes the full daily dose at bedtime. Many bothersome side effects limit its use in favor of newer, less toxic agents.

Valproic acid (divalproex, Depakene, Depakote) is effective in treating *petit mal* seizure disorders in children. It acts by augmenting the postsynaptic action of GABA. Valproic acid has a short half-life (about 6 to 12 hours); it must therefore be administered two or three times a day. Common side effects include sedation and cognitive impairments. Serious side effects are rare, but liver failure has been reported. Like many of the newer anticonvulsants, valproic acid is effective in people with bipolar disorder, posttraumatic stress disorder, borderline personality disorder, aggressive behaviors, schizophrenia, and alcohol and cocaine dependence. A long-acting, slow-release formulation (Depakote-ER) is approved for the treatment of migraine headache.

Carbamazepine (Tegretol, Equitro) is an antiepileptic drug with a sedative effect that is perhaps less intense than that of the other antiepileptic agents. The primary limitations of carbamazepine include serious alterations in the cellular composition of blood (reduced numbers of white blood cells), presumably secondary to a depressant effect on bone marrow. Carbamazepine also increases the production of drug-metabolizing enzymes in the liver, such that other drugs metabolized by the same enzymes are metabolized much faster than would normally be expected and these drugs become clinically "less effective" due to lower-than-expected blood concentrations.

For nonepileptic use, carbamazepine is used in the treatment of bipolar disorder, explosive behavioral disorders, pain syndromes, and alcohol withdrawal.

Gabapentin (Neurontin), a structural analogue of GABA (see Figure 7.7), was synthesized as a specific GABA-mimetic antiepileptic drug. In 1995, gabapentin was reported effective in treating both an anxiety disorder (phobia) and pain (reflex sympathetic dystrophy). Since then, gabapentin has been used in a wide variety of chronic pain states and psychiatric disorders, including bipolar disorder, and in the demented elderly to treat agitation and aggressive behavior. Gabapentin can be effective in treating alcohol withdrawal and for prevention of relapse. It also possesses significant anxiolytic efficacy, and therefore is used for treatment of a variety of anxiety disorders.

Lamotrigine (Lamictal), introduced into medicine in 1995, acts by inhibiting ion fluxes through sodium channels, stabilizing neuronal membranes, and inhibiting the presynaptic release of neurotransmitters, principally glutamate. First introduced as an antiepileptic drug, it has beneficial effects on mood, mental alertness, and social interactions in some epilepsy patients. An unusual and significant advantage of lamotrigine is that it improves cognitive functioning (Aldenkamp et al., 2003) and exerts antidepressant actions (Brown, 2009). Clinically, it has been used for the treatment of resistant depression (McIntyre and Morel, 2006)

Oxcarbazepine (Trileptal) is a structural derivative of carbamazepine. It differs in two ways: (1) it is rapidly metabolized by a process called *reduction* to an active molecule, and (2) it has not been associated with the white blood cell toxicity associated with carbamazepine. Oxcarbazepine is being increasingly used to treat bipolar illness (Hellewell, 2002) and other disorders for which carbamazepine is also effective (Gentry et al., 2002).

Tiagabine (Gabitril) became clinically available in 1998 as another antiepileptic drug. The drug acts by inhibiting neuronal and glial uptake of GABA, secondary to its irreversibly inhibiting one of the GABA reuptake transporters located on the presynaptic nerve terminals of GABA-releasing neurons. This action serves to prolong GABA's synaptic action. Tiagabine appears to be less useful in the treatment of bipolar illness than are other antiepileptic drugs. It has been shown effective in the treatment of generalized anxiety disorder, although its efficacy was limited (Pollack et al., 2008).

Several other new antiepileptic drugs have found use in the treatment of bipolar illness: *topiramate* (Topamax), *levetiracetam* (Keppra), and *zonisamide* (Zonegran). Topiramate is discussed in Chapter 13 for its use in treating alcoholism. Zonisamide has been shown to be effective as an antiobesity agent when combined with a balanced low-calorie diet (Gadde et al., 2003). It has also been used to treat binge-eating disorder.

Recently introduced is an antiepileptic agent called *lacosamide* (Vimpat). This new drug appears to act in a different way than do other anticonvulsants such as phenytoin. Traditional anticonvulsants affect a "fast action potential generation," while lacosamide interacts with sodium channels without affecting fast inactivation (Curia et al., 2009). It is therefore a "novel sodium channel modulator" (Bee and Dickenson, 2009) useful in the treatment of epilepsy (Kellinghaus, 2009). Lacosamide has also been shown to be effective in the treatment of neuropathic pain (Harris and Murphy, 2009) and anxiety disorders (Higgins et al., 2009). It may exert fewer cognitive-depressing side effects than other anticonvulsants (Higgins et al., 2010).

Antiepileptic Drugs in Pregnancy

Rates of stillbirth and infant mortality are higher for mothers with epilepsy. Children of epileptic mothers who received antiseizure medication during the early months of pregnancy have an increased incidence of a variety of birth defects. The risk is approximately 7 to 15 percent, compared with 2 to 3 percent for the general population. The effects of specific anticonvulsants as teratogenic agents is discussed in Chapter 18.

Antiepileptic Drugs and Risk of Suicidal Thoughts and Behavior

On December 16, 2008, the FDA notified manufacturers of antiepileptic medicines that it now requires a warning that the use of these drugs may increase the risk of suicidal thoughts and behaviors. Patients taking antiepileptic drugs should be carefully monitored for behavioral changes that could be precursors to emerging suicidality, including anxiety, agitation, hostility, and mania or hypomania. This warning applies whether these medicines are used to treat seizures, psychiatric disorders, migraine headaches, or other conditions. The exact risk appears to be small and was not considered sufficient to require a "black-box warning" (the FDA's strongest warning); however, both revised labeling and development of a medication guide were required.

STUDY QUESTIONS

1. What are the advantages of benzodiazepines over barbiturates?
2. Describe the mechanism of action of benzodiazepines.
3. Describe evidence for and against a natural anxiolytic in the brain.
4. Describe the structure and function of the benzodiazepine receptor.
5. How might you describe anxiety or panic in terms of receptors or neurochemicals (at this point)?
6. List some of the clinical uses of benzodiazepines.
7. List three processes that might prolong the half-life of a benzodiazepine.
8. Why should the elderly avoid using long-acting benzodiazepines?
9. Describe the most clinically significant drug interaction that involves benzodiazepines.
10. Discuss benzodiazepine withdrawal and its treatment.
11. What is flumazenil and for what purpose can it be used?
12. Compare and contrast the mechanisms of action and clinical uses of benzodiazepines and buspirone.
13. To what benzodiazepine is zolpidem most often compared? Why?
14. Compare and contrast zolpidem, zaleplon, and eszopiclone.
15. Discuss the future treatment of anxiety disorders with either benzodiazepines or serotonin agonists.

REFERENCES

Aldenkamp, A. P., et al. (2003). "Newer Antiepileptic Drugs and Cognitive Issues." *Epilepsia* 44, Supplement 4: 21–29.

Allain, H., et al. (2005). "Postural Instability and Consequent Falls and Hip Fractures Associated with Use of Hypnotics in the Elderly: A Comprehensive Review." *Drugs and Aging* 22: 749–765.

Arkowitz, H., and Lilienfeld, S. O. (2007). "A Pill to Fix Your Ills?" *Scientific American Mind* 18(1): 80–81.

Bee, L. A., and Dickenson, A. H. (2009). "Effects of Lacosamine, a Novel Sodium Channel Modulator, on Dorsal Horn Neuronal Responses in a Rat Model of Neuropathy." *Neuropsychopharmacology* 57: 472–479.

Bielski, R. J., et al. (2008). "Gepirone Extended-Release in the Treatment of Adult Outpatients with Major Depressive Disorder: A Double-Blind, Randomized, Placebo-Controlled, Parallel-Group Study." *Journal of Clinical Psychiatry* 69: 571–577.

Brown, E. S. (2009). "Effects of Glucocorticoids on Mood, Memory, and the Hippocampus. Treatment and Preventive Therapy." *Annals of the New York Academy of Science* 1179: 41–55.

Curia, G., et al. (2009). "Lacosamide: A New Approach to Target Voltage-Gated Sodium Currents in Epileptic Disorders." *CNS Drugs* 23: 555–568.

Eadie, M. J. (2008). "Antiepileptic Drugs as Human Teratogens." *Expert Opinion on Drug Safety* 7: 195–209.

Fuller, D. E., et al. (2004). "The Xyrem Risk Management Program." *Drug Safety* 27: 293–306.

Gadde, K. M., et al. (2003). "Zonisamide for Weight Loss in Obese Adults: A Randomized Controlled Trial." *Journal of the American Medical Association* 289: 1820–1825.

Gentry, J. R., et al. (2002). "New Anticonvulsants: A Review of Applications for the Management of Substance Abuse Disorders." *Annals of Clinical Psychiatry* 14: 233–245.

Harris, J. A., and Murphy, J. A. (2009). "Lacosamide: An Adjunctive Agent for Partial-Onset Seizures and Potential Therapy for Neuropathic Pain." *Annals of Pharmacotherapy* 43: 1809–1817.

Hartzler, B., and Fromme, K. (2003). "Fragmentary and En Bloc Blackouts: Similarity and Distinction Among Episodes of Alcohol-Induced Memory Loss." *Journal of Studies on Alcohol* 64: 547–550.

Hellewell, J. S. (2002). "Oxcarbazepine (Trileptal) in the Treatment of Bipolar Disorders: Review of Efficacy and Tolerability." *Journal of Affective Disorders* 72, Supplement 1: S23–S34.

Higgins, G. A., et al. (2009). "The Anti-Epileptic Drug Lacosamide (Vimpat) Has Anxiolytic Property in Rodents." *European Journal of Psychopharmacology* 624: 1–9.

Higgins, G. A., et al. (2010). "Comparative Study of Five Antiepileptic Drugs on a Translational Cognitive Measure in the Rat: Relationship to Antiepileptic Property." *Psychopharmacology* 207: 513–527.

Howland, R. H. (2009). "Prescribing Psychotropic Medications During Pregnancy and Lactation: Principles and Guidelines." *Journal of Psychosocial Nursing and Mental Health Services* 47: 19–23.

John, E. R., and Prichap, L. S. (2005). "The Anesthetic Cascade: A Theory of How Anesthesia Suppresses Consciousness." *Anesthesiology* 102: 447–471.

Kellinghaus, C. (2009). "Lacosamide as Treatment for Partial Epilepsy: Mechanisms of Action, Pharmacology, Effects, and Safety." *Therapeutics and Clinical Risk Management* 5: 757–766.

Lee, H., et al., (2009). "Alcohol-Induced Blackout." *International Journal of Environmental Research and Public Health* 6: 2783–2792.

McIntyre, J., and Morel, M. A. (2006). "Spotlight on Lamotrigine for Depression." *Drug News Perspectives* 19: 427–430.

Mizrak, A., et al. (2010). "Pretreatment with Desmedetomidine or Thiopental Decreases Myoclonus After Etomidate: A Randomized, Double-Blind Controlled Trial." *Journal of Surgical Research* 159(1): e11–e16.

Morgenthaler, T., et al. (2006). "Practice Parameters for the Psychological and Behavioral Treatment of Insomnia: An Update. An American Academy of Sleep Medicine Report." *Sleep* 29: 1415–1419.

Morin, C. M., et al. (2006). "Psychological and Behavioral Treatment of Insomnia: Update of the Recent Evidence (1998–2004)." *Sleep* 29: 1398–1414.

Nicholson, K. L., and Balster, R. L. (2001). "GHB: A New and Novel Drug of Abuse." *Drug and Alcohol Dependence* 63: 1–22.

Nurmi-Luthje, I., et al. (2006). "Use of Benzodiazepines and Benzodiazepine-Related Drugs Among 223 Patients with an Acute Hip Fracture in Finland: Comparison of Benzodiazepine Findings in Medical Records and Laboratory Assays." *Drugs and Aging* 23: 27–37.

Paine, M. F., et al (2006). "A Furanocoumarin-Free Grapefruit Juice Establishes Furanocoumarins as the Mediators of the Grapefruit Juice-Felodipine Interaction." *American Journal of Clinical Nutrition* 83: 1097–1105.

Pandi Perumal, S. R., et al. (2009). "Ramelteon: A Review of Its Therapeutic Potential in Sleep Disorders." *Advances in Therapeutics* 26: 613–626.

Paris, A., et al. (2007). "The Anesthetic Effects of Etomidate: Species-Specific Interaction with Alpha-2-Adrenoceptors." *Anesthesia and Analgesia* 105: 1644–1649.

Patat, A., et al. (2001). "Pharmacodynamic Profile of Zaleplon: A New Non-Benzodiazepine Hypnotic Agent." *Human Psychopharmacology* 16: 369–392.

Paterniti, S., et al. (2002). "Long-Term Benzodiazepine Use and Cognitive Decline in the Elderly: The Epidemiology of Vascular Aging Study." *Journal of Clinical Psychopharmacology* 22: 285–293.

Pollack, M. H. (2009). "Refractory Generalized Disorder." *Journal of Clinical Psychiatry* 70, Supplement 2: 32 38.

Pollack, M., et al. (2008). "Tiagabine in Adult Patients with Generalized Anxiety Disorder: Results from 3 Randomized, Double-Blind, Placebo-Controlled, Parallel-Group Studies." *Journal of Clinical Psychopharmacology* 28: 308–316.

Rambos, S., et al. (1998). "Serotonin Receptor 1A Knockout: An Animal Model of Anxiety-Related Disorder." *Proceedings of the National Academy of Sciences* 95: 14476–14481.

Rang, H. P., and Dale, M. M. (1991). *Pharmacology*, 2nd ed. Edinburgh: Churchill Livingstone.

Reynoldson, J. N., et al. (2008). "Ramelteon: A Novel Approach in the Treatment of Insomnia." *Annals of Pharmacotherapy* 42: 1262–1271.

Sateia, M. J., et al. (2008). "Efficacy and Clinical Safety of Ramelteon: An Evidence-Based Review." *Sleep Medicine Reviews* 12: 319–332.

Sigel, E. (2002). "Mapping of the Benzodiazepine Recognition Site on GABA(A) Receptors." *Current Topics in Medicinal Chemistry* 2: 833–839.

Simpson, D., and Curran, M. P. (2008). "Ramelteon: A Review of Its Use in Insomnia." *Drugs* 68: 1901–1919.

Sivertsen, B., et al. (2006). "Cognitive Behavioral Therapy vs. Zopiclone for Treatment of Chronic Primary Insomnia in Older Adults: A Randomized Controlled Trial." *Journal of the American Medical Association* 295: 2851–2858.

Srinivasan, V., et al. (2008). "Jet Lag: Therapeutic Use of Melatonin and Possible Application of Meletonin Analogs." *Travel Medicine and Infectious Disease* 6: 17–28.

Stewart, S. A. (2005). "The Effects of Benzodiazepines on Cognition." *Jounal of Clinical Psychiatry* 66, Supplement 2: 9–13.

Stocchi, F., et al. (2003). "Efficacy and Tolerability of Paroxetine for the Long-Term Treatment of Generalized Anxiety Disorder." *Journal of Clinical Psychiatry* 64: 250–258.

Timmermann, G., et al. (2008). "A Study of the Teratogenic and Fetotoxic Effects of Large Doses of Barbital, Hexobarbital, and Butobarbital Used for Suicide Attempts by Pregnant Women." *Toxicology and Industrial Health* 24: 109–119.

Timmermann, G., et al. (2009). "Congenital Abnormalities of 88 Children Born to Mothers Who Attempted Suicide with Phenobarbital During Pregnancy: The Use of a Disaster Epidemiological Model for the Evaluation of Drug Teratogenicity." *Pharmacoepidemiology and Drug Safety* 18: 815–825.

Uno, T., and Yasui-Furukori, N. (2006). "Effect of Grapefruit Juice in Relation to Human Pharmacokinetic Study." *Current Clinical Pharmacology* 1: 157–161.

Verster, J. C., et al. (2002a). "Effects of Alprazolam on Driving Ability, Memory Functioning, and Psychomotor Performance: A Randomized, Placebo-Controlled Study." *Neuropsychopharmacology* 27: 260–269.

Verster, J. C., et al. (2002b). "Residual Effects of Middle-of-the-Night Administration of Zaleplon and Zolpidem on Driving Ability, Memory Functions, and Psychomotor Performance." *Journal of Clinical Psychopharmacology* 22: 576–583.

Weston, A. L., et al. (2010). "Potentially Inappropriate Medication Use in Older Adults with Mild Cognitive Impairment." *Journal of Gerontology, Series A, Biological Sciences and Medical Sciences* 65A(3): 318–321 doi:10.1093/gerona/glq158.

White, A. M., et al. (2004). "Experimental Aspects of Alcohol-Induced Blackouts Among College Students." *American Journal of Drug and Alcohol Abuse* 30: 205–224.

Wu, C. S., et al. (2009). "The Association Between Dementia and Long-Term Use of Benzodiazepines in the Elderly: Nested Case-Control Study Using Claims Data." *American Journal of Geriatric Psychiatry* 17: 614–620.

Zammit, G. (2009). "Comparative Tolerability of Newer Agents for Insomnia." *Drug Safety* 32: 735–748.

Zitman, F. G., and Couvee, J. E. (2001). "Chronic Benzodiazepine Use in General Practice Patients with Depression: An Evaluation of Controlled Treatment and Taper-Off." *British Journal of Psychiatry* 178: 317–324.

Chapter 8

Herbal Medicines and Natural Treatments for Psychological Disorders

Many drugs derived from natural plant sources are covered elsewhere in this book (Table 8.1). Covered here are herbal products with CNS effects that are otherwise not addressed elsewhere in the book. These products are widely used by patients and recommended by alternative health practitioners for the treatment of various psychological disorders. We focus on herbal or natural medicines that may help alleviate psychological disorders (Wong et al., 1998). Included are discussions of St. John's wort, kava, ephedrine, omega-3 fatty acids, and other substances thought to affect the brain or behavior. A special edition of the *Physicians' Desk Reference* is devoted to herbal medicines, although it does not contain critical analysis of potential or claimed efficacy (*PDR for Herbal Medicines*, 2007). Such analysis is crucial, as some hold that such products are universally effective, while others (Guo et al., 2007) hold that "there is a sparsity of evidence regarding the effectiveness of individualized herbal medicine and no convincing evidence to support the use of individual herbal medicine in any indication" (p. 633).

Recently, Freeman and coworkers (2010a, b) with an editorial by Gelenberg (2010) critically reviewed the use of complimentary and alternative medicines in the treatment of major depressive disorder.

This chapter will attempt to address these disparate views. Each herb and natural product discussed here presumably contains an active

TABLE 8.1 Some of the naturally occurring psychoactive drugs covered in this book

Drug	Chapter	Used in therapeutics	Drug of abuse
Cocaine	12	Rarely	Yes
Caffeine	11	Occasionally	Probably
Nicotine	11	No	Yes
Lithium	6	Yes	No
Morphine	10	Yes	Yes
Codeine	10	Yes	Yes
Tetrahydrocannabinol	14	Rarely	Yes
Scopolamine	15	Occasionally	Occasionally
Mescaline	15	No	Yes
Myristicin/Elemicin	15	No	Yes
Psilocybin/Psilocin	15	No	Yes
Dimethyltryptamine	15	No	Yes
Bufotenine	15	No	Yes
Ololiuqui	15	No	Yes
Harmine	15	No	Yes
Omega-3 fatty acids	6	Possibly	No
Khat	12	No	Yes

ingredient that accounts for its claimed clinical effect. In some instances, the presumed active ingredient has not been conclusively identified, so discussion is oriented to the plant material and the safety, side effects, drug interactions, and efficacy in treating symptoms or diagnoses (Table 8.2).

The widespread, largely unregulated availability and promotion of herbal products is not new. Herbals have been used from the time of Hippocrates, and patent medicines were widely promoted in the United States until the early part of the twentieth century. Federal regulations in the 1920s severely restricted the sale and nonprescription use of such products, most of which contained large amounts of alcohol as well as "natural" drugs such as cocaine and opium. But passage of the Dietary Supplement Health Education Act of 1994 severely restricted the Food and Drug Administration's ability to exert control over herbal products. Thus, since 1994, any product can be labeled a "supplement" as long as the product makes no claim to cure a disease. Hence, a manufacturer cannot claim that a product "alleviates depression"; the manufacturer can, however, claim that it "promotes emotional balance." An herbal product cannot claim to alleviate the signs and symptoms of Alzheimer's disease; rather, it "enhances mental

TABLE 8.2 Herbal remedies commonly used to treat psychiatric symptoms*

Herb	Common usage	Quality of evidence category[†]	Adverse effects	Cautions/ contraindications	Drug interactions
Black cohosh	Menopause symptoms PMS Dysmenorrhea	I II III	GI upset (rare), headaches, CV depression	Pregnancy, lactation	Hormonal treatments (theoretical)
German chamomile	Insomnia Anxiety	III III	Allergy (rare)	Allergy to sunflower family of plants	None reported
Evening primrose	Schizophrenia ADHD Dementia	IV IV IV	None reported	Mania, epilepsy	Phenothiazines, NSAIDs, corticosteroids., ß blockers, anticoagulants
Ginkgo	"Cerebrovascular insufficiency" symptoms Dementia	I I	Headache. GI upset	Pregnancy, lactation, potential bleeding (e.g., PUD)	Anticoagulants
Hops	Insomnia	III	Allergy, menstrual irregularity	Depression, pregnancy, lactation	Sedative-hypnotics, alcohol (both theoretical)
Kava	Insomnia Anxiety Seizures	III III IV	Scaling of skin on extremities	Pregnancy, lactation	Benzodiazepines, alcohol
Lemon balm	Insomnia Anxiety	IV III	None reported	Thyroid disease, pregnancy, lactation	CNS depressants, thyroid medications

(continued)

TABLE 8.2 Herbal remedies commonly used to treat psychiatric symptoms* *(continued)*

Herb	Common usage	Quality of evidence category[†]	Adverse effects	Cautions/ contraindications	Drug interactions
Passion flower	Insomnia Anxiety	III ⎤ III ⎦	Hypersensitivity vasculitis, sedation	Pregnancy, lactation	Insufficient data
Skullcap	Insomnia Anxiety	IV ⎤ IV ⎦	Sedation, confusion, seizures	Pregnancy, lactation	Insufficient data
St. John's wort	Depression	I	Photosensitivity, GI upset, sedation, anticholinergic	CV disease, pregnancy, lactation, pheochromocytoma	Drugs that interact with MAOIs
Valerian	Insomnia Anxiety	III ⎤ III ⎦	Sedation	Pregnancy, lactation	CNS depressants

*PMS = premenstrual syndrome; GI = gastrointestinal; CV = cardiovascular; ADHD = attention deficit with hyperactivity disorder; NSAIDs = nonsteroidal anti-inflammatory drugs; PUD = peptic ulcer disease; CNS = central nervous system; MAOIs = monoamine oxidase inhibitors.
[†]Quality of evidence: I = evidence from at least two properly randomized controlled trials; II = evidence from well-designed trials without randomization; III = opinions of respected authorities based on clinical experience, descriptive studies, or reports of expert committees; IV = insufficient evidence to warrant conclusions about efficacy or safety.

From Wong et al. (1998), Table 1.

sharpness." Even though some herbal products can have significant adverse neuropsychiatric reactions, manufacturers must demonstrate neither safety nor efficacy. Promotion of many herbals addresses the fact that fatigue, headache, insomnia, depression, and anxiety—the symptoms and complaints most often underappreciated and untreated by medical doctors—are the most common reasons patients cite for seeking treatment from alternative practitioners.

The newly created National Center for Complementary and Alternative Medicine (NCCAM), one of the 27 institutes and centers that make up the National Institutes of Health within the U.S. Department of Health and Human Services, is the federal government's lead agency for scientific research on the diverse medical and health care systems, practices, and products that are not generally considered part of conventional medicine. It can be accessed online at www.nccam.nih.gov.

St. John's Wort

St. John's wort, *Hypericum perforatum*, is named after John the Baptist because it blooms around his feast day (June 24) and exudes a red color symbolic of his blood. It has many constituents with biological activity, including naphthodianthrones, flavonoids, and xanthones. *Hypericin* (Figure 8.1) (and possibly *pseudohypericin* and/or *hyperforin*) is generally considered to be the active ingredient, and dosage of the herb is based on its presumed hypericin content (Wurglics and Schubert-Zsilavecz, 2006). The term *hypericin* is from the Greek *hyper* and *eikon*, meaning "to overcome an apparition"; the ancients believed in its ability to ward off evil spirits.

Draves and Walker (2003) analyzed the summed total of hypericin and pseudohypericin in commercially available St. John's wort

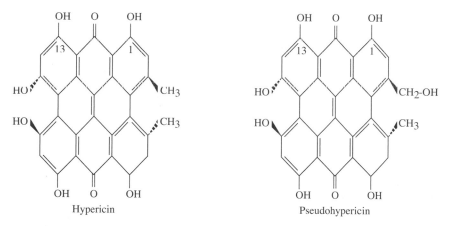

FIGURE 8.1 Structural formulas of hypericin and pseudohypericin.

preparations. The percentage of drug relative to the claimed amount varied from 0 to 108 percent for capsules and from 31 to 80 percent for tablets. Only two products had an amount within 10 percent of the label amount. Tinctures (alcohol extracts) varied from 0 to 118 percent of the label amount. On average, most labels overstated the amount by a factor of almost 2 (they thus contained only 50 percent of the labeled amount). St. John's wort is licensed in Germany for the treatment of anxiety, depression, and insomnia. In the United States, no claims of effectiveness in treating these disorders may be made; St. John's wort is sold only as a dietary supplement, perhaps to promote emotional balance. Currently, it is little utilized for alleviating anxiety; most use is for the treatment of depression. The efficacy of its use in treating depression is discussed later.

Pharmacokinetics

Hypericin has been shown to be absorbed following oral administration, with peak blood levels achieved in about 5 hours (Figure 8.2). Hypericin has an elimination half-life of about 25 hours; it thus achieves steady-state concentrations in the brain in about 4 to 6 days (Figure 8.3). Only about 15 to 20 percent of the administered hypericin reaches the central circulation and is available systemically. Of all the alkyloids in *Hypericum perforatum*, only hypericin appears to be detectable in brain tissue. Whether hypericin is metabolized, how it is metabolized, what its metabolites are, and how it is excreted are unknown.

St. John's wort contains bioflavonoids, one of which is *quercitin*. Quercitin inhibits the drug-metabolizing enzyme CYP-1A2. Hyperforin is a potent inhibitor of CYP-2D6 and CYP-2C9. The use of St. John's wort therefore results in numerous adverse interactions when combined with other drugs. For example, it may reduce the effectiveness of codeine (blocking conversion to morphine) and increase the blood levels of caffeine and several psychoactive medications, including tricyclic antidepressants and antipsychotic drugs. St. John's wort has also been reported to induce certain hepatic drug-metabolizing enzymes, increasing the activity of CYP-3A4, for example, and thus reducing the levels in the blood of certain cardiac and anti-inflammatory medicines. It has been reported to reduce the concentration (and presumably the efficacy) of oxycodone (Nieminen, et al., 2010), birth control hormones, protease inhibitors, and the anticoagulants warfarin and coumadin.

Pharmacodynamics

The mechanism of action of hypericin and hypericum extracts is unclear. Initially, it was thought that inhibition of monoamine oxidase (MAO; Chapter 5) increased the levels of norepinephrine, epinephrine, and dopamine. This would certainly account for the antidepressant action of St. John's wort. However, although MAO inhibition can be demonstrated

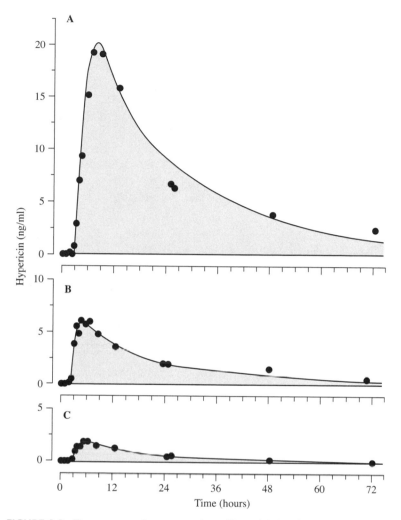

FIGURE 8.2 Time course of concentration of hypericin in plasma in three subjects after receiving a single dose of (**A**) 1800 milligrams, (**B**) 900 milligrams, or (**C**) 300 milligrams. [From B. Staffeldt et al., "Pharmacokinetics of Hypericin and Pseudohypericin After Oral Intake of the *Hypericum perforatum* Extract in Healthy Volunteers," *Journal of Geriatric Psychiatry and Neurology* 7 (1994), Supplement 1: S49.]

in vitro at high concentrations, the effect is too weak to account for clinical efficacy. Other reports hypothesize a hypericin-induced blockade of the presynaptic reuptake of serotonin, norepinephrine, and dopamine. Kasper and coworkers (2006), reviewing the work of others, stated:

> Experimental investigations have provided evidence that serotonin receptor expression is markedly reduced during treatment with hypericum extract, ultimately leading to enhanced synaptic availability of serotonin and norepinephrine. (p. 2)

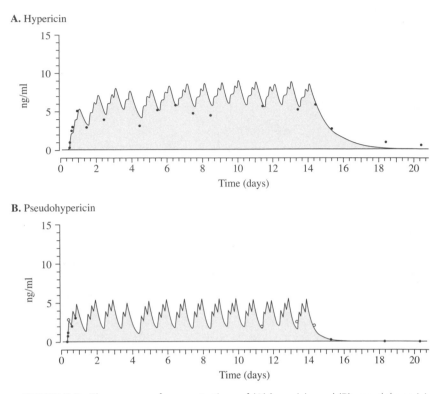

FIGURE 8.3   Time course of concentrations of (**A**) hypericin and (**B**) pseudohypericin in a subject taking one 300-milligram tablet of hypericum extract three times daily for 14 days. [From B. Staffeldt et al., "Pharmacokinetics of Hypericin and Pseudohypericin After Oral Intake of the *Hypericum perforatum* Extract in Healthy Volunteers," *Journal of Geriatric Psychiatry and Neurology* 7 (1994), Supplement 1: S50.]

Evidence for this statement is relatively weak. Other reported effects of hypericum extract include binding to GABA receptors, benzodi-azepine receptors, and glutaminergic NMDA-type receptors (Wong et al., 1998).

Sanchez-Reus and coworkers (2007) reported that, in studies of rats, a standardized extract of *Hypericum perforatum* exerted an antioxidant action, perhaps protecting neurons from oxidative damage. If correct, St John's wort might be indicated for depressed elderly patients with de-generative disorders exhibiting elevated oxidative stress status.

Clinical Efficacy

As early as 1996, Linde and coworkers conducted a meta-analysis of the clinical efficacy of St. John's wort for depression. They concluded that over a period of two to four weeks of treatment, hypericum extract was superior to placebo. However, data were less than convincing. Kim and coworkers (1999) conducted a similar meta-analysis. In a total of 651 patients, they concluded: "Hypericum perforatum was more effective than placebo and similar in effectiveness to low-dose tricyclic antidepressants in the short-term treatment of mild to moderately severe depression" (p. 532). However, they were careful to state that "serious questions remain regarding the research design of the studies analyzed."

Philipp and coworkers (2000) reported that hypericum extract (1 gram per day) was comparable in efficacy to imipramine (100 milligrams per day) and superior to placebo. Commenting, Linde and Berner (2000) noted that the study "confirms the existing evidence that hypericum extract is more effective than placebo in mild and moderate depression." Linde and Berner added, however, that the dose of hypericum was high, the dose of imipramine was low, and the superiority of both drug treatments over placebo was "not impressive," with placebo responses being quite robust.

In 2001, Shelton and coworkers conducted the first large-scale, multicentered, randomized, double-blind, placebo-controlled trial of St. John's wort extract and placebo in the treatment of major depression. In this study, St. John's wort (900 to 1200 milligrams per day) was no more effective than placebo (Figure 8.4). In 2002, results were reported of a multicentered, randomized, double-blind, placebo-controlled trial of St. John's wort extract versus both placebo and sertraline [a selective serotonin reuptake inhibitor (SSRI) antidepressant] in the treatment of major depression (Hypericum Depression Trial

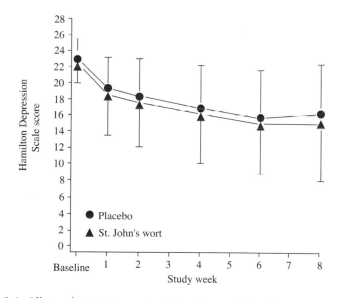

FIGURE 8.4 Effects of St. John's wort and placebo on the Hamilton Rating Scale for Depression over eight weeks of study. [From Shelton et al. (2001): 1983.]

Study Group, 2002). Neither St. John's wort nor sertraline was superior to placebo. The researchers concluded:

> This study fails to support the efficacy of *H. perforatum* in moderately severe major depression . . . the complete absence of trends suggestive of efficacy for *H. perforatum* is noteworthy. (p. 1807)

Findling and coworkers (2003) conducted an eight-week, open-label trial of St. John's wort (dosed to 900 milligrams per day) in 33 youths (mean age 10.5 years) with major depression. Twenty-five met the criteria for a positive response. The researchers stated that controlled trials in youths appear to be indicated.

More recent studies have continued to examine the clinical efficacy of St. John's wort. Anghelescu and coworkers (2006) compared hypericum extract (HE) with paroxetine (Paxil) in moderate to severe depression. The Hamilton Depression Scale scores were reduced by HE from 25 to 4 and by paroxetine from 25 to 5. Overall, 81 percent of HE-treated patients and 71 percent of paroxetine-treated patients achieved remission. These positive response rates are much higher than most researchers would predict. Kasper and coworkers (2006) reported that HE was superior to placebo in a six-week, placebo-controlled study of patients with mild to moderate depression (Figure 8.5). Moreno and

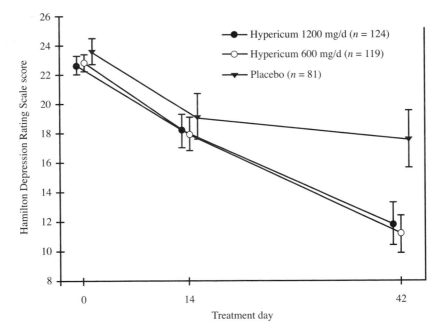

FIGURE 8.5 Change in mean total Hamilton Rating Scale for Depression score of patients suffering a major depressive episode over a six-week treatment period with hypericum extract (600 or 1200 milligrams per day) or placebo. Means and standard deviations are shown. [From Kasper et al. (2006), Figure 2.]

coworkers (2006), in a double-blind study, reported that HE was less effective than was either fluoxetine (Prozac) or placebo in treating mild to moderate depression.

Gastpar and coworkers (2006) compared HE and citalopram (Celexa) in moderate depression. They demonstrated the "noninferiority" of HE compared with citalopram and a superiority of HE over placebo. Overall, 54 percent of HE-treated patients, 55 percent of citalopram-treated patients, and 39 percent of placebo-treated patients responded positively.

Randlov and coworkers (2006) reported that HE was effective in treating nondysthymic patients with mild to moderate depression. It was ineffective in patients with comorbid depression and dysthymia or in patients with dysthymia alone.

Linde and coworkers (2008) performed a meta-analysis of St John's wort and concluded that, despite research inconsistencies, it appeared to be superior to placebo in patients with major depression, to be similar to "standard antidepressants," and to have few side effects. Rahimi and coworkers (2009) performed a similar analysis, concluding that HE was similar to standard antidepressants in efficacy and safety. Kasper and coworkers (2008) reanalyzed earlier data and concluded that St. John's wort extract "has a meaningful beneficial effect during acute treatment of patients suffering from mild depression and leads to a substantial increase in the probability of a remission" (p. 59).

Brattstrom (2009), in a study of 440 patients, reported efficacy in an open trial in mild to moderate depression, advocating use for relapse prevention. Shelton (2009) reported equivocal results, concluding that evidence does not support its use and that, because of potential drug interactions, "St John's wort is not a benign treatment" (p. 23).

Lavretsky (2009) reviewed the use of St. John's wort and other alternative medicines in elderly persons with late-life mood and cognitive disorders. Because this population has been little studied, no definitive conclusions were drawn.

Mannel and coworkers (2010) reported that use of HE approached statistical significance in the treatment of depression with atypical features. Finally, the National Center for Complementary and Alternative Medicine stated the following on its Web site:

- There is some scientific evidence that St. John's wort is useful for treating mild to moderate depression. However, two large studies, one sponsored by NCCAM, showed that the herb was no more effective than placebo in treating major depression of moderate severity.

- NCCAM is studying the use of St. John's wort in a wider spectrum of mood disorders, including minor depression.

In summary, have we learned anything more than we knew several years ago? Data are unclear. Perhaps hypericum extract has some efficacy in mild to moderate depression, an effect that may be comparable to that achieved by standard pharmacological agents, even though such effects are not "robust." This conclusion was reiterated in the recent review by Freeman and coworkers (2010a).

Side Effects

The side effects of St. John's wort are not insignificant. The extract has been shown to cause photosensitivity, especially in fair-skinned people who take large doses. Fortunately, the effect is reversible, usually within a few days. There are also several reports of St. John's wort precipitating a hypomanic state when used either with or without other antidepressant drugs. Used with SSRI-type antidepressants, a serotonin syndrome can occur (Chapter 5). Other (usually mild) side effects include sedation, lethargy, and gastrointestinal upset. The potential for involvement in potentially serious drug interactions was discussed earlier.

St. John's wort, at least until proved safe, should not be used during pregnancy or with other psychoactive agents. Klier and coworkers (2006) found little adverse effect of St. John's wort on the breast-feeding infants of mothers taking the product; very low levels of the herbal were found in the breast milk of the mother and the plasma of the infant. In 54 females exposed to St. John's wort during pregnancy, Moretti and coworkers (2009) found an incidence of major malformations similar to that in women not exposed to the product. This small study provided some evidence of fetal safety.

Since St. John's wort induces the CYP-450 enzymes that metabolize oral contraceptives, there continues to be concern about unwanted pregnancies; however, to date, this has not been a clinical problem.

Ginkgo

The ginkgo tree (*Ginkgo biloba*) is one of the oldest deciduous tree species on earth. The extract of ginkgo, referred to as *EGb-760*, is one of the most popular plant extracts used in Europe to alleviate symptoms associated with a range of cognitive disorders, including dementia. In the United States, the extract can be promoted not to treat cognitive dysfunctions but, for example, to provide "mental sharpness," provide antioxidant protection, maintain healthy circulatory perfusion, and so on. Purported medical indications for use include dementia, chronic cerebrovascular insufficiency (insufficient blood flow to the brain), and "brain protection."

The active ingredients in ginkgo extracts are not completely known. The standardized commercial preparation contains 24 percent ginkgo flavonoids and 6 percent terpenoids. As noted in the discussion of St. John's wort, flavonoids inhibit CYP-1A2 and set the stage for drug interactions with many medications.

Flavonoids and terpenoids are antioxidants that scavenge free radicals that have been implicated as the mediators of the cellular damage observed in Alzheimer's disease. Ginkgolide B (a terpenoid) inhibits a platelet-activating factor, interfering with platelet aggregation and slowing blood clotting (as does aspirin). This antiplatelet action by itself provides therapeutic effectiveness by limiting abnormal clot formation in small arteries (as aspirin does). Adversely, it may increase the tendency to bleed and it potentiates the actions of other blood thinners (again, as does aspirin). Presumed antioxidant effects have not been convincingly demonstrated for ginkgo, nor do they correlate well with efficacy in treating cognitive dysfunction.

Pharmacokinetics

Taken orally, *Ginkgo biloba* extracts appear to be readily absorbed, although blood levels of any of the substances found in the extract have not been reported. Concentrations of ginkgo flavonoids peak in plasma at 2 to 3 hours after ingestion. The mechanism of elimination of these substances from the body is not known. It is also not known whether any of the flavonoids or terpenoids are metabolized before excretion. The half-life is thought to be about 5 hours.

Pharmacodynamics

The EGb-761 extract of ginkgo contains several compounds that are thought by some people to act on unidentified processes involved in the homeostasis of inflammation and oxidative stress, presumably providing membrane protection and neurotransmission modulation. EEG studies demonstrate an activating effect with increased alpha wave activity, indicative of increased alertness and perhaps of improved cognitive performance (perhaps similar to the effects of caffeine on the EEG).

Clinical Efficacy

Most early studies on ginkgo extract were too poorly conducted to merit conclusions, despite a general conclusion that ginkgo may produce modest reduction in memory loss in patients severely affected with Alzheimer's disease. Wong and coworkers (1998) concluded that there is no clear evidence of efficacy in the treatment of depression, impotence, or brain injury. Van Dongen and colleagues (2000) reported on a 24-week study of EGb-761 in 214 elderly patients in the Netherlands. Ginkgo had no positive effects as a treatment for older people with mild to moderate dementia or age-related memory impairment. The authors' meticulous attention to detail set a new standard for the study of herbal preparations.

In 2002, Solomon and coworkers conducted a 6-week, randomized, placebo-controlled trial of the effects of ginkgo on 220 patients over the age of 60 to assess drug effects on memory function. The authors found that ginkgo had no beneficial effects on standard neuropsychological tests of learning, memory, attention, or concentration. They concluded that "ginkgo, when taken following the manufacturer's instructions, provides no measurable benefit in memory or related cognitive function" (p. 835).

In contrast to the results provided by Solomon and coworkers, Mix and Crews (2002) performed a nearly identical set of memory and cognitive experiments in 262 people aged 60 or older. These authors reported modest improvements in memory and cognition, evaluated both objectively and subjectively.

DeKosky and coworkers (2008) followed 3069 persons aged 75 or older with either normal cognition or mild cognitive impairments. Twice-daily doses of 120 mg extract of "*Ginkgo biloba* was ineffective in reducing the overall incidence of Alzheimer's disease" in either group of elderly people. Yancheva and coworkers (2009) compared *Ginkgo biloba*, an acetylcholinesterase inhibitor (donepezil; Chapter 19), or a combination in a small sample (96 patients) with probable Alzheimer's disease. With no placebo control group, both treatments demonstrated improvements in measures of activities of daily living, intellectual functioning, and emotional states. The combination of *Ginko biloba* and donepezil seemed most effective.

To summarize, ginkgo may have modest effects on cognitive functioning associated with cerebrovascular impairments (cases where blood flow to the brain is impaired, as in atherosclerotic vascular disease). This potential benefit can likely be accounted for solely by the herbal's action to reduce the "stickiness" of blood platelets (an action identical to that exerted by aspirin).

Side Effects and Precautions

Side effects of ginkgo include headache and gastrointestinal upset, but they are mild and infrequent. Headache is the most common and can be minimized by starting with a low dose and increasing it gradually. It is important to note that ginkgo blocks platelet function and increases bleeding time testing, increases spontaneous bleeding, causes interaction with aspirin and other anticoagulants, and has resulted in cases of spontaneous intracranial hemorrhage (Bent et al., 2005). Safety in pregnancy and during lactation has not been established; ginkgo preparations should likely be used with caution during pregnancy, especially around the time of delivery, when its antiplatelet action may put the fetus/newborn at risk of hemorrhage.

Kava

Preparations made from the roots of kava (*Piper methysticin*) have been used for ceremonial and social purposes by the peoples of the South Pacific for thousands of years. Captain James Cook first described kava in the account of his voyage in 1768. Scientific study was not conducted until the early days of pharmacology and pharmacognosy (the study of drugs in their natural state) in 1886. Kava is used by the Oceanic peoples as an antianxiety drug, similar to our use of ethyl alcohol. Kava induces relaxation, improves social interaction, promotes sleep, and plays an important role in the sociocultural life of the islanders of the South Pacific. At higher doses, kava produces sleep and stupor, again like alcohol. Extracts of kava have been widely used in Western countries for the therapy of anxiety, tension, restlessness, and insomnia.

Chemistry

Many agents in kava exhibit pharmacological activity. Most interest centers on the kava lactones, found in the fat-soluble portions of the plant root. Other compounds in kava contribute to efficacy, and the sedative activity of a crude preparation exceeds that of extracted kava lactones. However, because the kava lactone content of the root varies from 3 to 20 percent, preparations standardized for kava lactone content are preferred to crude preparations.

Pharmacokinetics

When taken as the extract, kava lactones appear to be well absorbed when the crude preparation is taken. Little is known about the distribution, metabolism, and excretion of the ingredients. Kava markedly inhibits the cytochrome P450 liver enzymes that metabolize many drugs, potentially increasing the blood concentrations and toxicity of these other drugs. Thus, multiple drug interactions may occur in users of Kava preparations.

Pharmacodynamics

The mechanism of action of ingredients in kava is poorly elucidated. Kava pyrones appear to bind to various GABA receptors or to the benzodiazepine-binding site, a likely action since kava produces effects similar to those produced by the benzodiazepines and alcohol. A kava lactone has been shown to block sodium channels, an anestheticlike effect. Kava has been shown in animals to be an anticonvulsant and a muscle relaxant and to be neuroprotective (much as are benzodiazepines and barbiturates). The EEG alterations induced by kava resemble those induced by benzodiazepines. Therefore, one can hypothesize that kava's action should closely resemble that of ethyl alcohol and the traditional sedative-hypnotic compounds.

Clinical Effects

At a dose of up to 70 milligrams of kava lactone, an anxiolytic effect is thought to occur. At higher doses (125 to 210 milligrams), drowsiness, sedation, and a feeling of intoxication are produced. In Oceanic cultures, doses of 250 milligrams are consumed, often more than once, and inebriation is quite rapidly induced. Saeed and coworkers (2007) summarized the efficacy of kava in the treatment of anxiety, showing modest efficacy, usually beginning after about eight weeks of therapy. They concluded that for persons with mild to moderate anxiety who wish to use natural remedies and are not using alcohol or taking other medications that are metabolized by the liver, kava appears to be acceptable for short-term use.

Recently, Sarris and coworkers (2009) studied the safety and efficacy of an aqueous extract of kava in 60 persons with generalized anxiety. They reported that kava was effective, with no serious adverse effects. Depressive symptoms also improved.

Side Effects and Complications

Side effects of kava are generally mild and include drowsiness, nausea, muscle weakness, blurred vision, and (with chronic use) yellow skin discoloration. Since kava is a sedative/intoxicant, it should not be combined with alcohol, benzodiazepines, barbiturates, THC, or other CNS depressants. Kava should not be taken before driving or operating machinery.

Campo and coworkers (2002) reported a case of fulminant liver failure (requiring liver transplantation) in a 14-year-old girl. Since this report, other cases of hepatotoxicity have been reported and the herbal has been banned in several Western countries, including Germany, France, Switzerland, Austria, and Canada. It continues to be available in the United States, despite evidence of adverse hepatic toxicity (Lim et al., 2007). Any use should be short term (i.e., up to 24 weeks) (Saeed et al., 2007).

Since kava is an intoxicant, it is interesting that barbiturates and benzodiazepines are restricted to prescription use, alcohol has age restrictions, marijuana is illegal, but kava is freely available in the United States. The chief deterrents to its more widespread use as an alcohol-like intoxicant are its expense and its potential for causing serious liver damage.

Ephedrine (Ma-Huang)

Ephedrine is the naturally occurring psychoactive drug found in *Ephedra sinica*, also called ma-huang. The medicinal parts are the young canes collected in autumn and the dried rhizome with roots. Ephedrine is a potent psychostimulant that acts by releasing the body's own stores of the catecholamine neurotransmitters epinephrine (adrenaline), norepi-nephrine, and dopamine.

Pharmacologically, ephedrine closely resembles the ampheta-mines, although ephedrine's duration of action is considerably shorter. Because of this, ephedrine-containing products should not be consid-ered as metabolic supplements, as dietary supplements, or for any other designation implying that it is not a drug.

Deaths from ephedrine now number in the dozens. The adrenaline and other catecholamines released by ephedrine increase blood pres-sure, heart rate, the force of cardiac contraction, and cardiac output of blood. Cardiac arrhythmias can be serious and potentially fatal. Like amphetamines, ephedrine temporarily reduces appetite, is a cardiovas-cular stimulant, and is a psychostimulant. Its disadvantages, however, far outweigh any therapeutic utility. In athletics, ephedrine is a "doping" substance. Numerous drug interactions occur, many of which are serious and potentially fatal. Several herbal preparations contain both ephedrine and caffeine: this is a combination that should be avoided be-cause caffeine increases the cardiovascular toxicity of ephedrine. In April 2004, the U.S. Food and Drug Administration (FDA), in response to 155 deaths and dozens of heart attacks and strokes, banned the sale of ephedrine-containing products as too dangerous for use. It was the U.S. government's first ban of a purported dietary supplement.

Omega-3 Fatty Acids

The major omega-3 fatty acids are eicosapentaenoic acid (EPA) and docosahexaenoic acid (DHA). These two substances are poorly synthe-sized in humans, and they are not herbal substances. However, they are found in large quantity in wild ocean fish such as wild salmon, swordfish, tuna, sardines, and mackerel. In the past few years, EPA and DHA have been noted to be not only generally deficient in Western diets, but deficient during pregnancy, in normal brain maturation in children and adolescents, and in several disorders in adults ranging from mood disorders, cardiovascular health, chronic pain syndromes. and even prevention of dementia. Here we address evidence for and against these uses.

Use During Pregnancy

Essential fatty acids are required for normal fetal development as well as for optimal maternal outcome. Acquiring these substances involves ingestion of oceanic fatty fish. However, ingestion of trace levels of mercury and other toxins found in fish has raised concern. Certainly omega-3 fatty acids are not synthesized in sufficient amounts by preg-nant women or by newborns, whether bottle- or breast-fed. Therefore, supplemental DHA and EPA are necessary, especially DHE. In the pregnant female, omega-3 fatty acids may help treat or prevent depressive symptoms (Su et al., 2008; Golding et al., 2009; Rees et al., 2009). In the fetus, omega-3 fatty acids are necessary for neural and retinal tissues, which are involved in cognitive and visual development (Cetin and Koletzko, 2008; Helland et al., 2008). These authors recommend a daily intake by the mother of about 200 mg/day. Finally, maternal use of omega-3 fatty acids may reduce susceptibility to allergic reactiveness in offspring; this effect perhaps persists into adolescence (Calder et al., 2010).

Use in Children and Adolescents

Chapter 18 discusses the use of omega-3 fatty acids in the treatment of bipolar disorder in children and adolescents; while efficacy is likely not robust, there is certainly little harm in administering modest doses. Because omega-3 fatty acids are involved in neural development (Ryan et al., 2010), there has been some efficacy in autism spectrum disorders (Meiri et al., 2009), in reduction of allergy risks (Kremmyda et al., 2009), and in developmental behaviors in children (Schuchardt et al., 2010). Regarding omega-3 fatty acids and symptoms of attention deficit/hyperactivity disorder (ADHD), results have been mixed (Raz and Gabis, 2009; Belanger et al., 2009); children with ADHD consume only about half the amount of fish/seafood, meat, and eggs than do children without ADHD (Ng et al., 2009). Finally, Amminger and coworkers (2010) found that in adolescents and young adults with subthreshold psychosis omega-3 intake correlated markedly with reduced transition to a psychotic disorder.

Antidepressant Use

Chapters 5 and 6 discuss the use of omega-3 fatty acids in the treatment of depression and bipolar disorder. In general, use in bipolar disorder is quite well supported, while use in unipolar depression is more controversial. Several studies have shown that the omega-3 fatty acids DHA and EPA alone or in combination can reduce depressive symptoms when used as adjuncts to antidepressant drugs (Chapter 5). Much less is known about their efficacy as monotherapy. In a small, 8-week study of patients with Hamilton Rating Scale for Depression (HAM-D) scores greater than 18, these patients received 1 gram per day of EPA or placebo (Mischoulon et al., 2009). Forty-five percent of treated patients versus 23 percent of placebo patients responded significantly. Remission rates (HAM-D < 7) were 36 percent versus 15 percent, respectively. Freeman and coworkers (2010a) state that "the low risks make omega-3 fatty acids a reasonable augmentation strategy for MDD" (pp. 670–671).

Analgesic Efficacy

For several years it has been recognized that omega-3 fatty acids have therapeutic utility in alleviating pain in patients with rheumatoid arthritis, inflammatory bowel disease, and other painful conditions (Shapiro, 2003; Goldberg and Katz, 2007; Ruggiero et al., 2009). Ko and coworkers (2010) recently reported the first case series suggesting that omega-3 fatty acids may be of benefit in the management of patients with neuropathic pain. Thus, omega-3 fatty acids may add to the utility of anticonvulsant drugs (e.g., gabapentin and pregabalin; Chapter 6) in managing neuropathic pain. Ko and coworkers (2008) extensively reviewed the mechanisms behind the efficacy of omega-3 fatty acids in alleviating neuropathic pain. The authors explained that omega-6 fatty acids (from vegetable oils such as safflower, sunflower, corn, cottonseed, soybean) promote the production of inflammatory mediators, while omega-3 fatty acids inhibit the production of these same mediators (Figure 8.6). In today's Westernized countries, our diets are extremely high in vegetable oils and low in omega-3 products. An ideal omega-6 to omega-3 ratio should be about 1:1. Our current ratio is estimated to be about 8:1, perhaps as high as 20–30:1 (Ko et al., 2008).

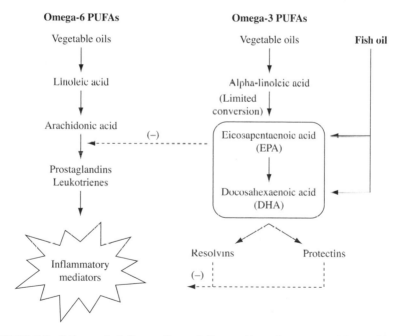

FIGURE 8.6 Pathways to inflammation as influenced by polyunsaturated fatty acids (PUFAs) of two types: omega-6 and omega-3. Omega-6 PUFAs increase the synthesis of arachidonic acid and inflammatory mediators. Omega-3 PUFAs reduce the conversion of arachidonic acid to prostaglandins and leukotrienes and inflammatory mediators. (−) and dotted line means inhibition. [From Ko et al. (2008), Figure 4.]

Is this one reason our society has such a high rate of chronic pain and chronic fatigue syndromes?

Cardiovascular Effects

Through a variety of mechanisms, omega-3 fatty acids exert beneficial effects on the cardiovascular system (Wierzbicki, 2008), reducing risk of cardiovascular deaths (Calder and Yaqoob, 2010). A healthy daily intake is about 500 mg/day (whether from oily fish or fish oil capsules) (Harris, 2010). Adding omega-3 fatty acids to low-dose aspirin therapy appears to confer added thrombotic protection by further reducing platelet adhesion (Lev et al, 2010). Finally, adding omega-3 fatty acids to weight-loss protocols provides additional cardiovascular protection by exerting positive benefits on triglycerides (McCombie et al., 2009). Several authors (Harris, 2009; Milte et al., 2009; Von Schacky, 2010) discuss an "omega-3 index" as a measure of cardiovascular risk. This index is the percentage of EPA + DHA in red blood cells (erythrocytes). A low omega-3 index can be considered a risk factor for sudden cardiac death and for nonfatal cardiovascular events. A high omega-3 index can be used as a therapeutic target. Currently, this index is being more fully evaluated for its prognostic use.

Omega-3 and Dementia Risk

In 2006, Johnson and Schaefer, in conjunction with the Framingham Heart Study in aging persons, made a shocking statement:

> 180 mg/day or more of dietary DHA (approximately 2.7 fish servings/ week) is associated with an approximately 50% reduction in dementia risk. At least this amount of DHA is generally found in one commercially available 1-gram fish oil capsule given daily. (p. 1494S)

Today, it is generally believed that omega-3 fatty acids, especially DHA, reduce the incidence of dementia, prevent cognitive decline, improve synaptic and neurotransmitter functioning, enhance learning and memory performances, and display neuroprotective properties (Carrie et al., 2009). DHA is not likely to become a sole agent for treatment of cognitive decline; it will instead be adjuvant therapy (Cederholm and Palmblad, 2010). DHA may be more effective if it is begun early or used in conjunction with other medications.

It is of note that several research articles have reported a negative association between omega-3 fatty acid use and dementia prevention (Kroger et al., 2009; Devore et al., 2009; Fotuhi et al., 2009). Obviously, much remains to be learned. However, at this point, any potential advantage appears to outweigh the risks of having older persons ingest reasonable doses of omega-3 fatty acids.

Other Herbals That Act on the Central Nervous System

A variety of other herbals have been used to treat signs and symptoms of CNS dysfunction. A few are described here. Complete descriptions may be found in the *PDR for Herbal Medicines* (2007) and in the review by Wong and coworkers (1998).

Valerian (*Valeriana officinalis*) has a long history of use as a mild sedative and anxiolytic as well as an antidepressant. The mechanism behind its action is obscure; some data indicate that it may affect GABA receptors, thus acting as a type of mild benzodiazepine. GABA itself is a component of valerian, leading some people to state that valerian is a source of naturally occurring GABA, which it is. The problem is that GABA only very poorly crosses the blood-brain barrier, and it is unlikely that this source of GABA affects the CNS.

Reported side effects of valerian include liver toxicity, headache, excitability, and uneasiness. There are potential drug interactions between valerian and SSRI-type antidepressants, perhaps precipitating a serotonin syndrome (Chapter 5). Nevertheless, valerian may produce CNS depression similar to that produced by benzodiazepines. There is no evidence to indicate that valerian is superior to existing sedative-hypnotic agents for the treatment of insomnia. The safety of valerian during pregnancy has not been delineated, so valerian probably should not be used by pregnant women. Valerian would be expected to potentiate the effects of other CNS depressants, such as ethyl alcohol, and caution is warranted. Valerian should not be taken before driving or in other situations when alertness is required. The usual precautions that apply to other sedatives apply to valerian. As does St. John's wort, valerian contains quercitin; this substance inhibits the drug-metabolizing enzyme CYP-1A2 and can possibly result in clinically significant drug interactions.

German chamomile (*Matricaria recutita*) is used to treat mild insomnia and anxiety. The herb contains flavinoids that are postulated to have affinity for the benzodiazepine receptor and perhaps for a histamine receptor, either perhaps inducing a sedative effect. In a recent eight-week, double-blind, placebo-controlled trial, Amsterdam and coworkers (2009) found that chamomile extract was modestly effective in reducing Hamilton Rating Scale for Anxiety scores in patients with mild to moderate generalized anxiety disorder (GAD). Doses were initiated at 220 mg and advanced to 1100 mg (once daily or in divided doses) if tolerated. The product reduced the anxiety scores, but self-rated scores for anxiety failed to improve. The authors did not recommend the substance as an alternative to established treatments for GAD.

Evening primrose (*Oenothera biennis*) has been promoted for the treatment of schizophrenia and ADHD, but little scientific evidence or cultural tradition backs up the claims. Primrose contains an omega-3 fatty acid called gamma-linolenic acid, which is felt to be the active ingredient. Objective research reporting efficacy is lacking.

Hops (*Humulus lupulus*) are used in the brewing industry as a component in beer. Hops also have a long history of use as a sedative-hypnotic agent. No clinical studies support the use of hops as a single agent to treat either insomnia or anxiety. When hops are used as a sedative, drug interactions can occur, especially potentiation of the effects of other sedatives such as alcohol and benzodiazepines. Use of hops should be avoided in depression, in pregnancy, and during lactation.

Lemon balm (*Melissa officinalis*), *passion flower* (*Passiflora incarnata*), and *skullcap* (*Scutellaria laterifolia*) are all thought to possess CNS sedative properties and are promoted for use as sedatives and anxiolytics. Data on efficacy are lacking, as is information on active ingredients and mechanisms of action. As sedatives, the usual precautions apply, including those concerning drug interactions and cognitive and motor impairments.

STUDY QUESTIONS

1. Describe the recent legislation changing the herbal industry. How has it helped society? How has it hurt?

2. What is hypericin? Describe its pharmacokinetics. What is the evidence for its efficacy?

3. What is ginkgo? What are its claimed actions? What evidence is there for efficacy to improve memory? For other uses?

4. What is kava? Does it have therapeutic potential? Does it have abuse potential? What drug does it appear to most resemble? Should there be legal restrictions on its use? Defend your answer.

5. What is ma-huang? What is its active ingredient? Does it have a potential for abuse? Might it induce toxicity? Should its use be regulated? Defend your answer.

6. What in valerian might result in drug interactions?

7. Are there any unaddressed concerns about the use of herbals during pregnancy or by women who might become pregnant? What about by breast-feeding women?

8. Discuss the variety of therapeutic uses of omega-3 fatty acids from conception to old age.

REFERENCES

Amminger, G. P., et al. (2010). "Long-Chain Omega-3 Fatty Acids for Indicated Prevention of Psychotic Disorders: A Randomized, Placebo-Controlled Trial." *Archives of General Psychiatry* 67: 146–154.

Amsterdam, J. D., et al. (2009). "A Randomized, Double-Blind, Placebo-Controlled Trial of Oral *Matricaria recutita* (Chamomile) Extract Therapy for Generalized Anxiety Disorder." *Journal of Clinical Psychopharmacology* 29: 378–382.

Anghelescu, I. G., et al. (2006). "Comparison of Hypericum Extract WS 5570 and Paroxetine in Ongoing Treatment After Recovery from an Episode of Moderate to Severe Depression: Results from a Randomized Multicenter Study." *Pharmacopsychiatry* 39: 213–219.

Belanger, S. A., et al. (2009). "Omega-3 Fatty Acid Treatment of Children with Attention-Deficit-Hyperactivity Disorder: A Randomized, Double-Blind, Placebo-Controlled Study." *Paediatrics and Child Health* 14: 89–98.

Bent, S., et al. (2005). "Spontaneous Bleeding Associated with *Ginkgo biloba:* A Case Report and Systematic Review of the Literature." *Journal of General Internal Medicine* 20: 657–661.

Brattstrom, A. (2009). "Long-Term Effects of St. John's Wort (*Hypericum perforatum*) Treatment: A 1-Year Safety Study in Mild to Moderate Depression." *Phytomedicine* 16: 277–283.

Calder, P. C., and Yaqoob, P. (2010). "Omega-3 (n-3) Fatty Acids, Cardiovascular Disease and Stability of Atherosclerotic Plaques." *Cell and Molecular Biology* 56: 28–37.

Calder, P. C., et al. (2010). "Is There a Role for Fatty Acids in Early Life Programming of the Immune System?" *Proceedings of the Nutrition Society* 13: 1–8.

Campo, J. V., et al. (2002). "Kava-Induced Fulminant Hepatic Failure." *Journal of the American Academy of Child & Adolescent Psychiatry* 41: 631–632.

Carrie, I., et al. (2009). "PUFA for Prevention and Treatment of Dementia?" *Current Pharmaceutical Design* 15: 4173–4185.

Cederholm, T. and Palmblad, J. (2010). "Are Omega-3 Fatty Acids Options for Prevention and Treatment of Cognitive Decline and Dementia?" *Current Opinion in Clinical Nutrition and Metabolic Care* 13: 150–155.

Cetin, I. and Koletzko, B. (2008). "Long-Chain Omega-3 Fatty Acid Supply in Pregnancy and Lactation." *Current Opinion in Clinical Nutrition and Metabolic Care* 11: 297–302.

DeKosky, S. T., et al. (2008). "*Ginkgo biloba* for Prevention of Dementia: A Randomized Controlled Trial." *Journal of the American Medical Association* 300: 2253–2262.

Devore, E. E., et al. (2009). "Dietary Intake of Fish and Omega-3 Fatty Acids in Relation to Long-Term Dementia Risk." *American Journal of Clinical Nutrition* 90: 170–176.

Draves, A. H., and Walker, S. E. (2003). "Analysis of the Hypericin and Pseudohypericin Content of Commercially Available St. John's Wort Preparations." *Canadian Journal of Clinical Pharmacology* 10: 114–118.

Findling, R. L., et al. (2003). "An Open-Label Pilot Study of St. John's Wort in Juvenile Depression." *Journal of the American Academy of Child & Adolescent Psychiatry* 42: 908–914.

Fotuhi, M., et al. (2009). "Fish Consumption, Long-Chain Omega-3 Fatty Acids and Risk of Cognitive Decline or Alzheimer's Disease: A Complex Association." *Nature Clinical Practice Neurology* 5: 140–152.

Freeman, M. P., et al. (2010a). "Complimentary and Alternative Medicine for Major Depressive Disorder: The American Psychiatric Association Task Force Report." *Journal of Clinical Psychiatry* 71: 669–681.

Freeman, M. P., et al. (2010b). "Complimentary and Alternative Medicine for Major Depressive Disorder: A Meta Analysis of Patient Characteristics, Placebo-Response Rates, and Treatment Outcomes Relative to Standard Antidepressants." *Journal of Clinical Psychiatry* 71: 682–688.

Gastpar, M., et al. (2006). "Comparative Efficacy and Safety of a Once-Daily Dosage of Hypericum Extract STW3-VI and Citalopram in Patients with Moderate Depression: A Double-Blind, Randomized, Multicentre, Placebo-Controlled Study." *Pharmacopsychiatry* 39: 66–75.

Gelenberg, A. J. (2010). "Complimentary and Alternative Medicine in Psychiatry." *Journal of Clinical Psychiatry* 71: 667–668.

Goldberg, R. J. and Katz, J. (2007). "A Meta-Analysis of the Analgesic Effects of Omega-3 Polyunsaturated Fatty Acid Supplementation for Inflammatory Joint Pain." *Pain* 129: 210–223.

Golding, J., et al. (2009). "High Levels of Depressive Symptoms in Pregnancy with Low Omega-3 Fatty Acid Intake from Fish." *Epidemiology* 20: 598–603.

Guo, R., et al. (2007). "A Systematic Review of Randomized Clinical Trials of Individualized Herbal Medicine in Any Indication." *Postgraduate Medical Journal* 83: 633–637.

Harris, W. S. (2009). "The Omega-3 Index: From Biomarker to Risk Marker to Risk Factor." *Current Atherosclerosis Reports* 11: 411–417.

Harris, W. S. (2010). "Omega-6 and Omega-3 Fatty Acids: Partners in Prevention." *Current Opinion in Clinical Nutrition and Metabolic Care* 13: 123–124.

Helland, I. B., et al. (2008). "Effect of Supplementing Pregnant and Lactating Mothers with n-3 Very-Long-Chain Fatty Acids on Children's IQ and Body Mass Index at 7 Years of Age." *Pediatrics* 122: e472–e479.

Hypericum Depression Trial Study Group. (2002). "Effect of *Hypericum perforatum* (St. John's Wort) in Major Depressive Disorder: A Randomized Controlled Trial." *Journal of the American Medical Association* 287: 1807–1814.

Johnson, E. J. and Schaefer, E. J. (2006). "Potential Role of Dietary n-3 Fatty Acids in the Prevention of Dementia and Macular Degeneration." *American Journal of Clinical Nutrition* 83: 1494S–1498S.

Kasper, S., et al. (2006). "Superior Efficacy of St. John's Wort Extract WS 5570 Compared to Placebo in Patients with Major Depression: A Randomized, Double-Blind, Placebo-Controlled, Multi-Center Trial." *BMC Medicine* 23(4): 1–13.

Kasper, S., et al. (2008). "Efficacy of St. John's Wort Extract WS 5570 in Acute Treatment of Mild Depression: A Reanalysis of Data from Controlled Clinical Trials." *European Archives of Psychiatry and Clinical Neuroscience* 258: 59–63.

Kim, H. L., et al. (1999). "St. John's Wort for Depression." *Journal of Nervous and Mental Disease* 187: 532–539.

Klier, C. M., et al. (2006). "St. John's Wort (*Hypericum perforatum*) and Breastfeeding: Plasma and Breast Milk Concentratons of Hyperforin for 5 Mothers and 2 Infants." *Journal of Clinical Psychiatry* 67: 305–309.

Ko, G. D., et al. (2008, September). "Omega-3 Fatty Acids and Neuropathic Pain." *Practical Pain Management*, pp. 21–31.

Ko, G. D., et al. (2010). "Omega-3 Fatty Acids for Neuropathic Pain: Case Series." *Clinical Journal of Pain* 26: 168–172.

Kremmyda, L. S., et al. (2009). "Atopy Risk in Infants and Children in Relation to Early Exposure to Fish, Oily Fish, or Long Chain Omega-3 Fatty Acids: A Systematic Review." *Clinical Reviews in Allergy and Immunology.* In press.

Kroger, E., et al. (2009). "Omega-3 Fatty Acids and Risk of Dementia: The Canadian Study of Health and Aging." *American Journal of Clinical Nutrition* 90: 184–192.

Lavretsky, H. (2009). "Complementary and Alternative Medicine Use for Treatment and Prevention of Late-Life Mood and Cognitive Disorders." *Aging and Health* 5: 61–78.

Lev, E. I., et al. (2010). "Treatment of Aspirin-Resistant Patients with Omega-3 Fatty Acids versus Aspirin Dose Escalation." *Journal of the American College of Cardiology* 55: 114–121.

Lim, S. T., et al. (2007). "Effects of Kava Alkaloid, Pipermethystine, and Kavalactones on Oxidative Stress and Cytochroma P450 in F-344 Rats." *Toxicological Sciences* 97: 214–221.

Linde, K., and Berner, M. (2000). "Commentary: Has Hypericum Found Its Place in Antidepressant Treatment?" *British Medical Journal* 319: 1534–1539.

Linde, K., et al. (1996). "St. John's Wort for Depression—An Overview and Meta-Analysis of Randomized Clinical Trials." *British Medical Journal* 313: 253–258.

Linde, K., et al. (2008). "St. John's Wort for Major Depression." *Cochrane Database of Systematic Reviews* CD000448.

Mannel, M., et al. (2010). "St. John's Wort Extract LI160 for the Treatment of Depression with Atypical Features—A Double-Blind, Randomized, and Placebo-Controlled Trial." *Journal of Psychiatric Research* 44: 760–767.

McCombie, G., et al. (2009). "Omega-3 Oil Intake During Weight Loss in Obese Women Results in Remodelling of Plasma Triclyceride and Fatty Acids." *Metabolomics* 5: 363–374.

Meiri, G., et al. (2009). "Omega 3 Fatty Acid Treatment in Autism." *Journal of Child and Adolescent Psychopharmacology* 19: 449–451.

Milte, C. M., et al. (2009). "Polyunsaturated Fatty Acid Status in Attention Deficit Hyperactivity Disorder, Depression, and Alzheimer's Disease: Towards an Omega-3 Index for Mental Health?" *Nutrition Review* 67: 573–590.

Mischoulon, D., et al. (2009). "A Double-Blind, Randomized, Controlled Trial of Ethyl-Eicosapentaenoate for Major Depressive Disorder." *Journal of Clinical Psychiatry* 70: 772–777.

Mix, J. A., and Crews, W. D. (2002). "A Double-Blind, Placebo-Controlled, Randomized Trial of *Ginkgo biloba* Extract Egb 761 in a Sample of Cognitively Intact Older Adults: Neuropsychological Findings." *Human Psychopharmacology* 17: 267–277.

Moreno, R. A., et al. (2006). "*Hypericum perforatum* versus Fluoxetine in the Treatment of Mild to Moderate Depression: A Randomized Double-Blind Trial in a Brazilian Sample." *Revista Brasileira Psiquiatria* 28: 29–32.

Moretti, M. E., et al. (2009). "Evaluating the Safety of St. John's Wort in Human Pregnancy." *Reproductive Toxicology* 28: 96–99.

Ng, K. H., et al. (2009). "Dietary PUFA Intakes in Children with Attention-Deficit/Hyperactivity Disorder Symptoms." *British Journal of Nutrition* 102: 1635–1641.

Nieminen, T. H., et al. (2010). "St. John's Wort Greatly Reduces the Concentrations of Oral Oxycodone." *European Journal of Pain.* In press.

PDR for Herbal Medicines, 4th ed. (2007). Montvale, NJ: Medical Economics Company.

Philipp, M., et al. (2000). "Hypericum Extract versus Imipramine or Placebo in Patients with Moderate Depression: Randomized Multicentre Study of Treatment for Eight Weeks." *British Medical Journal* 319: 1534–1539.

Rahimi, R., et al. (2009). "Efficacy and Tolerability of *Hypericum perforatum* in Major Depressive Disorder in Comparison with Selective Serotonin Reuptake Inhibitors: A Meta-Analysis." *Progress in Neuropsychopharmacology and Biological Psychiatry* 33: 118–127.

Randlov, C., et al. (2006). "The Efficacy of St. John's Wort in Patients with Minor Depressive Symptoms or Dysthymia—A Double-Blind Placebo-Controlled Study." *Phytomedicine* 13: 215–221.

Raz, R., and Gabis, L. (2009). "Essential Fatty Acids and Attention-Deficit-Hyperactivity Disorder: A Systematic Review." *Developmental Medicine & Child Neurology* 51: 580–592.

Rees, A. M., et al. (2009). "Omega-3 Deficiency Associated with Perinatal Depression: Case Control Study." *Psychiatry Research* 166: 254–259.

Ruggiero, C., et al. (2009). "Omega-3 Polyunsaturated Fatty Acids and Immune-Mediated Diseases: Inflammatory Bowel Disease and Rheumatoid Arthritis." *Current Pharmaceutical Design* 15: 4135–4148.

Ryan, A. S., et al. (2010). "Effects of Long-Chain Polyunsaturated Fatty Acid Supplementation on Neurodevelopment in Childhood: A Review of Human Studies." *Prostaglandins, Leukotrienes and Essential Fatty Acids* 82: 305–314.

Saeed, S. A., et al. (2007). "Herbal and Dietary Supplements for Treatment of Anxiety Disorders." *American Family Physician* 76: 549–556.

Sanchez-Reus, M. I., et al. (2007). "Standardized *Hypericum perforatum* Reduces Oxidative Stress and Increases Gene Expression of Antioxidant Enzymes on Rotenone-Exposed Rats." *Neuropharmacology* 52: 606–616.

Sarris, J., et al. (2009). "The Kava Anxiety Depression Spectrum Study (KADSS): A Randomized, Placebo-Controlled Crossover Trial Using an Aqueous Extract of *Piper methysticum*." *Psychopharmacology* 205: 399–407.

Schuchardt, J. P., et al. (2010). "Significance of Long-Chain Polyunsaturated Fatty Acids (PUFAs) for the Development and Behaviors of Children." *European Journal of Pediatrics* 169: 149–164.

Shapiro, H. (2003). "Could n-3 Polyunsaturated Fatty Acids Reduce Pathological Pain by Direct Actions on the Nervous System?" *Prostaglandins, Leukotrienes and Essential Fatty Acids* 68: 219–224.

Shelton, R. C. (2009). "St. John's Wort (*Hypericum perforatum*) in Major Depression." *Journal of Clinical Psychiatry* 70, Supplement 5: 23–27.

Shelton, R. C., et al. (2001). "Effectiveness of St. John's Wort in Major Depression: A Randomized Controlled Trial." *Journal of the American Medical Association* 285: 1978–1986.

Solomon, P. R., et al. (2002). "Ginkgo for Memory Enhancement: A Randomized Controlled Trial." *Journal of the American Medical Association* 288: 835–840.

Su, K. P., et al. (2008). "Omega-3 Fatty Acids for Major Depressive Disorder During Pregnancy: Results from a Randomized, Double-Blind, Placebo-Controlled Trial." *Journal of Clinical Psychiatry* 69: 644–651.

Van Dongen, M., et al. (2000). "The Efficacy of Ginkgo for Elderly People with Dementia and Age-Associated Memory Impairment: New Results of a Randomized Clinical Trial." *Journal of the American Geriatric Society* 48: 1183–1194.

Von Schacky, C. (2010). "Omega-3 Fatty Acids vs. Cardiac Disease—The Contribution of the Omega-3 Index." *Cell and Molecular Biology* 56: 93–101.

Wierzbicki, A. S. (2008). "A Fishy Business: Omega-3 Fatty Acids and Cardiovascular Disease." *International Journal of Clinical Practice* 62: 1142–1146.

Wong, A. H. C., et al. (1998). "Herbal Remedies in Psychiatric Practice." *Archives of General Psychiatry* 55: 1033–1044.

Wurglics, M., and Schubert-Zsilavecz, M. (2006). "*Hypericum perforatum:* A 'Modern' Herbal Antidepressant: Pharmacokinetics of Active Ingredients." *Clinical Pharmacokinetics* 45: 449–468.

Yancheva, S., et al. (2009). "Ginkgo biloba Extract EGb 761, Donepezil, or Both Combined in the Treatment of Alzheimer's Disease with Neuropsychiatric Features." *Aging & Mental Health* 13: 183–190.

Drugs Used to Treat Pain: Analgesic Medications

The two chapters in Part 3 deal with the pharmacology of drugs used to treat pain: Chapter 9 covers the nonnarcotic or nonopioid analgesics (such as aspirin); Chapter 10 concentrates on the pharmacology of opioid (narcotic) analgesics, the treatment of opioid dependency, and the uses of opioid receptor antagonists in medicine. The importance of the nonopioid analgesics is their ability to reduce the dose of coadministered opioid while contributing their own pain relief and anti-inflammatory effects (an "opioid-sparing" action).

Other drugs possess analgesic actions (the antidepressants and the mood stabilizers discussed previously), but the drugs discussed in these two chapters are primarily used therapeutically for the relief of both acute and chronic pain. However, as the reader is certainly aware, the opioid narcotics are subject to considerable and serious abuse. Therefore, these chapters cover not only their analgesic actions but also their propensity to produce compulsive abuse and dependence.

Chapter 9

Nonnarcotic Anti-Inflammatory Analgesics (NSAIDs)

Pain, anxiety, and depression are often inseparable, and all three need to be addressed during treatment of the patient with chronic pain syndromes (for example, fibromyalgia, chronic fatigue syndrome, and chronic back pain). Although opioid narcotics (Chapter 10) are effective in the treatment of severe acute pain (for example, pain caused by surgery or injury), they are much less effective in the treatment of chronic pain (for example, chronic lower-back pain) (Martell et al., 2007). In the treatment of chronic pain, therefore, efforts must be made to apply and optimize three kinds of medications before opioid narcotics are utilized (Wasan, 2005):

1. Analgesic/anti-inflammatory drugs (discussed in this chapter)
2. Antidepressant medications having a norepinephrine-potentiating action (Chapter 5)
3. Mood-stabilizing anticonvulsants with analgesic action (Chapter 6)

Only then is an opioid added, and then only when pain cannot be controlled by the first three types of drugs.

The value of antidepressants and mood stabilizers lies in their capacity to provide analgesic effect and to address symptoms that trigger, exacerbate, or compound the effects of pain, notably depression, anxiety, sleep disturbances, anger, and other states of neural excitation (Shanti et al., 2006). As discussed by Durie and McCarson (2006), antidepressants and nonopioid analgesic/anti-inflammatory drugs work synergistically to reduce nociceptive (pain-producing) sensory activation and to block both pain- and stress-evoked emotional responses that involve alterations in hippocampal and spinal cord gene expression.

The nonnarcotic analgesics are commonly called *nonsteroidal anti-inflammatory drugs* (NSAIDs). These drugs act at the local (peripheral) site of tissue injury both to reduce the inflammation commonly associated with tissue injury and to reduce the transmission of pain impulses to the central nervous system (CNS). The NSAIDs do not produce euphoria, and they are not considered to be drugs of abuse. NSAIDs do not bind to opioid receptors, but they exert a prominent morphine-sparing effect in improving pain relief in a variety of clinical situations. The historical development of NSAIDs and the future of anti-inflammarory drug therapy were recently reviewed by Rainsford (2007).

The NSAIDs are a group of chemically unrelated drugs (Figure 9.1) that block the generation of peripheral pain impulses by inhibiting the synthesis and release of chemical mediators called *prostaglandins*. Prostaglandins are body hormones that perform a variety of functions, including the production of local inflammatory responses. NSAIDs act by inhibiting the enzyme cyclooxygenase. *Cyclooxygenase* (also called *prostaglandin synthetase*) functions to convert a precursor substance (arachidonic acid) to prostaglandins. NSAIDs are therefore also called *cyclooxygenase* (COX) *inhibitors.*

There are two closely related forms of cyclooxygenase enzyme: COX-1 and COX-2. COX-1 primarily functions to mediate the production of prostaglandins that protect and regulate cell function in the gastrointestinal (GI) tract and in blood platelets during normal physiological conditions. Among other things, this action permits platelets to function normally as initiators of blood clotting. COX-2 has fewer roles under normal conditions; however, in response to stressors such as inflammation, COX-2 is markedly induced by chemical mediators associated with inflammation. Such induction by immune or inflammatory stimuli leads to the production of prostaglandins that mediate inflammation and pain. COX-2 (in contrast to COX-1) is therefore considered an *inducible enzyme.* It is induced in peripheral tissues and in the spinal cord in response to such immune instigators as autoimmune diseases (for example, osteoarthritis and rheumatoid arthritis), for which anti-inflammatory drugs are so effective therapeutically.

Classical NSAIDs, such as aspirin, nonselectively inhibit the cyclooxygenase enzymes (both COX-1 and COX-2). Therefore, they would be expected to adversely affect both the GI tract and platelet function, as well as reducing pain and inflammation. By 2004, three prescription-only selective inhibitors of the COX-2 enzyme were being marketed. Because of drug-induced complications, two were

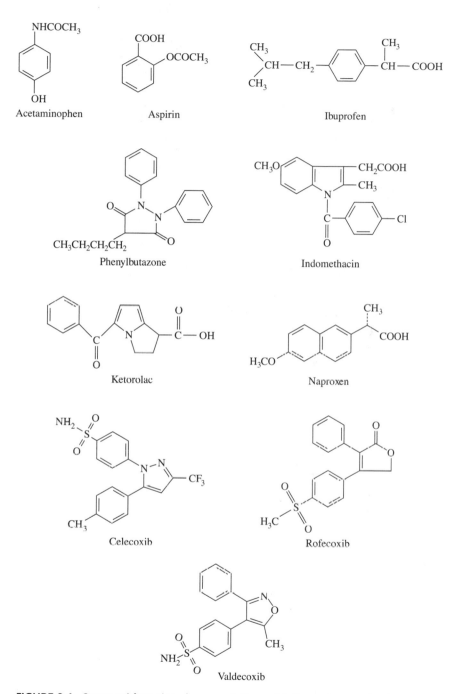

FIGURE 9.1   Structural formulas of representative anti-inflammatory analgesics.

removed from the market and only one (celecoxib, trade name Celebrex) remains. New COX-2 selective agents are in various stages of development. These include etoricoxib (Arcoxia), lumiracoxib (Prexige), and licofelone. Currently eterocoxib is approved in more than 60 countries worldwide, but not in the United States, where the Food and Drug Administration (FDA) requires additional safety and efficacy data for etoricoxib before it will issue approval. In April 2007, an FDA panel recommended against approving lumirocoxib because studies found the drug no more effective than naproxen (a nonselective COX inhibitor). Although lumiracoxib had been marketed in several countries, it was withdrawn in most of them due to liver toxicity concerns. It was never approved for use in the United States. The status of licofelone is pending; interestingly, it may possess analgesic/anti-inflammatory actions besides COX-2 inhibition (Sud'ina et al., 2008; Kulkarni and Singh, 2008).

The effects of anti-inflammatory analgesic drugs (selective or nonselective) include the following:

- Reduction of inflammation (an anti-inflammatory effect)
- Reduction in body temperature when the patient has a fever (an antipyretic effect)
- Reduction of pain without sedation (an analgesic effect)
- Inhibition of platelet aggregation (an anticoagulant effect)— nonselective drugs only

Nonselective Cyclooxygenase Inhibitors

Nonselective cyclooxygenase (COX) inhibitors are drugs that inhibit both COX-1 and COX-2 variants of the COX enzyme. The prototype nonselective NSAID is aspirin; hence, all nonselective NSAIDs can be referred to as aspirinlike drugs. Other nonselective NSAIDs include acetaminophen, ibuprofen, mefenamic acid (Ponstel), meclofenamate sodium (Meclomen), tolmetin (Tolectin), diclofenac (Voltaren), piroxicam (Feldene), and nabumetone (Relafen). These drugs are used as analgesics and for the long-term treatment of the pain and inflammation associated with arthritis. Nonselective COX inhibitors exert clinically significant effects on pain, inflammation, blood platelets, and the GI tract. These effects differentiate these drugs from the opioid analgesics, such as morphine, and from the selective COX-2 inhibitors. Opioid analgesics, although powerfully analgesic, do not exert anti-inflammatory effects, and they do not affect blood platelet function. The selective COX-2 inhibitors have the same analgesic and anti-inflammatory actions as the nonselective agents discussed here, but they do not affect platelet function.

Aspirin

Aspirin has been a commercial drug for over a century. In the United States, between 10,000 and 20,000 tons of aspirin are consumed each year. As an analgesic, aspirin is most effective for low-intensity pain, as increased doses rapidly reach a ceiling beyond which additional drug provides little more analgesia than do lower doses (all NSAIDs demonstrate this ceiling effect against pain). The ceiling is reached with doses of between about 650 and 1300 milligrams (a single, full-strength, regular aspirin contains 325 milligrams of drug).

Aspirin's antipyretic (fever-lowering) effect follows the inhibition of prostaglandin synthesis in the hypothalamus, a structure in the brain that modulates body temperature. However, one caution is necessary regarding the use of aspirin to reduce fever in children. An association exists between the use of aspirin for the fever that accompanies varicella (chicken pox) or influenza and the subsequent development of Reye's syndrome, including severe liver and brain damage and even death. Therefore, in children, aspirin use is precluded for the treatment of virus-induced febrile illness.

Aspirin exerts important effects on blood coagulation. For blood to coagulate, platelets must first be able to aggregate, an action requiring the presence of prostaglandins.[1] Aspirin binds to blood platelets, irreversibly inhibiting their function for the 8- to 10-day lifetime of the platelet. Homeostasis is inhibited, reducing the tendency for blood to clot. In daily low doses (usually only 80 to 160 milligrams per day), aspirin is used to prevent blood from clotting in diseased coronary arteries, markedly reducing the incidence of occlusive strokes and heart attacks secondary to the development of atherosclerotic plaques in the cerebral and coronary blood vessels (Patrono and Baigent, 2009).

Sohn and Krotz (2006) state, "Inhibition of platelet aggregation by aspirin . . . is a cheap, safe, and effective strategy to prevent myocardial infarction (heart attacks) or stroke and is thus the most established strategy of secondary prevention of atherothrombotic disease" (p. 1275). Karlikaya and coworkers (2006) state, "Daily low-dose aspirin has a protective effect in reducing the risk of early death in stroke" (p. 263). This protective effect exerted by reducing the ability of the blood to clot increases the risk of gastrointestinal bleeding, but the benefits in the prevention of heart attacks and thrombotic (occlusive) strokes outweigh the risks of serious bleeding in adults with coronary heart disease.

Because of the anticoagulant effect, it has been postulated that aspirin or other NSAIDs might be useful in reducing cognitive decline in

---

[1] Platelets are small components of the blood that adhere to vascular membranes after injury to a vessel. They form an initial plug, over which a blood clot eventually forms to limit bleeding from a lacerated blood vessel.

the elderly, perhaps even in reducing the incidence of late-life dementias. Recent studies, however, have reported that these drugs are ineffective in reducing cognitive decline or delaying the onset of Alzheimer's disease (Kang et al., 2007; Waldstein et al., 2010).

Side effects of aspirin include gastric upset that can range from mild upset and heartburn to severe bleeding of the stomach or upper intestine. Poisoning due to aspirin overdosage is not infrequent and can be fatal. The average lethal dose is 20–30 grams. Mild intoxication can produce ringing in the ears, auditory and visual difficulties, mental confusion, thirst, and hyperventilation. In aspirin-sensitive people, a single dose of aspirin can precipitate an asthma attack. In addition, aspirin increases oxygen consumption by the body, which increases the production of carbon dioxide, an effect that stimulates respiration. Therefore, an overdose of aspirin is often characterized by a marked increase in respiratory rate, which causes the overdosed person to appear to pant. This overdose effect results in other severe metabolic consequences that are beyond this discussion.

Acetaminophen

Acetaminophen (Tylenol) is an effective alternative to aspirin both as an analgesic and as an antipyretic agent. However, acetaminophen is less effective in reducing inflammation. As a pain-relieving agent, acetaminophen is as effective as aspirin. The usual oral dose of acetaminophen is 325 to 1000 milligrams, with daily doses averaging 1000 milligrams. Total daily doses should not exceed 4000 milligrams (2000 milligrams for alcoholics).

Acetaminophen has three advantages over aspirin. First, acetaminophen does not inhibit platelet function, so bruising easily is not a problem. (On the other hand, acetaminophen is not useful for preventing vascular clotting or for prophylaxis against heart attacks or stroke.) Second, no reports have associated acetaminophen with Reye's syndrome; therefore, it has an improved margin of safety in children. Third, acetaminophen generally produces less gastric distress and less ringing in the ears than does aspirin.

On the negative side, an acute overdose (either accidental or intentional) might produce severe liver damage. Alcoholics appear to be especially susceptible to the hepatotoxic effects of even moderate doses of acetaminophen and should avoid acetaminophen while they persist in heavy consumption of alcohol. Finally, there may be an association between the use of acetaminophen (and other NSAIDs except aspirin) and the development of hypertension (high blood pressure) in a small minority of women who consume these drugs nearly daily (Armstrong and Malone, 2003). Women who are hypertensive would be wise to discuss the use of acetaminophen with their physician before taking it.

In summary, acetaminophen has proved to be a reasonable substitute for aspirin when analgesic or antipyretic effectiveness is desired, especially in children and in patients who cannot tolerate aspirin.

Ibuprofen

Ibuprofen (Advil) and related drugs (Table 9.1) such as fenoprofen (Nalfon) and ketoprofen (Orudis) exert aspirinlike analgesic, antipyretic, and anti-inflammatory effects and are often better tolerated than aspirin. Their analgesic effectiveness is comparable to that of acetaminophen, aspirin, codeine, aspirin with codeine, and propoxyphene. Like other NSAIDs, ibuprofen's actions result from drug-induced inhibition of prostaglandin synthesis. The incidence and severity of side effects produced by ibuprofen are somewhat lower than those of aspirin, but gastric distress and the formation of peptic ulcers have occasionally been reported. Like aspirin (but unlike acetaminophen), ibuprofen and related drugs inhibit platelet aggregation. These drugs should be used with caution in patients who suffer from peptic ulcer disease or

TABLE 9.1 Ibuprofen and related drugs: Available formulations and recommendations for anti-inflammatory therapy

Nonproprietary name	Trade name	Formulation	Usual anti-inflammatory dose
Ibuprofen	Motrin, Advil, Nuprin, Medipren	Tablets	400 mg, three to four times a day
Naproxen	Naprosyn, Aleve, Anaprox	Tablets, suspension	250–500 mg, twice a day
Fenoprofen	Nalfon	Tablets, capsules	300–600 mg, three to four times a day
Ketoprofen	Orudis, Oravail	Capsules	150–300 mg, two to four times a day
Flurbiprofen	Ansaid, others	Tablets	50–75 mg, two to four times a day
Oxaprozin	Daypro	Tablets	600–1200 mg, once a day
Mefenamic acid	Ponstel	Tablets	250 mg, three to four times a day
Celecoxib	Celebrex	Capsules	100 mg, twice a day

bleeding abnormalities. Ibuprofen, unlike most other NSAIDs, is not secreted in breast milk, but in general, NSAIDs are not recommended for breast-feeding mothers or pregnant women.

FDA-approved indications for ibuprofen include use as an analgesic and use for the symptomatic treatment of various forms of arthritis, tendonitis, bursitis, and dysmenorrhea (painful menstrual cramps). The anti-inflammatory effect is comparable to that of aspirin. The generally lower level of gastrointestinal side effects (in comparison with aspirin) must be measured against its generally greater cost.

Clark and coworkers (2007) studied 300 children (ages 6 to 17) who presented for emergency room treatment with musculoskeletal pain. They were administered acetaminophen, ibuprofen, or codeine. At 60 minutes post administration, patients in the ibuprofen group had significantly better pain relief.

Indomethacin and Sulindac

Indomethacin (Indocin), available for over 40 years, is an effective anti-inflammatory drug that is used primarily for treating rheumatoid arthritis and similar disorders. However, its use is limited by its toxicity. Indomethacin is an analgesic, antipyretic, and anti-inflammatory agent. Its clinical effects closely resemble those of aspirin. Side effects occur in about 50 percent of the patients who take indomethacin; gastric upset is the most prominent. Paradoxically, drug-induced headache limits its use in about 50 percent of patients. Other side effects are rare but potentially serious.

Sulindac (Clinoril) is an NSAID that is structurally and pharmacologically related to indomethacin. Sulindac is itself inactive, but its metabolite (sulindac sulfide) is very active. Its efficacy is comparable to that of indomethacin but perhaps with a lower level of gastrointestinal toxicities (less than indomethacin but greater than many other NSAIDs).

Ketorolac

Ketorolac (Toradol) is an analgesic and anti-inflammatory agent available in both oral and intravenous formulations. Ketorolac is the only NSAID available for injection. Administered either intramuscularly or intravenously, ketorolac is effective in the short-term treatment of moderate to severe pain. Like the other NSAIDs, ketorolac inhibits prostaglandin synthesis. Its analgesic potency is comparable to that of low doses of morphine, and it offers an anti-inflammatory action not offered by morphine. Its concomitant use with morphine offers synergistic action, reducing the required analgesic dose of morphine by about 50 percent. In mid-2010, ketorolac was made available as a nasal spray (Sprix) for short-term outpatient management of moderate to severe pain.

Side effects of ketorolac include excessive bleeding (due to platelet inhibition) and renal failure; the latter is minimized by limiting the use of the drug to a few days after surgery. Used orally, analgesic efficacy differs little from that of other orally administered NSAIDs.

Diclofenac

Diclofenac (Voltaren, Zipsor) is another nonspecific NSAID, available since 1988 and indicated for treatment of acute and chronic pain of arthritis and for the mitigation of painful menstrual periods. The half-life of diclofenac is short (about two hours), so delayed-release preparations are commonly used. Diclofenac has recently become available as a topical solution (Pennsaid) and in a skin patch (Flector).

Nabumetone

Nabumetone (Relafen) is a nonspecific NSAID available since 1991 for the treatment of arthritis and other conditions treatable with similar drugs. Nabumetone itself is inactive; it is rapidly converted in the body to a pharmacologically active metabolite that is a potent inhibitor of prostaglandin synthetase. Its gastrointestinal toxicity appears to be somewhat lower than that of aspirin or indomethacin. The drug is primarily indicated for the long-term treatment of the pain and inflammation associated with arthritis.

Miscellaneous Nonspecific NSAIDs

Several other nonspecific cyclooxygenase inhibitors are available for use in treating various forms of arthritis or painful menstrual periods. These agents include *meloxicam* (Mobic), *naproxen* (Aleve, Anaprox), *oxaprozin* (Daypro), *piroxicam* (Feldene), and *tolmetin* (Tolectin). These drugs, as well as several of the drugs discussed earlier, were introduced in medicine in the late 1980s to early 1990s as alternatives to aspirin. Since the patent protection of most of these drugs has expired, they are available in generic form, and few manufacturers promote their use today. Naproxen appears to exert a cardioprotective effect of therapeutic significance (Ray et al., 2009).

Selective COX-2 Inhibitors

Only since the late 1990s have the roles of cyclooxygenase enzymes in health and disease been extensively explored, in particular, the role of "inducible" COX-2 in inflammation (O'Banion, 1999) and in the prevention of various cancers (Cuzick et al., 2009; Harris, 2009).[2] COX-2 enzyme is expressed in certain malignant cells of epithelial tissues such as

---

[2] *Inducible* means that the enzyme level of COX-2 in the body, normally low, increases markedly in response to inflammation.

colon, breast, prostate, bladder, lung, and pancreas, and it plays a role in tumor proliferation and growth. It is best demonstrated in cancers of the colon. COX-2 inhibitors reduce the risk of these cancers and therefore have a role in cancer chemoprotection, probably as an adjunct to more traditional anticancer medications. Whether COX-2 inhibitors will play a beneficial role in the treatment of noncarcinogenic inflammatory diseases of the colon is as yet unclear. It is interesting that the nonselective COX inhibitor aspirin is similarly effective in reducing the long-term risk of colorectal cancers and perhaps breast cancer. A dose of 300 milligrams or more daily for five years is effective in the primary prevention of colon cancers after a latent period of about ten years (Flossmann and Rothwell, 2007).

Selective COX-2 inhibitors are as effective as aspirin and other nonselective NSAIDs for the relief of pain and the reduction of inflammation while halving the rate of associated gastric ulcerations (Figure 9.2). Consequently, prior to September 2004 the selective COX-2 inhibitors

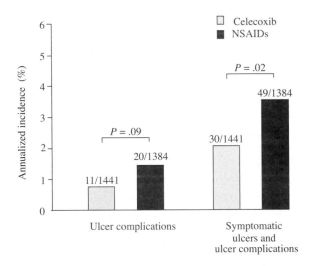

FIGURE 9.2 Annualized incidences of upper gastrointestinal tract ulcer complications alone and with symptomatic gastrointestinal ulcers. Left two bars represent ulcer complications for 1441 patient-years of celecoxib and 1384 patient-years of nonselective NSAIDs. The right two bars represent ulcer complications plus the presence of symptomatic ulcers in the same populations of patients. The numbers above the bars indicate events per patient-years of exposure. The annualized incidence of ulcer complications in celecoxib-treated patients was 0.76 percent (11 events per 1441 patient-years) versus an incidence of 1.45 percent (20 events per 1384 patient-years) in patients taking NSAIDs. When symptomatic ulcers were added, the percentage of complications in each group increased, but celecoxib patients still exhibited a 40 percent reduction in total complications. [From F. E. Silverstein et al., "Gastrointestinal Toxicity with Celecoxib vs. Nonsteroidal Anti-Inflammatory Drugs for Osteoarthritis and Rheumatoid Arthritis: The CLASS Study: A Randomized Controlled Study," *Journal of the American Medical Association* 284 (2000): 1251.]

became wildly popular as modern NSAIDs that were clinically effective while reducing the incidence of gastric ulcerations. Unfortunately, two of the three selective COX-2 inhibitors that were clinically available were withdrawn from the market because of adverse cardiac complications.

Celecoxib

Celecoxib (Celebrex) was the first selective COX-2 inhibitor; it became available clinically in 1998. The drug is as effective as aspirin in reducing the pain and inflammation of rheumatoid arthritis and osteoarthritis without the gastrointestinal toxicity and platelet blockade produced by aspirin. Celecoxib is associated with a 50 percent reduction in the occurrence of drug-induced gastric ulcerations and hemorrhages (see Figure 9.2). However, although the incidence of skin bruising is less frequent, the lack of effect on blood platelets causes loss of the protective effect of aspirin in reducing the incidence of heart attacks and strokes, although whether it increases the rate over that of placebo is unclear. Currently, celecoxib remains commercially available. Because it lacks antithrombotic action (it lacks a blocking action on platelet function), it might possibly slightly increase the incidence of heart attacks over the use of aspirin (while reducing the likelihood of gastrointestinal bleeding).

Rofecoxib

Rofecoxib (Vioxx), the second COX-2 inhibitor, was introduced into medicine in 2000. It was approved for the treatment of osteoarthritis, acute pain, and menstrual pain, with some superiority over naproxen in reducing the incidence of gastric ulcerations. Unfortunately, its use was associated with an increased risk of heart attacks (Baron et al., 2008), so the drug was removed from the market.

Valdecoxib

The third selective COX-2 inhibitor, *valdecoxib* (Bextra), was introduced into medicine in 2002. Like rofecoxib, valdecoxib was associated with an increased rate of cardiovascular side effects, so it, too, was voluntarily withdrawn from commercial sale.

Nonopioid Analgesics of the Future: Nitric Oxide-Donating Analgesics

Advances beyond COX-2 inhibition are being explored and are needed because the nonselective NSAIDs do not protect against gastrointestinal bleeding and ulcerations and because the COX-2 inhibitors do not block platelet action and therefore do not offer cardiac protection against atherothrombotic catastrophes. An interesting example of possible agents of the future is a class of drugs called nitroaspirins, or nitric oxide-donating aspirins. At least one has been submitted for FDA approval, but none have yet been approved for use in the United States. Agents include naproxcinod (for treating osteoarthritis), NCX-4016 (as an insulin-sensitizing agent for treating type 2 diabetes), and NCX-6560 (for treating cardiovascular disease). Other potential uses are for the treatment of asthma, ocular diseases, and allergic rhinitis (among others). These drugs are new chemical entities that are obtained by adding a nitric oxide-releasing moiety to aspirin, other analgesics, or even cholesterol-lowering agents. Each drug consists of a parent molecule (for example, aspirin) linked to a "spacer" via an ester linkage, which is in turn connected to the nitric oxide-releasing moiety.

Nitric oxide is normally found in the body and exerts a protective effect on the endothelium (cell lining) of blood vessels and the gastrointestinal tract. Therefore, the aspirin moiety contributes the analgesic, anti-inflammatory, and antiplatelet actions, while the nitric oxide protects both the GI tract and coronary blood vessels (Brzozowski et al., 2003). These drugs also protect against carcinomas of the GI tract (Rigas, 2007; Rigas and Williams, 2008). Nitric oxide-donating analgesics have potential for a wide range of therapeutic applications because of analgesic, anti-inflammatory, cardioprotective, and chemopreventive actions (Turnbull et al., 2006). They exhibit antiatherosclerotic and antioxidant damage in the walls of blood vessels, and they also reduce vascular injury in blood vessels, promoting vascular remodeling after injury.

STUDY QUESTIONS

1. What is an NSAID? What does this term mean?

2. List the various actions of aspirin. How might each action be used therapeutically? Which ones might present clinical problems?

3. What is meant by the term *COX inhibitor*?

4. Differentiate between COX-1 and COX-2.

5. How is the anticoagulant action of aspirin "good"? How is it "bad"?

6. Describe the theoretical advantages of COX-2 inhibitors over NSAIDs (nonselective COX inhibitors).

7. What is the correlation between COX enzyme and tumor genesis? How might COX inhibitors be of benefit?

8. What is a nitric oxide-releasing aspirin? What are its advantages? What might be its clinical uses?

REFERENCES

Armstrong, E. P., and Malone, D. C. (2003). "The Impact of Nonsteroidal Anti-Inflammatory Drugs on Blood Pressure, with an Emphasis on Newer Agents." *Clinical Therapeutics* 25: 1–18.

Baron, J. A., et al. (2008). "Cardiovascular Events Associated with Rofecoxib: Final Analysis of the APPROVe Trial." *Lancet* 372: 1756–1764.

Brzozowski, T., et al. (2003). "Implications of Reactive Oxygen Species and Cytokines in Gastroprotection Against Stress-Induced Gastric Damage by Nitric Oxide-Releasing Aspirin." *International Journal of Colorectal Diseases* 18: 320–329.

Clark, E., et al. (2007). "A Randomized, Controlled Trial of Acetaminophen, Ibuprofen, and Codeine for Acute Pain Relief in Children with Musculoskeletal Trauma." *Pediatrics* 119: 460–467.

Cuzick, J., et al. (2009). "Aspirin and Non-Steroidal Anti-Inflammatory Drugs for Cancer Prevention: An International Consensus Statement." *Lancet Oncology* 10: 501–507.

Durie, V., and McCarson, K. E. (2006). "Effects of Analgesic or Antidepressant Drugs on Pain- or Stress-Evoked Hippocampal and Spinal Neurokinin-1 Receptor and Brain-Derived Neurotrophic Factor Gene Expression in the Rat." *Journal of Pharmacology and Experimental Therapeutics* 319: 1235–1243.

Flossmann, E., and Rothwell, P. (2007). "Effect of Aspirin on Long-Term Risk of Colorectal Cancer: Consistent Evidence from Randomized and Observational Studies." *Lancet* 369: 1603–1613.

Harris, R. E. (2009). "Cyclooxygenase-2 (COX-2) Blockade in the Chemoprevention of Cancers of the Colon, Breast, Prostate, and Lung." *Inflammopharmacology* 17: 55–67.

Kang, J. H., et al. (2007). "Low Dose Aspirin and Cognitive Function in the Women's Health Study Cognitive Cohort." *British Medical Journal* 334: 987–997.

Karlikaya, G., et al. (2006). "Does Prior Aspirin Use Reduce Stroke Mortality?" *Neurologist* 12: 263–267.

Kulkarni, S. K., and Singh, V. P. (2008). "Licofelone: The Answer to Unmet Needs in Osteoarthritis Therapy?" *Current Rheumatology Reports* 10: 43–48.

Martell, B. A., et al. (2007). "Systematic Review: Opioid Treatment for Chronic Back Pain: Prevalence, Efficacy, and Association with Addiction." *Annals of Internal Medicine* 146: 116–127.

O'Banion, M. K. (1999). "Cyclooxygenase-2: Molecular Biology, Pharmacology, and Neurobiology." *Critical Reviews in Neurobiology* 13: 45–82.

Patrono, C., and Baigent, C. (2009). "Low-Dose Aspirin, Coxibs, and Other NSAIDs: A Clinical Mosaic Emerges." *Molecular Interventions* 9: 31–39.

Rainsford, K. D. (2007). "Anti-Inflammatory Drugs in the 21st Century." *Subcellular Biochemistry* 42: 3–27.

Ray, W. A., et al. (2009). "Cardiovascular Risks of Nonsteroidal Antiinflammatory Drugs in Patients After Hospitalization for Serious Coronary Heart Disease." *Circulation, Cardiovascular Quality and Outcomes* 2: 155–163.

Rigas, B. (2007). "The Use of Nitric Oxide-Donating Nonsteroidal Anti-Inflammatory Drugs in the Chemoprotection of Colorectal Neoplasia." *Current Opinions in Gastroenterology* 23: 55–59.

Rigas, B., and Williams, J. L. (2008). "NO-Donating NSAIDs and Cancer: An Overview with a Note on Whether NO is Required for Their Action." *Nitric Oxide* 19: 199–204.

Shanti, B. F., et al. (2006, April). "Adjuvant Analgesia for Management of Chronic Pain." *Practical Pain Management,* pp. 18–27.

Sohn, H. Y., and Krotz, F. (2006). "Cyclooxygenase Inhibition and Atherothrombosis." *Current Drug Targets* 7: 1275–1284.

Sud'ina, G. F., et al. (2008). "Cyclooxygenase (COX) and 5-Lipoxygenase (5-LOX) Selectivity of COX Inhibitors." *Prostaglandins, Leukotrienes, and Essential Fatty Acids* 78: 99–108.

Turnbull, C. M., et al. (2006). "Therapeutic Effects of Nitric Oxide-Aspirin Hybrids." *Expert Opinion on Therapeutic Targets* 10: 911–922.

Waldstein, S. R., et al. (2010). "Nonsteroidal Anti-Inflammatory Drugs, Aspirin, and Cognitive Function in the Baltimore Longitudinal Study of Aging." *Journal of the American Geriatrics Society* 58: 38–43.

Wasan, A. D. (2005). "Treating Depression and Anxiety in Chronic Pain Patients." *Pain Management Rounds* 2(2): 1–6. May be obtained as full text online at www.painmanagementrounds.org. Click on "archives" and choose issue 2–4.

Chapter 10

Opioid Analgesics

Pain is one of the most common of human experiences and one of the most common reasons people seek medical care. Pain is a major cause of disability and has enormous economic consequences. It exacts a tremendous physical, psychological, social, and vocational toll on the sufferer, family, friends, and health care workers.

Pain can be defined as a highly undesirable and unpleasant sensory and emotional experience often associated with actual or potential tissue damage. Pain is both a sensory event of the peripheral and central nervous systems and an emotional and cognitive experience. Acute pain is biologically desirable because it functions as a warning system against real or potential damage to the body. Chronic pain, however, serves no useful purpose, causes suffering, limits activities of daily living, and increases the costs of health care and disability. Pain also often occurs comorbidly with anxiety and depression, and all may need to be addressed during treatment.

Pain is modulated, enhanced, or diminished by both cerebral and peripheral mechanisms. Cerebral factors include the placebo response, psychological phenomena, and conscious cognitive activation. These factors are powerfully affected by the opioid analgesics, whereas the nonsteroidal anti-inflammatory drugs (NSAIDs; Chapter 9) mostly affect the peripheral inflammatory responses. In addition to invoking endogenous opioids (endorphins), central mechanisms activate pain-inhibiting pathways beginning in the limbic forebrain and relayed through the brain stem to primary pain input sites in the dorsal horn of the spinal cord, modulating the intensity of the incoming pain response.

When body tissues are damaged, tissue injury is accompanied by the activation of *nociceptive* (pain-sensing) neurons (Figure 10.1) in response

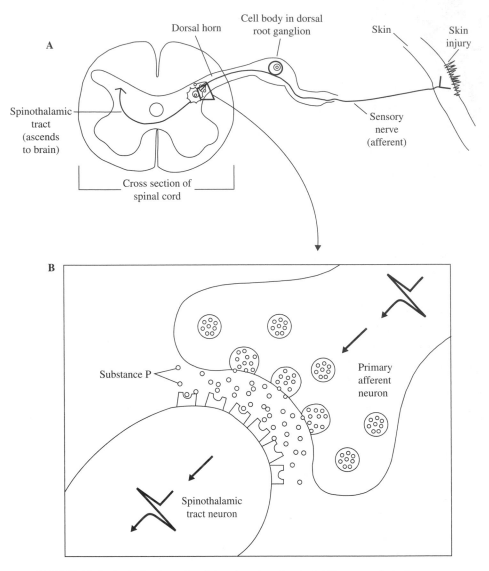

FIGURE 10.1 **A.** Activation of peripheral nociceptive (pain) fibers results in the release of substance P and other pain-signaling neurotransmitters from nerve terminals in the dorsal horn of the spinal cord. The cell body for the nerve is located in the dorsal root ganglion. **B.** Enlargement of synapse between afferent nociceptive neuron and a spinothalamic tract neuron. Substance P is thought to be a major nociceptive neurotransmitter.

to mechanical, thermal, or chemical injuries. With tissue injury or during inflammation, nociceptors become sensitized, discharge spontaneously, and produce ongoing pain. The cell bodies of the axons from these neurons are located in the dorsal root ganglia, and their bidirectional axon relays pain impulses to a synapse in the dorsal horn of the spinal cord

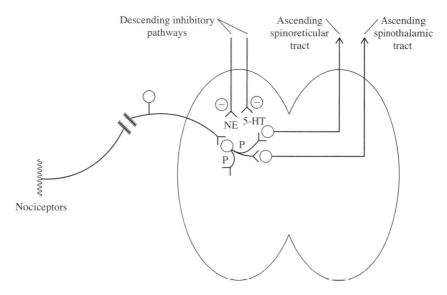

FIGURE 10.2 Release of substance P in the dorsal horn of the spinal cord with transmission of secondary relay pathways to higher centers. Descending inhibitory pathways (−) are also shown. NE = norepinephrine; 5-HT = serotonin.

and from there to the brain (Figure 10.2). In the brain, the mechanisms associated with the modulation and transfer of pain impulses are very complex: a host of different processes involve multiple neurotransmitters and neuromodulators. The ultimate perception of pain is thus dependent on both the activity in the afferent peripheral system and its modulation at multiple levels of the nervous system. Indeed, analgesic drugs therefore can modulate pain processes by the following actions:

- Reducing the peripheral inflammatory response to tissue injury (NSAIDs)
- Blocking glutaminergic NMDA receptors in the spinal cord (dextromethorphan and ketamine; Chapter 15)
- Reducing repetitive activity in injured neurons (anticonvulsant "neuromodulators")
- Modulating neuronal responsiveness in the dorsal horn of the spinal cord through activation of inhibitory endorphin-secreting neurons or inhibitory GABA-secreting neurons (opioid analgesics, neuromodulators)
- Activating descending inhibitory neurons projecting from the brain stem to the dorsal horn of the spinal cord (for example, opioids or antidepressants)
- Modulating the central processing of pain stimuli, reducing the sensory and affective components of pain (opioids)

Drugs that we call *opioids, opiates,* or *"narcotics"* mimic the actions of our intrinsic, or endogenous, *endorphins* (the normal biological neurotransmitter at opioid or endorphin receptors). Drugs that so act are called *opioid agonists,* since they mimic the analgesic actions both of our endogenous endorphins (acting on the same set of receptors) and of morphine, the major analgesic in the opium poppy. Endorphins and opioids exert much of their analgesic action by acting presynaptically on nociceptive afferent sensory neurons to inhibit the release of pain-inducing transmitters (such as substance P) in the dorsal horn of the spinal cord (Figure 10.3).

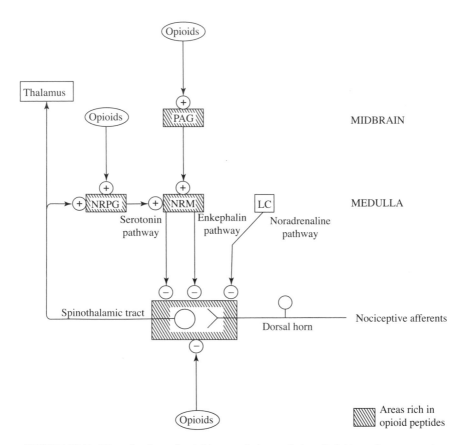

FIGURE 10.3 Sites of action of opioids on pain transmission. Opioids excite neurons in the periaqueductal gray matter (PAG) and in the midbrain and the nucleus raphe magnus (NRM) in the medulla. From there, serotoninergic and enkephalinergic neurons run to the dorsal horn and exert an inhibitory influence on transmission. Opioids also act directly on the dorsal horn. The locus coeruleus (LC) sends noradrenergic neurons to the dorsal horn, which also inhibits transmission. The pathways shown in this diagram represent a considerable oversimplification, but they depict the general organization of the supraspinal control mechanisms. NRPG = nucleus reticularis paragigantocellularis.

Chronic pain sets up ongoing spinal processes of neuroadaptation with associated physiological changes in spinal circuitry. Chronic pain is thought to be poorly responsive to opioids but quite responsive to anticonvulsants such as gabapentin (Chapter 6). For this reason, treatment of chronic pain with only opioid therapy is usually ill-advised because efficacy is limited and the risk of developing drug dependence is high. A new guideline for chronic pain management is available (American Society of Anesthesiologists, 2010).

Besides the physical component of pain, there are affective components (notably anxiety and depression) that determine a person's emotional response to real or perceived distress. Indeed, the affective component may be the underlying factor in the mechanism of chronic pain for which no objective cause can be identified. If depression or anxiety is present, opioids are ill advised; antidepressant/anxiolytic therapies, both pharmacological and behavioral, are preferable. For people with chronic pain, treatment focuses on behavior modification, hypnosis, cognitive-behavioral therapy, or self-management approaches that include biopsychosocial models of therapy (Cianfrini and Doleys, 2006).

History of Opioids

Opium is extracted from the opium poppy and has been used for thousands of years to produce euphoria, analgesia, sleep, and relief from diarrhea and cough. In ancient times, opium was used primarily for its constipating effect and later for its sleep-inducing properties (noted by writers such as Homer, Hippocrates, Dioscorides, Virgil, and Ovid). Even in those times, recreational abuse and addiction were common. From the early Greek and Roman days through the sixteenth and seventeenth centuries, the medicinal and recreational uses of opium were well established. Combined with alcohol, the mixture was called *laudanum* (named by Paracelsus in 1520), meaning "something to be praised," and it was referred to as the "stone of immortality." Thereafter, opium and laudanum were used for practically every known disease.

In the early 1800s, morphine was isolated from opium as its active ingredient. Since then, morphine has been used throughout the world as the premier agent for treating severe pain. Recognition of the addictive properties of opium, morphine, and other opioids has led to restrictions of their use, limiting them to the treatment of conditions for which they are known to be effective. After the invention of the hypodermic needle in 1856 and especially after the Civil War (when opioid addiction was referred to as "soldier's disease"), a new type of drug user appeared in the United States—one who self-administered opioids by injection. By about 1910, concern had begun to mount about the dangers of opioids and the dependence they could induce. In 1914 the Harrison Narcotic Act was passed, and the use of most opioid products was strictly controlled. Nonmedical uses of opioids were banned, although today nonmedical use continues, despite intense efforts to eradicate it.

The Controlled Substances Act was enacted in 1970 and has been modified several times. This legislation is the federal U.S. drug policy under which the manufacture, importation, possession, use, and distribution of certain substances is regulated. The legislation created five schedules (classifications), with varying qualifications for a substance to be included in each. Two federal agencies, the Drug Enforcement Administration and the Food and Drug Administration (FDA), now determine which substances are added to or removed from the various schedules, though the statute passed by Congress created the initial listing. Classification decisions must be made according to specific criteria, including potential for abuse (an undefined term), currently accepted medical use in treatment in the United States, and international treaties.[1]

The use of opioids is deeply entrenched in society; it is widespread and impossible to stop. Opioids exert pleasurable effects, produce tolerance and physiological dependence, and have a potential for compulsive misuse—all liabilities that are likely to resist any efforts at legal control. Also, the opioids will continue to be used in medicine because they are irreplaceable as pain-relieving agents. Opioids dramatically relieve emotional as well as physical pain. This property contributes to making them extremely seductive for self-administration. Savage (2005) stated:

> Therapeutic opioid use is increasing and greater volumes of prescriptions for opioid medications are being distributed through legitimate channels, from manufacturer to pharmacy to patient, creating greater opportunities for the diversion of opioids for non-therapeutic use. . . . [From] 1997 through 2001 . . . there has been a 1.5-fold to 4.3-fold increase in therapeutic opioid demand. (p. 1)

Savage illustrates his point in a figure reproduced here as Figure 10.4.

Furthermore, regarding the seeking of opioids for nontherapeutic purposes, the rates of involvement of prescription opioids in patients presenting to emergency rooms more than doubled between 1996 and 2001 (Figure 10.5), doubling again between 2004 and 2008. After marijuana, prescription pain pills are currently the drugs most often illicitly abused by people in the United States, far surpassing the numbers of people who abuse psychedelic drugs, cocaine, methamphetamine, inhalants, and even heroin. Figure 10.6 illustrates the increase through 2008 in the abuse of opioids, with short-acting preparations of hydrocodone (Vicodin and generic equivalents) and long-acting oxycodone (OxyContin) and methadone far exceeding abuse of other opioids.

---

[1] Specifics of the scheduling may be found at en.wikipedia.org/wiki/Controlled _Substances_Act

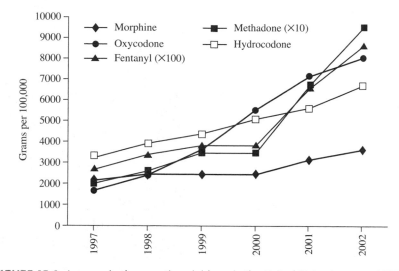

FIGURE 10.4   Increase in therapeutic opioid use in the United States between 1997 and 2002. [From Savage (2005), Figure 1.]

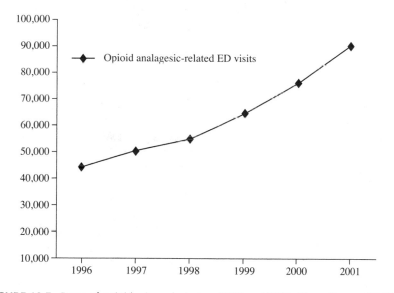

FIGURE 10.5   Rates of opioid misuse between 1996 and 2001. [From Savage (2005), Figure 2.]

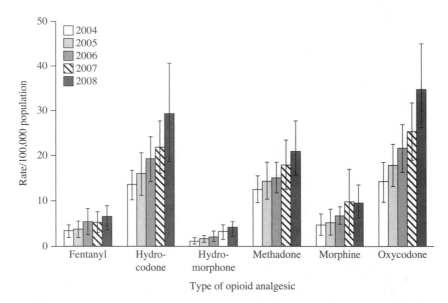

FIGURE 10.6 Rates of emergency department visits for nonmedical use of selected opioid analgesics by type in the United States during 2004–2008. Visit rates for opioid analgesics were highest for oxycodone, hydrocodone, and methadone during the entire study period. [Centers for Disease Control and Prevention (2010), figure 1.]

Terminology

Before proceeding, some terms need definition. *Opium* comes from a Greek word (*opion*) that means "juice"; more specifically, it refers to the juice or exudate from the poppy *Papaver somniferum*. An *opiate*, strictly defined, is a drug extracted from the exudate of the poppy. Therefore the term is restricted to two drugs that are naturally found in the exudates: *morphine* and *codeine*. An *opioid* is any exogenous drug (natural, semisynthetic, or synthetic) that binds to an opiate receptor and produces agonistic, or morphinelike, effects.

Endorphin is an all-inclusive term that applies to an endogenous substance (a substance naturally formed in the body) that exhibits the pharmacological properties of morphine. There are three families of endogenous opioid peptides—*enkephalins, dynorphins,* and *beta endorphins.* The topic of endogenous opioids is large and complex. The reader is referred to the review by Akil and coworkers (1998).

Opioids occur in nature in two places: in the juice of the opium poppy (morphine and codeine) and within our own bodies as any of the endorphins. All other opioids are either prepared from morphine (*semisynthetic opioids,* such as heroin) or synthesized from other precursor compounds (*synthetic opioids,* such as fentanyl).

The term *narcotic* is derived from the Greek word *narke,* meaning "numbness," "sleep," or "stupor." Originally referring to any drug that induced sleep, the term later became associated with opioids, such as morphine and heroin. Today, it is an imprecise term, sometimes used in a legal context to refer to a wide variety of abused substances that includes nonopioids, such as cocaine and marijuana. The term is not useful in a pharmacological context, and its use in referring to opioids is discouraged.

Opioid Receptors

Opioids are agonists at highly specific receptor sites, and the analgesic potency of the agonist correlates with the affinity of the agonist for the opioid receptor. There is general agreement on the existence of at least three types of opioid receptors: *mu, kappa,* and *delta.* The genes encoding these three families, as well as the receptors themselves, have been cloned, sequenced, and well studied. Receptors on which endorphins and exogenous opioids act are widely distributed throughout the central nervous system (CNS), and each type of opioid receptor is differentially distributed. Some regions of the CNS (for example, the spinal cord) have all three types of receptors; other regions have predominantly one type (the thalamus, for example, has primarily mu receptors). The clinical significance of this distribution is still unclear. However, overall, it seems that mu receptor agonists display not only the strongest analgesic actions but also the highest potential for abuse.

Mu receptors are located in the brain, in the spinal cord, and in the periphery. Morphine is the classic example of a mu agonist. It exerts powerful effects on the brain (especially in the thalamus and striatum), the brain stem (where it slows respiration), and the spinal cord (where it exerts a strong analgesic action). In contrast, the delta receptor agonists exhibit little addictive potential and are also poor analgesics. Delta receptors are thought to modulate the activity of mu receptors. Kappa agonists exert modest analgesic effects, little or no respiratory depression, miosis (pinpoint pupils), and little or no dependence effects. In fact, activation of kappa receptors may serve to antagonize mu receptor-mediated actions in the brain. The use of kappa agonists is limited by strong and unpleasant dysphoric responses that can accompany their use.

In the mid-1990s the opioid receptors were first isolated, purified, cloned, and sequenced, and their three-dimensional structures were modeled. All opioid receptors belong to a superfamily of G-protein-coupled receptors, all of which possess seven membrane-spanning regions (Figure 10.7) similar to the receptors discussed earlier. Each receptor type (mu, kappa, delta) arises from its own gene and is expressed through a specific messenger RNA (mRNA). Each receptor is a chain of

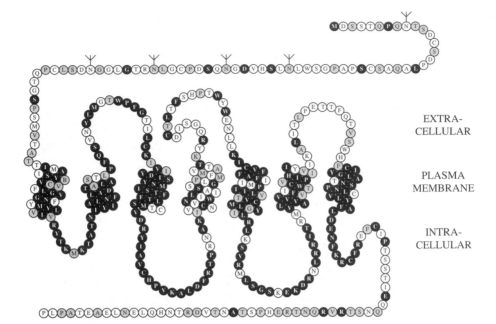

FIGURE 10.7 Two-dimensional model of the rat mu opioid receptor. The receptor is a chain of about 390 amino acids (the letter in each circle is the first letter of the individual amino acid), with seven transmembrane coils and a terminal chain both intracellular (linked to a G protein, not illustrated) and extracellular (binds the transmitter). Amino acids conserved in mu, delta, and kappa receptors are shown in black; amino acids conserved in mu and either delta or kappa receptors are shown in gray; amino acids preset only in the mu receptor (not in delta or kappa receptors) are shown in white. [From M. Satoh and M. Minami, "Molecular Pharmacology of the Opioid Receptors," *Pharmacology and Therapeutics* 68 (1995), Figure 1.]

approximately 400 amino acids, and the amino acid sequences are about 60 percent identical to one another and 40 percent different (see Figure 10.7). The diversity is responsible for the specific fit of an endogenous endorphin or an exogenous opioid to a specific receptor. A fit for a fentanyl derivative for a mu receptor is illustrated in Figure 10.8. In this figure, note that the flat, two-dimensional drawing of the receptor shown in Figure 10.7 is now depicted more realistically as a three-dimensional receptor with seven helical coils embedded in the membrane and three amino acid loops and a terminal chain (located in the extracellular, synaptic space) forming a fit with the opioid.

What is the consequence of the binding of an opioid agonist to a mu receptor? As discussed, the primary action of opioid receptor activation (by either an endorphin or an opioid) is reduction in or inhibition of neurotransmission, which occurs largely through opioid-induced presynaptic inhibition of neurotransmitter release (Figure 10.9). Changes are different for each receptor type and may explain the differences in receptor

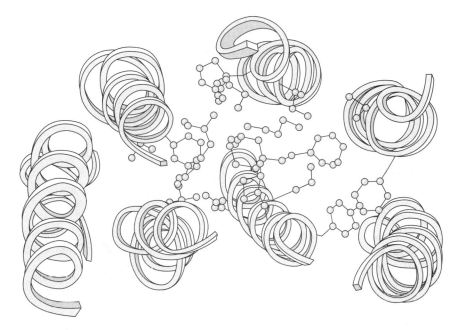

FIGURE 10.8   Speculative three-dimensional depiction of interaction of the mu opioid receptor with the potent pure mu agonist lofentanyl. Transmembrane helices are depicted by coils. The cell membrane within which the coils reside is not illustrated. Lofentanyl structure is shown by the connected small balls, which represent carbon molecules of the drug. Specific side chains of amino acids on the receptor helices bind with specific portions of the lofentanyl molecule. [Original details by H. Moereels, L. M. Kaymans, J. Leysen, and P. Janssen, Janssen Research Foundation, Beerse, Belgium.]

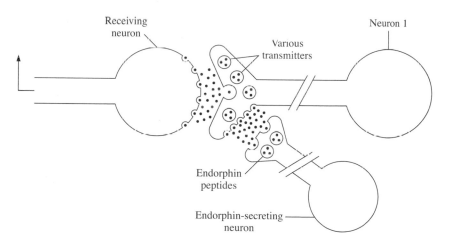

FIGURE 10.9   Simplified illustration demonstrating the presynaptic inhibition (exerted by an endorphin-secreting neuron) on neuron 1, inhibiting its release of transmitter. In the spinal cord, neuron 1 would be a primary afferent (sensory pain neuron), with enkephalin-inhibiting substance P release. In the ventral tegmentum, neuron 1 might be a GABA-secreting neuron, with an endorphin-inhibiting GABA release, disinhibiting a dopaminergic neuron, a mechanism of opioid-induced reward.

function (for example, mu receptor action induces euphoria and is a positive reinforcer, while kappa receptor activation causes dysphoria and is not reinforcing). Snyder and Pasternak (2003) present a historical review of the development of our knowledge about opioid receptors.

Mu Receptors

Mu opioid receptors are present in all structures in the brain and spinal cord involved in morphine-induced analgesia. The structures include the periaqueductal gray matter, spinal trigeminal nucleus, caudate and geniculate nuclei, thalamus, and spinal cord (dorsal horn). Mu receptors are also present in brain-stem nuclei involved in control of respiration (and in morphine's depression of respiration), in brain-stem structures involved in initiation of nausea and vomiting, and in the nucleus accumbens, an area involved in the compulsive abuse of opioids and other drugs subject to compulsive abuse (Trigo et al., 2010). Few or no mu receptors are found in the cerebral cortex or cerebellum.

Kappa Receptors

Kappa receptors are found in the basal ganglia, nucleus accumbens, ventral tegmentum, deep layers of the cerebral cortex, hypothalamus, periaqueductal gray matter, dorsal horn of the spinal cord, and the periphery. Binder and coworkers (2001) studied two experimental kappa agonists that do not cross the blood-brain barrier but act only in the periphery. They were both analgesic and anti-inflammatory. The researchers concluded that the agonists might potentiate centrally acting opioids or standard NSAIDs (Chapter 9).

As stated, kappa receptors in the CNS may actually antagonize mu receptor activity. Kappa receptors produce modest amounts of analgesia, dysphoria (as opposed to mu receptor-induced euphoria), disorientation, rare feelings of depersonalization, and only mild respiratory depression. The mixed agonist-antagonist drugs (discussed later), such as pentazocine (Talwin), are agonists at the kappa receptors. Dynorphin is the endorphin with the greatest affinity for the kappa receptor.

The hallucinogenic agent salvinorin A (from the psychedelic mint plant *Salvia divinorum*) is a potent agonist (stimulant) of the kappa opioid receptor (Chavkin et al., 2004). Salvinorin A is discussed further in Chapter 15. Therefore, kappa receptor activation may be related to the modulation of human perception. For example, bremazocine, a potent kappa-opioid receptor agonist, is more analgesic than is morphine, without inducing euphoria, dependence, or respiratory depression. Unfortunately, the perceptual side effects (space and time distortions, visual distortions, body image distortions, depersonalization, derealization, and loss of self-control) limit its use as a clinical analgesic (Dortch-Carnes and Potter, 2005).

Delta Receptors

The enkephalins are the endogenous endorphins for the delta receptors. These receptors have limited analgesic effects, but they do display a prominent effect on emotional states: they exert robust antidepressant and anxiolytic effects, suggesting potential as clinical antidepressants and anxiolytics (Jutkiewicz, 2006). In agreement with the discussion of the involvement of brain-derived neurotrophic factor in depression, delta opioid agonists increase the levels of this substance (Narita et al., 2006; Torregrossa et al., 2006).

Classification of Opioid Analgesics

Classification of opioids is usually according to the receptors to which they bind and the consequences of the binding. Thus, an individual opioid is called an *agonist,* a *partial agonist,* a *mixed agonist-antagonist,* or a *pure antagonist* at the given receptor (Table 10.1). All the strong opioids, such as morphine, primarily act as agonists at mu receptors, and their pharmacological effects, including analgesia, respiratory depression, miosis, euphoria, reward, and constipation, all follow from this action.

Pure Agonists

An agonist is a drug that has an affinity for (binds to) cell receptors and induces changes in the cell characteristic of the natural neurotransmitter chemical (for example, an endorphin) for the receptor. Morphine is the prototype opioid analgesic, but there are many others, including methadone, an orally active, long-acting opioid used to treat heroin dependency. All these strong opioids bind to mu receptors (Table 10.2). Therefore, a mu agonist produces analgesia, respiratory depression, and euphoria and has a propensity to cause dependence. So far, all attempts to separate analgesia from euphoria, dependence, and respiratory depression have been unsuccessful, and attempts in the foreseeable future are likely to be so as well.

Pure Antagonists

Pure antagonists have *affinity* for a receptor (here, the mu receptor), but after attaching they elicit no change in cellular functioning (they lack intrinsic activity). What they do is compete with the mu agonist for the receptor, precipitating withdrawal in an opioid-dependent person and reversing any analgesia caused by the agonist. One example is the clinical use of the opioid antagonist naltrexone in treatment programs for heroin addicts, where heroin taken after the antagonist elicits no analgesic or euphoric effects.

TABLE 10.1 Classification of opioid analgesics by analgesic properties

Pure agonists	Mixed agonist-antagonists	Pure antagonists	Partial agonists
Morphine	Nalbuphine (Nubain)	Naloxone (Narcan)	Buprenorphine (in Suboxone)
Codeine	Butorphanol (Stadol)	Naltrexone (Trexan,	Tramadol (Ultram)[a]
Heroin	Pentazocine (Talwin)	ReVia, Vivitrol)	Tapentadol (Nucynta)
Meperidine (Demerol)	Dezocine (Dalgan)	Nalmefene (Revex)	
Methadone (Dolophine)			
Oxymorphone (Numorphan)			
Hydromorphone (Dilaudid)			
Fentanyl (Sublimaze)			

[a] Tramadol also blocks reuptake of norepinephrine and serotonin.

TABLE 10.2 Classification of opioid analgesics by actions at opioid receptors

Compound	Receptor types[a]		
	Mu	**Kappa**	**Delta**
Morphine	+++	+	+
Naloxone	−	−	−
Pentazocine	+/0	+	NA
Butorphanol	+/0	+	NA
Nalbuphine	−	+	NA
Buprenorphine	++	+	+
Fentanyl	+++	+	+
Dezocine	+	+	+

[a] The mu receptor is thought to mediate supraspinal analgesia, respiratory depression, euphoria, and physical dependence; the kappa receptor, spinal analgesia, miosis, and sedation. Categorizations are based on best inferences about actions in humans. See text for further explanation. Agonists are indicated by one or more plus signs, antagonists by a minus sign, and agents that have no significant action at the receptor by zero. NA = data not available.

Mixed Agonist-Antagonists

A mixed agonist-antagonist drug produces an agonistic effect at one receptor and an antagonistic effect at another. Clinically useful mixed drugs are kappa agonists and weak mu antagonists (they bind to both kappa and mu receptors, but only the kappa receptor is activated). In contrast to a pure agonist, a mixed agonist-antagonist usually displays a ceiling effect for analgesia; in other words, it has decreased efficacy compared to a pure agonist and usually is not so effective in treating severe pain. Also, when a mixed agonist-antagonist is administered to an opioid-dependent person, the antagonistic effect at a mu receptor precipitates an acute withdrawal syndrome. *Pentazocine* (Talwin) is the prototype mixed agonist-antagonist.

Partial Agonists

A partial agonist binds to opioid receptors but has a low intrinsic activity (low efficacy). It therefore exerts an analgesic effect, but the effect has a ceiling at less than the maximal effect produced by a pure agonist. *Buprenorphine* (in Suboxone) is the prototype partial opioid agonist. When administered to a person who is not opioid dependent, analgesia is observed; when administered to an opioid-dependent person, however, blockade of the pure agonist can occur and withdrawal can be precipitated. Compared to a mixed agonist-antagonist, the partial agonist buprenorphine binds to all three types of opioid receptors with higher efficacy at mu receptors than do the mixed agonist-antagonist agents. Its potential for producing respiratory depression is lower than that of morphine.

Morphine: A Pure Opioid Agonist

Of the two analgesics found in the opium poppy, morphine and codeine, morphine (Figure 10.10) is the more potent and represents about 10 percent of the crude exudate. Codeine is much less potent and constitutes only 0.5 percent of the crude exudate. Despite decades of research, no other drug has been found that exceeds morphine's effectiveness as an analgesic, and no other drug is clinically superior for treating severe pain.

Pharmacokinetics

Morphine is usually administered by injection, but it may also be given orally or rectally. Under development is an intranasal delivery system for morphine (Rylomine). This product would have a rapid onset of action in situations where oral use is not desired. Orally, morphine is available in immediate-release formulation and as a long-acting, time-release product (MS-Contin). In general, absorption of morphine from the gastrointestinal tract is slow and incomplete compared to absorption following injection or inhalation. Absorption through the rectum is adequate, and several opioids (morphine, hydromorphone, and oxymorphone) are available in suppository form.[2]

The action of opioids in the spinal cord has led to the administration of morphine directly into the spinal canal (through small catheters), placing the drug right at its site of action and avoiding its effects both on higher CNS centers (maintaining wakefulness and avoiding respiratory depression) and in the periphery (avoiding drug-induced constipation). In medicine, this technique is used to control the pain of obstetric labor and delivery, to treat postoperative pain, and (for long-term use) to relieve otherwise intractable pain associated with terminal cancer and chronic pain. Morphine administered by any route must be given with great care to avoid potentially fatal respiratory depression.

For millennia, crude opium has been smoked for recreational purposes; the rapidity of onset of drug action rivals that following intravenous injection. Morphine itself is rarely abused in this manner; heroin is the preparation of choice. However, for therapeutic use, a nebulized form of morphine has been found to be effective, for example, in patients with terminal illnesses who cannot tolerate injections (Thipphawong et al., 2003). Nebulizer preparations of morphine have not yet been marketed.

---

[2] This kind of preparation might be indicated for patients suffering from muscle-wasting diseases who cannot tolerate other routes of administration.

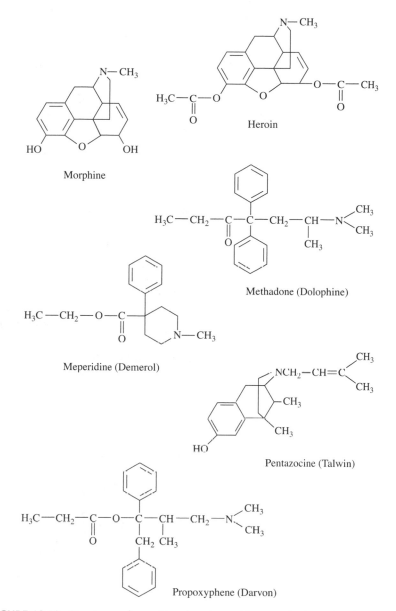

FIGURE 10.10 Structures of morphine, heroin, and four synthetic analgesics.

Morphine crosses the blood-brain barrier fairly slowly, as it is more water soluble than lipid soluble. Other opioids (such as heroin and fentanyl) cross the blood-brain barrier much more rapidly. Only about 20 percent of administered morphine reaches the CNS. This may explain why the "flash" or "rush" following intravenous injection of heroin is much more intense than that perceived after injecting morphine.

Opioids reach all body tissues, including the fetus; infants born to addicted mothers are physically dependent on opioids and exhibit withdrawal symptoms that require intensive therapy. The habitual use of morphine or other opioids during pregnancy does not seem to increase the risk of congenital anomalies; thus, these drugs are not considered to be teratogenic. However, there are increased risks of birth-related problems and fetal growth retardation. Other delays and impairments observed in the development of opioid-exposed children may relate more to environmental and social-developmental problems.

The liver metabolizes morphine, and one of its metabolites (morphine-6-glucuronide) is actually 10 to 20 times more potent as an analgesic than morphine. Much of the analgesic action of morphine is mediated by this active metabolite. The half-lives of morphine and morphine-6-glucuronide are both 3 to 5 hours. Patients with impaired kidney function tend to accumulate the metabolite and thus may be more sensitive to morphine administration.

Urine-screening tests can be used to detect codeine and morphine as well as their metabolites. Because heroin is metabolized to monoacetylmorphine and then to morphine, and because street heroin also contains acetylcodeine, heroin use is suspected when monoacetylmorphine, morphine, and codeine are present in urine. Frequently, urinalysis cannot accurately determine which specific drug (heroin, codeine, or morphine) has been used. Furthermore, codeine is widely available in cough syrups and analgesic preparations, and even poppy seeds contain small amounts of morphine. Depending on the drug that was taken, morphine and codeine metabolites may be detected in a patient's urine for two to four days.

Pharmacological Effects

Morphine produces a syndrome characterized by analgesia, relaxed euphoria, sedation, a sense of tranquility, reduced apprehension and concern, respiratory depression, suppression of the cough reflex, and pupillary constriction.

Analgesia. Morphine produces intense analgesia and indifference to pain, reducing the intensity of pain and thus reducing the associated distress by altering the central processing of pain. Morphine analgesia occurs without loss of consciousness and without affecting other sensory modalities. The pain may actually persist as a sensation, but patients feel more comfortable and are able to tolerate the pain. In other words, the perception of the pain is significantly altered.

Euphoria. Morphine produces a pleasant euphoric state, which includes a strong feeling of contentment, well-being, and lack of concern. This effect is part of the affective, or reinforcing, response to the drug. Use of exogenous opioids gives a person access to the reinforcement system, especially in the nucleus accumbens. Once opioids reach this positive reward system, normally reserved to reward the performance of species-specific survival behaviors, the user has a profoundly rewarding experience (Trigo et al., 2010).

Opioid use becomes an acquired drive state that permeates all aspects of human life. With acute use, all painful feelings, emotions, and physical discomforts become tolerable. Even the knowledge that withdrawal will follow, that life and livelihood are imperiled, that only more drug will prevent withdrawal, that legal apprehension or even death may follow—all become tolerable as long as the drug is present. Separate neural pathways that cause withdrawal events to be perceived as life-threatening and the subsequent physiological reactions often lead to renewed opioid consumption. As discussed in the section on the treatment of chronic alcoholism in Chapter 13, the drive to resume ingestion of the drug now appears to involve the endogenous cannabinoid system, as cannabinoid receptor antagonists can block the compulsion to return to drug use (Chapter 14). The same cannabinoid system that can propel a return to alcohol drinking is probably involved in a compulsion to return to opioid use.

Regular users of morphine describe the effects of intravenous injection in ecstatic and often sexual terms, but the euphoric effect becomes progressively less intense after repeated use. At this point, users inject the drug for one or more of several possible reasons: to try to reexperience the euphoria felt after the first few injections, to maintain a state of pleasure and well-being, to prevent mental discomfort that may be associated with reality, or to prevent withdrawal symptoms.

The mechanism of morphine's positive reinforcing and euphoria-producing action probably involves dopaminergic as well as mu receptors. Opioids activate mu receptors within the mesolimbic dopamine reward system by means of the dopaminergic ventral tegmental–nucleus accumbens pathway that is involved in the rewarding effects of cocaine and alcohol. As stated by Narita and coworkers (2001):

> Various studies provide arguments to support substantial roles for mu-opioid receptors and the possible involvement of delta-opioid receptors in the development of physical and psychological dependence on morphine. Noradrenergic transmission originating in the locus coeruleus is most likely to play the primary causal role in the expression of physical dependence on morphine. In contrast, many studies have pointed to the mesolimbic dopaminergic pathway projecting from the ventral tegmental area to the nucleus accumbens as a critical site for the initiation of psychological dependence on opioids. (p. 1)

In the ventral tegmental area, morphine inhibits GABA neurons via mu opioid receptors, thus disinhibiting dopaminergic neurons and increasing dopamine input in the nucleus accumbens and in other areas; this phenomenon may be involved in the mechanism of reward, that is, the positive reinforcement of opioid addiction.

Sedation and Anxiolysis. Morphine produces anxiolysis, sedation, and drowsiness, but the level of sedation is not so deep as that produced by the CNS depressants. Although people who are taking morphine doze, they can usually be awakened readily. During this state, cognitive slowing is prominent, accompanied by a lack of concentration, apathy, complacency, lethargy, reduced mentation, and a sense of tranquility. Obviously, in such a state, cognitive impairment results.

Depression of Respiration. Morphine causes a profound depression of respiration by decreasing the respiratory center's sensitivity to higher levels of carbon dioxide in the blood. Respiratory rate is reduced even at therapeutic doses; at higher doses, the rate slows even further, respiratory volume decreases, breathing patterns become shallow and irregular, and, at sufficiently high levels, breathing ceases. Respiratory depression is the single most important acute side effect of morphine and is the cause of death from acute opioid overdosage. The combination of morphine (or other opioid) with alcohol or other sedatives is especially dangerous.

Suppression of Cough. Opioids suppress the cough center, which is located in the brain stem. Opioids have historically been used as cough suppressants; codeine is particularly popular for this purpose. Today, however, less addicting drugs are used as cough suppressants, and opioids have become inappropriate choices for treating persistent cough.

Pupillary Constriction. Morphine (as well as other mu and kappa agonists) causes pupillary constriction (miosis). Indeed, pupillary constriction in the presence of analgesia is characteristic of opioid ingestion.

Nausea and Vomiting. Morphine stimulates receptors in an area of the medulla that is called the chemoreceptor trigger zone. Stimulation of this area produces nausea and vomiting, which are the most characteristic and unpleasant side effects of morphine and other opioids, but they are not life-threatening.

Gastrointestinal Symptoms. Morphine and the other opioids relieve diarrhea as a result of their direct actions on the intestine, the most important action of opioids outside the CNS. Opioids cause intestinal tone to increase, motility to decrease, feces to dehydrate, and intestinal spasm (and cramping) to occur. This combination of decreased propulsion, increased intestinal tone, decreased rate of movement of food, and dehydration hardens the stool and further retards the advance of fecal material. Nothing more effective than the opioids has yet been developed for treating severe diarrhea. Two opioids have been developed that only very minimally cross the blood-brain barrier into the CNS. One is *diphenoxylate* (the primary active ingredient in Lomotil), and the other is *loperamide* (Imodium). These two drugs are exceedingly effective opioid antidiarrheals. Later, we will discuss two new peripherally acting opioid antagonists effective in treating opioid-induced constipation.

Endocrine Effects. Morphine and other opioids exert subtle but important effects on the functioning of the endocrine system (Katz, 2005). Effects include reduced libido in men and menstrual irregularities and infertility in women. These effects occur secondary to drug-induced reductions in sex hormone-releasing agents from the hypothalamus. As a result, testosterone levels in males fall, as do the levels of luteinizing and follicle-stimulating hormones in females. If a person is taking an opioid for chronic pain, both the reduction in sex hormones and the chronic pain may result in loss of sexual desire and impaired performance, alterations in gender role, fatigue, mood alterations, loss of muscle mass and strength, abnormal menses, infertility, and osteoporosis and fractures (Katz, 2005). Therefore, it may be unclear whether the opioid-induced hypogonadism or the chronic pain was responsible.

Other Effects. Morphine can release histamine from its storage sites in mast cells in the blood, which can result in localized itching or more severe allergic reactions, including bronchoconstriction (an asthmalike constriction of the bronchi of the lungs). Opioids also affect white blood cell function, perhaps producing complex alterations in the immune system. It is advisable, perhaps, to avoid the use of morphine in patients with compromised immune function.

Tolerance and Dependence

The development of tolerance and dependence with repeated use is a characteristic feature of all opioid drugs, including morphine. The use of all mu agonist opioids is severely limited because of the development of tolerance, the presence of uncomfortable side effects, and the potential for compulsive abuse.

The molecular basis of tolerance and drug-seeking behaviors are thought to involve glutaminergic mechanisms (Xu et al., 2007; LaLumiere and Kalivas, 2008). It appears that glutaminergic receptors may regulate mu receptor mRNA, accounting for the development of tolerance to the continuous presence of opioid. The rate at which tolerance develops varies widely. When morphine or other opioids are used only intermittently, little, if any, tolerance develops, and the opioids retain their initial efficacy. When administration is repeated, tolerance may become so marked that massive doses have to be administered to either maintain a degree of euphoria or prevent withdrawal discomfort (avoidance of discomfort is more common). The degree of tolerance is illustrated by the fact that the dose of morphine can be increased from clinical doses (50 to 60 milligrams per day) to 500 milligrams per day over as short a period as 10 days.

Tolerance to one opioid leads to cross-tolerance to all other natural and synthetic opioids, even if they are chemically dissimilar. Cross-tolerance, however, does not develop between the opioids and the sedative hypnotics. In other words, a person who has developed a tolerance for morphine will also have a tolerance for heroin but not for alcohol or benzodiazepines.

Physical dependence was described in Chapter 1 as an altered state of biology induced by a drug whereby withdrawal of a drug is followed by a complex set of biological events typical for that class of drugs. Acute withdrawal from opioids has been well studied since it can be easily precipitated in a drug-dependent person by injecting the opioid antagonist naloxone (Narcan). Withdrawal results in a profound reduction in the release of dopamine in the nucleus accumbens and a threefold increase in the release of norepinephrine in various structures, including the hippocampus, nucleus accumbens, and locus coeruleus. The firing rate of neurons located in the locus coeruleus is actively inhibited by morphine, returns to baseline levels with tolerance, and rises dramatically during withdrawal; these phenomena may be involved in the mechanism of dependence.

Symptoms of withdrawal are, in general, the opposite of pharmacological effects (Table 10.3) and include restlessness, dysphoria, drug craving, sweating, extreme anxiety, depression, irritability, fever, chills, retching and vomiting, increased respiratory rate (panting), cramping, insomnia, explosive diarrhea, and intense aches and pains. The magnitude of these acute withdrawal symptoms depends on the dose of opioid that had been used, the frequency of previous drug administration, and the duration of drug dependence. Acute opioid withdrawal is not considered to be life-threatening, although it can seem unbearable to the person experiencing it.

To help alleviate the symptoms of acute withdrawal, several approaches have been tried, none with great success (O'Connor, 2005). These approaches include clonidine-assisted detoxification, buprenorphine-assisted detoxification, and rapid anesthesia-aided detoxification. Clonidine is a drug that acts on the sympathetic nervous system to reduce

TABLE 10.3 Acute effects of opioids and rebound withdrawal symptoms	
Acute action	**Withdrawal sign**
Analgesia	Pain and irritability
Respiratory depression	Hyperventilation
Euphoria	Dysphoria and depression
Relaxation and sleep	Restlessness and insomnia
Tranquilization	Fearfulness and hostility
Decreased blood pressure	Increased blood pressure
Constipation	Diarrhea
Pupillary constriction	Pupillary dilation
Hypothermia	Hyperthermia
Drying of secretions	Lacrimation, runny nose
Reduced sex drive	Spontaneous ejaculation
Peripheral vasodilation; flushed and warm skin	Chilliness and "gooseflesh"

From R. S. Feldman, J. S. Meyer, and L. F. Quenzer, *Principles of Neuropsychopharmacology* (Sunderland, MA: Sinauer, 1997), Table 12.8, p. 533.

some of the physical manifestations of withdrawal. Buprenorphine will be discussed later in this chapter.

In *rapid anesthesia-aided detoxification* (RAAD), a pure opioid antagonist, such as naloxone or naltrexone, and the sympathetic blocker clonidine are administered intravenously to the opioid-dependent person while he or she is asleep under general anesthesia. The procedure goes on for about 72 hours, during which time the withdrawal signs are blunted. The objective is to enable the patient to tolerate high doses of an opioid antagonist and thus undergo complete detoxification while unconscious. After awakening, the patient is maintained on naltrexone to reduce opioid craving and undergoes supportive psychotherapy and group therapies for relapse prevention and to address the underlying causes of addiction. The RAAD technique is controversial, in part because it is expensive, it involves the risks of anesthesia, and it focuses only on short-term dependence rather than on long-term cravings and social adjustments. One study compared the three techniques of detoxification and concluded that RAAD was no less safe or effective than other techniques (Collins et al., 2005).

No matter the method of opioid withdrawal, following acute withdrawal focus is directed toward a protracted *abstinence syndrome*, beginning when the acute phase of opioid withdrawal ends and persisting for up to six months. Symptoms of this syndrome include depression, abnormal responses to stressful situations, drug hunger, decreased self-esteem, anxiety, and other psychological disturbances.

Complicating the diagnosis of prolonged abstinence syndrome is the high prevalence of other psychiatric disorders (for example, affective and personality disorders) in opioid-dependent patients; antisocial personality disorder and major depression are the most common co-morbidities. Antidepressants such as imipramine or desipramine (Chapter 5) can be effective.

　　Several behavioral theories have been posited to account for continued opioid use:

- Continued use prevents the distress and dysphoria associated with withdrawal (a negative reinforcing effect).
- The euphoria produced by the opioids leads to their continued use (a positive reinforcing effect).
- Preexisting dysphoric or painful affective states are alleviated (presuming that the opioids were initially used as a type of self-medication to treat these symptoms and that dependence developed gradually).
- Preexisting psychopathology may be the basis for initial experimentation and euphoria, but repeated use is prompted by the desire to avoid withdrawal.
- Some people have deficient endorphin systems that are corrected by the use of opioids.
- Because repeated use of opioids leads to permanent dysfunction in the endorphin system, normal function eventually requires the continued use of exogenous opioids.
- Drug effects and drug withdrawal can become linked through environmental cues and internal mood states. Emotions and external cues recall the distress of withdrawal or the memory of opioid euphoria or opioid reduction of dysphoria or painful affective states.

To varying degrees, all these theories are probably involved in a given person's use of opioids. Opioid tolerance and dependence exist not merely in a few predisposed people; they can develop in anyone who uses the drugs repeatedly, not necessarily people who are abusing them. A patient in the chronic pain of terminal illness should not be denied opioids, despite the inevitable development of tolerance and dependence.

Other Pure Opioid Agonists

As stated earlier, another naturally occurring opioid found in the opium poppy is codeine. Several synthetic and semisynthetic opioids are also agonists of the mu opioid receptor.

Codeine

Codeine is one of the most commonly prescribed opioids; it is usually combined with aspirin or acetaminophen for the relief of mild to moderate pain. These combination products are frequently sought drugs of abuse. About 40 percent of people who use them meet the criteria for codeine dependence (Sproule et al., 1999), and the use of codeine-containing products is strongly associated with endogenous depression—a dual-diagnosis problem. The plasma half-life and duration of action is about three to four hours.

Pharmacokinetically, codeine is metabolized by the hepatic drug-metabolizing enzyme CYP-2D6 to morphine, and many of the clinical effects attributed to codeine (for example, pain relief and euphoria) may, in fact, result from the actions of morphine. Four of the six selective serotonin reuptake inhibitor (SSRI) antidepressants (fluoxetine, fluvoxamine, sertraline, and paroxetine; Chapter 5) can block the pain relief of codeine because they block the conversion of codeine to morphine. For patients taking one of these drugs, an analgesic drug other than codeine may be necessary.

Heroin

Heroin (diacetylmorphine) is three times more potent than morphine and is produced from morphine by a slight modification of chemical structure (see Figure 10.10). The increased lipid solubility of heroin leads to faster penetration of the blood-brain barrier, producing an intense rush when the drug is either smoked or injected intravenously. Heroin is metabolized to monoacetylmorphine and morphine; morphine is eventually metabolized and excreted. Heroin is legally available in Great Britain, where it can be used clinically. The drug is not legal in the United States, but it is widely used illicitly. When heroin is smoked together with crack cocaine, euphoria is intensified, the anxiety and paranoia associated with cocaine are tempered, and the depression that follows after the effects of cocaine wear off seems to be reduced. Unfortunately, this combination creates a multidrug addiction that is extremely difficult to treat.

Hydromorphone and Oxymorphone

Hydromorphone (Dilaudid) and oxymorphone (Numorphan, Opana-ER) are both structurally related to morphine. Both drugs are as effective as morphine, and they are six to ten times more potent than morphine. Somewhat less sedation but equal respiratory depression are observed.

Palladone (not to be confused with *paliperidone;* Chapter 4) and Exalgo are trade names for two new, long-acting formulations of hydromorphone that are taken once daily for treatment of chronic pain in patients who have developed a tolerance to opioids and thus can tolerate the high doses of 10–32 milligrams per day (the dose of short-acting hydromorphone is about 1–2 milligrams). The half-life of both Palladone and Exalgo is about 18 hours. Palladone is formulated as an immediately dissolving capsule containing controlled-release pellets. Exalgo contains hydromorphone in the OROS osmotic delivery system similar to that used for Concerta (Chapter 18).

Meperidine

Meperidine (Demerol) is a synthetic opioid whose structure differs from that of morphine (see Figure 10.10). Because of this structural difference, meperidine was originally thought to be free of many of the undesirable properties of the opioids. However, meperidine is addictive; it can be substituted for morphine or heroin in addicts and is widely prescribed medically. It is one-tenth as potent as morphine, produces a similar type of euphoria, and is equally likely to cause dependence. Meperidine's side effects differ from morphine's and include more excitatory effects, such as tremors, delirium, hyperreflexia, and convulsions. These effects are produced by a metabolite of meperidine (normeperidine) that appears to be responsible for the CNS excitation. Meperidine and normeperidine can accumulate in people who have kidney dysfunction or who use only meperidine for their opioid addiction. Following discontinuation, withdrawal symptoms develop more rapidly than with morphine because of meperidine's shorter duration of action.

Methadone

Methadone (Dolophine) is a synthetic mu agonist opioid (see Figure 10.10), the pharmacological activity of which is very similar to that of morphine. Methadone was first shown to cover for and block the effects of heroin withdrawal in 1948. In 1965 it was introduced as a substitute treatment for opioid dependency, and since then it has become the principal pharmacological agent for prevention of abstinence symptoms and signs. The outstanding properties of methadone are its effective analgesic activity, its efficacy by the oral route, its extended duration of action in suppressing withdrawal symptoms in physically dependent people, and its tendency to show persistent effects with repeated administration.

Today, methadone has two primary legitimate uses: (1) as an orally administered substitute for heroin in methadone maintenance treatment programs and (2) as a long-acting analgesic for the treatment of chronic pain syndromes. Federal prescription regulations clearly separate these two uses. Physicians who do not practice in federally licensed methadone treatment programs may not prescribe the drug for the maintenance of opioid dependency; the drug may be prescribed only through licensed methadone maintenance treatment program centers. However, office-based physicians may prescribe methadone for the treatment of either acute pain or chronic pain.

The main objectives of methadone maintenance treatment programs are rehabilitation of the dependent person and reduction of needle-associated diseases, illicit drug use, and crime. Randomized controlled trials of methadone maintenance programs have shown that they generally fulfill these aims. Although there are a number of predictors of the success of a program, the most important is the magnitude of the daily methadone dose. Programs that prescribe average daily doses exceeding 100 milligrams have higher retention rates and lower illicit drug use rates than those in which the average dose is less.

Even where liberal doses are used (sometimes up to 160 milligrams per day or higher), about one-third of the clients regularly experience withdrawal (they are called *nonholders*) and two-thirds (called *holders*) do not on a once-daily dosing schedule. Thus, to maintain compliance, prescribers must be free to regulate doses to meet individual requirements. (The generally accepted half-life of methadone is 24 hours.)

Methadone requires multiple CYP hepatic enzymes to metabolize the drug. Therefore, methadone is the opioid most susceptible to serious drug interactions resulting from drug-induced enzyme inhibition. For example, some sedatives and antidepressants inhibit methadone's metabolism, resulting in large elevations in blood concentrations, often resulting in unexpected fatalities (Tennant, 2010).

As well as some methadone maintenance programs may work, they reach only 170,000 of the estimated 810,000 opioid-dependent people in the United States. Fiellin and coworkers (2001) studied stable methadone maintenance program clients and offered data showing that they can be well cared for by community physicians; the researchers suggest steps to take in order to do so.

In recent years, diversion of methadone (from methadone clinic programs and from physicians' prescriptions for analgesic effects) has become a major problem. When the large doses prescribed for an opioid-dependent person (40 to 100 milligrams) are taken by a nonopioid-dependent person, severe respiratory depression and death frequently result.

LAAM

Levo-alpha acetylmethadol (LAAM) is related to methadone. It is an oral opioid analgesic that was approved in mid-1993 for the clinical management of opioid dependence in heroin addicts. It is currently not available due to possible serious cardiac complications (Wedam et al., 2007;

Wieneke et al., 2009). LAAM has a slow onset and a long duration of action (about 72 hours). Its primary advantage over methadone is its long duration of action; in maintenance therapy it is administered by mouth three times a week.

With LAAM, controversy relates both to dose-related efficacy and to comparative efficacy with methadone (Wolstein et al., 2009). In general, LAAM and methadone are of equal efficacy, as measured by opioid-free urine samples in heroin-dependent persons. LAAM is administered three times a week; methadone, daily. Higher doses of methadone (60 to 100 milligrams) and 75- to 115-milligram doses of LAAM both substantially reduced the use of heroin (Johnson et al., 2000). Because of cardiac concerns, the use of LAAM has not been widespread.

Oxycodone

Oxycodone (Percodan, OxyContin) is another semisynthetic opioid similar in action to morphine. The short-acting preparation (Percodan) is primarily prescribed for the treatment of acute pain. Usual doses are about 5 milligrams every 4 to 6 hours. Percodan has been associated with widespread abuse, dependence, and deaths from overdosage. OxyContin is a long-acting product intended for the treatment of chronic or long-lasting pain, such as the pain that often accompanies cancer and persistent musculoskeletal problems. Drug tolerance usually develops, and doses are high (tablets of OxyContin contain from 10 to 80 milligrams).

OxyContin goes by many street names: poor man's heroin, hillbilly heroin, oxy, OC, killer, and oxycotton, among others. Street prices are ten times the prescription price, usually about $1 per milligram of drug. Abusers crush the pills, destroying the time-release mechanisms, and either snort the powder, smoke the drug, or dilute it in water and inject it. Thus, while chronic pain patients are certainly physically dependent on the drug, high-dose abusers are true addicts. Today there is immense abuse of OxyContin, much of it through diversion (see Figure 10.6), which has been responsible for untold numbers of deaths. Drastically needed are immediate efforts to add the opioid antagonist naloxone to OxyContin so that use by smoking or injection would precipitate withdrawal.[3] To date, the manufacturer has been slow to respond to the problem of widespread abuse, possibly because yearly sales of OxyContin easily exceed $1 billion!

---

[3] If the oxycodone/naloxone product were taken as intended (orally), the naloxone would not be absorbed and the oxycodone would be an effective analgesic. However, if injected, the naloxone would precipitate withdrawal.

Propoxyphene

Propoxyphene (Darvon) is an analgesic compound that is structurally similar to methadone (see Figure 10.10). As an analgesic for treating mild to moderate pain, it is less potent than codeine but more potent than aspirin. When propoxyphene is taken in large doses, opioidlike effects are seen; when it is used intravenously, addicts recognize it as an opioid. Taken orally, propoxyphene does not have much potential for abuse. Some cases of drug dependence have been reported, but to date they have not been of major concern. Because commercial intravenous preparations of propoxyphene are not available, intravenous abuse is encountered only when someone attempts to inject solutions of the powder that is contained in capsules intended for oral use.

Darvon was marketed in 1957 when there were few alternatives for treating pain, except aspirin and strong opioids, like morphine. In early 2009, an FDA advisory panel recommended that the FDA ban the drug from commercial sale because of concerns about drug suicide, drug dependence, and overdoses. The drug, however, remains commercially available. Now mainly marketed as Darvocet, which includes a dose of acetaminophen, the drug continues to be commonly prescribed.

Fentanyl and Its Derivatives

Fentanyl (Sublimaze) and three related compounds, *sufentanil* (Sufenta), *alfentanil* (Alfenta), and *remifentanil* (Ultiva), are short-acting, intravenously administered opioid agonists that are structurally related to meperidine. These four compounds are intended to be used during and after surgery to relieve surgical pain.

As stated earlier, fentanyl is available in intravenous formulation. It is also available in a transdermal skin patch (Durapatch), as a dissolvable buccal tablet (to be placed above a molar tooth, between the upper cheek and gum; trade name Fentora), and as an oral lozenge on a stick (a "lollipop," marketed under the trade name Actiq). The transdermal route of drug delivery offers prolonged, rather steady levels of drug in blood; the buccal tablet and lollipop are used for the treatment of unrelieved pain in opioid-dependent chronic pain patients who are intolerant of injections. In Europe, a nasal spray form of fentanyl (trade name Instanyl) has been approved.

Fentanyl and its three derivatives are 80 to 500 times as potent as morphine as analgesics and profoundly depress respiration. Death from these agents is invariably caused by respiratory failure. In illicit use, fentanyl is known by several nicknames including "china white." Numerous derivatives (such as *methylfentanyl*) have been manufactured illegally; they emerge periodically and have been responsible for many fatalities.

Partial Opioid Agonists

Pure agonists (such as morphine) have strong activity at mu opioid receptors. In contrast to morphine, a few—such as buprenorphine, tramadol, and tapentadol—have a somewhat lower level of agonist activity at these same receptors. Since they retain some of the analgesic activity of morphine, they have been referred to as *partial opioid agonists*.

Buprenorphine

Buprenorphine (Subutex) is a semisynthetic partial opioid agonist whose action is characterized by a limited stimulation of mu receptors, which is responsible for its analgesic properties. As a partial agonist, however, there is a ceiling to its analgesic effectiveness as well as to its potential for inducing euphoria and respiratory depression. Buprenorphine has a prolonged duration of action (about 24 hours) because it binds very strongly to mu receptors; this characteristic also limits its reversibility by naloxone should reversal be considered necessary. The most common side effects are flulike symptoms, headache, sweating, sleeping difficulties, nausea, and mood swings.

Johnson and coworkers (2000) found buprenorphine comparable to methadone and LAAM for treatment of opioid-dependent people. Kakko and coworkers (2003) reported that buprenorphine was safe and effective as a maintenance medication in treating heroin addiction. As an agonist, however, the use of buprenorphine has been associated with considerable abuse throughout the world, as the drug exerts morphinelike effects.

The abuse problem can be largely solved through the addition of the opioid antagonist naloxone to the buprenorphine (Alho et al., 2007). The combination is trade-named Suboxone and is marketed and approved for the office-based maintenance treatment of heroin or other opioid dependence. Suboxone is FDA classified as a Schedule III agent, intended for office-based opioid dependency treatment under the Federal Drug Addiction Treatment Act of 2000. Therefore, unlike methadone, a physician in his or her office can prescribe Suboxone for the treatment of opioid dependence. Also, patients can take the drug home instead of appearing at a clinic every day. Sullivan and Fiellin (2008) and Barry and coworkers (2009) discuss the role of Suboxone as an office-based treatment option. Allen (2006) discusses physician requirements for prescribing Suboxone for opioid dependence.

In Suboxone treatment programs, the preparation can be used to maintain opioid dependency or as part of an opioid withdrawal program. Umbricht and coworkers (1999) used buprenorphine as a tapering medication for rapid opioid detoxification; they followed buprenorphine with successful naltrexone therapy. The researchers concluded that the combination was an acceptable and safe treatment for shortened opioid detoxification and induction of naltrexone maintenance. Kakko and coworkers (2007) compared the efficacy of methadone maintenance with Suboxone maintenance for heroin dependence. Overall, the two treatments were equally efficacious: urine samples free of illicit opioids reach approximately 80 percent with either treatment. The authors concluded that "broad implementation of strategies using buprenorphine as first-line treatment should be considered" (p. 797). An accompanying editorial by Brady (2007) expands on the success of this treatment.

Marsch and coworkers (2005) reported that, in adolescents 13 to 18 years old with opioid dependency, combining Suboxone with behavioral interventions was quite effective in preventing relapse to opioid use. As yet, Suboxone has not been associated with significant diversionary problems and illicit use.

Tramadol

Tramadol (Ultram) became available for use as an analgesic in the United States in 1995. The drug exhibits a unique dual analgesic action: (1) it is a partial agonist at mu receptors, and (2) it blocks the presynaptic reuptake of norepinephrine and serotonin, both contributing to its analgesic action. In the United States, tramadol is available only for oral use. Well absorbed orally, the drug undergoes a two-step metabolism, and the first metabolite (monodemethyl tramadol) is as active or more active than the parent compound. As a partial agonist, the drug exhibits a ceiling effect on analgesia (it is not as analgesic as morphine), which limits respiratory depression and abuse potential. Side effects are considerable and include drowsiness and vertigo, nausea, vomiting, constipation, and headache. Additive sedation with CNS depressants is observed. Reports of the use of tramadol in treating opioid dependency are not available.

There has been concern about the combination of tramadol and serotonin-type antidepressant drugs: the combination may increase the toxicity of the antidepressants (causing a serotonin syndrome; Chapter 5). This drug combination should probably be avoided if possible.

Tapentadol

In 2009, tapentadol became commercially available under the trade name Nucynta. Tapentadol is considered to have a potency between tramadol and morphine. Structurally, tapentadol is similar to tramadol (Ultram); there is some question about whether it has the abuse potential of morphine or the somewhat lesser abuse potential of tramadol (Guay, 2009; Wade and Spruill, 2009). Currently, it is FDA scheduled like morphine (a Schedule II drug) rather than tramadol (a Schedule III drug that has lesser requirements for prescription). This may limit its clinical utility.

Similar to tramadol, tapentadol has opioid and nonopioid activity, with a dual mode of action as an agonist at the mu opiod receptor and as a norepinephrine reuptake inhibitor. Tapentadol has been approved by the FDA for the treatment of moderate to severe acute pain (Hartrick, 2009). Due to the dual mechanism of action as an opioid agonist and norepinephrine reuptake inhibitor, there is potential for off-label medical use in chronic pain disorders such as in the treatment of chronic low back pain (Etropolski et al., 2010).

As discussed earlier, inhibition of norepinephrine reuptake provides analgesic efficacy; in practice, this should reduce the dose of opioid necessary to relieve pain. Antidepressants such as milnacipran (Savella), duloxetine (Cymbalta), and reboxetine (Strattera, Edronax) share this norepinephrine reuptake blocking action, but without opioid agonism.

Mixed Agonist-Antagonist Opioids

Four commercially available drugs are classified as mixed agonist-antagonist opioids: pentazocine, butorphanol, nalbuphine, and dezocine (Figure 10.11). Each of these drugs binds with varying affinity to the mu

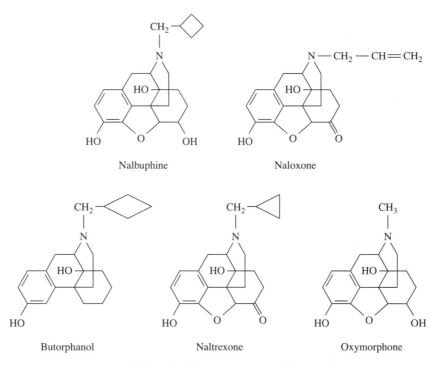

FIGURE 10.11 Structural formulas of oxymorphone and four analogues. Oxymorphone is a pure mu agonist. Nalbuphine and butorphanol have mixed agonistic and antagonistic properties. Naloxone and naltrexone are pure antagonists.

and kappa receptors. The drugs are weak mu agonists; most of their analgesic effectiveness (which is limited) results from their stimulation of kappa receptors (see Table 10.2). Low doses cause moderate analgesia; higher doses produce little additional analgesia. In opioid-dependent people, these drugs precipitate withdrawal. A high incidence of adverse psychotomimetic side effects (dysphoria, anxiety reactions, hallucinations, and so on) is associated with the use of these agents, limiting their therapeutic use but increasing their attraction for illicit use.

Pentazocine (Talwin) and *butorphanol* (Stadol) are prototypical mixed agonist-antagonists. Neither has much potential for producing respiratory depression or physical dependence. In 1993 butorphanol, previously available for use by injection, became available as a nasal spray (Stadol NS), the first analgesic so formulated. After it is sprayed into the nostrils, peak plasma levels (and maximal effect) are achieved in 1 hour, with a duration of 4 to 5 hours. Use of the nasal spray can result in euphoria, and abuse of butorphanol spray appears to be increasing.

The abuse of pentazocine has also been increasing, particularly in combination with tripelennamine, an antihistamine. This combination of drugs, called "Ts and blues," has caused serious medical complications, including seizures, psychotic episodes, skin ulcerations, abscesses, and muscle wasting. (The latter three effects are caused by the repeated injections rather than by the drugs themselves.)

Nalbuphine (Nubain) is primarily a kappa agonist of limited analgesic effectiveness. Because it is also a mu antagonist, it is not likely to produce either respiratory depression or patterns of abuse.

Dezocine (Dalgan) was introduced in 1990 as the newest of the agonist-antagonist drugs. As a moderate mu agonist and a weak delta and kappa agonist, dezocine can substitute for morphine. Its clinical efficacy and potential for abuse appear limited.

Pure Opioid Antagonists

Three pure opioid antagonists are clinically available: naloxone, naltrexone, and nalmefene. Each is a structural derivative of oxymorphone, a pure opioid agonist (see Figure 10.11). All three have an affinity for opioid receptors (especially mu receptors), but after binding they exert no agonistic effects of their own. Therefore, they antagonize the effects of opioid agonists.

Naloxone (Narcan) is the prototype pure opioid antagonist: it has no effect when injected into non-opioid-dependent people, but it rapidly precipitates withdrawal when injected into opioid-dependent people. Naloxone is neither analgesic nor subject to abuse. Because naloxone is neither absorbed from the gastrointestinal tract nor absorbed across the oral mucosa, it must be given by injection. Its duration of action is very brief, in the range of 15 to 30 minutes. Thus, for continued opioid antagonism, it must be reinjected at short intervals to avoid return of the depressant effects caused by the longer-acting agonist opioid. Naloxone is used to reverse the respiratory depression that follows acute opioid intoxication (overdoses) and to reverse opioid-induced respiratory depression in newborns of opioid-dependent mothers. The limitations of naloxone include its short duration of action and its parenteral route of administration.

Naltrexone (Trexan, ReVia) became clinically available in 1985 as the first orally absorbed, pure opioid antagonist approved for the treatment of heroin dependence. The actions of naltrexone resemble those of naloxone, but naltrexone is well absorbed orally and has a long duration of action, necessitating only a single oral daily dose of about 40 to 100 milligrams. Naltrexone is used clinically in treatment programs when it is desirable to maintain a person on chronic therapy with an opioid antagonist rather than with an agonist such as methadone. In people who take naltrexone daily, any injection of an opioid agonist such as heroin is ineffective. Naltrexone can cause nausea (which can be quite severe in some people) and dose-dependent liver toxicity, which can be a problem in patients with preexisting liver disease.

One problem with naltrexone is that the drug must be taken in order to be effective. Trite as that sounds, the opioid-dependent person must choose between taking naltrexone or returning to heroin use. Therefore, treatment compliance is poor and only highly motivated addicts take the drug. In 2006, the FDA approved a new long-acting preparation of injectable naltrexone (Vivitrol) for the maintenance of sobriety in withdrawn alcoholics. The success of this preparation is still open to question, primarily because of its expense. However, Vivitrol set an example for the type of product that might be useful in opioid-dependent people who are motivated to maintain abstinence from opioids—for example, professional people who have more to gain by being off opioids (maintaining their occupational employment) than by remaining on them.

More recently, under development and in non-FDA-approved use are implanted naltrexone pellets, or slow-release tablets that are placed under the skin (subcutaneously) and release naltrexone over a period of several months (variable, depending on the preparation). These can reduce opioid use (they block the effects of opioids) and do not necessitate the dependent person's taking a daily tablet (Hulse et al., 2009; Kunoe et al., 2009).

As discussed in Chapter 13, both oral and long-acting injectable formulations of naltrexone are approved by the FDA for use in the treatment of alcoholism to reduce the craving for alcohol during the maintenance period of treatment. It is thought that such action follows from the antagonism of endorphin action rather than from an as yet unidentified action outside the opioid system. Whether therapy is useful or not is unclear. Ceasing to take naltrexone would certainly be expected to result in loss of any positive effects. Carroll and coworkers (2001) reported that contingency management (mainly voucher rewards) significantly improved the response to naltrexone.

Naltrexone may have a specific preventive role in reducing self-injurious behaviors (White and Schultz, 2000). It is thought that self-injurious behavior can be used to maintain a high level of endogenous opioids, either to prevent decreases in endorphins or to experience the euphoric effect of opioid stimulation following injury.

Jayaram-Lindstrom and coworkers (2008) discuss an anticraving action of naltrexone in amphetamine dependence.

Nalmefene (Revex), introduced in 1996, is an injectable pure opioid antagonist with a half-life of about 8 to 10 hours, in contrast to the short half-life of injected naloxone. The drug is useful by injection for the treatment of acute opioid-induced respiratory depression caused by overdosage. Because of its long half-life, the incidence of its wearing off and the depressant action of the agonist opioid returning is greatly reduced. If administered to an addict, however, the precipitation of withdrawal can be prolonged and require additional medical treatment. Mason and coworkers (1999) studied the effects of orally administered nalmefene as an alternative to naltrexone in alcoholic patients.[4] Treatment for 12 weeks was effective in preventing relapse. The oral preparation is not available commercially.

There has been some discussion about whether or not nalmefene or naltrexone therapy might be a treatment for gambling addiction (pathological gambling) either alone or as part of therapy involving Gamblers Anonymous. Grant and coworkers (2008), in a multicentered trial, demonstrated the effectiveness of the drug in 284 men and women diagnosed with pathological gambling. A positive family history of alcoholism was the variable most strongly associated with treatment response, lending support to a close relationship between pathological gambling and consideration of pathological gambling as a behavioral addiction.

Finally, two specialized opioid antagonists, *methylnaltrexone* (Relistor) and *alvimopan* (Entereg), have recently been introduced and marketed for their ability to reduce opioid-induced constipation. Because these two drugs do not cross the blood-brain barrier, they block opioid agonist actions in the periphery (e.g., in the bowel) but do not block opioid-induced analgesia in the brain or spinal cord; thus, they do not precipitate withdrawal symptoms. Alvimopan is intended to restore normal bowel function in hospitalized patients who have

---

[4] Nalmefene is currently available only in injectable form. For this study, experimental tablets of nalmefene were supplied by the manufacturer.

undergone bowel surgery (McNicol et al., 2008; Webster et al., 2008). Methylnaltrexone is intended as an injectable medication to restore bowel function in adults with advanced illnesses who are receiving opioids on a continuous basis and suffer from their constipating effects (Thomas et al., 2008).

Opioid Combinations to Reduce Abuse

Opioids are irreplaceable as strong and effective pain-relieving agents. However, their dependency potential is enormous, as is the problem of diversion of the drug to illicit users. The major problems, therefore, are twofold: (1) how to maintain efficacy while reducing dependence potential and (2) how to reduce diversion, or use of the drug by others than those for whom the drug was intended.

The first problem has been addressed for years, first by developing analgesics thought to have less dependency potential. Unfortunately, most attempts have failed. For example, heroin was initially developed as a semisynthetic alternative to morphine, which occurs naturally from opium. Meperidine and numerous other drugs were similarly developed. As yet, it has been impossible to separate analgesia, dependence, and respiratory depression, and abuse continues to be a huge problem.

Another approach was to combine the opioid with an analgesic that did not induce dependency. The second analgesic is used to potentiate opioid-induced analgesia using less opioid. For example, for decades, codeine has been combined with aspirin or acetaminophen as a less addicting analgesic product. A few years ago, a combination of morphine and dextromethorphan was evaluated for the treatment of moderate to severe pain, but development has not been pursued.

Other morphine-sparing analgesic regimens combine morphine (or another opioid) with an anticonvulsant neuromodulator (Chapter 6) such as gabapentin or pregabalin. The latest attempt has been the introduction of tapentadol (Nucynta), a single compound that both acts as an opioid agonist and blocks norepinephrine reuptake.

As discussed, diversion and abuse of opioids persist, as shown by the wide abuse of oxycodone, fentanyl, morphine, and methadone. Many years ago, abuse of an opioid called pentazocine (Talwin) was widespread. Naloxone was added to the pill (the product was called Talwin NX) such that, should it be injected, the naloxone would precipitate withdrawal reactions. This essentially ended abuse of Talwin. A second attempt at combining an opioid with an antagonist occurred with *Suboxone* (the combination of buprenorphine and naltrexone). When buprenorphine was first developed as a partial opioid agonist in the late 1990s, abuse of the drug ensued. However, combining the drug with naloxone in 2003 (as Suboxone) maintained analgesic efficacy while reducing diversion. The reason is as follows. Buprenorphine is effective given orally, sublingually, or by injection. Naloxone is not absorbed orally or sublingually and is effective as an antagonist only when it is injected. Therefore, when Suboxone is taken sublingually, the buprenorphine is absorbed (and is effective), but the naloxone is not absorbed and is ineffective. However, when this product is crushed, dissolved, and injected, the naloxone is placed in the bloodstream and precipitates withdrawal. Therefore, it is not attractive as a product of abuse.

In late 2009, the FDA approved a combination of morphine and naltrexone (trade name *Embeda*). Here, pellets of an extended-release oral formulation of morphine surround a core of naltrexone. As reported by Katz and coworkers (2010), the naltrexone does not interfere with the analgesic action of the morphine, but abuse potential is considerably reduced. At this time, different dosing regimes are commercially available, all with a morphine-to-naltrexone ratio of 100:4. These products are available in six dosage strengths (20 mg/0.8 mg, 30 mg/1.2 mg, 50 mg/2 mg, 60 mg/2.4 mg, 80 mg/3.2 mg, and 100 mg/4 mg). Embeda is the first FDA-approved long-acting opioid designed to reduce enjoyment of the drug and euphoria when tampered with by crushing or chewing.

Today, one of the major forms of opioid abuse (besides heroin) is the diversionary use of OxyContin, a long-acting formulation of oxycodone. Adding naloxone or naltrexone to OxyContin would help to end much of the abuse of oxycodone. Indeed, a combination product using extended-release oxycodone (OxyContin) and extended-release naloxone was recently marketed in Europe under the trade name Targin. Promotion of the drug emphasizes the fact that the oxycodone provides analgesic action, but the naloxone remains in the intestine (not being absorbed when taken orally) and blocks the constipating effect of the oxycodone. A combination of oxycodone and ultra-low-dose naltrexone (proposed trade name Oxytrex) is under development in the United States (Largent-Milnes et al., 2008). If the dose of naltrexone in the product is sufficient and if the drug is abused by injection, the naloxone would precipitate withdrawal symptoms. If the dose of naloxone is only 1 or 2 *micrograms*, this would likely not be sufficient to precipitate withdrawal. A combination product with sufficient naloxone or naltrexone to precipitate withdrawal if injected or smoked is urgently needed in the United States to help stem the abuse catastrophes associated with OxyContin preparations.

Pharmacotherapy of Opioid Dependence

Opioid dependence is a brain-related medical disorder (characterized by predictable signs and symptoms) that can be effectively treated with significant benefits for the patient and for society. However, society must make a commitment to offer effective treatment for opioid dependence to all who need it. Everyone dependent on opioids should have access to agonist maintenance therapy (methadone), agonist-antagonist therapy (Suboxone or Embeda), or antagonist therapy (for example, naltrexone). Not only must government policies ensure availability of the programs, but insurance coverage for the programs should be a required benefit in public and private insurance. In any treatment of opioid dependence, pharmacotherapy is the foundation. Medicines are used for the following functions:

- To maintain dependence on orally administered medications (methadone or Suboxone), thus reducing the use of heroin or other injected agonists
- To maintain detoxification in predisposed people (oral or implanted naltrexone), combined with random urine checks and vouchers to ensure compliance
- To maintain detoxification in less compliant people (intramuscular injections of Vivitrol or use of naltrexone implants) and eliminate the positive reinforcement effects of heroin should that drug be smoked or injected
- To treat comorbid disorders, especially affective disorders such as depression, that complicate recovery

An important area of concern is the marked increase in prescription opioids for nonmalignant chronic pain (Boudreau et al., 2009). These increases are most marked in persons with mental health and substance use disorders (Edlund et al., 2010), especially persons suffering from mood disorders such as depression (Braden et al., 2009) and persons with prior substance use disorders (Weisner, et al., 2009). Interestingly, nonabusers of opioids such as oxycodone self-administer active doses of opioids only when they are in pain, whereas abusers of opioids self-administer regardless of the pain condition (Comer et al., 2010). In addition to using opioids when not in pain, abusers also tend to overuse sedatives such as benzodiazepines, with concurrent use being unexpectedly common (Boudreau et al., 2009).

In addition to appropriate pharmacotherapy, nonpharmacological support services are pivotal to successful therapy, whether the therapy is agonist maintenance or detoxification. How much nonpharmacological support is optimal? Can there be too little? Can there be too much? Likely, the answer is in the middle. Avants and coworkers (1999) reported that intensive day treatment programs for unemployed, inner-city methadone patients cost twice as much and were no more effective than a program of enhanced methadone maintenance services, which consisted of standard methadone maintenance plus a weekly skills training group and referral to on-site and off-site services.

Doran (2008) further reviews the economic benefits and limitations of various treatments of opioid dependence.

Should the goal of methadone, Suboxone, or Embeda maintenance be eventual withdrawal from agonist therapy? Although data are poor, it is felt that total abstinence from all opioids need not be an objective for all addicts. Goals, however, must include prevention of major relapse to the use of illicitly obtained injectable or smoked opioids (such as heroin). Continuing medically managed supportive opioid therapy may be necessary for many addicts, an approach that follows models of medical illness. Certainly, in the presence of chronic pain syndromes, continuous opioid therapy may be necessary. Accomplishing pain relief in the face of opioid dependence or excess usage is difficult; this is well discussed by Tennant and Reinking (2008).

Until recently, the objective has been medically managed withdrawal to an opioid-free state. This goal can be reached successfully in patients who are highly motivated to remain opioid-free. Examples include addicted medical personnel whose continued licensure to practice their profession is contingent on complete abstention from opioids. The continued presence of naltrexone in the blood implies that an opioid agonist will be ineffective if taken. In many addicts, however, naltrexone therapy is unacceptable, and continued opioid therapy is needed. For these patients, the benefits of maintenance therapy, including significant reductions in illicit opioid use, are increases in treatment retention and improved psychosocial functioning, which have been clearly demonstrated within the methadone maintenance model.

Many years ago, Goldstein (1994) reviewed more than 20 years of administering methadone maintenance therapy to 1000 heroin addicts in New Mexico. More than half the patients were traced and analyzed. Of these 500+ patients, more than one-third had died; causes included violence, overdosage, and alcoholism. About one-quarter were still enmeshed in the criminal justice system. Another one-quarter had gone on and off methadone maintenance. Data indicated that opioid dependence is a lifelong condition for a considerable fraction of the addict population.

Hser and coworkers (2001) reported a remarkable 33-year follow-up of 581 male heroin addicts who were first identified in the early 1960s. At follow-up in 1996–1997, 284 were dead and 242 were interviewed; the mean age at interview was 57 years. Of the 242, 20 percent tested positive for heroin (an additional 9.5 percent refused to provide a urine sample, and 14 percent were incarcerated, so urinalysis was unavailable); 22 percent were daily alcohol drinkers; 67 percent smoked; many reported illicit drug use (heroin, cocaine, marijuana, amphetamines). The group also reported high rates of physical health, mental health, and criminal justice problems. Long-term heroin abstinence was associated with less criminality, morbidity, and psychological distress and with higher employment.

It therefore appears that setting a goal of total abstinence is seldom accompanied by a positive outcome and leads to a productive life-style in only a minority of people who were dependent on opioids. If detoxification to a drug-free state is chosen, as soon as opioid-withdrawn people relapse, they must be readmitted to agonist maintenance programs immediately and receive both adequate doses and the necessary supportive therapies. The most interesting data now support prolonged agonist/antagonist maintenance (with Suboxone or Embeda) as a treatment goal. Availability of implanted naltrexone products may provide another option in antagonist-only therapy.

STUDY QUESTIONS

1. Describe the location of opioid receptors in the brain and in the spinal cord.

2. How are pain impulses modulated as they enter the spinal cord?

3. What is substance P and how is it influenced by opioid analgesics?

4. What might be the effects of the endorphins?

5. What is an opioid agonist? What is an opioid antagonist? What is a mixed agonist-antagonist? A partial agonist? Give an example of each.

6. What might lead a person to misuse or abuse opioids? What are the signs of opioid misuse/abuse?

7. Differentiate between naloxone and naltrexone. How might each one be used?

8. Describe the various ways that opioid dependence might be handled or treated.

9. Why are tricyclic antidepressants analgesic?

10. Differentiate between the opioid modulation of afferent pain impulses and the affective component of pain.

11. Give your thoughts for and against the existence of endogenous opioid peptides (endorphins) that serve as natural opioids.

12. If a patient suffers from chronic pain, what two classes of drugs should be optimized before starting opioid therapy? If opioid therapy is started, how should the opioids be administered?

13. Differentiate the use of opioids for people with chronic, nonmalignant pain and the use of opioids for people with pain due to a terminal malignancy.

14. What is buprenorphine? What are its potential uses? Why combine it with naloxone?

15. What allows this drug to be used in medical clinics located in the community and outside licensed methadone clinics?

16. Discuss the various options in the pharmacological management of opioid withdrawal and in the prevention of relapse.

REFERENCES

Akil, H., et al. (1998). "Endogenous Opioids: Overview and Current Issues." *Drug and Alcohol Dependence* 51: 127–140.

Alho, H., et al. (2007). "Abuse Liability of Buprenorphine-Naloxone Tablets in Untreated IV Drug Users." *Drug and Alcohol Dependence* 88: 75–78.

Allen, J. (2006). "Office-Based Treatment of Opioid Dependence: New Hope for Patients with Concomitant Pain and Addiction Issues." *Practical Pain Management* 6: 52–55.

American Society of Anesthesiologists (2010). "Practice Guidelines for Chronic Pain Management. *Anesthesiology* 112: 810–833.

Avants, S. K., et al. (1999). "Day Treatment versus Enhanced Standard Methadone Services for Opioid-Dependent Patients: A Comparison of Clinical Efficacy and Cost." *American Journal of Psychiatry* 156: 27–33.

Barry, D. T., et al. (2009). "Integrating Buprenorphine Treatment into Office-Based Practice: A Qualitative Study." *Journal of General Internal Medicine* 24: 218–225.

Binder, W., et al. (2001). "Analgesic Antiinflammatory Effects of Two Novel Kappa-Opioid Peptides." *Anesthesiology* 94: 1034–1044.

Boudreau, D., et al. (2009). "Trends in Long-Term Opioid Therapy for Chronic Non-Cancer Pain." *Pharmacoepidemiology and Drug Safety* 18: 1166–1175.

Braden, J. B., et al. (2009). "Trends in Long-Term Opioid Therapy for Noncancer Pain Among Persons with a History of Depression." *General Hospital Psychiatry* 31: 564–570.

Brady, K. T. (2007). "Medical Treatment of Opiate Dependence: Expanding Treatment Options." *American Journal of Psychiatry* 164: 702–704.

Carroll, K. M., et al. (2001). "Targeting Behavioral Therapies to Enhance Naltrexone Treatment of Opioid Dependence: Effects of Contingency Management and Significant Other Involvement." *Archives of General Psychiatry* 58: 755–761.

Centers for Disease Control and Prevention (2010, June 18). "Emergency Department Visits Involving Nonmedical Use of Selected Prescription Drugs—United States, 2004–2008." *Morbidity and Mortality Weekly Report* 59(23): 705–709.

Chavkin, C., et al. (2004). "Salvinorin A, an Active Component of the Hallucinogenic Sage *Salvia divinorum*, Is a Highly Efficacious Kappa-Opioid Receptor Agonist: Structural and Functional Considerations." *Journal of Pharmacology and Experimental Therapeutics* 308: 1197–1203.

Cianfrini, L. R., and Doleys, D. M. (2006). "The Role of Psychology in Pain Management." *Practical Pain Management* 6: 18–28.

Collins, E. D., et al. (2005). "Anesthesia-Assisted vs Buprenorphine- or Clonidine-Assisted Heroin Detoxification and Naltrexone Induction: A Randomized Trial." *Journal of the American Medical Association* 294: 903–913.

Comer, S. D., et al. (2010). "Abuse Liability of Oxycodone as a Function of Pain and Drug Use History." *Drug and Alcohol Dependence* 109: 130–138.

Doran, C. M. (2008). "Economic Evaluation of Interventions to Treat Opiate Dependence: A Review of the Evidence." *Pharmacoeconomics* 26: 371–393.

Dortch-Carnes, J., and Potter, D. E. (2005). "Bremazocine: A Kappa-Opioid Agonist with Potent Analgesic and Other Pharmacologic Properties." *CNS Drug Reviews* 11: 195–212.

Edlund, M. J., et al. (2010). "Trends in Use of Opioids for Chronic Noncancer Pain Among Individuals with Mental Health and Substance Use Disorders: The TROUP Study." *Clinical Journal of Pain* 26: 1–8.

Etropolski, M. S., et al. (2010). "Dose Conversion Between Tapentadol Immediate and Extended Release for Low Back Pain." *Pain Physician* 13: 61–70.

Fiellin, D. A., et al. (2001). "Methadone Maintenance in Primary Care: A Randomized Controlled Trial." *Journal of the American Medical Association* 286: 1724–1731.

Goldstein, A. (1994). *Addiction: From Biology to Drug Policy.* New York: Freeman.

Grant, J. E., et al. (2008). "Predicting Response to Opiate Antagonists and Placebo in the Treatment of Pathological Gambling." *Psychopharmacology* 200: 521–527.

Guay, D. R. (2009). "Is Tapentadol an Advance on Tramadol?" *The Consultant Pharmacist* 24: 833–840.

Hartrick, C. T. (2009). "Tapentadol Immediate Release for the Relief of Moderate-to-Severe Acute Pain." *Expert Opinion on Pharmacotherapy* 10: 2687–2696.

Hser, Y.-I., et al. (2001). "A 33-Year Follow-Up of Narcotic Addicts." *Archives of General Psychiatry* 58: 503–508.

Hulse, G. K., et al. (2009). "Improving Clinical Outcomes in Treating Heroin Dependence: Randomized, Controlled Trial of Oral or Implant Naltrexone." *Archives of General Psychiatry* 66: 1108–1115.

Jayaram-Lindstrom, N., et al. (2008). "Naltrexone for the Treatment of Amphetamine Dependence: A Randomized, Placebo-Controlled Trial." *American Journal of Psychiatry* 165: 1442–1448.

Johnson, R. E., et al. (2000). "A Comparison of Levomethadyl Acetate, Buprenorphine, and Methadone for Opioid Dependence." *New England Journal of Medicine* 343: 1290–1297.

Jutkiewicz, E. M. (2006). "The Antidepressant-Like Effects of Delta-Opioid Receptor Agonists." *Molecular Interventions* 6: 162–169.

Kakko, J., et al. (2003). "1-Year Retention and Social Function After Buprenorphine-Assisted Relapse Prevention Treatment for Heroin Dependence in Sweden: Randomized, Placebo-Controlled Trial." *Lancet* 361: 662–668.

Kakko, J., et al. (2007). "A Stepped Care Strategy Using Buprenorphine versus Conventional Methadone Maintenance in Heroin Dependence: A Randomized Controlled Trial." *American Journal of Psychiatry* 164: 797–803.

Katz, N. (2005). "The Impact of Opioids on the Endocrine System." *Pain Management Rounds* 1 (9): 1–6. Available online at www.painmanagement-rounds.org.

Katz, N., et al. (2010). "ALO-01 (Morphine Sulfate and Naltrexone Hydrochloride) Extended-Release Capsules in the Treatment of Chronic Pain of Osteoarthritis of the Hip or Knee: Pharmacokinetics, Efficacy, and Safety." *Journal of Pain* 11: 303–311.

Kunoe, N., et al. (2009). "Naltrexone Implants After In-Patient Treatment for Opioid Dependence: Randomized Controlled Trial." *British Journal of Psychiatry* 194: 541–546.

LaLumiere, R. T., and Kalivas, P. W. (2008). "Glutamate Release in the Nucleus Accumbens Core Is Necessary for Heroin Seeking." *Journal of Neuroscience* 28: 3170–3177.

Largent-Milnes, T. M., et al. (2008). "Oxycodone plus Ultra-Low-Dose Naltrexone Attenuates Neuropathic Pain and Associated Mu-Opioid Receptor-Gs Coupling." *Journal of Pain* 9: 700–713.

Marsch, L. A., et al. (2005). "Comparison of Pharmacological Treatments for Opioid-Dependent Adolescents: A Randomized Controlled Trial." *Archives of General Psychiatry* 62: 1157–1164.

Mason, B. J., et al. (1999). "A Double-Blind, Placebo-Controlled Study of Oral Nalmefene for Alcohol Dependence." *Archives of General Psychiatry* 56: 719–724.

McNicol, E. D., et al. (2008). "Mu-Opioid Antagonists for Opioid-Induced Bowel Dysfunction." *Cochrane Database of Systematic Reviews* 16: CD006332.

Narita, M., et al. (2001). "Regulations of Opioid Dependence by Opioid Receptor Types." *Pharmacology and Therapeutics* 89: 1–15.

Narita, M., et al. (2006). "Role of Delta-Opioid Receptor Function in Neurogenesis and Neuroprotection." *Journal of Neurochemistry* 97: 1494–1505.

O'Connor, P. G. (2005). "Methods of Detoxification and Their Role in Treating Patients with Heroin Dependence." *Journal of the American Medical Association* 294: 961–963.

Savage, S. R. (2005). "Critical Issues in Pain and Addiction." *Pain Management Rounds* 2(9): 1–6. Available online at www.painmanagementrounds.org.

Snyder, S. H., and Pasternak, G. W. (2003). "Historical Review: Opioid Receptors." *Trends in Pharmacological Sciences* 2: 198–204.

Sproule, B. A., et al. (1999). "Characteristics of Dependent and Nondependent Regular Users of Codeine." *Journal of Clinical Psychopharmacology* 19: 367–372.

Sullivan, L. E., and Fiellin, D. A. (2008). "Narrative Review: Buprenorphine for Opioid-Dependent Patients in Office Practice." *Annals of Internal Medicine* 148: 662–670.

Tennant, F. (2010). "Making Practical Sense of Cytochrome P450." *Practical Pain Management* 10 (4): 12–18.

Tennant, F., and Reinking, J. (2008). "Appropriate Opioid Dosing for Activities of Daily Living." *Practical Pain Management* 8(9): 12–18.

Thipphawong, J. B., et al. (2003). "Analgesic Efficacy of Inhaled Morphine in Patients After Bunionectomy Surgery." *Anesthesiology* 99: 693–700.

Thomas, J., et al. (2008). "Methylnaltrexone for Opioid-Induced Constipation in Advanced Illness." *New England Journal of Medicine* 358: 2332–2343.

Torregrossa, M. M., et al. (2006). "Peptic Delta Opioid Receptor Agonists Produce Antidepressant-Like Effects in the Forced Swim Test and Regulate BDND mRNA Expression in Rats." *Brain Research* 1069: 172–181.

Trigo, J. M., et al. (2010). "The Endogenous Opioid System: A Common Substrate in Drug Addiction." *Drug and Alcohol Dependence* 108: 183–194.

Umbricht, A., et al. (1999). "Naltrexone-Shortened Opioid Detoxification with Buprenorphine." *Drug and Alcohol Dependence* 56: 181–190.

Wade, W. E., and Spruill, W. J. (2009). "Tapentadol Hydrochloride: A Centrally Acting Oral Analgesic." *Clinical Therapeutics* 31: 2804–2818.

Webster, L., et al. (2008). "Alvimopan, a Peripherally Acting Mu-Opioid Receptor (PAM-OR) Antagonist for the Treatment of Opioid-Induced Bowel Dysfunction: Results from a Randomized, Double-Blind, Placebo-Controlled, Dose-Finding Study in Subjects Taking Opioids for Chronic Non-Cancer Pain." *Pain* 137: 428–440.

Wedam, E. F., et al. (2007). "QT-Interval Effects of Methadone, Levomethadyl, and Buprenorphine in a Randomized Trial." *Archives of Internal Medicine* 167: 2469–2475.

Weisner, C. M., et al. (2009). "Trends in Prescribed Opioid Therapy for Non-Cancer Pain for Individuals with Prior Substance Use Disorders." *Pain* 145: 287–293

White, T., and Schultz, S. K. (2000). "Naltrexone Treatment for a 3-Year-Old Boy with Self-Injurious Behavior." *American Journal of Psychiatry* 157: 1574–1580.

Wieneke, H., et al. (2009). "Levo-Alpha-Acetylmethadol (LAAM) Induced QTc-Prolongation: Results from a Controlled Clinical Trial." *European Journal of Medical Research* 14: 7–12.

Wolstein, J., et al. (2009). "A Randomized, Open-Label Trial Comparing Methadone and Levo-Alpha-Acetylmethadol (LAAM) in Maintenance Treatment of Opioid Addiction." *Pharmacopsychiatry* 42: 1–8.

Xu, T., et al. (2007). "Role of Spinal Metabotropic Glutamate Receptor Subtype 5 in the Development of Tolerance to Morphine-Induced Antinociception in Rat." *Neuroscience Letters* 420: 155–159.

PART 4

Pharmacology of Drugs of Abuse

This section is composed of seven chapters that cover the pharmacology of drugs commonly considered primarily as drugs subject to considerable amounts of compulsive use, abuse, and dependency. Some have no recognized medical use (for example, LSD and alcohol), while others have well-recognized therapeutic uses (for example, methylphenidate and amphetamines for the treatment of attention deficit/hyperactivity disorder).

The psychostimulants are discussed in two chapters. Chapter 11 details the pharmacology of caffeine and nicotine, the most widely used recreational drugs. Neither drug has much therapeutic value, but both are attractive to users because of their psychostimulant properties. Their overuse can result in moderate to extreme degrees of habituation or dependence. The toxicities associated with smoking cigarettes and the treatment of nicotine dependence are discussed as well. Chapter 12 describes the psychostimulants classically thought to act through potentiation of dopaminergic neurotransmission, thus directly activating the reward system involving the nucleus accumbens, the limbic system, and the frontal cortex. These drugs include cocaine, amphetamine, methamphetamine, and several amphetamine-related psychostimulants. These drugs have historical and continuing uses in medicine and significant abuse issues as well.

Chapter 13 presents the pharmacology of ethyl alcohol, a sedative-hypnotic quite similar in its pharmacology to the sedatives discussed earlier in Chapter 7. Alcohol differs, however, in that it has few or no medical indications and is used as a recreational intoxicant.

Chapter 14 presents the pharmacology of of tetrahydrocannabinol and other compounds found in the marijuana plant. Current research is uncovering medical uses of psychedelic cannabinoids (for example, THC), nonpsychedelic marijuana alkaloids (for example, cannabadiol), and cannabinoid antagonists (for example, rimonabant). Medical and abuse issues related to these products are discussed.

Chapter 15 presents the pharmacology of drugs characterized by their ability to produce altered states of consciousness, the so-called psychedelic drugs, including those found in nature as well as those synthetically produced. Included in this chapter are drugs considered to be "club drugs" because of their ability to increase energy (an amphetaminelike action) and produce altered states of consciousness.

Chapter 16 presents the pharmacology of anabolic steroids. Although indicated for specific medical disorders, they are often used by physically healthy persons to improve muscle mass, conferring "unfair" athletic advantages as well as providing a more muscular or lean appearance in nonathletes.

Finally, Chapter 17 addresses the overall picture of drug abuse, its etiology, and principles of treatment.

Chapter 11

Caffeine and Nicotine

CAFFEINE

Caffeine is the most commonly consumed psychoactive drug in the world; in the United States, it is consumed daily by up to 80 percent of the adult population. Caffeine is found in significant concentrations in coffee, tea, cola drinks, chocolate candies and ice creams, fortified waters, and cocoa (Table 11.1). Caffeine is probably one of the most widely used stimulants in sports, with documented efficacy and safety (Magkos and Kavouras, 2005).

The average cup of coffee contains about 100 milligrams of caffeine.[1] A 12-ounce bottle of cola contains about 40 milligrams. The caffeine content of chocolate may be as high as 25 milligrams per ounce. Over-the-counter (OTC) wakefulness-promoting drugs (for example, NoDoz, Vivarin) contain as much as 200 milligrams of caffeine per tablet. Excedrin contains 75 milligrams of caffeine per tablet, Anacin about half that amount, and NoDoz 100 milligrams (the same as a cup of brewed coffee). Many herbal-based OTC products contain fairly large amounts of caffeine. Among regular caffeine users, daily intake

---

[1] The caffeine content of coffee varies widely. One hundred milligrams is often used as an average. However, among popular "gourmet" coffees, one company's coffee averages 200 milligrams per 8 fluid ounces. Thus, a 12-ounce cup of black coffee has 300 milligrams; the 16-ounce "grande" has 400 milligrams. Mixed coffee drinks have less caffeine because of added milk or flavorings. Another company's coffee averages 80 to 90 milligrams; the coffee of a third company has 100 to 125 milligrams of caffeine per 8 ounces. McCusker and coworkers (2003) found wide variances in caffeine content (260 to 564 milligrams) in the same 16-ounce beverage at the same outlet on six consecutive days.

TABLE 11.1 Caffeine content in beverages, foods, and medicines

Item	Caffeine content	
	Average (mg)	Range
Coffee (5 ounces)	100	50–150
Tea (5 ounces)	50	25–90
Cocoa (5 ounces)	5	2–20
Chocolate (semisweet, baking) (1 ounce)	25	15–30
Chocolate milk (1 ounce)	5	1–10
Cola drink (12 ounces)	40	35–55
OTC stimulants (NoDoz, Vivarin)[a]	100+	
OTC analgesics (Excedrin)	65	
(Anacin, Midol, Vanquish)	33	
OTC cold remedies (Coryban-D, Triaminic)	30	
OTC diuretics (Aqua-ban)	100	

[a]OTC=over the counter.

averages between 200 and 500 milligrams, correlating with two to five cups of coffee daily. Regulatory agencies impose no restrictions on the sale or use of caffeine, nor is the human consumption of caffeine-containing beverages commonly considered to be drug abuse.

"Energy drinks" are fortified with extra-large amounts of caffeine and may put imbibers at risk. Aimed primarily at younger people, these "ergogenic aids" are intended to enhance athletic performance and aid cognitive functioning, although high doses can result in tremors, insomnia, gastrointestinal upset, agitation, panic, and tachycardia. One of these products, Rocketstar Zero Carb, purports to be "bigger, faster, and stronger" and to enable the imbiber to "party like a rock star." One 24-ounce can is fortified with 320 milligrams of caffeine, equivalent to about four cups of coffee.

Pharmacokinetics

Taken orally, caffeine is rapidly and completely absorbed. Significant blood levels of caffeine are reached in 30 to 45 minutes; complete absorption occurs over the next 90 minutes. Levels in plasma peak at about 2 hours and decrease thereafter.

Caffeine is freely and equally distributed throughout the total water in the body. Thus, caffeine is found in almost equal concentrations in all parts of the body and the brain. Like all psychoactive drugs, caffeine freely crosses the placenta to the fetus.

The liver metabolizes most caffeine before the kidneys excrete it. Only about 10 percent of the drug is excreted unchanged. Caffeine's half-life of elimination varies from about 2.5 hours to 10 hours (Magkos and Kavouras, 2005). In predisposed people, a long half-life can account for nighttime wakefulness. Caffeine's half-life is extended in infants, pregnant women, and the elderly. During the latter part of pregnancy, the half-life of caffeine increases from 3 to 10 hours. In cigarette smokers, caffeine's half-life is shortened; however, when smoking is terminated, caffeine's half-life increases. The reduced metabolism of caffeine can result in an increase in plasma caffeine levels and may contribute to cigarette withdrawal symptoms in heavy coffee drinkers, particularly since caffeine can induce or intensify anxiety disorders, such as panic disorder (Lambert et al., 2006).

It now appears that some coffee drinkers are "slow metabolizers" and some are more rapid metabolizers. Cornelis and coworkers (2006) studied these two populations in a group of Costa Rican caffeine users and found a genetic basis for the differences in metabolism; they also found isoenzyme differences in their CYP-1A2 drug-metabolizing enzymes. In addition, slow metabolizers under the age of 50 who were moderate- to high-level coffee drinkers were several times more likely to suffer nonfatal heart attacks than were matched controls who drank little coffee.

The structure and metabolism of caffeine are shown in Figure 11.1. The two major metabolites of caffeine, theophylline and paraxanthine,

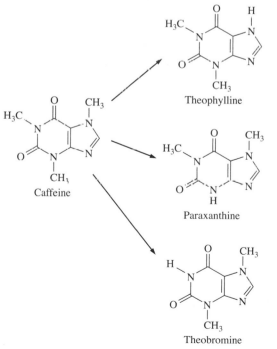

FIGURE 11.1 Metabolism of caffeine to three end products.

behave similarly to caffeine; a third metabolite, theobromine, does not. Caffeine is metabolized by the CYP-1A2 subgroup of hepatic drug-metabolizing enzymes. Certain selective serotonin reuptake inhibitor (SSRI) antidepressants, such as fluoxetine and fluvoxamine (Chapter 5), are potent inhibitors of CYP-1A2, and people taking these antidepressants can exhibit unexpected toxicity or intolerance to caffeine as plasma levels of caffeine rise, including de novo production of "caffeinism" (defined in the next section) with severe anxiety reactions.

Pharmacological Effects

The CNS-stimulant, cardiac, respiratory, and diuretic effects of caffeine have been known for many years. Therapeutically, these effects have been used to treat a variety of disorders, including asthma, narcolepsy, and migraine, and as an adjunct to aspirin or other analgesics in treating headache and other pain syndromes.

Caffeine is an effective psychostimulant, ingested to obtain a rewarding effect, usually described as feeling more alert and competent. Behavioral effects seen at lower doses of caffeine include increased mental alertness, a faster and clearer flow of thought, and wakefulness. Fatigue is reduced and the need for sleep is delayed. This increased mental awareness results in sustained intellectual effort for prolonged periods of time without significant disruption of coordinated intellectual or motor activity. Tasks that involve delicate muscular coordination and accurate timing or arithmetic skills may be adversely affected. These effects occur after oral doses as small as 100 or 200 milligrams (1 to 2 cups of coffee). Most people adjust, or titrate, their intake of caffeine to achieve these beneficial effects while minimizing undesirable effects. Heavy consumption of coffee (12 or more cups per day, or 1.5 grams of caffeine) can cause agitation, anxiety, tremors, rapid breathing, and insomnia. The lethal dose of caffeine is about 10 grams, equivalent to 100 cups of coffee.

People with anxiety disorders tend to be sensitive to the anxiogenic properties of caffeine, especially if they usually avoid caffeinated products and do not develop a tolerance to caffeine's effect. In general, people with anxiety disorders are wise to totally avoid caffeinated products.

Caffeinism is a clinical syndrome, characterized by both central nervous system (CNS) and peripheral symptoms, produced by the overuse or overdoses of caffeine. CNS symptoms include increases in anxiety, agitation, and insomnia as well as mood changes. Peripheral symptoms include tachycardia, hypertension, cardiac arrhythmias, and gastrointestinal disturbances. Caffeinism is usually dose related, with doses higher than about 500 to 1000 milligrams (1 gram, or 5 to 10 cups of coffee) causing the most unpleasant effects. Cessation of caffeine ingestion resolves these symptoms. Much lower doses of caffeine produce this syndrome in sensitive people, such as people who have an underlying anxiety disorder. The usually ingested doses of caffeine do not induce panic attacks in normal people, but in people predisposed to panic disorders, the peripheral and the CNS effects of caffeine are exaggerated.

Outside the CNS, caffeine exerts significant effects, some beneficial and some adverse. Caffeine has a slight stimulant action on the heart. It increases both cardiac contractility (increases the workload of the heart) and cardiac output. Although this effect might predispose a person to hypertension (caffeine does raise blood pressure in adults prone to hypertension), caffeine also dilates the coronary arteries, providing more oxygen to the harder-working heart. As stated earlier, slow metabolizers of caffeine who are moderate to heavy caffeine users have an increased risk of nonfatal heart attacks. Whether others can suffer cardiac problems as a result of caffeine ingestion is unclear. Boiled or unfiltered coffee is associated with increased blood cholesterol levels and may increase the risk of coronary artery disease (Cornelis and El-Sohemy, 2007), although moderate levels of coffee brewed otherwise may be beneficial, perhaps due to the antioxidants found in coffee. Thus, it remains controversial whether or not caffeine increases the incidence of heart disease and deaths due to cardiac disease. Certainly, people with hypertension or heart disease might do well to minimize exposure to caffeinated products, especially boiled, "French press," or unfiltered coffee. Currently, there is no evidence that coffee consumption increases the rates or risks of cancers (Higdon and Frei, 2006).

It should be noted that caffeine exerts an opposite effect on cerebral blood vessels; it constricts these vessels, thus decreasing blood flow to the brain by about 30 percent and reducing pressure within the brain. This action can effect striking relief from headaches, especially migraines. Other physical actions of caffeine include bronchial relaxation (an antiasthmatic effect), increased secretion of gastric acid, and increased urine output.

Caffeine consumption has been associated with improved glucose tolerance and a lower risk of type 2 diabetes. The same effect has been found for decaffeinated coffee, indicating that some substance in coffee other than caffeine may be responsible. Even caffeine-induced weight loss may be responsible (Greenberg et al., 2006).

Mechanism of Action

Caffeine exerts a variety of effects on the CNS. In Figure 11.2, note the close structural resemblance of caffeine and a naturally occurring substance in the brain called adenosine. It should therefore not be surprising

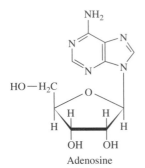

FIGURE 11.2 Structure of adenosine. Note the similarity of adenosine to caffeine (shown in Figure 11.1).

that caffeine might bind to any receptors to which adenosine binds. Caffeine does have a strong affinity for adenosine receptors, but binding is not accompanied by adenosinelike action; caffeine blocks access of adenosine to its receptors, and thus caffeine is classified as an adenosine antagonist at least at physiological concentrations comparable to one or more cups of coffee.

Since caffeine is an adenosine antagonist, a pharmacological effect of caffeine would not be expected unless adenosine receptors were tonically active under stimulation by adenosine (Magkos and Kavouras, 2005). Adenosine is a *neuromodulator* that influences the release of several neurotransmitters in the CNS. There do not appear to be discrete adenosinergic pathways in the CNS; rather, adenosinergic neurons form a diffuse system that appears to exert sedative actions. Adenosine levels usually increase during the day and exert a sleep-inducing effect in the brain. By blocking adenosine receptors, caffeine promotes wakefulness. Blockade of adenosine receptors accounts for the actions of caffeine that provide modest rewards and increase vigilance and mental acuity.

The positive stimulatory effects of caffeine appear to be due in large measure to blockade of the adenosine receptors that stimulate GABAergic neurons of inhibitory pathways to the dopaminergic reward system of the striatum. Therefore, caffeine may produce its behavioral effects by removing the negative modulatory effects of adenosine from dopamine receptors, thus indirectly stimulating dopaminergic activity. Caffeine does not induce a release of dopamine in the nucleus accumbens; it leads to a release of dopamine in the prefrontal cortex, which is consistent with caffeine's alerting effects with only mild behavioral reinforcing properties. In fact, caffeine appears to fulfill some of the criteria for drug dependency and shares with amphetamines and cocaine a certain specificity of action on the cerebral dopaminergic system. However, it does not act on the dopaminergic structures related to reward, motivation, and addiction. Satel (2006) reviewed the addictive potential of caffeine and concluded that it does not fit the common perception of drug dependency.

Reproductive Effects

Is caffeine safe during pregnancy? Caffeine, the most widely used psychotropic drug in the world, is consumed by at least 75 percent of pregnant women via caffeinated beverages, but whether ingesting caffeine during pregnancy is safe is an unresolved question. As early as 1980, the U.S. Food and Drug Administration (FDA) cautioned pregnant women to minimize their intake of caffeine. Wisborg and coworkers (2003) reported a study of over 18,000 pregnancies in Denmark that attempted to determine whether there was an association between coffee consumption during pregnancy and the risks of either stillbirth or infant death in the first year of life. Pregnant women who drank 8 or more cups of coffee per day during pregnancy had an increased risk of having a stillbirth compared with women who did not consume caffeine. Adjusting for smoking habits and alcohol consumption modestly reduced the risk. There was no association between caffeine consumption and infant deaths during the first year of life. The overall risk of stillbirth increased from 4 per 1000 births in nonusers of caffeine to 12 per 1000 in drinkers of 8 or more cups of coffee per day. At 4 to 7 cups per day, the risk was 7 per 1000 births. More recent reports have explored the connection between caffeine intake and rates of miscarriage (Weng et al., 2008; Pollack et al., 2010), fetal growth restriction (CARE Study Group, 2008), birth weight, and length of gestation (Jahanfar and Sharifah, 2009). In general, while data are limited and controversial, caffeine, at least in reasonable doses, seems to cause a modest degree of fetal growth restriction (Figure 11.3), in very large doses may slightly increase the risk of miscarriage, has little or no effect on birth weight or length of gestation, and does not appear to increase the incidence of later presentation of attention deficit/hyperactivity disorder (ADHD) in offspring of women exposed to caffeine during pregnancy (Linnet et al., 2009).

Caffeine itself does not appear to be a human teratogen, nor does it appear to affect the course of normal labor and delivery. Browne (2006) reviewed literature on possible adverse fetal effects and concluded that "there is no evidence to support a teratogenic effect of caffeine in humans" (p. 324). Higdon and Frei (2006) stated: "Currently available evidence suggests that it may be prudent for pregnant women to limit coffee consumption to 3 cups per day, ingesting no more than 300 milligrams per day of caffeine to exclude any increased probability of spontaneous abortion or impaired fetal growth" (p. 101). Kuczkowski (2009) stated that "reproductive-aged and pregnant women are 'at risk' subgroups of the population who may require specific advice on moderating their daily caffeine intake" (p. 695). This seems like reasonable advice.

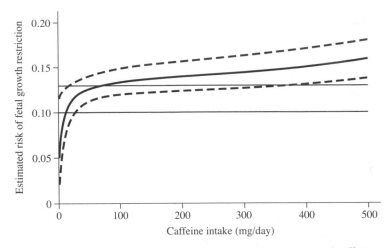

FIGURE 11.3 Relation between the risk of fetal growth restriction and caffeine intake (milligrams per day) during pregnancy. The graph is restricted to less than 500 mg/day (about 5 cups of coffee) for clarity. Thin horizontal lines mark the average risk of fetal growth restriction (10 percent) and average risk in a study cohort (13 percent). The solid curve represents the average, with 95 percent confidence levels shown above and below it by the dashed curves. [From CARE Study Group (2008), Figure 1.]

Tolerance and Dependence

Chronic use of caffeine, even in regular daily doses as low as 100 milligrams, is associated with habituation and tolerance, and discontinuation may produce low-grade withdrawal symptoms. People who drink a great deal of coffee complain of headache (the most common symptom), drowsiness, fatigue, and a generally negative mood state on withdrawal from caffeine. Withdrawal symptoms typically begin slowly, maximize after one or two days, and cease within a few days; readministering caffeine rapidly relieves withdrawal symptoms. Other reported withdrawal signs include impaired intellectual and motor performance, difficulty with concentration, drug (caffeine) craving, and other psychological complaints. Greden and Walters (1997) wrote:

> Caffeine . . . will continue to be the norm in most people. However, caffeinism and caffeine withdrawal also continue to be common and clinically important but unrecognized, underdiagnosed even when recognized, and untreated in many treatment settings. . . . Clinicians who actively consider the diagnosis of caffeinism in their patients will be surprised at how many afflicted subjects are identified, impressed at how many are helped by removal of the offending agent, and pleased to know that almost all are grateful. (p. 305)

NICOTINE

Nicotine is one of the three most widely used psychoactive drugs in our society; the others are caffeine and ethyl alcohol. Despite the fact that nicotine has no therapeutic applications in medicine, its widespread use and its well-defined toxicity give it immense importance. Nicotine and the other ingredients in tobacco are responsible for a wide variety of health problems, including the deaths of more than 1100 Americans every day. Every year, 443,000 Americans die from nicotine-related causes, accounting for 5.1 million years of lost potential life (Morbidity and Mortality Weekly Report, 2009a). Worldwide, 4.3 million people die prematurely as a result of cigarette smoking. Approximately 900,000 people in the United States become addicted to smoking each year. Smoking is now the leading cause of preventable death in the United States and the single most important cause of morbidity and premature mortality worldwide. Interestingly, nicotine-dependent people who are psychiatrically ill consume about 70 percent of all cigarettes smoked, at least in the United States (Grant et al., 2004). Cigarette smoking is also common in people of low socioeconomic classes: indeed, Medicaid recipients are disproportionately affected by tobacco-related disabilities and diseases (Centers for Disease Control and Prevention, 2006). In 2008, adults with a General Educational Development (GED) certificate had a smoking rate of 41.3 percent; those with less than a high school diploma, who comprise about half of current smokers, 27.5 percent; and those with a college degree, 5.7 percent (Morbidity and Mortality Weekly Report, 2009b).

Prior to about the mid-1960s, cigarette smoking was considered chic. Today, after more than 45 years of U.S. government reports on the adverse health consequences of cigarettes, cigarette smoking is being increasingly shunned as unhealthy and unwise. Nevertheless, each day 6000 American teenagers try their first cigarette and 3000 children become regular smokers; almost 1000 of them will eventually die from diseases related to smoking. Also, 9 in 10 smokers become addicted before age 21. Today, in the United States, 3 million adolescents are smokers. Advertisements for cigarettes still appeal to children, and, in subtle ways, the depiction of smoking as okay continues.

Indeed, widely promoted today are "dissolvable tobacco" products that place several milligrams of purified nicotine tobacco into the buccal cavity of the mouth (as strips, sticks, or pellets that dissolve completely, leaving no wad to spit out). These preparations are widely promoted to young people as products that involve no spitting; are useful in smoke-free areas; are discreet; and have no odor, no mess, no secondhand smoke, and "no boundaries." They range in nicotine content from less than 1 milligram to about 4 milligrams of drug (normal nicotine cigarettes have about 1 milligram of nicotine); brands include Ariva, Stonewall, Camel Strips, Camel Sticks, and Camel Orbs. Obviously, with this much nicotine, development of dependence is a considerable concern. The use of these buccal snuffs is associated with oral cancers, but their potential for producing other cancers or cardiovascular disease is unclear. Obviously, these are intended to be chic. Hopefully, the Tobacco Products Scientific Advisory Committee of the FDA will address the safety of these products and their promotion. Finally, Santa Fe Natural Tobacco Company has marketed additive-free cigarettes (Natural American Spirit cigarettes), which still contain almost 2 milligrams of nicotine and almost 20 milligrams of tars per cigarette.[2]

In an interesting study, Strandberg and coworkers (2008) examined the quality of life as smokers and nonsmokers aged. In a remarkable 26-year prospective study, beginning in 1974, they found that nonsmokers lived a mean of 10 years longer than heavy smokers (more than two packs a day) and their extra years were of better quality.

On the positive side, half of all people who have ever smoked cigarettes have quit, and the proportion of American adults who smoke fell from 50 percent in 1965 to 25 percent in 1998. This reduction, unfortunately, has now leveled off (Morbidity and Mortality Weekly Report, 2009b). About 1 million potential deaths have been averted or postponed by people who have quit smoking. Millions more deaths will be avoided or postponed in the twenty-first century. More than 30 years ago, the Surgeon General of the United States identified smoking as the major preventable cause of death and disability, and this finding will probably continue to be the case. In this discussion, it is important to note the following:

- Nicotine is the primary active ingredient in tobacco.
- Nicotine is only one of about 4000 compounds released by the burning of cigarette tobacco.
- Nicotine accounts only for the acute pharmacological effects of smoking and for the dependence on cigarettes. The adverse, long-term cardiovascular, pulmonary, and carcinogenic effects of cigarettes are related to other compounds contained in the product.
- Although nicotine itself may have some adverse effects, its delivery device (the tobacco cigarette) is responsible for much of its toxicity.

Pharmacokinetics

Nicotine is readily absorbed from every site on or in the body, including the lungs, buccal and nasal mucosa, skin, and gastrointestinal tract. Easy and complete absorption forms the basis for the recreational

---

[2] Recently, car-enthusiast magazines included manufacturer's coupons for $20 toward purchase of these "natural" cigarettes to induce persons to smoke the product.

abuse of smoked or chewed tobacco as well as the medical use of nicotine (in treating nicotine dependency) in chewing gums, nasal sprays, transdermal skin patches, and smokeless inhalers.

Nicotine is suspended in cigarette smoke in the form of minute particles (tars), and it is quickly absorbed into the bloodstream from the lungs when the smoke is inhaled, although absorption is much slower than once thought and arterial concentrations of nicotine rise rather slowly. It is likely that blood rapidly saturates with nicotine, and blood leaving the lungs (to the left side of the heart) can carry only a modest amount of drug. Thus, the arterial concentration rises slowly, even though blood carried to the brain at the initiation of smoking is nearly saturated with nicotine, accounting for the early "rush" perceived with the first cigarette.

Most cigarettes contain between 0.5 and 2.0 milligrams of nicotine, depending on the brand. Only about 20 percent (between 0.1 and 0.4 milligram) of the nicotine in a cigarette is actually inhaled and absorbed into the smoker's bloodstream; the hepatic enzyme CYP-2A6 rapidly metabolizes the remainder. People in whom the CYP-2A6 enzyme is absent (or inhibited by certain drugs) have higher blood levels of nicotine and lower levels of its metabolite. One study reported that because of improved cigarette design, "smoke nicotine yield" had increased by about 11 percent over the prior seven years, increasing the addictive potential of cigarettes (Harvard School of Public Health, 2007). Whether this will continue with the new smokeless, dissolvable nicotine products is unclear.

A smoker can readily avoid acute toxicity because inhalation as a route of administration offers exceptional controllability of the dose. The user-controlled frequency of breaths, the depth of inhalation, the time the smoke is held in the lungs, and the total number of cigarettes smoked all allow the smoker to regulate the rate of drug intake and thus control the blood level of nicotine. The pharmacokinetic goals of nicotine administration were summarized by Sellers (1998):

> Tobacco smoking is a complex but highly regulated behavior that has as its goal the maintenance of steady-state brain levels of the highly addictive psychoactive agent nicotine. Smokers "self-regulate" the level of nicotine in their system to produce desired effects (e.g., relaxation, increased concentration) and to avoid unpleasant adverse effects associated with too high (e.g., dizziness) or too low concentrations (e.g., desire to smoke or withdrawal). (p. 179)

Smokers wake in the morning in a state of nicotine deficiency. Characteristically, they will smoke one or more cigarettes fairly rapidly to achieve a blood level of about 15 milligrams per liter and continue smoking through the day to maintain this level. The smoker does not behave this way consciously, but the behavior occurs nevertheless. The

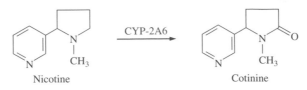

FIGURE 11.4 Structures of nicotine and its metabolite cotinine.

elimination half-life of nicotine in a chronic smoker is about 2 hours, necessitating frequent administration of the drug to avoid withdrawal symptoms or drug craving. When nicotine is administered in the form of snuff, chewing tobacco, or gum, blood levels of nicotine are comparable to the levels achieved by smoking.

Nicotine is quickly and thoroughly distributed throughout the body, rapidly penetrating the brain, crossing the placental barrier, and appearing in all bodily fluids, including breast milk. There are no barriers in the body to the distribution of nicotine.

The liver metabolizes approximately 80 to 90 percent of the nicotine administered to a person either orally or by smoking before the kidneys excrete it. The primary metabolite of nicotine is *cotinine* (Figure 11.4); this substance serves as a marker of both tobacco use and exposure to environmental smoke.

Pharmacological Effects

Nicotine is the only pharmacologically active drug in tobacco smoke apart from carcinogenic tars. It exerts powerful effects on the brain, the spinal cord, the peripheral nervous system, the heart, and various other body structures.

Effects on the Brain

In the early stages of smoking, nicotine causes nausea and vomiting by stimulating both the vomiting center in the brain stem and the sensory receptors in the stomach. Tolerance to this effect develops rapidly. Nicotine stimulates the hypothalamus to release a hormone, antidiuretic hormone, which causes fluid retention. Nicotine reduces the activity of afferent nerve fibers coming from the muscles, leading to a reduction in muscle tone. This action may be involved (at least partially) in the relaxation a person may experience as a result of smoking. Nicotine also reduces weight gain, probably by reducing appetite and altering taste bud sensitivity.

Nicotine produces multiple actions in the CNS, resulting in increases in psychomotor activity, cognitive functioning, sensorimotor performance, attention, and memory consolidation. Rose and coworkers

(2003) reported that nicotine increases blood flow to the CNS structures that mediate arousal and reward, suggesting a link between activation of these structures and the positive motivational effects of nicotine. Brody and coworkers (2002) reported that exposure to cues related to cigarette smoking increased brain activity in areas associated with arousal, compulsive behaviors, sensory integration, and episodic memory. Areas included the orbitofrontal cortex, prefrontal cortex, and anterior insula (a region of brain implicated in conscious urges). Naqvi and coworkers (2007) demonstrated that smokers with brain damage involving the insula were more likely than smokers with brain injury not involving the insula to undergo a disruption of smoking addiction. Damage involving the insula was characterized by the "ability to quit smoking easily, immediately, without relapse, and without persistence of the urge to smoke," suggesting that "the insula is a critical neural substrate in the addiction to smoking" (p. 531).

Nicotine improves performance in a variety of cognitive tasks, such as vigilance and rapid information processing, probably a reflection of activation of frontal cortical executive functioning (Rose et al., 2003). The beneficial effects of nicotine seem to be greatest for tasks requiring working memory rather than long-term memory. Smokers often state that they will smoke a cigarette before doing a complex task that requires attention and arousal, perhaps combining the drug's anxiolytic action with its stimulant action.

Several reports note an antidepressant effect of nicotine as well as the comorbidity of depression and cigarette use. Salin-Pascual and coworkers (1996), who first noted a high frequency of cigarette smoking among people with major depression, found that, in nonsmokers, transdermal nicotine patches produced a remarkable reduction in depression (Figure 11.5). They postulated that the high rate of smoking among depressed people might, in part, represent an attempt at self-medication to assist in dealing with some of their depressive symptoms. In agreement with this concept, Fergusson and colleagues (1996), in a study of 16-year-olds, reported:

> There was evidence of clear comorbidity between depressive disorders and nicotine dependence in this cohort of 16-year-olds; subjects with depression had odds of nicotine dependence that were more than 4.5 times the odds for those without depression. This relationship was similar for male and female subjects. These results suggest that comorbidities between nicotine dependence and depression are well established by the age of 16 years. (p. 1047)

Riggs and coworkers (1999) noted that most of the risk for adolescent smoking, as well as the subsequent development of nontobacco substance involvement, is mediated through the presence of conduct disorder. Additional comorbidity, such as ADHD and depression, adds to

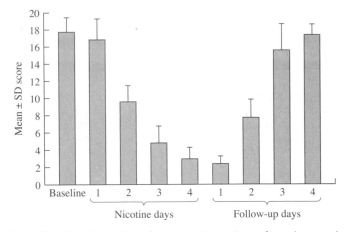

FIGURE 11.5 Hamilton Rating Scale for Depression ratings of ten depressed patients before, during, and after administration of nicotine patches. A significant reduction was observed on the second day of nicotine patches and continued until the second follow-up day. [From Salin-Pascual et al. (1996), p. 388.]

the already high risk of smoking imparted by conduct disorder. This study highlights the contribution of comorbidity to smoking initiation and the need for coordinated assessment and treatment of smoking cessation along with concurrent treatment of other drug use and psychiatric comorbidity such as ADHD and major depression in adolescents.

Anda and coworkers (1999), in a retrospective survey of over 9000 adults, found a strong relationship between smoking behaviors and adverse childhood experiences, including emotional, physical, and sexual abuse; spouse abuse; parental separation or divorce; and growing up with a substance-abusing, mentally ill, or incarcerated household member. At least one of these experiences was listed by 63 percent of respondents. As the number of adverse experiences increased, the likelihood of being an early and a current smoker increased, as did the likelihood of being currently depressed. The authors speculated that for these people cigarette smoking may provide a mood-elevating effect and that "unconscious selection of cigarette use could occur in situations of chronic distress, such as depression" (p. 1657). How conduct disorder and adult ADHD fit into this pattern was not addressed.

Since depression and a propensity to smoke nicotine-containing cigarettes may be closely linked, does cessation of smoking in patients with a history of depression lead to relapse to depressive episodes? Tsoh and coworkers (2000) and Glassman and coworkers (2001) addressed this issue and noted that cessation of smoking placed depressed patients at risk of relapse, at least over a one-year period postcessation (Figure 11.6). This risk needs to be kept in mind during treatment for smoking cessation in patients with a history of depression or dysthymia.

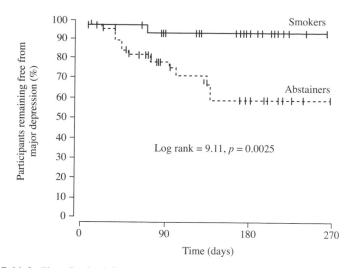

FIGURE 11.6 Time (in days) for people who were smokers and had a history of major depression to relapse to an episode of depression. Two groups of depressed patients were studied. One group (solid line) of 34 smokers continued to smoke and few relapsed. The second group of 42 patients (dashed line) abstained from smoking, and almost 50 percent experienced a depressive episode within 4 months of smoking cessation. [From Glassman et al. (2001), p. 1931.]

Nicotine exerts a potent behavior-reinforcing action, especially in the early phases of drug use. The reinforcing action of nicotine involves indirect activation of midbrain dopamine neurons. In the veteran smoker, this reinforcing action diminishes, and the user smokes primarily to relieve or avoid withdrawal symptoms. Spring and coworkers (2003) studied the rewarding effects of cigarette smoking in schizophrenic patients, depressed patients, and controls. While all three groups of patients recognized the drawbacks associated with smoking, schizophrenic and depressed smokers perceived more benefits than did controls and found cigarettes more appealing than alternative rewards. Thus, these two groups of patients found that smoking offered ongoing rewards while patients without a mental health history did not. This may be important for the tailoring of smoking withdrawal programs to different patient populations.

Some of the acute effects and motivational responses elicited by nicotine can be modulated by the endogenous cannabinoid system (Chapter 14), which argues for the existence of a physiological interaction between the nicotine and the cannabinoid systems (Gonzalez et al., 2002). Similarly, there is close association between the nicotine and the opioid narcotic receptor systems, particularly in the context of nicotine addiction (McGehee, 2006). Much remains to be learned about these interactions.

Effects on the Body

In addition to its effects on the CNS, normal doses of nicotine can increase heart rate, blood pressure, and cardiac contractility. In nonatherosclerotic coronary arteries, nicotine initiates vasodilation, increasing blood flow to meet the increased oxygen demand of the heart muscle. In atherosclerotic coronary arteries (which cannot dilate), however, cardiac ischemia can result when the oxygen supply fails to meet the oxygen demand created by the drug's cardiac stimulation. This occurrence can precipitate angina or myocardial infarction (heart attack). Importantly, cessation of smoking reduces long-term cardiac mortality.

> A substantial progressive decrease in the mortality rates among nonsmokers over the past half century (due to prevention and improved treatment of disease) has been wholly outweighed among cigarette smokers by a progressive increase in the smoker vs. nonsmoker death rate ratio due to earlier and more intensive use of cigarettes. Among men born around 1920, prolonged cigarette smoking from early adult life tripled age-specific mortality rates, but cessation at age 50 halved the hazard, and cessation at age 30 avoided almost all of it. (Doll et al., 2004, p. 1519)

Mechanism of Action

Nicotine exerts virtually all its CNS and peripheral effects by activating certain specific acetylcholine receptors (nicotinic receptors). In the peripheral nervous system, activation of these receptors causes an increase in blood pressure and heart rate, causes release of epinephrine (adrenaline) from the adrenal glands, and increases the activity of the gastrointestinal tract.

In the CNS, the nicotine-sensitive acetylcholine receptors are widely distributed and may be located on the presynaptic nerve terminals of dopamine-, acetylcholine-, and glutamine-secreting neurons. Activation of nicotinic receptors by nicotine facilitates the release of these transmitters and increases their actions in the brain.

Nicotine increases dopamine levels in the mesocorticolimbic system involving the ventral tegmentum, nucleus accumbens, and forebrain. This increase accounts for the behavioral reinforcement, stimulant, antidepressant, and addictive properties of the drug.

The increased acetylcholine resulting from nicotine administration contributes to the cognitive potentiation and memory facilitation properties of the drug. It may also be responsible for the arousal effects commonly seen with smoking. It is at least theoretically possible that nicotine (if administered other than by cigarette smoking) might have some use in delaying the onset of some of the cognitive deficits seen in Alzheimer's disease. Finally, the facilitation of glutaminergic neurotransmission might contribute to the improvement in memory functioning seen in nicotine users.

Tolerance and Dependence

Nicotine does not appear to induce any pronounced degree of biological tolerance. On the other hand, nicotine clearly induces both physiological and psychological dependence in a majority of smokers (Breslau et al., 2001; Hughes, 2001). Only a minority of smokers appear capable of abrupt cessation of smoking without abstinence symptoms, and even they are prone to craving and relapse. As early as 1988, the Surgeon General of the United States (U.S. Department of Health and Human Services, 1988) came to the following conclusions:

- Cigarettes and other forms of tobacco are addicting.
- Nicotine is the drug in tobacco that causes addiction.
- The pharmacological and behavioral processes that determine tobacco addiction are similar to those that determine addiction to drugs such as heroin and cocaine.
- More than 300,000 cigarette-addicted Americans die yearly as a consequence of their addiction. (Today this number approaches 440,000 per year.)

Despite all the verbal exchanges among public, regulatory, medical, political, and industry sources, the scientific case that nicotine is addictive is overwhelming:

> Patterns of use by smokers and the remarkable intractability of the smoking habit point to compulsive use as the norm. Studies in both animal and human subjects have shown that nicotine can function as a reinforcer, albeit under a more limited range of conditions than with some other drugs of abuse. In drug discrimination paradigms, there is some cross generalization between nicotine on the one hand, and amphetamine and cocaine on the other. A well-defined withdrawal syndrome has been delineated which is alleviated by nicotine replacement. Nicotine replacement also enhances outcomes in smoking cessation, roughly doubling success rates. In total, the evidence clearly identifies nicotine as a powerful drug of addiction, comparable to heroin, cocaine, and alcohol. (Stolerman and Jarvis, 1995, p. 2)

Withdrawal from cigarettes is characterized by an abstinence syndrome that is usually not life-threatening. Abstinence symptoms include a severe craving for nicotine, irritability, anxiety, anger, difficulty in concentrating, restlessness, impatience, increased appetite, weight gain, and insomnia. The period of withdrawal may be intense and persistent, often lasting for many months. The difficulty in handling cigarette dependence is illustrated by the fact that cigarette smokers who seek treatment for other drug and alcohol problems often find it harder to quit cigarette smoking than to give up the other drugs. Even Sigmund Freud continued his cigar habit (20 per day) until death, in spite of an endless series of operations for mouth and jaw cancer (the jaw was eventually totally removed), persistent heart problems that were exacerbated by smoking, and numerous attempts at quitting.

Abstinent smokers displaying signs of withdrawal often tend to increase their caffeine (coffee) consumption; blood caffeine levels increase and remain elevated for as long as six months. The symptoms of nicotine withdrawal, caffeine withdrawal, and caffeine toxicity are similar enough to be confused; symptoms of nicotine withdrawal may be a mixture of nicotine withdrawal and caffeine toxicity.

A report from the Harvard School of Public Health (2007) clearly documents that cigarette manufacturers have increased the nicotine content in all types and brands of cigarettes by about 11 percent over a recent seven-year period. The increased amount of drug in the delivery product (cigarettes) undoubtedly creates an increased addictive potential of continued smoking. This may also be happening with the new dissolvable nicotine products discussed earlier.

Toxicity

As previously discussed, both the acute pharmacological effects and the withdrawal signs seen on cessation of smoking result from the nicotine in tobacco. The tar in tobacco is mainly responsible for the diseases associated with long-term tobacco use. Of the 440,000 people in the United States who die prematurely each year from tobacco use, 82,000 deaths are caused by noncancerous lung diseases, 115,000 are caused by lung cancer, 30,000 are caused by cancers of other body organs, and more than 200,000 result from heart and vascular diseases. A person's life is shortened 14 minutes for every cigarette smoked. In other words, a person who smokes two packs of cigarettes a day for 20 years loses about 13 or 14 years of his or her life.

More than 50 million people (one out of every five Americans) alive today will die prematurely from the effects of smoking cigarettes. Cigarette smoking, the nation's greatest public health hazard, is also the nation's most preventable cause of premature death, illness, and disability. For each of the approximately 22 billion packs of cigarettes sold yearly in the United States, $3.45 was spent on medical care attributable to smoking and $3.73 in productivity losses were incurred, for a total cost of $7.18 for each and every pack smoked. The total economic toll exceeds $157 billion each year in the United States—$75 billion in direct medical costs and $82 billion in lost productivity (Centers for Disease Control and Prevention, 2006).

Cardiovascular Disease

The carbon monoxide in smoke decreases the amount of oxygen delivered to the heart muscle, while nicotine increases the amount of work the heart must do (by increasing the heart rate and blood pressure). Both carbon monoxide and nicotine increase the incidence of

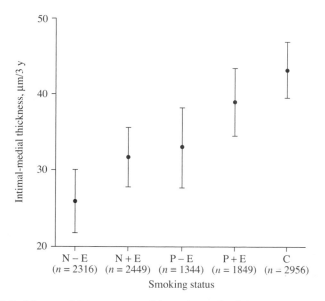

FIGURE 11.7 Mean and 95 percent confidence intervals of three-year progression in the wall thickness of the carotid artery, shown by smoking status category, after adjustment for demographic characteristics, cardiovascular risk factors, and life-style variables. N − nonsmoker. P = past smoker; C = current smoker; +E = with exposure to environmental tobacco smoke; −E = without exposure to environmental tobacco smoke. [From G. Howard et al., "Cigarette Smoking and Progression of Atherosclerosis: The Atherosclerosis Risk in Communities (ARIC) Study," *Journal of the American Medical Association* 279 (1998): 122.]

atherosclerosis (narrowing) and thrombosis (clotting) in the coronary arteries. These three actions (and others as well) seem to underlie the dramatic increase in the risk of death from coronary heart disease in smokers compared to nonsmokers (Teo et al., 2006). Cigarette smokers manifest a 50 percent increase in the progression of atherosclerosis when compared with people who have never smoked (Figure 11.7).

Besides occurring in the coronary arteries, atherosclerosis occurs in other arteries as well, most notably the aorta (in the abdomen), the carotid arteries (in the neck), and the femoral and other arteries of the legs. Cigarette-induced occlusion of these vessels blocks the blood flow to important body organs and results in ischemic damage, strokes, and other disorders, causing great discomfort and disability and necessitating continuing and often futile surgical interventions. Bhat and coworkers (2008) reported cigarette smoking as a causative factor in the risk of stroke in young women.

Pulmonary Disease

In the lungs, chronic smoking results in a smoker's syndrome, characterized by difficulty in breathing, wheezing, chest pain, lung congestion, and increased susceptibility to infections of the respiratory tract. Cigarette smoking impairs ventilation and greatly increases the risk of emphysema (a form of irreversible lung damage). Smoke exposure also reduces the efficacy of the immune defense mechanisms in the lungs. About 9 million Americans suffer from cigarette-induced chronic bronchitis and emphysema. In fact, 70 percent of pulmonary diseases and deaths are tobacco related; 57,000 deaths per year result from emphysema alone.

Cancer

Although nicotine itself is not carcinogenic, the relationship between smoking and cancer is now beyond question. Cigarette smoking is the major cause of lung cancer in both men and women, causing approximately 112,000 deaths in the United States every year. More women today die from cigarette-induced lung cancer than die from breast cancer, a remarkable testament to the carcinogenicity of cigarettes. Harris and coworkers (2004) followed 940,000 male and female smokers and nonsmokers for six years and concluded that the risk of dying from lung cancer was the same for smokers of very low-tar, low-tar, and medium-tar cigarettes. Risk increased only in smokers of very high-tar, nonfiltered cigarettes. Only smokers who quit smoking and people who never smoked had a significantly lower risk of lung cancer. Interestingly, smokers who switch from cigarettes to spit (chewing) tobacco continue to have higher risks of dying from major tobacco-related diseases than do former smokers who quit using tobacco entirely (Henley et al., 2007). Certainly, smoking "natural," "organic," or "green" cigarettes will not reduce the incidence of cancers.

Smoking is also a major cause of cancers of the mouth, voice box, and throat. Concomitant alcohol ingestion greatly increases the incidence of these problems. In addition, cigarette smoking is a primary cause of more than 50 percent of the nearly 10,000 deaths every year that result from bladder cancer; it is a primary cause of pancreatic cancer; and it increases the risk of cancer of the uterine cervix twofold. Of all cancer deaths in the United States, 30 percent (154,000 annually) would be prevented if no one smoked.

There has been thought that early screening for lung cancer [using computerized tomography (CT) scans] might identify cigarette-induced lung cancers at an early stage, allowing for early diagnosis and surgical treatment. Bach and coworkers (2007) recently demonstrated that while this may be true, such early detection and lung removal surgery did not result in any meaningful reduction in the risk of death from the cancer.

Effects of Passive Smoke

In 1986, the Surgeon General of the United States (C. Everett Koop, M.D.) released the first Surgeon General's report on the health consequences of being exposed to the smoke of cigarettes smoked by other people (U.S. Department of Health and Human Services, 1986). Twenty years later, a second report was released (U.S. Department of Health and Human Services, 2006). It documents that in 2005, exposure to secondhand smoke killed more than 3000 adult nonsmokers from lung cancer, 46,000 adult nonsmokers from coronary heart disease, and 430 newborns from sudden infant death syndrome. Secondhand smoke also causes nonfatal health concerns such as coughing, phlegm, and reduced lung function. Most nonsmokers feel that secondhand smoke is harmful and that nonsmokers should be protected in the workplace.

Policies prohibiting workplace smoking have many benefits: they protect nonsmokers from environmental exposure, they reduce tobacco use by smokers, and they change public attitudes about tobacco use from acceptable to unacceptable.

Effects During Pregnancy

About 1 million babies in the United States are born each year after prenatal cigarette smoke exposure from maternal smoking; this number does not include involuntary maternal exposure to passive smoke (Ng and Zelikoff, 2007). Cigarette smoking adversely affects the developing fetus, leading to two- to threefold increases in being small for gestational age (SGA) or being born preterm (McCowan et al., 2009). Stopping smoking early in pregnancy appears to reverse the SGA and preterm risks. Also, the weight of a smoker's SGA offspring usually returns to normal at about 18 months of age.

Even women exposed to passive smoke inhalation have low-birth-weight children. More than 2000 infant deaths per year are attributed to maternal smoking. Respiratory diseases, such as asthma, are commonly observed in offspring. Sudden infant death syndrome (SIDS), various immunological diseases, and other medical problems have all been implicated, with various levels of confirmatory data (U.S. Department of Health and Human Services, 2006, Chapter 5).

Cigarette smoking reduces oxygen delivery to the developing fetus, causing a variable degree of fetal hypoxia. This condition may underlie the reported increases in irritability and increased muscle tone in the neonate (Stroud et al., 2009) and even longer-term intellectual and physical deficiencies. It has long been presumed that school-age children born of mothers who smoked during pregnancy are at risk for lower intelligence quotients (IQs) and an increased prevalence of ADHD when compared with children born of nonsmoking mothers. Thus, maternal smoking is postulated to cause persistent neurobehavioral deficits. Recent reports, however, suggest that future neurodevelopmental problems, including ADHD, may reflect maternal ADHD, suggesting that this disorder is due to an inherited predisposition rather than being a direct consequence of maternal cigarette smoking (Thapar et al., 2009; Agrawal et al., 2010).

Smoking cessation programs designed to reduce smoking behaviors and nicotine dependence during pregnancy offer special challenges (Oncken and Kranzler, 2009). The safety of pharmacological interventions (bupropion, nicotine replacement therapies, varenicline) has not been established. Therefore, psychosocial interventions should likely be the first treatment option for pregnant smokers.

Pharmacological Therapies for Nicotine Dependence

The mid-1990s saw dramatic advances in the recognition of nicotine dependence as a biological reality and in its treatment. Perhaps the first and most important advance at that time was the development and clinical application of *nicotine replacement therapies*, specifically nicotine-containing gum, transdermal nicotine-containing patches, and nicotine-containing nasal sprays and inhalers. Later in the 1990s came the identification of the antidepressant drug *bupropion* (Wellbutrin, Zyban) as a substance that could reduce cigarette cravings and relieve the distress of comorbid depression; however, its long-term efficacy is being questioned (Hajek et al., 2009). The most recent advance has been the introduction of a new *partial nicotine receptor agonist*, varenicline (trade name Chantix).

In 1996, the first clinical practice guidelines for the treatment of nicotine-dependent people was published. This was followed in 2000 by a guideline titled "A Clinical Practice Guideline for Treating Tobacco Use and Dependence, a U.S. Public Health Service Report" (Tobacco Use and Dependence Clinical Practice Guideline Panel, 2000). This report came to the following conclusions:

- Tobacco dependence is a chronic condition that warrants repeated treatment until long-term or permanent abstinence is achieved.

- Effective treatments for tobacco dependence exist and all tobacco users should be offered those treatments.

- Clinicians and health care delivery systems must institutionalize the consistent identification, documentation, and treatment of every tobacco user at every visit.

- Brief tobacco dependence treatment is effective and every tobacco user should be offered at least brief treatments.

- There is a strong dose-response relationship between the intensity of tobacco dependence counseling and its effectiveness.

- Three types of counseling were found to be especially effective: practical counseling, social support as part of treatment, and social support arranged outside treatment.

- Tobacco dependence treatments are cost effective relative to other medical and disease prevention interventions; as such, all health insurance plans should include as a reimbursed benefit the counseling and pharmacotherapeutic treatments identified as being effective.

- Six first-line pharmacotherapies for tobacco dependence are effective: nicotine gum, nicotine inhaler, nicotine nasal spray, nicotine patch, sustained-release bupropion, and varenicline. The first four are replacement therapy and the last two are drugs to reduce craving and relapse. At least one of these six medications should be prescribed in the absence of contraindications.

Rigotti (2002) reviewed the efficacy of both nicotine replacement therapies and bupropion. She first noted that a combination of any pharmacotherapy and counseling was more effective than either alone. The efficacy of behavioral interventions combined with pharmacotherapy has been verified by other researchers, including Ranney and colleagues (2006) and Stead and coworkers (2006). Unfortunately, interventional therapies have only modest effects for people who smoke (Grimshaw and Stanton, 2006) and in preventing relapse following initial cessation (Hajek et al., 2009).

The objective of nicotine replacement therapy is to replace smoking cigarettes as a source of the nicotine and replace the cigarette with a patch, gum, inhaler, or nasal spray. Once the cigarette is replaced, the dose of nicotine in the replacement product can be slowly reduced and then eliminated. Each product has demonstrable efficacy in randomized, controlled trials. Nicotine-containing patches double the long-term smoking cessation rate, while nicotine gum increases cessation rates by 50 to 70 percent. For heavy smokers, gum containing 4 milligrams of nicotine per piece is more effective than gum containing 2 milligrams. All forms of replacement therapy indicate similar efficacy at 12 weeks; compliance is highest for the patch, intermediate for the gum, and lowest for the vapor inhaler and nasal spray. Figure 11.8 illustrates the plasma nicotine levels achieved after a smoker has smoked a cigarette, received nicotine nasal spray, begun chewing nicotine gum, or applied a nicotine patch.

Although nicotine-containing medications are known to help people stop smoking, not everyone is helped by them or wants to use them. This prompted the evaluation of antidepressant drugs as smoking cessation agents. Hughes and coworkers (2007) concluded that the antidepressants bupropion (Wellbutrin, Zyban) and nortriptyline (Pamelor) double a person's chances of giving up smoking and have an

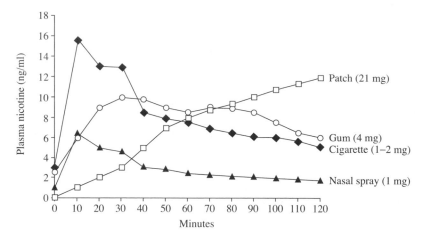

FIGURE 11.8 Plasma nicotine levels after a smoker has smoked a cigarette, received nicotine nasal spray, begun chewing nicotine gum, or applied a nicotine patch. The amount of nicotine in each product is shown in parentheses. The pattern produced by use of a nicotine inhaler (not shown) is similar to that for nicotine gum. [From Rigotti (2002), p. 510.]

acceptable rate of side effects. SSRI antidepressants such as fluoxetine (Prozac) are not effective. Of the two shown to be effective, bupropion is the most studied and most widely used. Bupropion delays smoking relapse and also results in less weight gain. Interestingly, bupropion and nortriptyline appear to work equally well in both depressed and nondepressed smokers; this suggests that these drugs help smokers quit in some way other than through their action as antidepressants. The norepinephrine reptake inhibitor atomoxetine (Strattera) has been shown to be efficacious in reducing cravings to smoke among smokers who use nicotine to increase stimulation (Ray et al., 2009). Figure 11.9 offers a smoking cessation strategy that may be used by health care workers in compliance with the recommendations of the U.S. Public Health Service.

Varenicline

In late 2006, a new approach to treating nicotine dependence was introduced (Cahill et al., 2007). Varenicline (Chantix; Figure 11.10) is pharmacologically classified as a *partial nicotine receptor agonist*. The drug binds weakly to the receptor, which normally binds nicotine strongly. It is therefore weaker than nicotine, partially stimulating the receptor: it reduces withdrawal symptoms but blocks the access of nicotine to the receptor, making nicotine less of a stimulant. Since nicotine indirectly induces the release of dopamine (whence follows its stimulant and behaviorally reinforcing action), varenicline enables a low-level release of

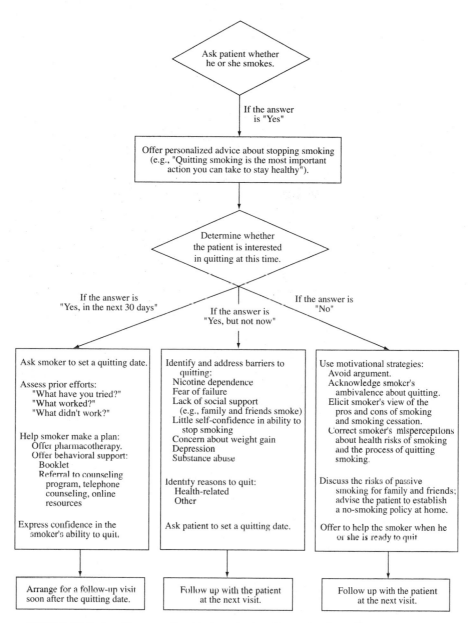

FIGURE 11.9 Smoking cessation strategy for health care workers. The strategy uses the steps recommended in Public Health Service guidelines: ask, advise, assess, assist, and arrange follow-up. [From Rigotti (2002), p. 508.]

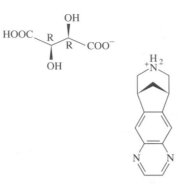

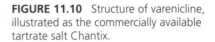

Varenicline (Chantix)

FIGURE 11.10 Structure of varenicline, illustrated as the commercially available tartrate salt Chantix.

dopamine, offering some agonist effect at dopamine receptors. However, by blocking nicotine's access to its receptors, continued smoking is less satisfying, which reduces a person's need to smoke and may help the person to quit completely and maintain abstinence (Tonstad et al., 2006; Oncken et al., 2006; Zierler-Brown and Kyle, 2007).

Compared with bupropion, varenicline is significantly more effective in maintaining abstinence (Jorenby et al., 2006; Gonzales et al., 2006). In one study of over 1000 smokers, Jorenby and colleagues (2006) compared varenicline titrated to a dose of 1 milligram twice daily with bupropion titrated to a dose of 150 milligrams twice daily (Figures 11.11 and 11.12). As shown, varenicline was significantly more effective than bupropion in achieving initial abstinence from smoking at 12 weeks and maintained this superiority through 52 weeks of treatment. Pooling of the available data indicates that varenicline increases the odds of quitting and maintaining abstinence for 12 months or longer about threefold compared with placebo and one and a half times compared with patients treated with bupropion (Figure 11.13). More recent literature also supports the superiority of varenicline over bupropion (Garrison and Dugan, 2009; Cahill et al., 2009). Note that unlike with bupropion, nicotine replacement therapy is not indicated with varenicline, since varenicline is a partial blocker of nicotine's receptors; excess nicotine might overcome the partial block caused by varenicline.

Nausea is the primary side effect of varenicline, occurring in 30 to 40 percent of varenicline users (Cahill et al., 2009). In 2008, however, some observations of varenicline users noted adverse events, including serious neuropsychiatric disturbances in mood (depressed), agitation, hostility, changes in behavior, suicidal ideation, and suicide. It is unclear whether the association of varenicline with these adverse events is causal, coincidental, or related to smoking cessation (Jimenez-Ruiz et al., 2009). Nevertheless, in July 2009 the FDA required the manufacturer

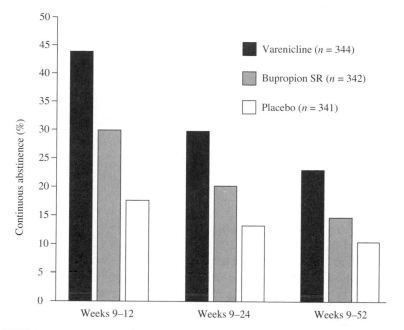

FIGURE 11.11   Percentage of smokers maintaining continuous smoking abstinence at periods 9–12 weeks, 9–24 weeks, and 9–52 weeks during treatment with varenicline (1 milligram twice daily), bupropion-SR (150 milligrams twice daily), or placebo. [From Jorenby et al. (2006), Figure 2.]

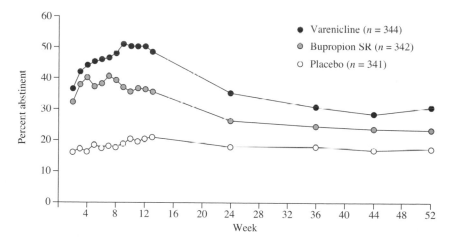

FIGURE 11.12   Percentage of smokers maintaining abstinence over a 52-week period of treatment with varenicline (1 milligram twice daily), bupropion-SR (150 milligram twice daily), or placebo. [From Jorenby et al. (2006), Figure 3.]

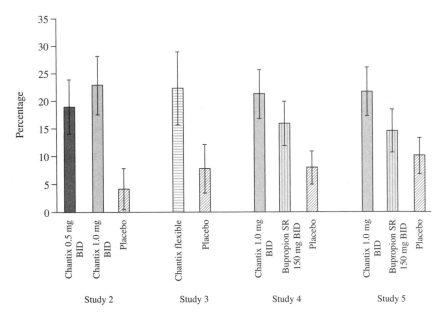

FIGURE 11.13   Manufacturer-supplied pooled data from five studies comparing rates of continuous smoking abstinence in weeks 9 through 52 with treatment with varenicline (0.5 or 1.0 milligram twice daily), bupropion (150 milligrams twice daily), or placebo. [From Pfizer Laboratories monograph LAB-0327-2.0, May 2006.]

of varenicline to add a black box warning highlighting the risk of the serious mental health events listed above. A similar warning was required of bupropion. Cahill and coworkers (2009) put this in perspective:

> In view of the potential, if unproven, risk that varenicline may be associated with serious adverse outcomes, patients attempting to quit smoking with varenicline, and their families and caregivers, should be alerted about the need to monitor for neuropsychiatric symptoms, including changes in behavior, agitation, depressed mood, suicidal ideation, and suicidal behavior, and to report such symptoms immediately to the patient's healthcare provider. (p. 126)

Therapy with varenicline is indicated for 12 weeks; positive responders undergo a second 12 weeks of therapy to support continued abstinence. Patients taking the drug are offered a behavioral modification program called GETQUIT.[3] This program uses cognitive-behavioral principles to help educate smokers about managing cravings and behavioral triggers. A "habit changer" identifies and addresses personal triggers to smoke, and daily communications help patients track their progress.

---

[3] Visit www.get-quit.com for information.

Vaccine Therapy

An interesting investigational therapy in development is a nicotine vaccine (similar to a cocaine vaccine; Chapter 12), administered by repeated intramuscular injections. Nicotine itself is a nonimmuno- genic molecule and must be conjugated (attached) to a carrier pro- tein to induce antibodies. Three of these vaccines are currently under clinical development, two of them termed NicQbeta and NicVAX. Here, several intramuscular injections of the vaccine induce suffi- cient nicotine-specific antibodies that sequester nicotine in the blood with the goal of binding the nicotine to a larger molecule and pre- venting the nicotine from entering the brain (Cerny and Cerny, 2009; Moreno et al., 2010). In this way, the addictive properties of cigarettes are eliminated and smokers attempting to quit may be able to smoke one or two cigarettes without effect, since the nicotine is sequestered.

In a randomized, controlled trial, Cornuz and coworkers (2008) reported that the vaccine induced nicotine antibodies in all subjects but was clinically effective only in people who produced a high num- ber of antibodies (Figure 11.14). Therefore, for a nicotine vaccine to

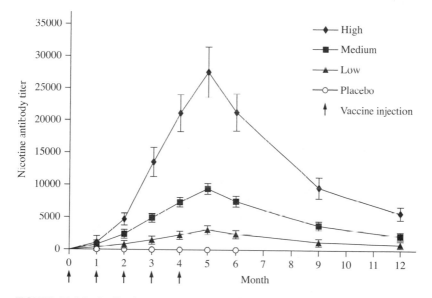

FIGURE 11.14 Antibody titers in subjects who received four injections of NicQbeta vaccine (upper three traces) in 229 persons or placebo vaccine (lowest trace) in 111 persons, administered intramuscularly at one-month intervals. Active vaccine produced antibodies in all subjects but was clinically effective only in persons who developed high vaccine titers. Note that titers reached maximal levels about one month following the last injection and declined thereafter. [From Cornuz et al. (2008), p. e2547, Figure 3.]

be effective, the following principles should be borne in mind when the vaccine is administered:

1. The vaccine must induce sufficient antibody to bind all nicotine in the blood and reduce the amount of nicotine entering the brain to subpharmacological levels.
2. The smoker must not smoke enough to overwhelm the amount of antibodies in blood.
3. The vaccine will not address withdrawal symptoms or craving (Cornuz et al., 2008).
4. The vaccine may have to be repeatedly administered to be effective.

In sum, a nicotine vaccine is not intended to address all aspects of nicotine dependence. However, antibodies sequestering nicotine in blood may help smokers quit, despite the fact that the vaccine can be 'beaten" by increasing nicotine intake to levels above which the vaccine can sequester. Optimal therapy for long-term smoking cessation remains to be elucidated.

STUDY QUESTIONS

1. Differentiate the CNS stimulant actions of caffeine from those of amphetamine and cocaine.
2. Describe the mechanism of action of caffeine. How does this mechanism explain the clinical effects of the drug?
3. What is the relationship between panic attacks and caffeine?
4. Discuss the effects of caffeine in the cardiovascular system.
5. What evidence is there for and against the use of caffeine by women who are pregnant or breast-feeding?
6. Discuss the political, health, and economic issues related to tobacco. Should the FDA regulate nicotine as a drug?
7. List some of the statistics about the health effects of cigarettes.
8. Discuss the antidepressant property of nicotine. Might this property contribute to cigarette dependence? Why?
9. Are cigarettes addicting or are they merely habit forming? Defend your position.
10. Discuss the clinical uses and limitations of nicotine replacement devices. How might their efficacy be boosted?
11. If nicotine exerts an antidepressant action, what drugs or therapies might assist in withdrawal and relapse prevention?

12. Should tobacco products be banned in our society? Defend your views.

13. Compare and contrast varenicline with bupropion for smoking cessation.

REFERENCES

Agrawal, A., et al. (2010). "The Effects of Maternal Smoking During Pregnancy on Offspring Outcomes." *Preventive Medicine* 50: 13–18.

Anda, R. F., et al. (1999). "Adverse Childhood Experiences and Smoking During Adolescence and Adulthood." *Journal of the American Medical Association* 282: 1652–1658.

Bach, P. B., et al. (2007). "Computed Tomography Screening and Lung Cancer Outcomes." *Journal of the American Medical Association* 297: 953–961.

Bhat, V. M., et al. (2008). "Dose-Response Relationship Between Cigarette Smoking and Risk of Ischemic Stroke in Young Women." *Stroke* 39: 2439–2443.

Breslau, N., et al. (2001). "Nicotine Dependence in the United States: Prevalence, Trends, and Smoking Persistence." *Archives of General Psychiatry* 58: 810–816.

Brody, A. L., et al. (2002). "Brain Metabolic Changes During Cigarette Craving." *Archives of General Psychiatry* 59: 1162–1172.

Browne, M. L. (2006). "Maternal Exposure to Caffeine and Risk of Congenital Abnormalities: A Systematic Review." *Epidemiology* 17: 324–331.

Cahill, K., et al. (2007). "Nicotine Receptor Partial Agonists for Smoking Cessation." *Cochrane Database of Systematic Reviews*, Issue 1, CD006103.

Cahill, K., et al. (2009). "A Preliminary Benefit-Risk Assessment of Varenicline in Smoking Cessation." *Drug Safety* 32: 119–135.

CARE Study Group. (2008). "Maternal Caffeine Intake During Pregnancy and Risk of Fatal Growth Restriction: A Large Prospective Observational Study." *British Medical Journal* 337: a2332.

Centers for Disease Control and Prevention. (2006). "The Health Consequences of Smoking: A Report of the Surgeon General." Office of Smoking and Health, United States Department of Health and Human Services, Washington, DC. www.cdc.gov/tobacco or www.surgeongeneral.gov

Cerny, E. H., and Cerny, T. (2009). "Vaccines Against Nicotine." *Human Vaccinations* 5: 200–205.

Cornelis, M. C., and El-Sohemy, A. (2007). "Coffee, Caffeine, and Coronary Heart Disease." *Current Opinions in Lipidology* 18: 13–19.

Cornelis, M. C., et al. (2006). "Coffee, CYP1A2 Genotype, and Risk of Myocardial Infarction." *Journal of the American Medical Association* 295: 1135–1141.

Cornuz, J., et al. (2008). "A Vaccine Against Nicotine for Smoking Cessation: A Randomized Controlled Trial." *PLoS One* 3: e2547.

Doll, R., et al. (2004). "Mortality in Relation to Smoking: 50 Years' Observations on Male British Doctors." *British Medical Journal* 328: 1519–1528.

Fergusson, D. M., et al. (1996). "Comorbidity Between Depressive Disorders and Nicotine Dependence in a Cohort of 16-Year-Olds." *Archives of General Psychiatry* 53: 1043–1047.

Garrison, G. D., and Dugan, S. E. (2009). "Varenicline: A First-Line Treatment Option for Smoking Cessation." *Clinical Therapeutics* 31: 463–491.

Glassman, A. H., et al. (2001). "Smoking Cessation and the Course of Major Depression: A Follow-Up Study." *Lancet* 357: 1929–1932.

Gonzales, D., et al. (2006). "Varenicline, an α4β2 Nicotinic Acetylcholine Receptor Partial Agonist, vs. Sustained-Release Bupropion and Placebo for Smoking Cessation: A Randomized Controlled Trial." *Journal of the American Medical Association* 296: 47–55.

Gonzalez, S., et al. (2002). "Changes in Endocannabinoid Contents in the Brain of Rats Chronically Exposed to Nicotine." *Brain Research* 954: 73–81.

Grant, B. F., et al. (2004). "Nicotine Dependence and Psychiatric Disorders in the United States." *Archives of General Psychiatry* 61: 1107–1115.

Greden, J. F., and Walters, A. (1997). "Caffeine." In J. H. Lowinson, P. Ruiz, R. B. Millman, and J. G. Langrod, eds., *Substance Abuse: A Comprehensive Textbook*, 3rd ed. (pp. 294–307). Baltimore: Williams & Wilkins.

Greenberg, J. A., et al. (2006). "Coffee, Diabetes, and Weight Control." *American Journal of Clinical Nutrition* 84: 682–693.

Grimshaw, G. M., and Stanton, A. (2006). "Tobacco Cessation Interventions for Young People." *Cochrane Database of Systematic Reviews*, Issue 4, CD003289.

Hajek, P., et al. (2009). "Relapse Prevention Interventions for Smoking Cessation." *Cochrane Database of Systematic Reviews* 21: CD03999.

Harris, J. E., et al. (2004). "Cigarette Tar Yields in Relation to Mortality from Lung Cancer in the Cancer Prevention Study II Prospective Cohort, 1982–8." *British Medical Journal* 328: 72–76.

Harvard School of Public Health. (2007). "Trends in Smoke Nicotine Yield and Relationship to Design Characteristics Among Popular U.S. Cigarette Brands, 1997–2005." A Report of the Tobacco Research Program, Division of Public Health Practice, Harvard School of Public Health.

Henley, S. J., et al. (2007). "Tobacco-Related Disease Mortality Among Men Who Switched from Cigarettes to Spit Tobacco." *Tobacco Control* 16: 22–28.

Higdon, J. V., and Frei, B. (2006). "Coffee and Health: A Review of Recent Human Research." *Critical Reviews in Food Science and Nutrition* 46: 101–123.

Hughes, J. R. (2001). "Distinguishing Nicotine Dependence from Smoking: Why It Matters to Tobacco Control and Psychiatry." *Archives of General Psychiatry* 58: 817–818.

Hughes, J. R., et al. (2007). "Antidepressants for Smoking Cessation." *Cochrane Database of Systematic Reviews*, Issue 1, CD000031.

Jahanfar, S. and Sharifah, H. (2009). "Effects of Restricted Caffeine Intake by Mother on Fetal, Neonatal and Pregnancy Outcome." *Cochrane Database of Systematic Reviews* 15: CD006965.

Jimenez-Ruiz, C., et al. (2009). "Varenicline: A Novel Pharmacotherapy for Smoking Cessation." *Drugs* 69: 1319–1338.

Jorenby, D. E., et al. (2006). "Efficacy of Varenicline, an α4β2 Nicotinic Acetylcholine Receptor Partial Agonist, vs Placebo or Sustained-Release

Bupropion for Smoking Cessation: A Randomized Controlled Trial." *Journal of the American Medical Association* 296: 56–63.

Kuczkowski, K. M. (2009). "Caffeine in Pregnancy." *Archives of Gynecology and Obstetrics* 280: 695–698.

Lambert, R.A., et al. (2006). "A Pragmatic, Unblinded, Randomized, Controlled Trial Comparing an Occupational Therapy-Led Lifestyle Approach and Routine GP Care for Panic Disorder Treatment in Primary Care." *Journal of Affective Disorders* 99: 63–71.

Linnet, K. M., et al. (2009). "Coffee Consumption During Pregnancy and the Risk of Hyperkinetic Disorder and ADHD: A Prospective Cohort Study." *Acta Pediatrica* 98: 173–179.

Magkos, F., and Kavouras, S. A. (2005). "Caffeine Use in Sports, Pharmacokinetics in Man, and Cellular Mechanisms of Action." *Critical Reviews in Food Science and Nutrition* 45: 535–562.

McCowan, L. M. E., et al. (2009). "Spontaneous Preterm Birth and Small for Gestational Age Infants in Women Who Stop Smoking Early in Pregnancy: Prospective Cohort Study." *British Medical Journal* 338: b1081.

McCusker, R. R., et al. (2003). "Caffeine Content of Specialty Coffees." *Journal of Analytical Toxicology* 27: 520–522.

McGehee, D. S. (2006). "Nicotinic and Opioid Receptor Interactions in Nicotine Addiction." *Molecular Interventions* 6: 311–314.

Morbidity and Mortality Weekly Report. (2009a, January 23). "State-Specific Smoking-Attributable Mortality and Years of Potential Life Lost—United States, 2000–2004." *MMWR Weekly* 58: 29–33. Available at www.cdc.gov/mmwr

Morbidity and Mortality Weekly Report. (2009b, November 13). "Cigarette Smoking Among Adults and Trends in Smoking Cessation—United States, 2008." *MMWR Weekly* 58: 1227–1232. Available at www.cdc.gov/mmwr

Moreno, A. Y., et al (2010). "A Critical Evaluation of a Nicotine Vaccine Within a Self-Administration Behavioral Model." *Molecular Pharmaceutics*. 7: 431–441.

Naqvi, N. H., et al. (2007). "Damage to the Insula Disrupts Addiction to Cigarette Smoking." *Science* 315: 531–534.

Ng, S. P., and Zelikoff, J. T. (2007). "Smoking During Pregnancy: Subsequent Effects on Offspring Immune Competence and Disease Vulnerability in Later Life." *Reproductive Toxicology* 23: 428–437.

Oncken, C. A., and Kranzler, H. R.. (2009). "What Do We Know About the Role of Pharmacotherapy for Smoking Cessation Before or During Pregnancy?" *Nicotine and Tobacco Research* 11: 1265–1273.

Oncken, C. A., et al. (2006). "Efficacy and Safety of the Novel Selective Nicotinic Acetylcholine Receptor Partial Agonist, Varenicline, for Smoking Cessation." *Archives of Internal Medicine* 166: 1571–1577.

Pollack, A. Z., et al. (2010). "Caffeine Consumption and Miscarriage: A Prospective Cohort Study." *Fertility and Sterility* 93: 304–306.

Ranney, L., et al. (2006). "Systematic Review: Smoking Cessation Intervention Strategies for Adults and Adults in Special Populations." *Annals of Internal Medicine* 145: 845–856.

Ray, R., et al. (2009). "Effects of Atomoxetine on Subjective and Neurocognitive Symptoms of Nicotine Abstinence." *Journal of Psychopharmacology* 23: 168–176.

Riggs, P. D., et al. (1999). "Relationship of ADHD, Depression, and Non-Tobacco Substance Use Disorders to Nicotine Dependence in Substance-Dependent Delinquents." *Drug and Alcohol Dependence* 54: 195–205.

Rigotti, N. A. (2002). "Treatment of Tobacco Use and Dependence." *New England Journal of Medicine* 346: 506–512.

Rose, J. E., et al. (2003). "PET Studies of the Influence of Nicotine on Neural Systems in Cigarette Smokers." *American Journal of Psychiatry* 160: 323–333.

Salin-Pascual, R. J., et al. (1996). "Antidepressant Effect of Transdermal Nicotine Patches in Nonsmoking Patients with Major Depression." *Journal of Clinical Psychiatry* 57: 387–389.

Satel, S. (2006). "Is Caffeine Addictive? A Review of the Literature." *American Journal of Drug and Alcohol Abuse* 32: 493–502.

Sellers, E. M. (1998). "Pharmacogenetics and Ethnoracial Differences in Smoking." *Journal of the American Medical Association* 280: 179–180.

Spring, B., et al. (2003). "Reward Value of Cigarette Smoking for Comparably Heavy Smoking Schizophrenic, Depressed, and Nonpatient Smokers." *American Journal of Psychiatry* 160: 316–322.

Stead, L. F., et al. (2006). "Telephone Counseling for Smoking Cessation." *Cochrane Database of Systematic Reviews*, Issue 13, CD002850.

Stolerman, I. P., and Jarvis, M. J. (1995). "The Scientific Case That Nicotine Is Addictive." *Psychopharmacology* 117: 2–10.

Strandberg, A. Y., et al. (2008). "The Effect of Smoking in Midlife on Health-Related Quality of Life in Old Age: A 26-Year Prospective Study." *Archives of Internal Medicine* 168: 1946–1947.

Stroud, L. R., et al. (2009). "Maternal Smoking During Pregnancy and Neonatal Behavior: A Large-Scale Community Study." *Pediatrics* 123: e842–e848.

Teo, K. K., et al. (2006). "Tobacco Use and Risk of Myocardial Infarction in 52 Countries in the INTERHEART Study: A Case-Controlled Study." *Lancet* 368: 642–658.

Thapar, A., et al. (2009). "Prenatal Smoking Might Not Cause Attention-Deficit/Hyperactivity Disorder: Evidence from a Novel Design." *Biological Psychiatry* 66: 722–727.

Tobacco Use and Dependence Clinical Practice Guideline Panel, Staff, and Consortium Representatives. (2000). "A Clinical Practice Guideline for Treating Tobacco Use and Dependence, a U.S. Public Health Service Report." *Journal of the American Medical Association* 283: 3244–3254.

Tonstad, S., et al. (2006). "Effect of Maintenance Therapy with Varenicline on Smoking Cessation: A Randomized Controlled Trial." *Journal of the American Medical Association* 296: 64–71.

Tsoh, J. Y., et al. (2000). "Development of Major Depression After Treatment for Smoking Cessation." *American Journal of Psychiatry* 157: 368–374.

U.S. Department of Health and Human Services. (1986). "The Health Consequences of Involuntary Smoking: A Report of the Surgeon General." Centers for Disease Control and Prevention, Office of Smoking and Health. U.S. Government Printing Office. www.cdc.gov/tobacco

U.S. Department of Health and Human Services. (1988). "The Health Consequences of Smoking—Nicotine Addiction: A Report of the Surgeon

General." Centers for Disease Control and Prevention, Office of Smoking and Health. U.S. Government Printing Office. www.cdc.gov/tobacco

U.S. Department of Health and Human Services. (2006). "The Health Consequences of Involuntary Exposure to Tobacco Smoke: A Report of the Surgeon General." Centers for Disease Control and Prevention, Office of Smoking and Health. U.S. Government Printing Office. www.cdc.gov/tobacco

Weng, X., et al. (2008). "Maternal Caffeine Consumption During Pregnancy and the Risk of Miscarriage: A Prospective Cohort Study." *American Journal of Obstetrics and Gynecology* 198: 279.e1–e8.

Wisborg, K., et al. (2003). "Maternal Consumption of Coffee During Pregnancy and Stillbirth and Infant Death in the First Year of Life: Prospective Study." *British Medical Journal* 326: 420–422.

Zierler-Brown, S. L., and Kyle, J. A. (2007). "Oral Varenicline for Smoking Cessation." *Annals of Pharmacotherapy* 41: 95–99.

Chapter 12

Cocaine, the Amphetamines, and Nonamphetamine Behavioral Stimulants

Cocaine and the amphetamines are powerful psychostimulants that markedly affect mental functioning and behavior. In exerting their acute behavioral stimulant effects, these drugs augment the action of several neurotransmitters, the most important of which is dopamine. Cocaine and the amphetamines, in addition to other actions, increase dopaminergic activity on the nucleus accumbens, other limbic structures, and the limbic cortex associated with behavioral reinforcement, compulsive abuse, drug dependency, and cue-induced drug craving. Cocaine and the amphetamines are therefore widely recognized as important drugs of compulsive abuse. Paradoxically, these drugs also have a variety of therapeutic uses, although today reasonable alternatives are available for most of them. All psychostimulants have significant side effects, toxicities, and patterns of abuse.

In low doses, cocaine and other psychostimulants evoke an alerting, arousing, or behavior-activating response that is not unlike a normal reaction to an emergency or stress. Physiologically, blood pressure and heart rate increase, pupils dilate, blood flow shifts from skin and internal organs to muscle, and oxygen levels rise, as does the level of glucose in the blood. In the central nervous system (CNS), psychostimulants produce positive and attractive effects that include an elevation of mood, induction of euphoria, increased alertness, reduced fatigue, a sense of increased energy, decreased appetite, improved task performance, and relief from boredom.

These positive effects, however, are offset by many negatives. Anxiety, insomnia, and irritability are common side effects. As doses increase, irritability and anxiety become more intense, and a pattern of psychotic behavior may appear. Eventually, intense dependence develops, a dependence that so far has resisted treatment and rehabilitation.

COCAINE

The leaves of *Erythroxylon coca* have been used since ancient times in their native South America for religious, mystical, social, euphoriant, and medicinal purposes—most notably to increase endurance, promote a sense of well-being, reduce fatigue, increase stamina, induce euphoria, and alleviate hunger (Calatayud and Gonzalez, 2003). Chewing the leaves as an endurant produces a usual total daily dose of cocaine of up to about 200 milligrams, a point that will become more important later in this discussion. Today, the relevant clinical issues related to cocaine's history have to do largely with the changes over time in dosage, route of administration, patterns of use, and technology of production.

The active alkaloid in *E. coca* was isolated in 1855 and purified and named cocaine in 1860. At the same time, the introduction of the syringe and hypodermic needle led to many attempts to use cocaine to produce local anesthesia for surgery. Perhaps the first medical report of cocaine's local anesthetic action was made in 1880.[1] Further identification of cocaine's local anesthetic properties was made by several surgeons, and cocaine became widely used for topical anesthesia, spinal anesthesia, and nerve blocks from about 1884 until about 1918, when procaine (Novocaine) was developed as the first synthetic local anesthetic. Procaine is devoid of psychological and dependence-producing effects.

In 1884, Sigmund Freud advocated the use of cocaine to treat depression and to alleviate chronic fatigue. He described cocaine as a magical and marvelous drug with the ability even to cure opioid (morphine and heroin) addiction. While using cocaine to relieve his own depression, Freud described the drug as inducing exhilaration and lasting euphoria that in no way differs from the normal euphoria of

---

[1] At that time, no other anesthetics (general or local) had been discovered. Surgery was limited to brief procedures conducted without anesthetic or with the patient under alcohol intoxication.

the healthy person. However, he did not immediately perceive its side effects—tolerance, dependence, a state of psychosis, and withdrawal depression. In his later writings, Freud called cocaine the "third scourge" of humanity, after alcohol and heroin, perhaps an appropriate description.

Around the end of the nineteenth century in the United States, there were no restrictions on the sale or consumption of cocaine. Thus, the drug was incorporated into numerous patent medicines and the beverage Coca-Cola, which contained approximately 60 milligrams of cocaine per 8-ounce serving. In the late 1800s, however, concern about cocaine's toxicities increased, with several hundred reports of cocaine intoxication and several reported deaths. About 1910, President Taft proclaimed cocaine to be Public Enemy Number 1, and in 1914 the Harrison Narcotic Act banned the incorporation of cocaine into patent medicines and beverages. With enforcement of the Narcotic Act, cocaine use decreased during the 1930s, largely replaced by the newly available amphetamines, which were cheaper and produced longer-lasting yet similar effects. Cocaine all but disappeared until the late 1960s, when tight federal restrictions on their distribution raised the cost of amphetamines, once again making cocaine attractive.

In the 1980s, a new epidemic of cocaine use began with the widespread availability of crack cocaine, intended for use by inhalation (smoking) rather than injection. This cocaine epidemic continues today, although the relatively inexpensive and widely available methamphetamine is currently more widely encountered. Cocaine users today are characterized by three patterns of use:

- Occasional users usually nasally "snort" (inhale) "lines" of powder containing cocaine hydrochloride; each line usually contains about 25 milligrams of the drug.
- Frequent, heavy users either snort the drug or smoke the freebase form for a recreational high.
- Regular users have developed tolerance to cocaine; they either inject water-soluble solutions of cocaine hydrochloride in doses of 100 milligrams to 1 gram or more or they smoke the freebase form in similar doses. These users usually continue to abuse the drug until their money runs out.

The use of high doses of either cocaine hydrochloride or the base form of cocaine is characterized by high-dose, rapid-onset effects and the rapid development of both toxicity and dependency. One of the most addictive and reinforcing of the abused drugs, cocaine has been used at some time by about 25 million people in the United States. The estimated U.S. cocaine market exceeded $70 billion in street value in 2005, exceeding revenues by corporations such as Starbucks. There is a tremendous demand for cocaine in the U.S. market, particularly among single adults and professionals with discretionary income. Cocaine's status as a club drug shows its immense popularity among the "party crowd." With the increased availability of lower-cost methamphetamine, the number of cocaine users has stabilzed. Its use, however, continues, and, as with methamphetamine, is associated with a range of violent and premature deaths, including homicides, suicides, and accidents. This toxicity is discussed below.

Forms of Cocaine

The leaf of *E. coca* contains about 1 percent cocaine. When the leaves are soaked and mashed, cocaine is extracted in the form of coca paste (60 to 80 percent cocaine). Coca paste is usually treated with hydrochloric acid to form the less potent, water-soluble salt *cocaine hydrochloride* before it is exported. The powdered hydrochloride salt can be absorbed through the nasal mucosa (snorted) and, because this salt form is water soluble, it can be injected intravenously. However, in the hydrochloride form, cocaine decomposes when it is heated and is destroyed at the temperature of smoke, making it unsuitable for use by inhalation. In contrast, cocaine base, also known as *freebase* or *crack cocaine*, is insoluble in water but is soluble in alcohol, acetone, or ether. Heating the freebase converts cocaine to a stable vapor that can be inhaled. The name *crack* is derived from the sound of cocaine crystals popping when smoked.

Cocaine hydrochloride ("crystal" or "snow"), when snorted as a line of drug, provides a dose of about 25 milligrams; a user might sniff about 50 to 100 milligrams of drug at a time. The smoking of crack cocaine yields average doses in the range of 250 milligrams to 1 gram (Table 12.1). The consequences of these higher doses are severe and are discussed later in this chapter.

Pharmacokinetics

Absorption

Cocaine is absorbed from all sites of application, including mucous membranes, the stomach, and the lungs. Thus, cocaine can be snorted, smoked, taken orally, or injected intravenously. Table 12.1 presents some pharmacokinetic data for common methods of administration. Snorted intranasally, cocaine hydrochloride poorly crosses the mucosal membranes since the drug is a potent vasoconstrictor (one of its defining pharmacological actions), constricting blood vessels and limiting its own absorption. As a consequence, only about 20 to 30 percent of the snorted drug is absorbed through the nasal mucosa into blood,

TABLE 12.1 Effects of cocaine administration

Administration		Initial onset of action	Duration of "high" (min)	Average acute dose (mg)	Peak plasma levels (ng/ml)	Purity (%)	Bioavailability (% absorbed)
Route	Mode						
Oral	Coca leaf chewing	300–600	45–90	20–50	150	0.5–1	25
Oral	Cocaine HCl	600–1800		100–200	150–200	20–80	20–30
Intranasal	Snorting cocaine HCl	120–180	30–45	5–30	150	20–80	20–30
Intravenous	Cocaine HCl	30–45	10–20	25–50	300–400	10–100	100
				>200	1000–1500		
Smoking	Coca paste	8–10	5–10	60–250	300–800	40–85	6–32
	Free base	8–10	5–10	250–1000	800–900	90–100	6–32
	Crack	8–10	5–10	250–1000	?	50–95	6–32

From M. S. Gold, "Cocaine (and Crack): Clinical Aspects," in J. H. Lowinson, P. Ruiz, R. B. Millman, and J. G. Langrod, eds., *Substance Abuse: A Comprehensive Textbook,* 3rd ed. (Baltimore: Williams & Wilkins, 1997), p. 185.

with plasma levels not peaking for 30 to 60 minutes. The time course of the pharmacological effects (the subjective "high") parallels the plasma levels as well as the amount of drug actually in brain tissue. With nasal inhalation, the euphoric effect is prolonged (because the drug is absorbed slowly) and the drug may persist in plasma for up to 6 hours.

When cocaine base is vaporized and smoked, drug molecules pass through the pharynx into the trachea and onto lung surfaces, from which absorption is rapid and quite complete. Onset of effects is within seconds, peaks at 5 minutes, and persists for about 30 minutes. Only about 6 to 32 percent of the initial amount vaporized ever reaches plasma.

Intravenous injection of cocaine hydrochloride bypasses all the barriers to absorption, placing the total dose of drug immediately into the bloodstream. The 30- to 60-second delay in onset of action simply reflects the time it takes the drug to travel from the site of injection through the pulmonary circulation and into the brain.

Distribution

Cocaine penetrates the brain rapidly; initial brain concentrations far exceed the concentrations in plasma. After it penetrates the brain, cocaine is rapidly redistributed to other tissues. Cocaine freely crosses the placental barrier, achieving levels in the fetus equal to those in the mother.

Metabolism and Excretion

Cocaine has a biological half-life in plasma of only about 50 minutes; it is rapidly and almost completely metabolized by enzymes located both in plasma and in the liver. Although it is rapidly removed from plasma, it is more slowly removed from the brain, in which it can be detected for 8 or more hours after initial use. Urine can test positive for cocaine for up to 12 hours. The major metabolite of cocaine is the inactive compound *benzoylecgonine* (BE; Figure 12.1), which can be detected in the urine for about 48 hours and much longer (up to 2 weeks) in chronic users. Urine detection of BE forms the primary basis of drug testing for cocaine use. The persistence of BE in urine implies that high-dose, long-term users might accumulate drug in their body tissues. Recently, Garcia-Bournissen and coworkers (2009) studied the identification of cocaine and BE in human hair following cessation of drug use. They concluded that cocaine and BE could be detected for several months; hair closest to the scalp took 3 to 4 months to become negative.

The metabolic interaction between cocaine and ethanol is interesting and important. In people who use cocaine and concurrently drink

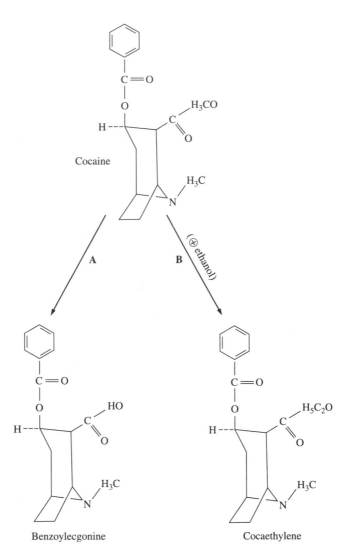

FIGURE 12.1 Structures of cocaine and the products of cocaine metabolism.
A. Normal metabolism to benzoylecognine. **B.** Metabolism to the abnormal, active
metabolite cocaethylene, formed from the interaction between cocaine and alcohol.
Cocaethylene is the ethyl ester of benzoylecognine.

alcohol, a unique ethyl ester of benzoylecgonine is produced by the
liver enzymes that metabolize the two drugs. This metabolite (called
cocaethylene; see Figure 12.1) is pharmacologically as active as cocaine
in blocking the presynaptic dopamine reuptake transporter, potentiating the euphoric effect of cocaine, increasing the risk of dual dependency, and increasing the severity of withdrawal with chronic patterns
of use (Bunney et al., 2001). The cocaethylene metabolite is actually

more toxic than cocaine and exacerbates cocaine's toxicity (Farooq et al., 2009; Wilson et al., 2009). The half-life of cocaethylene is about 150 minutes, outlasting cocaine in the body.

Mechanism of Action

Pharmacologically, cocaine has three prominent actions that account for virtually all its physiological and psychological effects; cocaine is the only drug that possesses these three characteristics.

1. It is a potent *local anesthetic.*
2. It is a *vasoconstrictor,* strongly constricting blood vessels and raising blood pressure.
3. It is a powerful *psychostimulant* with strong behavioral reinforcing qualities.

The psychostimulant property leads to compulsive abuse of and dependence on the drug. Therefore, this section focuses on the actions that lead to its psychostimulation and its behavior-reinforcing properties. Its vasoconstrictive and cardiac depressant actions contribute to severe cardiovascular and cerebrovascular toxicities (Phillips et al., 2009).

For 25 years, cocaine has been known to potentiate the synaptic actions of dopamine and serotonin. The potentiation occurs as a result of cocaine's ability to block the active reuptake of these neurotransmitters into the presynaptic nerve terminals from which they were released (Figure 12.2). Currently, most focus is on cocaine's blockade of the presynaptic transporter for dopamine as being crucial to its behavior-reinforcing and psychostimulant properties; there is also possible serotonin involvement, as discussed later.

Blockade of the dopamine transporter markedly increases the levels of dopamine within the synaptic cleft, an observation well documented in animal and human studies. Increased dopamine levels in the nucleus accumbens (NA) and other components of the dopaminergic reward system seem to be responsible for the euphoric/psychostimulant effects of the drug. This is discussed further in Chapter 17.

Thomsen and coworkers (2009a, 2009b) compared behavioral responsiveness to cocaine in normal mice and in mice lacking either the dopamine reuptake transporter or the serotonin reuptake transporter. Normal mice easily acquired the tendency to self-administer cocaine upon exposure to the drug, as did mice lacking the serotonin transporter. Mice lacking the dopamine reuptake transporter failed to reliably self-administer cocaine. This suggests a less significant role for serotonin on the direct rewarding effects of cocaine. However, serotonin may play a more substantial role in effects that lead to relapse to cocaine following detoxification.

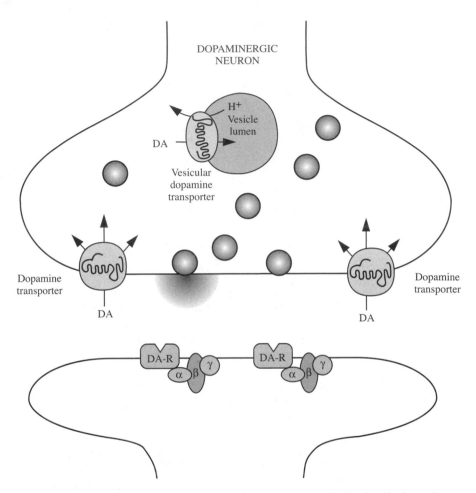

FIGURE 12.2 Dopamine nerve terminal and transporter proteins involved in the active uptake of dopamine (DA). Two transporters are shown. The first is a vesicular DA transporter located in the cytoplasm of the presynaptic neuron, bound to DA-containing storage vesicles. This transporter carries DA from the cytoplasm into storage. The second type of DA transporter is found on the synaptic membrane of the presynaptic neuron and functions to transport DA from the synaptic cleft into the presynaptic nerve terminal, recycling the transmitter and ending the process of synaptic transmission. It is the second transporter that is blocked by cocaine, prolonging the action of DA in the synaptic cleft. Amphetamines function to induce the release of increased amounts of DA from the storage vesicles into the synaptic cleft. The result is the same: increased amounts of DA at the postsynaptic receptor (DA-R).

Pharmacological Effects in Human Beings

Effects of Short-Term, Low-Dose Use

Low-dose (25 to 75 milligrams) nontoxic *physiological responses* to cocaine include increased alertness, motor hyperactivity, tachycardia, vasoconstriction, hypertension, bronchodilation, increased body temperature, pupillary dilation, increased glucose availability, and shifts in blood flow from the internal organs to the muscles. *Psychological effects* of low doses include immediate euphoria, giddiness, enhanced self-consciousness, and forceful boastfulness that last only about 30 minutes. This period is followed by one of milder euphoria mixed with anxiety, which can last for 60 to 90 minutes, followed by a more protracted anxious state that spans hours.

During acute and subacute intoxication, thoughts typically race and speech becomes rapid, often pressured, even garrulous, and sometimes tangential and incoherent. Appetite is markedly suppressed but later rebounds. Sleep is delayed; fatigue is postponed but later rebounds. Conscious awareness and mental acuity are increased but are followed by depression. Motor activity is increased, with agitation, restlessness, and a feeling of the need to be in constant motion. Perhaps most important, cocaine promotes one's desire to take more cocaine, even instead of such important reinforcers as food.

Low-dose acute effects of cocaine are difficult to maintain either (1) because the perceived effects promote increased use or (2) because tolerance develops and higher doses must be taken to perceive continued effects or avoid withdrawal. Thus, a person "graduates" rapidly to the use of higher doses and the onset of increased risks and toxicities.

Effects of Moderate-Dose Use

As the dose of cocaine or its duration of use increases, all the effects are intensified, and a rebound depression follows. There is a progressive loss of coordination, followed by tremors and eventually seizures. CNS activation is followed by depression, dysphoria, anxiety, somnolence, and drug craving. Although sexual interest may be heightened by using cocaine, and high doses (injected or smoked) are sometimes described as orgasmic, cocaine is not an aphrodisiac. Sexual dysfunction is common in heavy users, since they lose interest in interpersonal and sexual interactions. Further, when social and sexual dysfunction is combined with the isolation that a cocaine-dependent person experiences, normal interpersonal, sensual, and sexual interactions are further compromised.

Organ-specific medical and physiological risks as well as complications of cocaine use are listed in Table 12.2. In the CNS, acute use of cocaine may cause movement disorders, seizures, local depletions of oxygen (cerebral ischemia), vascular thrombosis, intracranial hemorrhage and hemorrhagic strokes.

TABLE 12.2 Organ-specific medical and physiological risks and complications of cocaine use

Central nervous system
Ischemic or hemorrhagic strokes
Seizures
Movement disorders
Intracranial hemorrhage

Cardiac complications
Acute myocardial infarction (heart attack)
Cardiac arrhythmias
Sudden cardiac arrest and death
Heart failure
Myocarditis (infections of the heart)
Ruptured aorta

Pulmonary complications
Nasal-septal perforations
Inhalation injuries
Immunity-related diseases
Pulmonary edema, hemorrhage
Bronchiolitis (inflammation of the bronchial tree)

Gastrointestinal complications
Ulcers, perforations of the stomach and upper intestine
Bowel ischemia (lack of oxygen)
Intestinal infarction

Renal complications
Renal failure
Renal ischemia

Maternal, fetal, and neonatal complications
Maternal
    Spontaneous abortion, abruptio placentae
    Placenta previa, stillbirth
Fetal
    Growth retardation, premature delivery
    Congenital anomalies
    Cerebral infarction and/or hemorrhage
Neonatal
    Drug withdrawal, seizure disorders
    Cardiovascular system complications

Cardiac complications associated with moderate use include hypertensive crises, cardiac ischemia (lack of oxygen), cardiac arrhythmias, heart failure, infected heart tissue or valves, heart attacks, rupture of the aorta, and sudden death. Complications can occur during prolonged use or with single use. Indeed, the cardiac side effects comprise the single greatest cause of premature deaths due to cocaine (Phillips et al., 2009).

Nasal and pulmonary complications include nasal-septal perforation, pulmonary lesions, hemorrhage, edema, and infections. Gastrointestinal and renal complications can also be seen (see Table 12.2).

With or without alcohol, cocaine plays a role in fatal automobile crashes. The mechanisms are unclear but probably involve visual deficits, alterations in judgment, incoordination, and feeling of power. Finally, morbidity and mortality in cocaine-positive persons admitted to emergency rooms is most commonly due to violence-related injury, as opposed to other medical conditions resulting from their cocaine use. In cocaine-positive emergency room patients, 24 percent of chief complaints were related to violent trauma, and an autopsy study found that the most common cause of death among cocaine-positive patients (37 percent) was violent injury (Walton et al., 2009).

Effects of Long-Term, High-Dose Use

Although low doses of cocaine can cause CNS stimulation that is pleasurable and euphoric, higher doses produce toxic symptoms, including anxiety, sleep deprivation, hypervigilance, suspiciousness, paranoia, and persecutory fears. A person taking cocaine may become hyperreactive, paranoid, and impulsive and may display a repetitive, compulsive pattern of behavior. The person can have a markedly altered perception of reality and become aggressive or homicidal in response to imagined persecution. These behaviors make up what is called a *toxic paranoid psychosis.*

Other high-dose, long-term effects of cocaine use include interpersonal conflicts (resulting from the sense of isolation and paranoia), depression, dysphoria, and bizarre and violent psychotic disorders that can last days or weeks after a person stops using the drug. In its most extreme form, a cocaine psychosis is characterized by paranoia; impaired reality testing; anxiety; a stereotyped, compulsive, repetitive pattern of behavior; and vivid visual, auditory, and tactile hallucinations. More subtle changes in behavior may include irritability, hypervigilance, extreme psychomotor activation, paranoid thinking, impaired interpersonal relations, and disturbances of eating and sleeping. An acutely toxic dose of cocaine has been estimated to be about 2 milligrams per kilogram of body weight. Thus, 150 milligrams of cocaine is a toxic one-time dose for a 150-pound (70-kilogram) person. Serious physiological toxicity follows higher doses.

Comorbidity

Cocaine-dependent people are typically young (12 to 39 years of age), dependent on at least three drugs, and male (75 percent). Like persons dependent on alcohol and heroin, cocaine addicts often show a certain profile on personality tests—they are reckless, rebellious, and have a low tolerance for frustration and a craving for excitement. They tend to have coexisting psychopathology (30 percent have anxiety disorders, 67 percent suffer from clinical depression, and 25 percent exhibit paranoia).

Other comorbidities include bipolar disorder, antisocial personality disorder, posttraumatic stress disorder, and attention deficit/hyperactivity disorder. Many have been or will be alcoholics or heroin addicts as well. They use opiates and alcohol either to enhance the effects of cocaine or to medicate themselves for unwanted side effects—calming jitters, dulling perceptions, and reducing paranoia to indifference. Intravenous drug users often take cocaine and heroin together in a mixture known as a speedball. Probably more than half of people treated for cocaine abuse are also alcoholic, and the rate of alcoholism in the families of cocaine addicts is high.

Cocaine and Pregnancy

One of the tragedies of the late twentieth century was the birth of thousands of infants who were thought to have been injured in utero by cocaine taken by their mothers while pregnant. Figure 12.3 outlines the effects of cocaine on the fetus. Indirect effects result from cocaine's vasoconstrictive action on the mother's blood vessels, decreasing blood flow to the uterus and placenta and reducing oxygen delivery to the fetus. Vasoconstriction in either the mother or the fetus can increase blood pressure in the fetus, leading to intracerebral hemorrhage, thickening of heart muscle, and various vascular and structural abnormalities.

In humans, the most common consequences to the infant of cocaine abuse during pregnancy include premature birth, respiratory distress, bowel infarctions, cerebral infarctions, reduced head circumference, and increased risk of seizures. Other adverse effects may include neurodevelopmental aberrations (Derauf et al., 2009) and basic alterations in gene expression leading to infant behavioral dysregulation, poor behavioral control and emotional dysregulation, and vulnerability to substance use in adolescence (Lester and Padbury, 2009). Obviously, cocaine use during pregnancy should be considered to be fetotoxic.

In Figure 12.3, note that cocaine also exerts adverse direct effects on the fetus. Cocaine easily crosses the placental barrier, and fetal concentrations can equal those in the mother. Direct organ toxicity can involve the heart, the urinary system, the gastrointestinal (GI) tract, and

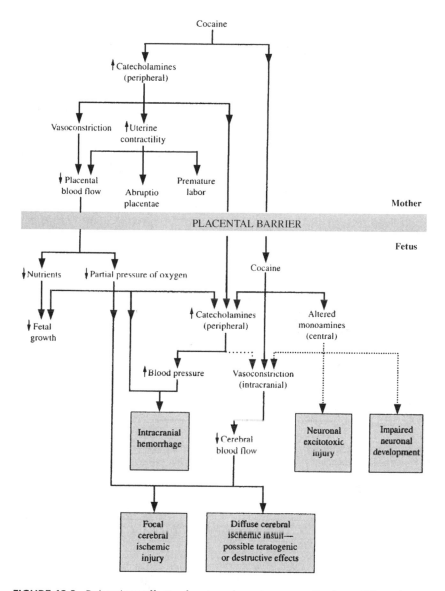

FIGURE 12.3   Deleterious effects of maternal cocaine use on the fetus. Effects that appear plausible on the basis of current information but whose confirmation requires more supporting evidence are indicated by dotted lines.

the CNS. As the brain develops, exposure of the fetus to cocaine may promote serious destructive lesions, leading to a neonatal neurological syndrome typified by abnormal sleep patterns, tremors, poor feeding, irritability, occasional seizures, and an increased risk or incidence of sudden infant death syndrome (SIDS).

Some have tried to define a fetal cocaine syndrome. However, because of the wide spectrum of indirect and direct effects on the fetus, any such syndrome is not as clearly defined as the fetal alcohol syndrome, and cocaine use by the mother is usually only one of many undesirable influences in the children's lives. Babies born into a drug-using environment that may also include poverty experience little physical or emotional nurturing, so bonding may be incomplete or absent. Cocaine's effects on the unborn and newborn may also be related to poor nutrition, poor hygiene, and neglect. Cocaine compromises the mother's or any caregiver's ability to respond to the baby through talking, eye contact, and tactile stimulation. The specific interactional behavior of cocaine-using mothers is still under investigation.

Singer and colleagues (2004) assessed the effects of maternal cocaine use on cognitive functioning in offspring at 4 years of age. Prenatal exposure to cocaine was associated with an increased risk for specific cognitive impairments; by age 4, cocaine-exposed offspring were less likely than their peers to have above-average IQs. The researchers also concluded that environmental intervention through foster or adoptive care was associated with a lower likelihood of mental retardation among cocaine-exposed children, even those with heavier drug exposure. Therefore, considering the role of environment and a slow, progressive recovery (about 4 years), the effects of prenatal cocaine exposure hopefully may diminish over time, especially in the context of environmental interventions (Williams and Ross, 2007).

Neurotoxicity of Cocaine

The possible neurotoxic effects of cocaine are difficult to measure by the persistence of neurological abnormalities for a period following cessation of drug use. Cocaine is a short-acting drug and is not present in the body if the drug is not repeatedly ingested, smoked, or injected. Toomey and coworkers (2003) conducted a twin study (all males) in which only one member had experienced heavy stimulant abuse (cocaine and/or methamphetamine). Subjects underwent a comprehensive battery of neuropsychological tests. Timed tests demonstrated evidence of long-term residual neuropsychological impairments in the abusers consistent with persistent psychomotor slowing and slowed reactions associated with cocaine abuse.

Drug-abstinent users may show persistent detrimental changes in their brains with associated alterations in memory function. Bartzokis and colleagues (1999) demonstrated that in men who were cocaine dependent, doses of cocaine usually caused a "subclinical" form of brain damage of the kind usually caused by vascular insufficiency. It is possible that this kind of injury could predispose to early-onset dementia and other neurological syndromes as subtle brain damage accumulates and adds to the effects of normal aging.

It now appears that *cocaine* can induce acute hyperthermia, which disrupts the blood-brain barrier, causing some degree of neurotoxicity secondary to this disruption. Sharma and coworkers (2009) state that "cocaine was able to enhance cellular stress as seen by upregulation of heat shock protein expression and resulted in marked neuronal and glial cell damage at the time of blood-brain-barrier disruption, . . . [thus,] cocaine-induced blood-brain-barrier disruption is instrumental in precipitating brain pathology" (p. 297).

Pharmacological Treatment of Cocaine Dependency

At the outset, it should be stated that there are no pharmacotherapies for cocaine addiction that have been proven or approved by the Food and Drug Administration (FDA; Sofuoglu and Kosten, 2006). Cognitive-behavioral therapy and contingency management strategies have been somewhat useful in preventing relapse (Vocci and Montoya, 2009), and pharmacotherapy can fortify cognitive regulation of behavior (Vocci and Elkashef, 2005). Pharmacological strategies include blocking euphoria, reducing withdrawal and negative mood symptoms (for example, depression), ameliorating craving, and enhancing the prefrontal cortical projections that seem to be impaired in cocaine-dependent patients. Since frontal cortical projections to the ventral tegmentum and nucleus accumbens are glutaminergic, compounds regulating glutaminergic transmission are in early clinical trials. Agents include such drugs as topiramate and lamotrigine (Gonzalez et al., 2007; Uys and LaLumiere, 2008).

Since cocaine as a euphoriant acts indirectly by blocking the presynaptic reuptake of dopamine, agents that can substitute for cocaine as either direct or indirect dopaminergic agonists might be thought to ameliorate not only withdrawal symptoms but also craving and relapse. Disulfiram (Antabuse), used as an aversion agent in the treatment of alcoholism, has dopaminergic effects and has been shown to be somewhat effective (Malcolm et al., 2008; Gavel-Cruz and Weinshenker, 2009; Haile et al., 2009; Pani et al., 2010). McCann (2008) suggested use of buprenorphine/naloxone (Suboxone; Chapter 10). Other dopaminergic agents include methylphenidate (Ritalin) and bupropion (Wellbutrin). Finally, significant attention is being focused on modafinil (Provigil) (Martinez-Raga, et al, 2008; Anderson et al., 2009) as a potential therapy that does not serve as a reinforcer in cocaine abusers (Vosburg et al., 2010).

In common with other classes of abused drugs, cocaine dependence has been shown to be strongly associated with depression (Rounsaville, 2004). Therefore, antidepressant drugs appear indicated. Of these, serotonin reuptake inhibitors are relatively ineffective, but agents such as bupropion (Wellbutrin, discussed earlier) are effective. Other comorbid psychiatric disorders are anxiety disorders, bipolar disorder, borderline personality disorder, and/or antisocial personality disorder. Each requires treatment in order for cocaine abuse treatment to be effective.

Anticraving or antirelapse agents are an area of intense study. Studies are currently focusing on two areas: antiepileptic neuromodulators and cannabinoid antagonists. Gabapentin (Neurontin; Chapter 6), a neuromodulator, has been reported to be effective in the treatment of cocaine dependence, although Gonzalez and coworkers (2007) found it to be without effect.

Gamma-vinyl-GABA (Vigabatrin, an antiepileptic drug available in Europe) exhibits anticraving effects against abused drugs, including cocaine (Brodie et al., 2009). Vigabatrin is an irreversible inhibitor of the enzyme *GABA transaminase;* it increases GABA activity and attenuates drug-induced increases in extracellular nucleus accumbens dopamine as well as the behaviors associated with this dopamine increase. Vigabatrin is being studied for use in treating cocaine dependence; its use is limited by a drug-induced loss of some portion of the visual field (peripheral vision), although a recent study demonstrated that short-term use of Vigabatrin is less damaging to visual fields than originally thought (Fechtner et al., 2006).

Cannabinoid antagonists (e.g., rimonabant) may be remarkably effective anticraving agents (Fattore et al., 2007). Unfortunately, rimonabant was removed from commercial sale in 2009. Future cannabinoid antagonists might have similar efficacy without unfortunate side effects (Chapter 14).

Many cocaine abusers seeking treatment have a history of childhood attention deficit/hyperactivity disorder (ADHD), and approximately 15 percent of cocaine abusers seeking treatment may have adult ADHD. Early studies of the efficacy of long-acting *methylphenidate* (Ritalin SR) on people with comorbid cocaine dependence and adult ADHD reported that the combined intervention of the drug plus relapse prevention therapy reduced both the ADHD and the cocaine dependency. Levin and coworkers (2007), in a placebo-controlled study of 106 people with comorbid ADHD and cocaine dependency, reported that methylphenidate-induced reductions in ADHD symptoms were accompanied by reductions in cocaine use. Volkow and coworkers (2008) reported that methylphenidate did not elicit cocaine craving unless it was coupled with cocaine cues. Therefore, the efficacy of methylphenidate appears to be context dependent.

Cocaine Vaccine for Cocaine Addiction

In a unique approach to dependency treatment, vaccines to treat cocaine and nicotine are being separately studied. Here, we discuss the status of the cocaine vaccine; the nicotine vaccine is discussed in Chapter 11. The idea behind both vaccines is to stimulate antibodies to the drug such that should the drug appear in the bloodstream, it would bind to the previously formed antibody and this complex would be too bulky to cross the blood-brain barrier, thus rendering the drug inactive.

The cocaine vaccine (termed TA-CD) is a cocaine derivative (succinylnorcocaine) coupled to recombinant cholera toxin B. It is designed to generate drug-specific antibodies that bind to cocaine and prevent it from travelling to the brain from the blood, thereby neutralizing its psychoaffective effect. While the concept is intriguing and promising, several important factors must be considered:

1. The vaccine must stimulate the production of sufficient antibodies to bind all the cocaine that might be snorted, smoked, or injected.
2. The induced antibodies must persist for sufficient time so that the vaccine need not be readministered at short intervals.
3. Cocaine users using the vaccine must not be able to override the amount of induced antibodies by taking very large quantities of cocaine.
4. The vaccine must be reasonably well tolerated

Two recent studies have investigated the relationship of efficacy to induction of sufficient antibody levels (Martell et al., 2009; Haney et al., 2010). In both studies, TA-CD vaccinations (five vaccine injections in one study and eight in the other) generated plasma antibody levels that varied greatly. The amount of antibody produced predicted clinical effectiveness. Antibody levels of 43 μg/ml or higher resulted in more cocaine-free urine samples than those with levels less than 43 μg/ml. Cocaine users with high antibody levels had robust reductions of good drug effect and cocaine quality. Discouraging was the observation that only 38 percent of the vaccinated cocaine users attained antibody levels greater than 43 μg/ml, and even those had only two months of adequate cocaine blockade. The most common adverse effect was local injection site irritation.

An interesting question is whether cocaine users who have been administered vaccine and have developed antibodies will be able to snort, smoke, or inject additional amounts of cocaine in order to overwhelm the amount of antibodies present and achieve a euphoriant effect (because the antibodies are saturated).

Even if the vaccine is successful, a cocaine-dependent person who has these antibodies in the blood may move to another drug or use large amounts of cocaine unless comorbid psychological issues are addressed. Stitzer and coworkers (2010) employed motivational (monetary) incentives to improve efficacy of the vaccine.

AMPHETAMINES

The amphetamines (Figure 12.4) are a structurally defined group of drugs that produce a variety of effects on both the CNS and the autonomic nervous system.[2] Amphetamines are also called *sympathomimetic agents* because they mimic the actions of adrenaline (epinephrine, one of the transmitters of our "sympathetic" nervous system). Amphetamines produce vasoconstriction, hypertension, tachycardia, and other signs and symptoms of our normal alerting response. These drugs also stimulate the CNS, producing tremor, restlessness, increased motor activity, agitation, insomnia, and loss of appetite. These actions result from an indirect action involving the presynaptic release of dopamine and norepinephrine and, to a lesser extent, direct stimulation of postsynaptic catecholamine receptors. Amphetamines have limited yet appropriate clinical use; they are widely abused, with significant personal and public health consequences. Representative amphetamines for clinical use in treating ADHD (Chapter 18) include *amphetamine* (Adderall) and *dextroamphetamine* (Dexedrine, DextroStat).

Amphetamines have long been used to treat a variety of disorders. Between 1935 and 1946, a list of 39 conditions for which amphetamines could be used in treatment was developed. The list included schizophrenia, morphine addiction, tobacco smoking, head injury, radiation sickness, hypotension, seasickness, severe hiccups, and caffeine dependence. During World War II, amphetamines were used to fight fatigue and enhance the performance of people in the armed services. In the 1960s, amphetamines were used as diet pills. Today, legitimate use is largely restricted to the clinical treatment of ADHD and occasionally in the treatment of narcolepsy.

---

[2] The *autonomic nervous system* (ANS) is frequently called the visceral nervous system because it regulates and maintains the homeostasis of the body's internal organs. It controls the function of the heart, the flow of blood, and the functioning of the digestive tract, and it regulates other internal functions that are essential for maintaining the balance necessary for life. The ANS comprises two subdivisions—the *sympathetic* and the *parasympathetic*. The function of the parasympathetic nervous system can be viewed as maintaining our "vegetative" functions, while the sympathetic nervous system handles the body's reaction to stress, fright, fear, and other responses that demand an immediate alerting response. Neurotransmitters in the sympathetic division of the ANS include epinephrine (adrenaline), norepinephrine, and dopamine.

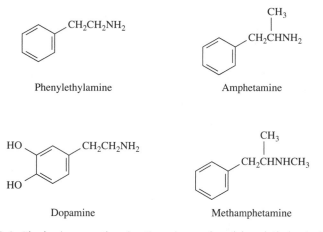

FIGURE 12.4 The basic sympathomimetic amine nucleus (phenylethylamine), the neurotransmitter dopamine (dihydroxyphenylethylamine), and the structures of amphetamine and methamphetamine.

Large-scale abuse (usually oral ingestion of amphetamine tablets) began in the late 1940s, primarily by students and truck drivers in efforts to maintain wakefulness, temporarily increase alertness, and delay sleep. Amphetamines continued to be used (and abused) as appetite suppressants, despite the fact that the anorectic effect persists only over the first two weeks of treatment, after which time it diminishes. In the late 1960s, the abuse pattern of amphetamines changed with the advent of injectable forms of the drug. These injectable products (by legitimate manufacturers) have been discontinued, so injection of methamphetamine today is illicit. Interest in the amphetamines today involves three areas:

- FDA-approved use in the treatment of narcolepsy and ADHD
- Off-label use as a "neuroenhancer" to improve memory, attention, and focus
- Compulsive abuse, especially with methamphetamine

Mechanism of Action

The amphetamines exert virtually all their physical and psychological effects by causing the release of norepinephrine and dopamine from presynaptic storage sites in nerve terminals. Other minor actions augment this releasing action, and all actions add up so that amphetamines act as highly potent releasers of dopamine (Barr et al., 2006). The behavioral stimulation and increased psychomotor activity appear to follow from the resulting stimulation of the dopamine receptors in the mesolimbic system, including the nucleus accumbens. The high-dose stereotypical behavior (including constant repetition of meaningless acts) appears to involve dopamine neurons in the basal ganglia.

The actions leading to an increase in aggressive behavior are complex. Clinically, this behavioral stimulant action is seen primarily in adults suffering from psychostimulant toxicity and consists of increases in stereotypical, repetitive behaviors. In children, low doses of amphetamines are used therapeutically to reduce aggressive behavior and activities characteristic of ADHD; in adults with a history of ADHD, behavioral calming can also occur.

Pharmacological Effects

As stated, amphetamines exert their peripheral and central actions largely by causing the release of norepinephrine and dopamine from presynaptic nerve terminals (see Figure 12.2). All the physical and behavioral effects of the amphetamines appear to follow from this action. Note that the release of dopamine increases the amount of dopamine available to the postsynaptic receptor, much as does cocaine. Both drugs have the net effect of increasing the amount of dopamine available (although through two different mechanisms), so cocaine abusers have difficulty distinguishing between the subjective effects of 8 to 10 milligrams of cocaine and 10 milligrams of dextroamphetamine when the doses are administered intravenously.

The pharmacological responses to amphetamines vary with the specific drug, the dose, and the route of administration. In general, with amphetamine itself, effects may be categorized as those observed at low to moderate doses (5 to 50 milligrams), usually administered orally, and those observed at high doses (more than approximately 100 milligrams), often administered intravenously. These dose ranges are not the same for all amphetamines. For example, dextroamphetamine is three to four times more potent than amphetamine. Low to moderate doses of dextroamphetamine range from 2.5 to 20 milligrams, while high doses are 50 milligrams or more. Because methamphetamine is even more potent, dose ranges must be lowered even more, although massive doses are taken by methamphetamine-dependent people who have developed a tolerance to the drug.

At low doses, all amphetamines increase blood pressure and heart rate, relax bronchial muscle, and produce a variety of other responses that follow from the body's alerting response. In the CNS, amphetamine is a potent psychomotor stimulant, producing increased alertness, euphoria, excitement, wakefulness, a reduced sense of fatigue, loss of appetite, mood elevation, increased motor and speech activity, and a feeling of power. Although task performance is improved, dexterity may deteriorate. When short-duration, high-intensity energy output is desired, such as during an athletic competition, a user's performance may be enhanced, despite the fact that his or her dexterity and fine motor skills may be impaired. Amphetamine metabolites are excreted in the urine and are detectable for up to 48 hours.

At moderate doses (20 to 50 milligrams), additional effects of amphetamines include stimulation of respiration, slight tremors, restlessness, a greater increase in motor activity, insomnia, and agitation. In addition, amphetamines prevent fatigue, suppress appetite, promote wakefulness, and cause sleep deprivation. As doses increase, this reaction is accompanied by the worsening or de novo production of anxiety disorders. Indeed, any drug that increases dopamine levels in the brain can worsen anxiety, possibly progressing from restlessness and nonspecific anxiety to obsessive behaviors, panic disorders, paranoia, and eventually a paranoid psychosis. Even compulsive gambling can be related to dopaminergic augmentation (Zack and Poulos, 2009).

A person who chronically uses high doses of amphetamines suffers from a different set of drug effects. Stereotypical behaviors include continual, purposeless, repetitive acts; sudden outbursts of aggression and violence; paranoid delusions; and severe anorexia. The harmful effects that are seen in the high-dose user include psychosis and abnormal mental conditions, weight loss, skin sores, infections resulting from neglected health care, and a variety of other consequences that occur both because of the actions of the drug itself and because of poor eating habits, lack of sleep, or the use of unsterile equipment for intravenous injections. Most high-dose users show a progressive deterioration in their social, personal, and occupational affairs. Also seen is amphetamine psychosis with paranoid ideation; many addicts must be hospitalized intermittently for treatment of episodes of psychosis. Today, psychosis is especially seen in people who abuse methamphetamine.

Cognitive Effects

Numerous studies have shown that daily or even one-time therapeutic doses of amphetamines can improve cognitive processing speed, attention, concentration, and psychomotor performance. This property underlies the use of amphetamine (Adderall, for example) and amphetaminelike drugs (for example, methylphenidate) as therapeutic treatments for child and adult ADHD as well as off-label use as a "neuroenhancer" to improve memory, attention, and focus.[3] However, high-dose amphetamine abuse, especially with methamphetamine, is associated with cognitive impairments secondary to severe anxiety

---

[3] Drugs considered to be cognitive enhancers are referred to as "neuroenhancers" or as "nootropics."

as well as profound neuropsychological deficits and toxicity (discussed below).

The toxic dose of amphetamine varies widely. Severe reactions can occur even from low doses (20 to 30 milligrams). On the other hand, people who have not developed tolerance have survived doses of 400 to 500 milligrams. Even larger doses are tolerated by chronic users. The slogan "Speed kills" refers not only to a direct fatal effect of single doses of amphetamine but also to the deteriorating mental and physical condition that occurs in the addicted user.

Effects in Pregnancy

The possible adverse effects of methamphetamine (MA) abuse during pregnancy have been studied. There is no clear-cut pattern of congenital abnormalities, although infants born to MA-abusing mothers exhibit growth retardation and lower birth weights (Smith et al., 2006). An increased rate of intracerebral hemorrhage can be observed. There is evidence of psychometric deficits, poor academic performance, behavioral problems, cognitive slowing, and general maladjustment. Sowell and colleagues (2010) reported that brain structures known to be sites of neurotoxicity in adult MA abusers are more vulnerable to prenatal MA exposure than to alcohol exposure and more severe cortical damage is associated with more severe cognitive deficits in offspring.

Dependence and Tolerance

As potent psychomotor stimulants and behavior-reinforcing agents, the amphetamines are prone to compulsive abuse. Physical dependence is readily induced in both humans and laboratory animals and follows a classical positive conditioning model (the positive reward leads to further drug use). Once drug use is stopped, a person experiences a withdrawal syndrome, although it is less dramatic than the withdrawal associated with either opioids (Chapter 10) or barbiturates (Chapter 7). Withdrawal symptoms associated with the amphetamines include increased appetite, weight gain, decreased energy, and increased need for sleep. Patients may develop a voracious appetite and sleep for several days after amphetamines are discontinued. Paranoid symptoms may persist during drug withdrawal but generally do not develop as a result of withdrawal. The patient suddenly discontinuing amphetamine use may develop severe depression and become suicidal. Management of amphetamine withdrawal does not require detoxification, but it does require appropriate and cautious clinical observation of the patient, recognition of depression, and treatment with an appropriate antidepressant drug if clinically necessary. Antipsychotic drugs, such as risperidone, quetiapine, or aripiprazole (Chapter 4), may be necessary to treat paranoid or psychotic reactions or behaviors (Shoptaw et al., 2009).

Tolerance rapidly develops and can necessitate higher and higher doses, which starts a vicious cycle of drug use and withdrawal. At this point, tolerance to the euphoriant effects develops, and periods of prolonged binge drug use begin. This tolerance, combined with the memory of drug-induced highs, leads to further drug intake, social withdrawal, and a focus on procuring drugs. Comer and coworkers (2001) studied the effects of 5 and 10 milligrams of methamphetamine twice daily on nonusers in a controlled setting. Positive feelings toward the drug were experienced only on day 1; on subsequent days, the subjects felt a loss of positive effects and increases in negative feelings (dizziness, nausea, depression, and so on). This rapid development of tolerance to the positive effects may lead to the psychotic consequences seen in long-term use. There has been concern about the long-term outcomes of amphetamine and methylphenidate use for treatment of ADHD. Poulton (2006) reviews this topic and concludes:

> It would appear that the medical complications associated with amphetamine addiction are not relevant to the therapeutic use of stimulant medication in the treatment of ADHD, although there is limited information on extended periods of treatment lasting 10 years or more. (p. 551)

Methamphetamine

Methamphetamine is a more potent drug than dextroamphetamine. Generally considered to be an illicit drug, manufactured in clandestine laboratories, methamphetamine was originally an approved drug, effective in the treatment of ADHD. Today, however, after so much negative publicity, it is rarely used legitimately and illicit use dominates. Methamphetamine is easily synthesized from readily obtainable chemicals, including pseudoephedrine. Methamphetamine has now been clearly demonstrated to be a neurotoxic agent.

Like cocaine hydrochloride, methamphetamine (the hydrochloride salt) is broken down at the temperatures that must be achieved for it to be vaporized for smoking. However, when converted to its crystalline form, methamphetamine can be effectively vaporized and inhaled in smoke. As a drug of abuse, crystalline methamphetamine is also known as ice, speed, crystal, crank, and go, with considerable overlap in nomenclature with other amphetamines except for "ice," which refers to the smokable form of methamphetamine. The speed of crystalline methamphetamine's absorption through the lungs and mucous membranes is as rapid as or even more rapid than that experienced with intravenous injection. Thus, ice is to methamphetamine as crack is to cocaine: the crystalline, smokable form of the parent compound. However, unlike cocaine, methamphetamine has an extremely long half-life (about 12 hours), resulting in an intense, persistent drug action.

Pharmacokinetics

Smoking ice results in its near-immediate absorption into plasma, with additional absorption continuing over the next 4 hours. The blood level then progressively declines. The biological half-life of methamphetamine is more than 11 hours. After distribution to the brain, about 60 percent of the methamphetamine is slowly metabolized in the liver, and the end products are excreted through the kidneys, along with unmetabolized methamphetamine (about 40 percent is excreted unchanged) and small amounts of its pharmacologically active metabolite, amphetamine.

Pharmacological Effects

The effects of methamphetamine closely resemble the effects produced by cocaine. Both drugs are potent psychomotor stimulants and positive reinforcers; self-administration is extremely difficult to control and modify, especially in abusers who either inject or smoke the drug. Repeated high doses of methamphetamine are associated with violent behavior and paranoid psychosis. Such doses cause long-lasting decreases in dopamine and serotonin in the brain. These changes appear to be persistent, at best. Just as prolonged cocaine use can result in psychoses resembling paranoid schizophrenia, smoking crystalline methamphetamine produces a pattern of acute delusional and psychotic behavior. However, unlike that of cocaine, ice-induced psychosis can persist for days or weeks. Fatalities have resulted from cardiac toxicity.

Neurotoxicity

As noted, prolonged use of methamphetamine is associated with a variety of toxicities, including psychosis. The etiology of these persistent, if not irreversible, toxicities is now being elucidated. These neurotoxicities include damage to serotonin and dopamine nerve terminals as well as neuronal death and replacement with astroglial and microglial cells in the brain (Sekine et al., 2008; Cadet and Krasnova, 2009). The serotonergic injuries have been implicated in the regulation of mood (e.g., depression), anxiety, and aggressive disorders (Sekine et al., 2006). Dopaminergic defects have been associated with slower motor function and memory deficits in users, perhaps with predisposition to future development of neurodegenerative disorders such as Parkinson's disease, depending on the degree of reversal with drug discontinuation (Volkow et al., 2001).

Thompson and coworkers (2004) first identified the structural defects in the human brain associated with chronic methamphetamine abuse (Figure 12.5). The authors noted an 11 percent reduction in gray matter (neurons), an 8 percent reduction in hippocampal volume, a 7 percent increase in white matter volume, and a 20 percent increase in ventricular (fluid chamber) volumes. These data indicate neuronal loss with scar replacement (white matter) and compensatory increase in ventricle size. The hippocampal losses can account for persistent mood and memory alterations.

The molecular basis of this neurotoxic effect of methamphetamine is becoming more clear. Overall, these mechanisms include "oxidative stress (metabolic activation), activation of genetically-based transcription factors, DNA damage, excitotoxicity, blood-brain barrier (BBB) breakdown, glial cell activation, and neuronal degeneration" (Cadet and

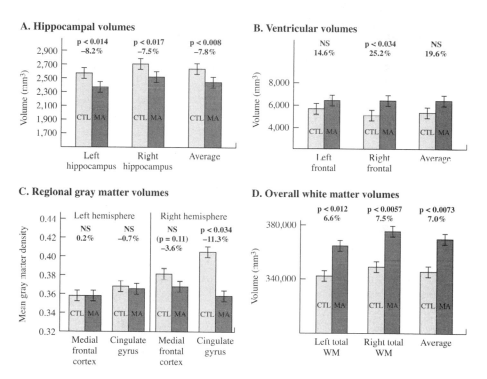

FIGURE 12.5 Comparison of brain structure volumes in methamphetamine abusers (MA) and healthy control persons (CTL). Mean values and mean percentage gains/losses (%) are shown for the volumes of the hippocampus (**A**), ventricles (**B**), total cerebral gray matter (**C**), and white matter (**D**). In general, hippocampal and gray matter volumes decrease and are compensated for by increases in ventricle and white matter volumes. NS = nonsignificant increase/decrease. The hippocampal volume deficits correlate with word recall (memory) performance. [Figure modified from Thompson et al. (2004), p. 6032, Figure 3.]

Krasnova, 2009, p. 101). Very importantly, acute and chronic methamphetamine intoxication "induces robust, widespread, but structure-specific leakage of the BBB, acute glial cell activation, and increased water content (edema), which are related to drug-induced brain hyperthermia (elevated temperature)" (Kiyatkin and Sharma, 2009, p. 65). Here, the damage mechanisms are similar to those seen in traumatic brain injuries (Gold et al., 2009), and BBB disruptions are most severe in limbic structures, including the amygdala, the hippocampus, and the caudate-putamen areas of the basal ganglia (Bowyer and Ali, 2006; Bowyer et al., 2008). The hippocampal damage should be sufficient to compromise learning and memory (Bowyer and Ali, 2006). Ramirez and coworkers (2009) explored the underlying mechanisms leading to BBB disruptions. Methamphetamine, through a hyperthermic-stress action, diminishes the DNA expression of cell-membrane-associated tight junction proteins, which diminishes the tightness of the cells that compose the tight junction of the BBB. This increases the porosity of the BBB and ultimately increases the migration of reactive oxygen molecules, such as white blood cells, into the brain, initiating the neuronal damage. Brain temperature appears critical to BBB disruption, and methamphetamine intoxication raises brain temperature, leading to BBB disruption, brain edema, and pathological injuries as described (Kiyatkin et al., 2007). This same action (and potential for brain injury) is also caused by methamphetamine derivatives, including MDMA (ecstasy) and 5-MeO-DiPT (Foxy) (Nakagawa and Kaneko, 2008; Gouzoulis-Mayfrank and Daumann, 2009).

Treatments of methamphetamine psychosis have been disappointing and are primarily "supportive." Akiyama (2006) studied 32 incarcerated females suffering from methamphetamine-induced psychosis. Psychotic relapses following discontinuation were common, sometimes persisting for over 30 months. Auditory and visual hallucinations, delusions of persecution, thought broadcasting, depression, and suicidal ideation were all common. Of currently available drugs, both traditional and atypical antipsychotic drugs seem most useful (Shoptaw et al., 2009). One experimental compound (H-290/51, an antioxidant inhibitor of lipid peroxidase), tested in a rat model of hyperthermia, blocked the hyperthermia-induced heat stress that can induce BBB impairment, brain edema formation, and neurotoxicity (Sharma et al., 2010).

NONAMPHETAMINE BEHAVIORAL STIMULANTS

An amphetamine is any drug with the basic amphetamine nucleus (see Figure 12.4). A *nonamphetamine behavioral stimulant* does not have this basic nucleus (Figure 12.6), but it shares the same action of potentiating the sympathomimetic actions of the neurotransmitter dopamine.

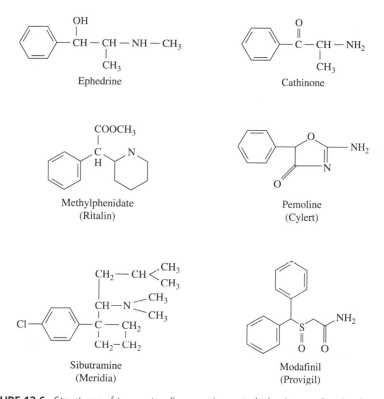

FIGURE 12.6 Structures of two naturally occurring catecholamine psychostimulants— ephedrine (from *Ephedra*, or ma-huang) and cathinone (from *Catha edulis*, or khat)— and four synthetic noncatecholamine psychostimulants—methylphenidate (Ritalin), pemoline (Cylert), sibutramine (Meridia), and modafinil (Provigil).

Nonamphetamine stimulants include ephedrine (found in nature in the Chinese herb ma-huang), pseudoephedrine, methylphenidate, pemoline, sibutramine, modafinil (Provigil), armodafinil (Nuvigil), and the herbal substance *khat*.

Ephedrine today has little use in medicine other than IV use in anesthesiology to transiently increase blood pressure. Most use of ephedrine has been in herbal medicine (Chapter 8). Ephedrine acts by transiently releasing body epinephrine, a normal adrenal hormone that causes elevations in blood pressure and heart rate. Ephedrine also transiently reduces appetite. It has been incorporated into numerous herbal and dietary supplements for both energy increase and weight loss. Unfortunately, the drug can be toxic or even fatal when combined with other stimulant drugs such as caffeine. Pseudoephedrine is used in cough and cold medicines to relieve nasal congestion. However, as a compound used in the illicit manufacture of methamphetamine, its use has been placed under prescription-only restriction.

Methylphenidate (Ritalin) is a nonamphetamine behavioral stimulant in which the regular-release formulation has a half-life of 2 to 4 hours. Its primary medical use is in the treatment of ADHD (Chapter 18). Mechanistically, methylphenidate increases the synaptic concentration of dopamine by blocking the presynaptic dopamine transporter (a cocainelike action) and also perhaps by slightly increasing the release of dopamine (an amphetaminelike or ephedrinelike action). When methylphenidate is injected intravenously, experienced cocaine users can perceive a cocainelike or amphetaminelike rush, an action not usually experienced with oral dosage. At clinically relevant doses, methylphenidate blocks more than 50 percent of the dopamine transporters 60 minutes after oral administration. A slow uptake of methylphenidate into the brain after oral administration accounts for the low rate of positive reinforcement effects seen with use of the drug.

Pemoline (Cylert) is a CNS stimulant structurally dissimilar to either methylphenidate or amphetamine (see Figure 12.6). Pemoline is presumed to reduce ADHD symptoms by potentiating CNS dopaminergic transmission. It is thought to have a lower abuse potential than does either methylphenidate or amphetamine. Its use is limited by reports of rare instances of hepatitis, necessitating close monitoring of liver function. Indeed, the risks of pemoline outweigh its usefulness in treating ADHD, and it has been removed from the market.

Sibutramine (Meridia) is a serotonin, norepinephrine, and (to a lesser extent) dopamine reuptake inhibitor (it blocks their presynaptic transporter proteins). Sibutramine, formerly marketed as an antiobesity agent, is structurally related to amphetamine (see Figure 12.6), but it is not literally an amphetamine. Sibutramine is rapidly metabolized in the liver to active metabolites that are responsible for the drug's pharmacological actions. These metabolites reach a peak concentration in plasma in 3 to 4 hours; their half-life is 14 to 16 hours. Modest weight losses for up to a year have been reported, and the drug does not appear to have a potential for compulsive misuse. Significant increases in heart rate and blood pressure have been reported and may limit the use of the drug. Since the drug is a serotonin and norepinephrine reuptake inhibitor, it is probably an antidepressant drug, although it is not marketed for this purpose. However, in combination with other serotonin-type antidepressants, it may predispose to development of serotonin syndrome (Chapter 5). A higher number of cardiovascular events have been observed in people taking sibutramine. In 2010 the FDA noted the concern that sibutramine increases the risk of heart attacks and strokes in patients with a history of cardiovascular disease. The drug has been removed from the commercial market in Great Britian and Europe, and the FDA is considering removing it from the U.S. market.

Modafinil (Provigil; see Figure 12.6) is a nonamphetamine psychostimulant whose mechanism of psychostimulant action has recently been shown to block dopamine transporters in the human brain (including the nucleus accumbens) in a manner similar to that exerted by cocaine (Volkow et al., 2009). Modafinil does, however, appear to have a lower potential for abuse, although this potential should be considered in at-risk populations. Indeed, modafinil does not serve as a positive reinforcer in cocaine abusers (Vosburg et al., 2010) and has been used in the treatment of cocaine dependence (Martinez-Raga et al., 2008; Anderson et al., 2009). A potentially serious skin rash limits its use.

Modafinil has been approved by the FDA for treatment of three disorders: narcolepsy, shift-work sleep disorder, and obstructive sleep apnea with residual excessive sleepiness despite use of a continuous positive airway pressure (CPAP) device (Kumar, 2008). Modafinil has also been used in the treatment of ADHD, although the FDA has not approved it for this use. More recently, it has been used for enhancing cognitive performance, even in the absence of a therapeutic need. Used in this manner, modafinil and related drugs are referred to as nootropics, and this use has become both controversial and widespread among college students and others (Cakic, 2009).

Armodafinil (Nuvigil) is the active (R)-isomer of the racemic drug modafinil. As was the case with citalopram/escitalopram, methylphenidate/desmethylphenidate, and amphetamine/dextroamphetamine, when an older racemic medicine goes generic and therefore becomes less expensive, a manufacturer can market the active "half" of the drug under a new patent (making it more expensive). That seems to be the situation with armodafinil, making it twice as "potent" as the racemic counterpart (therefore, one uses half of the milligram dosage). Nuvigil is protected by a U.S. patent that expires in 2023.

Armodafinil has the same FDA indications as does modafinil (Krystal et al., 2010), which can become generic in 2012. Provigil sales were about $1 billion in 2008, accounting for half of its manufacturer's revenue. As of January 2010, armodafinil was being considered as the first FDA-approved medication for combating jet lag, an additional indication for wakefulness-promoting medicines. The consumer will once again have a choice of less expensive or more expensive versions of the same medicine.

Catha edulis is a flowering shrub in East Africa. The leaves and fresh shoots are commonly known as *khat*. Khat can be chewed (like loose tobacco) or brewed as a tea at a daily dose of up to several hundred grams. Khat has stimulant properties and is said to cause excitement, loss of appetite, and euphoria, similar to the effects of amphetamine or cocaine. The active components of khat are cathinone (see Figure 12.6) and cathine (closely related in structure). Khat must be used fresh because cathinone, the pharmacologically more active substance, deteriorates within about 48 hours after harvest. Cathinone increases the levels of dopamine in the CNS and therefore is considered to be the primary psychostimulant in khat (al-Hebshi and Skaug, 2005). The cathine appears to be a mild psychostimulant, comparable to caffeine in potency. Khat is being increasingly encountered as a substance of abuse in the United States and elsewhere.

STUDY QUESTIONS

1. Compare and contrast cocaine and amphetamine.

2. What is crack? What is ice?

3. Describe the three major actions of cocaine.

4. Discuss the effects of cocaine on the fetus.

5. What are some of the issues in and therapeutic approaches to treating cocaine dependence?

6. Describe the behavioral states that are observed in high-dose amphetamine users.

7. Describe the effects of amphetamine on neurotransmission, neurotransmitters, and the CNS reward system.

8. Discuss the evidence for and against methamphetamine neurotoxicity.

9. Compare and contrast psychostimulants with clinical antidepressants.

10. What is meant by the phrase "Speed kills"?

11. What is modafinil? How does it differ from amphetamine? What are its potential uses? How does it differ from armodafinil?

REFERENCES

Akiyama, K. (2006). "Longitudinal Clinical Course Following Pharmacological Treatment of Methamphetamine Psychosis Which Persists After Long-Term Abstinence." *Annals of the New York Academy of Sciences* 1074: 125–134.

Anderson, A. L., et al. (2009). "Modafinil for the Treatment of Cocaine Dependence." *Drug and Alcohol Dependence* 104: 133–139.

Barr, A. A., et al. (2006). "The Need for Speed: An Update on Methamphetamine Addiction." *Journal of Psychiatry and Neuroscience* 31: 301–313.

Bartzokis, G., et al. (1999). "Magnetic Resonance Imaging Evidence of 'Silent' Cerebrovascular Toxicity in Cocaine Dependence." *Biological Psychiatry* 45: 1203–1211.

Bowyer, J. F., and Ali, S. (2006). "High Doses of Methamphetamine That Cause Disruption of the Blood-Brain Barrier in Limbic Regions Produce Extensive Neuronal Degeneration in Mouse Hippocampus." *Synapse* 60: 521–532.

Bowyer, J. F., et al. (2008). "Neurotoxic-Related Changes in Tyrosine Hydroxylase, Microglia, Myelin, and the Blood-Brain Barrier in the Caudate-Putamen from Acute Methamphetamine Exposure." *Synapse* 62: 193–204.

Brodie, J. D., et al. (2009). "Randomized, Double-Blind, Placebo-Controlled Trial of Vigabatrin for the Treatment of Cocaine Dependence in Mexican Parolees." *American Journal of Psychiatry* 166: 1269–1277.

Bunney, E. B., et al. (2001). "Electrophysiological Effects of Cocaethylene, Cocaine, and Ethanol on Dopaminergic Neurons of the Ventral Tegmental Area." *Journal of Pharmacology and Experimental Therapeutics* 297: 696–703.

Cadet, J. L., and Krasnova, I. N. (2009). "Molecular Basis of Methamphetamine-Induced Neurodegeneration." *International Review of Neurobiology* 88: 101–119.

Cakic, V. (2009). "Smart Drugs for Cognitive Enhancement: Ethical and Pragmatic Considerations in the Era of Cosmetic Neurology." *Journal of Medical Ethics* 35: 611–615.

Calatayud, J., and Gonzalez, A. (2003). "History of the Development and Evolution of Local Anesthesia Since the Coca Leaf." *Anesthesiology* 98: 1503–1508.

Comer, S. D., et al. (2001). "Effects of Repeated Oral Methamphetamine Administration in Humans." *Psychopharmacology* 155: 397–404.

Derauf, C., et al. (2009). "Neuroimaging of Children Following Prenatal Drug Exposure." *Seminars in Cell and Developmental Biology* 20: 441–454.

Farooq, M. U., et al. (2009). "Neurotoxic and Cardiotoxic Effects of Cocaine and Ethanol." *Journal of Medical Toxicology* 5: 134–138.

Fattore, L., et al. (2007). "An Endocannabinoid Mechanism in Relapse to Drug Seeking: A Review of Animal Studies and Clinical Perspectives." *Brain Research—Brain Research Reviews* 53: 1–16.

Fechtner, R. D., et al. (2006). "Short-Term Treatment of Cocaine and/or Methamphetamine Abuse with Vigabatrin: Ocular Safety Pilot Results." *Archives of Ophthalmology* 124: 1257–1262.

Garcia-Bournissen, F., et al. (2009). "Pharmacokinetics of Disappearance of Cocaine from Hair After Discontinuation of Drug Use." *Forensic Science International* 189: 24–27.

Gaval-Cruz, M., and Weinshenker, D. (2009). "Mechanisms of Disulfiram-Induced Cocaine Abstinence: Antabuse and Cocaine Relapse." *Molecular Interventions* 9: 175–187.

Gold, M. S., et al. (2009). "Methamphetamine- and Trauma-Induced Brain Injuries: Comparative Cellular and Molecular Neurobiological Substrates." *Biological Psychiatry* 66: 118–127.

Gonzalez, G., et al. (2007). "Clinical Efficacy of Gabapentin versus Tiagabine for Reducing Cocaine Use Among Cocaine Dependent Methadone-Treated Patients." *Drug and Alcohol Dependence* 87: 1–9.

Gouzoulis-Mayfrank, E., and Daumann, J. (2009). "Neurotoxicity of Drugs of Abuse—The Case of Methylenedioxyamphetamines (MDMA, Ecstasy) and Amphetamines." *Dialogues in Clinical Neuroscience* 11: 305–317.

Haile, C. N., et al. (2009). "Pharmacogenetic Treatments for Drug Addiction: Cocaine, Amphetamine and Methamphetamine." *American Journal of Drug and Alcohol Abuse* 35: 161–177.

Haney, M., et al. (2010). "Cocaine-Specific Antibodies Blunt the Subjective Effects of Smoked Cocaine in Humans." *Biological Psychiatry* 67: 59–65.

Hebshi, N. N. al-, and Skaug, N. (2005). "Khat (*Catha edulis*): An Updated Review." *Addiction Biology* 10: 299–307.

Kiyatkin, E. A., and Sharma, H. S. (2009). Acute Methamphetamine Intoxication: Brain Hyperthermia, Blood-Brain Barrier, Brain Edema, and Morphological Cell Abnormalities." *International Review of Neurobiology* 88: 65–100.

Kiyatkin, E. A., et al. (2007). "Brain Edema and Breakdown of the Blood-Brain Barrier During Methamphetamine Intoxication: Critical Role of Brain Hyperthermia." *European Journal of Neuroscience* 26: 1242–1253.

Krystal, A. D., et al. (2010). "A Double-Blind, Placebo-Controlled Study of Armodafinil for Excessive Sleepiness in Patients with Treated Obstructive Sleep Apnea and Comorbid Depression." *Journal of Clinical Psychiatry* 71: 32–40.

Kumar, R. (2008). "Approved and Investigational Uses of Modafinil: An Evidence-Based Review." *Drugs* 68: 1803–1839.

Lester, B. M., and Padbury, J. F. (2009). "Third Pathophysiology of Prenatal Cocaine Exposure." *Developmental Neuroscience* 31: 23–35.

Levin, F. R., et al. (2007). "Treatment of Cocaine Dependent Treatment Seekers with Adult ADHD: Double-Blind Comparison of Methylphenidate and Placebo." *Drug and Alcohol Dependence* 87: 20–29.

Malcolm, R., et al. (2008). "The Safety of Disulfiram for the Treatment of Alcohol and Cocaine Dependence in Randomized Clinical Trials: Guidance for Clinical Practice." *Expert Opinion on Drug Safety* 7: 459–472.

Martell, B. A., et al. (2009). "Cocaine Vaccine for the Treatment of Cocaine Dependence in Methadone-Maintained Patients: A Randomized, Double-Blind, Placebo-Controlled Efficacy Trial." *Archives of General Psychiatry* 66: 1116–1123.

Martinez-Raga, J., et al. (2008). "Modafinil: A Useful Medication for Cocaine Addiction? Review of the Evidence from Neuropharmacological, Experimental and Clinical Studies." *Current Drug Abuse Reviews* 1: 213–221.

McCann, D. J. (2008). "Potential of Buprenorphine/Naltrexone in Treating Polydrug Addiction and Co-Occurring Psychiatric Disorders." *Clinical Pharmacology and Therapeutics* 83: 627–630.

Nakagawa, T., and Kaneko, S. (2008). "Neuropsychotoxicity of Abused Drugs: Molecular and Neural Mechanisms of Neuropsychotoxicity Induced by Methamphetamine, 3,4-Methylenedioxymethamphetamine (Ecstasy) and 5-Methoxy-N,N-Diisopropyltryptamine (Foxy)." *Journal of Pharmaceutical Sciences* 106: 2–8.

Pani, P. P., et al. (2010). "Disulfiram for the Treatment of Cocaine Dependence." *Cochrane Database of Systematic Reviews* CD007024.

Phillips, K., et al. (2009). "Cocaine Cardiotoxicity: A Review of the Pathophysiology, Pathology, and Treatment Options." *American Journal of Cardiovascular Drugs* 9: 177–196.

Poulton, A. (2006). "Long-Term Outcomes of Stimulant Medication in Attention-Deficit Hyperactivity Disorder." *Expert Review of Neurotherapy* 6: 551–561.

Ramirez, S. H., et al. (2009). "Methamphetamine Disrupts Blood-Brain Barrier Function by Induction of Oxidative Stress in Brain Endothelial Cells." *Journal of Cerebral Blood Flow & Metabolism* 29: 1933–1945.

Rounsaville, B. J. (2004). "Treatment of Cocaine Dependence and Depression." *Biological Psychiatry* 56: 803–809.

Sekine, Y., et al. (2006). "Brain Serotonin Transporter Density and Aggression in Abstinent Methamphetamine Abusers." *Archives of General Psychiatry* 63: 90–100.

Sekine, Y., et al., (2008). "Methamphetamine Causes Microglial Activation in the Brains of Human Abusers." *Journal of Neuroscience* 28: 5756–5761.

Sharma, H. S., et al. (2009). "Cocaine-Induced Breakdown of the Blood-Brain Barrier and Neurotoxicity." *International Review of Neurobiology* 88: 297–334.

Sharma, H. S., et al. (2010). "A New Antioxidant Compound H-290/51 Attenuates Nanoparticle Induced Neurotoxicity and Enhances Neurorepair in Hyperthermia." *Acta Neurochirurgica Supplementum* 106: 351–357.

Shoptaw, S. J., et al. (2009). "Treatment for Amphetamine Psychosis." *Cochrane Database of Systematic Reviews* CD003026.

Singer, L. T., et al. (2004). "Cognitive Outcomes of Preschool Children with Prenatal Cocaine Exposure." *Journal of the American Medical Association* 291: 2448–2456.

Smith, L. M., et al. (2006). "The Infant Development, Environment, and Lifestyle Study: Effects of Prenatal Methamphetamine Exposure, Polydrug Exposure, and Poverty on Intrauterine Growth." *Pediatrics* 118: 1149–1156.

Sofuoglu, M., and Kosten, T. R. (2006). "Emerging Pharmacological Strategies in the Fight Against Cocaine Addiction." *Expert Opinion on Emerging Drugs* 11: 91–98.

Sowell, E. R., et al. (2010). "Differentiating Prenatal Exposure to Methamphetamine and Alcohol versus Alcohol and Not Methamphetamine Using Tensor-Based Brain Morphometry and Discriminant Analysis." *Journal of Neuroscience* 30: 3876–3885.

Stitzer, M. L., et al. (2010). "Drug Users' Adherence to a 6-Month Vaccination Protocol: Effects of Motivational Incentives." *Drug and Alcohol Dependence* 107: 76–79.

Thompson, P. M., et al. (2004). "Structural Abnormalities in the Brains of Human Subjects Who Use Methamphetamine." *Journal of Neuroscience* 24: 6028–6036.

Thomsen, M., et al. (2009a). "Dramatically Decreased Cocaine Self-Administration in Dopamine but Not Serotonin Transporter Knock-Out Mice." *Journal of Neuroscience* 29: 1087–1092.

Thomsen, M., et al. (2009b). "Lack of Cocaine Self-Administration in Mice Expressing a Cocaine-Insensitive Dopamine Transporter." *Journal of Pharmacology and Experimental Therapeutics* 331: 204–211.

Toomey, R., et al. (2003). "A Twin Study of the Neuropsychological Consequences of Stimulant Abuse." *Archives of General Psychiatry* 60: 303–310.

Uys, J. D., and LaLumiere, R. T. (2008). "Glutamate: The New Frontier in Pharmacology for Cocaine Addiction." *CNS & Neurological Disorders—Drug Targets* 7: 482–491.

Vocci, F. J., and Elkashef, A. (2005). "Pharmacotherapy and Other Treatments for Cocaine Abuse and Dependence." *Current Opinions in Psychiatry* 18: 265–270.

Vocci, F. J., and Montoya, I. D. (2009). "Psychological Treatments for Stimulant Misuse, Comparing and Contrasting Those for Amphetamine Dependence and Those for Cocaine Dependence." *Current Opinions in Psychiatry* 22: 263–268.

Volkow, N. D., et al. (2001). "Loss of Dopamine Transporters in Methamphetamine Abusers Recovers with Protracted Abstinence." *Journal of Neuroscience* 21: 9414–9418.

Volkow, N. D., et al. (2008). "Dopamine Increases in Striatum Do Not Elicit Craving in Cocaine Abusers Unless They Are Coupled with Cocaine Cues." *Neuroimage* 39: 1266–1273.

Volkow, N. D., et al. (2009). "Effects of Modafinil on Dopamine and Dopamine Transporters in the Male Human Brain: Clinical Implications." *Journal of the American Medical Association* 301: 1148–1154.

Vosburg, S. K., et al. (2010). "Modafinil Does Not Serve as a Reinforcer in Cocaine Abusers." *Drug and Alcohol Dependence* 106: 233–236.

Walton, M. A., et al. (2009). "Predictors of Violence Following Emergency Department Visit for Cocaine-Related Chest Pain." *Drug and Alcohol Dependence* 99: 79–88.

Williams, J. H., and Ross, L. (2007). "Consequences of Prenatal Toxin Exposure for Mental Health in Children and Adolescents: A Systematic Review." *European Child & Adolescent Psychiatry* 16: 243–253.

Wilson, L. D., et al. (2009). "Cocaine and Ethanol: Combined Effects on Coronary Artery Blood Flow and Myocardial Function in Dogs." *Academic Emergency Medicine* 16: 646–655.

Zack, M., and Poulos, C. X. (2009). "Parallel Roles for Dopamine in Pathological Gambling and Psychostimulant Addiction." *Current Drug Abuse Reviews* 2: 11–25.

Chapter 13

Ethyl Alcohol and the Inhalants of Abuse

ETHYL ALCOHOL

The term *alcohol* applies socially to *ethyl alcohol* (ethanol)—a psychoactive drug that is similar in most respects to all the other sedative-hypnotic compounds that were discussed in Chapter 7. The main difference from the other depressants is that ethanol is used primarily for recreational rather than medical purposes. Because ethanol is the second most widely used psychoactive substance in the world (after caffeine), its use as a sedative and intoxicant has created special problems for both individual users and society in general.

Ethyl alcohol is not merely a recreational beverage; it is a drug that, like any other psychoactive agent, affects the brain and behavior. Therefore, in discussing alcohol, we need to address its basic pharmacology (pharmacokinetics and pharmacodynamics) as well as its side effects, teratogenic effects, and toxicities. In addition, since alcohol ingestion is widely associated with drug dependence, treatment of alcohol dependence must be addressed.

Pharmacokinetics of Alcohol

Since alcohol is so rapidly and well absorbed orally, its major route of administration is the drinking of beverages containing the drug. Alcoholic beverages include beer, wine, and hard liquors; hard liquors, such as gin and whiskey, are fortified to alcohol levels beyond those achievable with fermentation.

Absorption

Ethyl alcohol is a simple two-carbon molecule (Figure 13.1). It is rarely drunk in its pure form; rather, it is found in 12 to 14 percent concentrations in wines and usually about 5 percent in beers (as much as 7 to 10 percent in some "microbrews," and as high as 10 to 12 percent in 16- and 24-ounce cans of fortified and caffeine-containing beverages). In "hard" liquors, alcohol is present in concentrations of 40 to 50 percent. In the latter, concentration is usually expressed as alcohol "proof," which is twice the percent concentration (for example, 80 proof = 40 percent ethanol). The appendix at the end of this chapter addresses the amount of alcohol that is present in representative forms of alcohol-containing beverages.

Alcohol is soluble in both water and fat, and it diffuses easily across all biological membranes. Thus, after it is drunk, alcohol is rapidly and completely absorbed from the entire gastrointestinal tract, although most is absorbed from the upper intestine because of its large surface area. The time from the last drink to maximal concentration in blood ranges from 30 to 90 minutes. In a person with an empty stomach, approximately 20 percent of a single dose of alcohol is absorbed directly from the stomach, usually quite rapidly. The remaining 80 percent is absorbed rapidly and completely from the upper intestine; the only limiting factor is the time it takes to empty the stomach.

Distribution

After absorption, alcohol is evenly distributed throughout all body fluids and tissues. The blood-brain barrier is freely permeable to alcohol. When alcohol appears in the blood and reaches a person's brain, it crosses the blood-brain barrier almost immediately. Alcohol is also freely distributed across the placenta and easily enters the brain of a developing fetus. Fetal blood alcohol levels are essentially the same as those of the drinking mother.

Metabolism and Excretion

Approximately 95 percent of the alcohol a person ingests is enzymatically metabolized by the enzyme *alcohol dehydrogenase*. The other 5 percent is excreted unchanged, mainly through the lungs.[1]

---

[1] Small amounts of alcohol are excreted from the body through the lungs; most of us are familiar with "alcohol breath." This excretion forms the basis for the breath analysis test because alcohol equilibrates rapidly across the membranes of the lung. In the "breathalyzer" test, a ratio of 1:2300 exists between alcohol in exhaled air and alcohol in venous blood. The blood alcohol concentration is easily extrapolated from the alcohol concentration in the expired air.

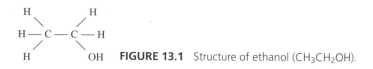

FIGURE 13.1   Structure of ethanol (CH_3CH_2OH).

About 85 percent of the metabolism of alcohol occurs in the liver. Up to 15 percent of alcohol metabolism is carried out by a gastric alcohol dehydrogenase enzyme, located in the lining of the stomach, which can decrease the blood level of alcohol by about 15 percent, obviously attenuating alcohol's systemic toxicity. The metabolism of alcohol by gastric alcohol dehydrogenase is part of what was called *first-pass metabolism* in Chapter 1. Rapid gastric emptying (as by drinking on an empty stomach) reduces the time that alcohol is susceptible to first-pass metabolism and results in increased blood levels. Drinking on a full stomach retains alcohol in the stomach, increases its exposure to gastric alcohol dehydrogenase, and reduces the resulting blood level of the drug.

Several years ago, Frezza and coworkers (1990) reported that whenever women and men consume comparable amounts of alcohol (after correction for differences in body weight), women have higher blood ethanol concentrations than men. The reasons appear to be threefold:

1. Women have about 50 percent less gastric metabolism of alcohol than men because women, whether alcoholic or nonalcoholic, have a lower level of gastric alcohol dehydrogenase enzyme. Since the gastric enzyme metabolizes about 15 percent of ingested alcohol, the blood alcohol concentration (BAC) is increased by about 7 percent over that in a male drinking the same weight-adjusted amount of alcohol.

2. Men may have a greater ratio of muscle to fat than do women. Men thus have a larger vascular compartment (fat has little blood supply). Therefore, alcohol is somewhat more diluted in men, again decreasing blood alcohol levels in men compared to women.

3. Women, with higher body fat than men (fat contains little alcohol), concentrate alcohol in plasma, drink for drink, more than men, raising the apparent blood level.

The metabolism of alcohol by alcohol dehydrogenase is only the first step in a three-step metabolic process involved in the breakdown of alcohol (Figure 13.2):

1. Alcohol dehydrogenase functions to convert alcohol to acetaldehyde. A coenzyme called *nicotinamide adenine dinucleotide* (NAD) is required for the activity of this enzyme. The availability of NAD is the rate-limiting step in this reaction; enough is present so that the

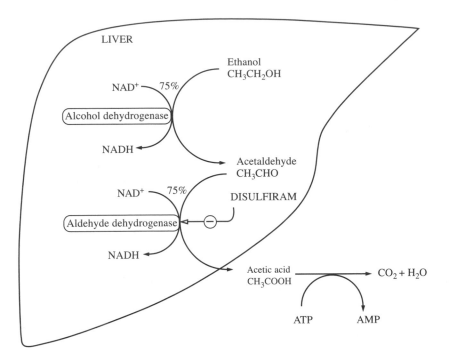

FIGURE 13.2 Metabolism of ethanol. Ethanol is oxidized by the enzyme alcohol dehydrogenase using NAD^+ (nicotinamide adenine dinucleotide) as a cofactor to form acetaldehyde. A second oxidative step converts acetaldehyde to acetic acid, which, in turn, is broken down to carbon dioxide and water. The first step involving alcohol dehydrogenase is the rate-limiting step. The drug disulfiram (Antabuse) blocks the second step by blocking the activity of aldehyde dehydrogenase. ATP = adenosine phosphate; AMP = adenosine monophosphate.

maximum amount of alcohol that can be metabolized in 24 hours is about 170 grams.

2. The enzyme *aldehyde dehydrogenase* converts acetaldehyde to acetic acid. The drug *disulfiram* (Antabuse) irreversibly inhibits this enzyme.

3. Acetic acid is broken down into carbon dioxide and water, thus releasing energy (calories).

The average person metabolizes about 10 to 14 milliliters of 100 percent alcohol per hour, independent of the blood level of alcohol. This rate is fairly constant for different people.[2] Figure 13.3 illustrates

---

[2] In biochemical terms, this is called zero-order metabolism. Virtually all other drugs are metabolized by first-order metabolism, which means that the amount of drug metabolized per unit time depends on the amount (or concentration) of drug in blood (see Chapter 1). Perhaps zero-order metabolism occurs because the amount of enzyme (or a cofactor required for activity of the enzyme) is limited and becomes saturated with only small amounts of alcohol in the body.

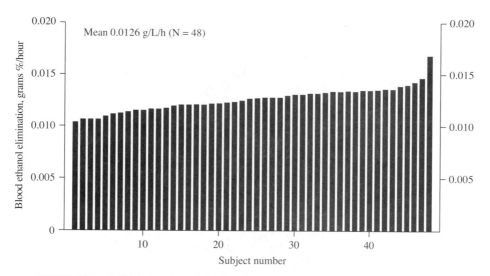

FIGURE 13.3 Individual variations in the elimination rate of ethanol as measured in 48 healthy males after they drank 0.68 gram of ethanol per kilogram of body weight. Neat whisky was ingested on an empty stomach. Values are expressed as grams of alcohol metabolized per liter of blood per hour. If expressed as grams%, 0.10 g/L/h would equate to a 0.01 grams% per hour fall in blood concentration; 0.15 g/L/hr would equal a 0.015 grams% per hour fall in blood concentration. [Reproduced from A. W. Jones, "Disposition and Fate of Ethanol in the Body." In J. C. Garriott, ed., *Medical-Legal Aspects of Alcohol*, 4th ed. Tucson, AZ: Lawyers & Judges Publishing Company, 2003, p. 73, Figure 3.9.]

the rate of alcohol elimination for a group of 48 healthy men administered a standard dose of ethanol. Here, the blood alcohol concentration falls at a rate of about 0.010 and 0.015 grams%/hour.[3] It takes an adult 1 hour to metabolize the amount of alcohol that is contained in a 1-ounce glass of 80 proof (40 percent) whiskey, a 4-ounce glass of 12 percent wine, a 12-ounce bottle of 5 percent beer, or a 6-ounce glass of 8 to 10 percent microbrew or fortified beer. Of note, commercially poured (for example, by bartenders) alcoholic drinks usually exceed these amounts by about 45 percent (Kerr, 2008).

Consumption of 4 to 5 ounces of wine, 12 ounces of 5 percent beer, or 1.0 to 1.5 ounces of 80 proof whiskey per hour would keep the blood levels of alcohol in a person fairly constant. If a person ingests more alcohol in any given hour than is metabolized, his or her blood concentrations increase. Consequently, there is a limit to the amount of alcohol a person can consume in an hour without becoming drunk. The appendix at the end of this chapter expands on the topic of drink equivalents.

[3] Grams% is the number of grams of ethanol that would be contained in 100 milliliters of blood.

These kinetics permit not only estimation of BAC after drinking a known amount of alcoholic beverage, but also estimation of the fall in blood concentration over time after drinking ceases. The following may serve to explain the relationship between the amounts of alcohol consumed, the resulting BAC, and the impairment of motor and intellectual functioning (here, driving ability): Most states define a BAC of 0.08 grams% as intoxication, and a person who drives with a BAC above this amount can be charged with driving while under the influence of alcohol. Thus, one might assume that a level of 0.07 grams% is acceptable but a level of 0.09 grams% is not. However, the behavioral effects of alcohol are not all or none; alcohol (like all sedatives) progressively impairs a person's ability to function. Thus, the 0.08 grams% blood level is only a legally established, arbitrary value. A person whose BAC is under 0.08 grams% yet functions with impairment detrimental to operation of a motor vehicle can still suffer criminal penalties. Driving ability is minimally impaired at a BAC of 0.01 grams%, but at 0.04 to 0.08 grams%, a driver has increasingly impaired judgment and reactions and becomes less inhibited. As a result, the risk of an accident quadruples. The deterioration of a person's driving ability continues at a BAC of 0.10 to 0.14 grams%, leading to a sixfold to sevenfold increase in the risk of having an accident. At 0.15 grams% and higher, a person is 25 times more likely to become involved in a serious accident.

Figure 13.4 illustrates the correlation between the number of drink equivalents imbibed, gender, body weight, and the resulting blood alcohol concentration. First choose the correct chart (male or female). Then find the number that is closest to your body weight in pounds. Look down the left column to find the number of drinks consumed. BAC is found by matching body weight with number of drinks ingested. Then note that BAC falls about 0.015 grams% every hour since the first drink was ingested. From the total number of drinks ingested, subtract the amount of alcohol that has been metabolized from the number of hours since drinking began (remember that approximately 1 drink equivalent is metabolized in 1 hour). The final figure is the approximate BAC. By calculating this number, the degree to which driving ability is impaired can be predicted.

Some agencies and organizations have even more stringent BAC standards than the states. For example, the Federal Department of Transportation regulations prohibit truck drivers from driving at 0.04 grams% and airline pilots from flying at 0.02 grams% after 8 hours of abstinence.

Factors that may alter the predictable rate of metabolism of alcohol are usually not clinically significant. With long-term use, however, alcohol can induce drug-metabolizing enzymes in the liver, increasing the liver's rate of metabolizing alcohol (and so inducing *tolerance*) as

Blood Alcohol Concentration – A Guide

One drink equals 1 ounce of 80 proof alcohol; 12-ounce bottle of beer; 2 ounces of 20% wine; 3 ounces of 12% wine.

Men

Drinks	Approximate blood alcohol percentage (grams%)								
	Body weight (pounds)								
	100	120	140	160	180	200	220	240	
0	.00	.00	.00	.00	.00	.00	.00	.00	Only safe driving limit
1	.04	.03	.03	.02	.02	.02	.02	.02	Impairment begins
2	.08	.06	.05	.05	.04	.04	.03	.03	Driving skills significantly affected
3	.11	.09	.08	.07	.06	.06	.05	.05	
4	.15	.12	.11	.09	.08	.08	.07	.06	Possible criminal penalties
5	.19	.16	.13	.12	.11	.09	.09	.08	
6	.23	.19	.16	.14	.13	.11	.10	.09	
7	.26	.22	.19	.16	.15	.13	.12	.11	Legally intoxicated
8	.30	.25	.21	.19	.17	.15	.14	.13	
9	.34	.28	.24	.21	.19	.17	.15	.14	
10	.38	.31	.27	.23	.21	.19	.17	.16	Criminal penalties

Alcohol is "burned up" by the body at .015 grams% per hour as follows:

Number of hours since starting first drink 1 2 3 4 5 6
Percent alcohol burned up .015 .030 .045 .060 .075 .090

Calculate BAC

Example:
180 lb. man? — 6 drinks in 4 hours
BAC = .130 grams% on chart
Subtract .060 grams% metabolized in 4 hours
BAC = .070 grams% DRIVING IMPAIRED

Women

Drinks	Approximate blood alcohol percentage (grams%)									
	Body weight (pounds)									
	90	100	120	140	160	180	200	220	240	
0	.00	.00	.00	.00	.00	.00	.00	.00	.00	Only safe driving limit
1	.05	.05	.04	.03	.03	.03	.02	.02	.02	Impairment begins
2	.10	.09	.08	.07	.06	.05	.05	.04	.04	Driving skills significantly affected
3	.15	.14	.11	.10	.09	.08	.07	.06	.06	
4	.20	.18	.15	.13	.11	.10	.09	.08	.08	
5	.25	.23	.19	.16	.14	.13	.11	.10	.09	Criminal penalties
6	.30	.27	.23	.19	.17	.15	.14	.12	.11	
7	.35	.32	.27	.23	.20	.18	.16	.14	.13	Legally intoxicated
8	.40	.36	.30	.26	.23	.20	.18	.17	.15	
9	.45	.41	.34	.29	.26	.23	.20	.19	.17	
10	.51	.45	.38	.32	.28	.25	.23	.21	.19	Criminal penalties

Alcohol is "burned up" by the body at .015 grams% per hour, as follows:

Number of hours since starting first drink 1 2 3 4 5 6
Percent alcohol burned up .015 .030 .045 .060 .075 .090

Calculate BAC

Example:
140 lb woman – 6 drinks in 4 hours
BAC = .190 grams% on chart
Subtract .060 grams% metabolized in 4 hours
BAC = .130 grams% – LEGALLY INTOXICATED

FIGURE 13.4 Relation between blood alcohol concentration, body weight, and the number of drinks ingested for men and women. See text for details.

well as its rate of metabolizing other compounds that are similar to alcohol (termed *cross-tolerance*).

Finally, biological markers that detect alcohol use even when BAC levels are reported as zero have been recently developed. Because alcohol is cleared fairly rapidly from the body, these biomarkers detect minor metabolites of alcohol and are usually positive for about 80 hours following drinking (Hoiseth et al., 2008, 2009). Such biomarkers are proving to be valuable tools to improve verification of abstention in alcohol-dependent persons (Junghanns, 2009). These minor metabolites include ethyl glucuronide and ethyl sulfate. A third biomarker being developed is a ratio between different serotonin metabolites (Hoiseth et al., 2008), although this latter marker has a shorter detection time. The ethyl glucuronide and ethyl sulfate comprise about 0.02 and 0.010 percent of the ethanol dose, but they can be reliably detected in blood, urine, and hair samples (Palmer, 2009).

Pharmacodynamics

Identifying the mechanism of the action of alcohol continues to be difficult (Vengeliene, et al., 2008). For many years, it was presumed that alcohol acted through a general depressant action on nerve membranes and synapses. Because it is both water soluble and lipid soluble, ethanol dissolves into all body tissues. This property led to a unitary hypothesis of action—that the drug dissolves in nerve membranes, distorting, disorganizing, or "perturbing" the membrane, similar to the action of general anesthetics (Chapter 7). The result is a nonspecific and indirect depression of neuronal function. This mechanism would account for the nonspecific and generalized depressant behavioral effects of the drug. The hypothesis, however, does not explain the evidence that alcohol may disturb both the synaptic activity of various neurotransmitters, especially major excitatory (glutamate) and inhibitory (GABA) systems, and various intracellular transduction processes.

Glutamate Receptors

Ethanol is a potent inhibitor of the function of the NMDA subtype of glutamate receptors. Ethanol disrupts glutaminergic neurotransmission by depressing the responsiveness of NMDA receptors to released glutamate. This attenuation of glutamate responsiveness may be exacerbated by alcohol's known enhancement of inhibitory GABA neurotransmission. With chronic alcohol intake and persistent glutaminergic suppression, there is a compensatory up regulation of NMDA receptors. Thus, on removal of ethanol's inhibitory effect (as would occur during alcohol withdrawal), these excess excitatory receptors would result in withdrawal signs, including seizures. Excess glutamate

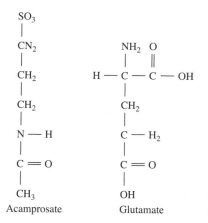

FIGURE 13.5 Structures of acamprosate and glutamate.

release during withdrawal may also be responsible for excitatory neuronal nerve damage and loss (Heinz et al., 2009).

The drug *acamprosate*, a structural analogue of glutamate (Figure 13.5), is an anticraving drug used to maintain abstinence in alcohol-dependent patients, an action thought to be produced by interaction with glutaminergic NMDA receptors, attenuating neuronal hyperexcitability induced by chronic alcohol ingestion and withdrawal (Mann et al., 2008). The use of acamprosate in the treatment of alcoholism is discussed later in this chapter.

GABA Receptors

Ethanol activates the GABA-mediated increase in chloride ion flows, resulting in neuronal inhibition. The behavioral results of this inhibition include sedation, muscle relaxation, and inhibition of cognitive and motor skills. A GABAergic antianxiety effect was illustrated as early as 1996 by Kushner and coworkers, who demonstrated that low doses of ethanol act acutely to reduce both panic and the anxiety surrounding panic. This finding lends support to the view that drinking by those with panic disorder, stress, and anxiety is reinforced by this GABAergic agonistic effect. Thus, the use of alcohol to self-medicate one's panic or anxiety disorder may contribute to the high rate at which alcohol use disorders occur with anxiety and panic disorders. Matsuzawa and Suzuki (2002) discuss the interaction between ethanol and stress in the mechanism of psychological dependence on ethanol. They invoke a mechanism in which GABAergic inhibition results in activation of opioid receptors that ultimately activates behaviorally rewarding dopaminergic neurons. Boehm and coworkers (2002) demonstrate that alcohol's behavioral effects may be exerted through modulation of GABA receptors on dopamine cell bodies in the ventral tegmental area. Johnson and colleagues (2005) review the role of GABAergic actions in the pharmacology of alcohol.

Ethanol binds to a different subunit on the $GABA_A$ receptor than do other GABA agonists. A chronic adaptive effect seems to involve changes in intracellular mRNA, suggesting that chronic alcoholism can affect gene expression. As a result of the GABAergic agonistic action, the activity of other transmitter systems is affected. The GABA agonistic action of ethanol has been linked to the positive reinforcing effects of the drug (Matsuzawa and Suzuki, 2002). The abuse potential of alcohol follows from an ultimate action to augment dopamine neurotransmitter systems, particularly the dopaminergic projection from the ventral tegmental area to the nucleus accumbens and to the frontal cortex (Chapter 3). This action is probably an indirect effect rather than a direct action exerted on dopamine-secreting neurons.

Opioid Receptors

Wand and coworkers (1998) present data consistent with a dysfunctional brain opioid system as part of a neurocircuitry involved in heavy alcohol drinking and alcohol dependence. Alcohol-dependent people and their offspring may have a deficit in brain opioid activity. Ethanol may induce opioid release, which in turn triggers dopamine release in the brain reward system (van der Zwaluw et al., 2007; Kohnke, 2008). Administration of *naltrexone* (ReVia, Vivatrol) blocks opioid release and may reduce alcohol craving. Naltrexone has been approved by the Food and Drug Administration (FDA) for the treatment of alcohol dependency; its use in treating alcohol dependency is discussed later in this chapter.

Serotonin Receptors

There is some literature on the role of serotonin in the actions of alcohol. Chronic alcohol consumption results in augmentations in serotonergic activity, and serotonin dysfunction has been postulated to play a role in the pathogenesis of some types of alcoholism. Today, emphasis is on the role of serotonin 5-HT_2 and 5-HT_3 receptors in the central effects of ethanol; these receptors are located on dopaminergic neurons in the nucleus accumbens. Serotonin reuptake-inhibiting antidepressants such as *sertraline* (Zoloft; Chapter 5) reduce alcohol drinking in alcoholics of lower risk and/or severity. Interestingly, sertraline is more effective in reducing alcoholic behaviors in lower-risk alcohol-dependent males than in lower-risk alcohol-dependent females (Pettinati et al., 2004).

Cannabinoid Receptors

Within the past few years, important information has been gathered on the probable role of cannabinoid receptors (Chapter 14) in the actions of alcohol, especially in postwithdrawal cravings and in the relapse to drinking. Chronic ingestion of ethanol stimulates the formation of the endogenous neurotransmitter for cannabinoid receptors, a substance called *anandamide*. This neurotransmitter activates the cannabinoid receptors and, with continued ethanol ingestion, eventually leads to down regulation of these receptors. Removal of ethanol by cessation of drinking leads to a hyperactive endocannabinoid reaction, which appears to result in a craving for alcohol and a return to drinking.

Mice that are genetically inbred to lack cannabinoid receptors do not voluntarily consume alcohol and also lack alcohol-induced dopamine-mediated reward responses in the nucleus accumbens (Hungund et al., 2003). Similarly, administration of drugs that block cannabinoid receptors (cannabinoid antagonists) prevents relapse to alcohol ingestion (Serra et al., 2002). Therefore, it now appears that ethanol and cannabinoid agonists (for example, tetrahydrocannabinol in marijuana) activate the same reward system. Down regulation of cannabinoid receptors may be involved in the development of tolerance to and dependence on ethanol, and an active response from cannabinoid receptors after alcohol detoxification may lead to alcohol craving and eventual compulsion to relapse (Wang et al., 2003). The effects of the cannabinoid antagonists in the treatment of alcohol dependence are discussed later in this chapter.

Pharmacological Effects

The graded, reversible depression of behavior, mental functioning, and cognition is the primary pharmacological effect of alcohol (Oscar-Berman and Marinkovic, 2007). Respiration is transiently stimulated at low doses, but as blood concentrations of alcohol increase, respiration becomes progressively depressed; at very high doses, respiration ceases, causing death. Alcohol is also anticonvulsant, although it is not clinically used for this purpose. On the other hand, withdrawal from alcohol ingestion is accompanied by a prolonged period of hyperexcitability, and seizures can occur: seizure activity peaks approximately 8 to 12 hours after the last drink.

In the central nervous system (CNS), the effects of alcohol are additive with those of other sedative-hypnotic compounds, resulting in more sedation and greater impairment of motor and cognitive abilities. Other sedatives (especially the benzodiazepines) and marijuana are the sedative-hypnotic drugs most frequently combined with alcohol, and they increase its deleterious effects on motor and intellectual skills (for example, driving ability) as well as alertness. Patients suffering from insomnia find alcohol to be an effective hypnotic agent.

Alcohol also affects the circulation and the heart. Alcohol dilates the blood vessels in the skin, producing a warm flush and a decrease in body temperature. Thus, it is pointless and possibly dangerous to drink alcohol to keep warm when one is exposed to cold weather. Long-term use of high doses of alcohol is associated with diseases of the heart muscle, which can result in heart failure. However, recent observations have demonstrated that *low* doses of alcohol consumed daily (up to 2 drink equivalents per day for men and 0.5 to 1.0 daily drink equivalent for women) *reduce* the risk of coronary artery disease and peripheral artery disease. This protective effect on coronary and peripheral blood vessels occurs because of an alcohol-induced increase in high-density lipoprotein in blood, with a corresponding decrease in low-density lipoprotein. (The higher the concentration of high-density lipoprotein and the lower the concentration of low-density lipoprotein, the lower is the incidence of development of arteriosclerosis and occlusive vascular disease.) Unfortunately, the cardioprotective effect of low doses of alcohol is lost on people who also smoke cigarettes.

Light to moderate doses of alcohol have also been shown to reduce the incidence of ischemic strokes (Figure 13.6). Ischemic strokes are strokes due to loss of oxygen delivery to specific areas of the brain. This protective action can reduce the risk of dementia among older adults (Solfrizzi et al., 2007). The mechanisms responsible for the protective effect of low doses of alcohol on ischemic stroke appear to

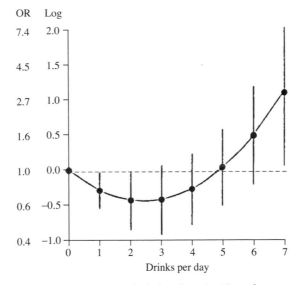

FIGURE 13.6 Relationship between alcohol and stroke. The reference group (indicated by the dashed horizontal line) is those not drinking during the past year. Analysis is matched for age, sex, and race/ethnicity and adjusted for hypertension, diabetes, heart disease, cigarette use, and education. OR = odds ratio for having a stroke; Log = logarithmic scale of stroke incidence. Vertical lines indicate 95 percent confidence intervals. [From R. L. Sacco et al., "The Protective Effect of Moderate Alcohol Consumption on Ischemic Stroke," *Journal of the American Medical Association* 281 (1999): 57.]

involve alcohol-induced increases in (protective) high-density cholesterol and an aspirinlike decrease in platelet aggregation. Higher amounts of alcohol (more than 14 drinks per week) were associated with an increased risk of stroke.

Alcohol (like all depressant drugs) is not an aphrodisiac. The behavioral disinhibition induced by low doses of alcohol may appear to cause some loss of restraint, but alcohol depresses body function and interferes with sexual performance. As Shakespeare says in *Macbeth*: "It provokes the desire, but it takes away the performance."

Psychological Effects

The short-term psychological and behavioral effects of alcohol are primarily restricted to the CNS, where a mixture of stimulant and depressant effects is seen after low doses of the drug. Figure 13.7 correlates the effects of alcohol with levels of the drug measured in the blood. The behavioral reaction to disinhibition, which occurs at low doses, is largely determined by the person, his or her mental expectations, and the environment in which drinking occurs. In one setting a person may become relaxed and euphoric; in another, withdrawn or violent. Mental expectations and the physical setting become progressively less

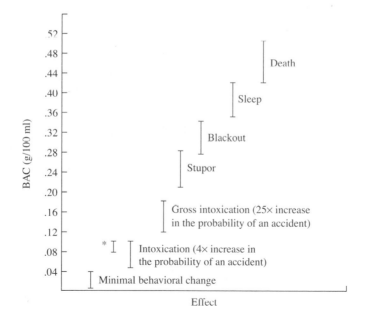

FIGURE 13.7 *Correlation of the blood level of ethanol with degrees of intoxication. The legal level of intoxication (*) varies according to state law; the range of BAC values is shown. BAC = blood alcohol concentration.*

important at increasing doses because the sedative effects increase and behavioral activity decreases.

As doses increase, a person may still function (although with less coordination) and attempt to drive or otherwise endanger self and others. Perceptual speed is an important component of task performance and is markedly impaired by ethanol (Schweizer et al., 2004). At BAC values of about 0.05 to 0.09 grams%, some common clinical symptoms are sociability; talkativeness; decreased inhibitions; diminution of attention, judgment, and control; slowed information processing; and loss of efficiency in critical performance testing. As the BAC increases, the drinker becomes progressively more incapacitated. Memory, concentration, and insight are progressively dulled and lost. At a BAC of about 0.25 to 0.30 grams%, the ability to transcribe (form) memory proteins from genetic material is impaired and "blackout"—a state closely related to organic dementia with severe cognitive dysfunction—eventually occurs (Lee et al., 2009).

Alcohol intoxication, with its resulting disinhibition, plays a major role in a large percentage of violent crimes, including fighting, rape, sexual assault, and certain kinds of deviant behaviors. Alcohol is implicated in more than half of all homicides and assaults; about 40 percent of violent offenders in jail were drinking at the time of the offense for which they were incarcerated. Many of these offenses probably would not have occurred if the offender, the victim, or both had not been intoxicated. Martin (2001) studied how alcohol use by men affects intimate-partner violence. She states that alcohol intoxication may contribute to aggressive and criminal behavior through its mediating effects on the physiological, cognitive, affective, or behavioral functioning of the drinker. Through effects on the GABA system, alcohol reduces anxiety about the consequences of aggressive behavior. Through dopaminergic activation, impulse control is reduced, which increases the likelihood of aggression. Through glutamate depression, cognitive functioning is impaired, reducing the drinker's ability to find peaceful (nonviolent) solutions to difficult situations. Many drinkers develop a type of "alcohol myopia," defined as shortsightedness in which superficially understood, immediate aspects of experience have a disproportionate influence on behavior and emotion. Cognitive and attentional deficits cause a focus on the present, reduce fear and anxiety, and impair problem-solving ability. Finally, alcohol use increases concerns with power and dominance, which are linked to male violence generally and to intimate-partner interactions in particular. The effect can be an inappropriate sense of mastery, control, or power (Abbey et al., 2002). This issue of violence and crime applies to women as well as to men. In fact, the effects of ethanol on aggression and violence, in the absence of cocaine, are more then three times as great for female as for male arrestees.

Hindson and coworkers (2001) surveyed 42,000 adults as part of a U.S. Census Bureau survey about alcohol use/abuse and physical fighting. Relative to those who did not begin drinking until age 21 or older, those who started drinking before age 17 were three to four times more likely ever in their lives and at least three times more likely in the past year to have been in a fight after drinking. Thus, early-age onset of drinking is associated with alcohol-related violence not only among people under 21 but among adults as well.

More than 50 percent of all motor vehicle highway accidents are alcohol related, a number that has changed little in 20 years. More than 10 million people in the United States currently suffer the consequences of their alcohol abuse, which include arrests, traffic accidents, occupational injuries, violence, and health and occupational losses. This number does not include the 10 million people considered to be alcohol dependent (and suffering their own negative consequences). About 10 percent of our society is personally afflicted with (or suffers the consequences of) another's alcohol use. Untreated alcohol problems lead to death, disability, and $185 billion each year in avoidable health, business, and criminal justice costs.

Noel and colleagues (2001) studied 30 recently detoxified male alcoholics (with matched controls) to assess "frontal lobe" or "executive" functioning and the vulnerability of the frontal lobes to alcohol abuse. In all tests of executive function, nondrinking alcoholics performed poorly compared with controls. The researchers stated:

> Chronic alcohol consumption is associated with severe executive function deficits, still present after a protracted period of alcohol abstinence. This supports the idea that cognitive deficit in detoxified, sober alcoholics is due, at least partly, to frontal lobe dysfunction. (p. 1152)

Furthermore:

> These findings could have important implications, particularly concerning relapse. Since drug use is largely controlled by automatic processes, executive functions are needed to block this and maintain abstinence. Thus, the existence of persistent executive function deficits could affect the capacity to maintain abstinence. (p. 1152)

Persistent alcohol use harms adolescents. Brown and coworkers (2000) studied alcohol-dependent adolescents (who developed dependency in early adolescence) and found that recent detoxification was associated with poor visuospatial functioning (as might be expected), whereas alcohol withdrawal early in life was associated with persistence of poor retrieval of verbal and nonverbal information. This finding reflects long-term effects on working memory.

Long-term effects of alcohol may also involve many different organs of a person's body. Long-term ingestion of only moderate amounts of alcohol seems to produce few physiological alterations. As noted earlier, low to moderate doses can even be protective to the heart and vascular system. On the downside, long-term ingestion of larger amounts of alcohol leads to a variety of serious neurological, mental, and physical disorders. These disorders are described in the section on alcoholism and its pharmacological treatment.

Alcohol is high in calories but has little nutritional value; consumption of a high-alcohol diet (and little else!) slowly leads to vitamin deficiencies and nutritional diseases, which may result in physical deterioration. Alcohol abuse has been suggested as the most common cause of vitamin and trace element deficiencies in adults.

Tolerance and Dependence

The patterns and mechanisms for the development of tolerance to, physical dependence on, and psychological dependence on alcohol are similar to those for other CNS depressants (Chapter 7). The extent of tolerance depends on the amount, pattern, and extent of alcohol ingestion. People who ingest alcohol only intermittently on sprees or more regularly but in moderation develop little or no tolerance. People who regularly ingest large amounts of alcohol develop marked tolerance. The tolerance is of three types:

1. *Metabolic tolerance,* whereby the liver increases its amount of drug-metabolizing enzyme. This type accounts for at most 25 percent of the tolerance to alcohol.

2. *Tissue, or functional, tolerance,* whereby neurons in the brain adapt to the amount of drug present. Drinkers who develop this type of tolerance characteristically display blood alcohol levels about twice those of nontolerant drinkers at a similar level of behavioral intoxication. Note, however, that despite behavioral adaptation, impairments in cognitive function are similar at similar blood levels in both tolerant and nontolerant drinkers. In other words, at a BAC of 0.15 grams%, both tolerant and nontolerant drinkers display marked deficits in insight, judgment, cognition, and other executive functions. The tolerant person may just *appear* less intoxicated. As discussed, memory formation and severe cognitive impairments occur at a BAC of about 0.25 grams% and higher. A "tolerant" person does not develop tolerance to these memory/cognitive effects but behaviorally may appear to function reasonably normally (for example, be able to drive home in a "blackout," although this activity is illegal).

3. *Associative, contingent, or homeostatic tolerance.* A variety of environmental manipulations can counter the effects of ethanol, and counterresponses are a possible mechanism of tolerance.

When physical dependence develops, withdrawal of alcohol results, within several hours, in a period of rebound hyperexcitability that may eventually lead to convulsions. Alcohol abuse is one of the most common causes of adult-onset seizures; seizures occur in about 10 percent of adults during alcohol withdrawal. Alcohol withdrawal seizures are a life-threatening consequence of alcohol cessation in alcoholics. The period of seizure activity is relatively short, usually 6 hours or less, but seizures can be very severe. Blocking seizure activity during withdrawal is a major goal of detoxification and usually involves two classes of agents: the benzodiazepines and the anticonvulsants. As early as 1978, Ballenger and Post noted that the severity of alcohol withdrawal seizures is correlated with the number of years of alcohol abuse and perhaps with the number of detoxifications.

A "kindling" model of alcohol withdrawal seizures suggests that repeated alcohol withdrawals may lead to an increase in the severity of subsequent withdrawals and a greater likelihood of withdrawal seizures with each detoxification. Indeed, the number of detoxifications is an important variable in the predisposition to withdrawal seizures. Malcolm and coworkers (2000) applied this concept to the postulate that repeated detoxifications might also cause neurobehavioral alterations that in turn may affect alcohol craving. Patients who had experienced multiple detoxifications had higher scores on tests that measure obsessive thoughts about alcohol, drink urges, and drinking behaviors. Thus, recurrent detoxifications may lead to increased rates of relapse due to a "kindling" of behaviors and thoughts leading to a compulsion to return to drinking. The researchers added that the kindling effect persists despite treatment with benzodiazepines or other traditional sedative-hypnotic drugs. In fact, the medical management of alcohol detoxification may be better achieved with anticonvulsant "mood stabilizers" (Chapter 6) than with benzodiazepines (Becker et al., 2006; Martinotti et al., 2010).

In addition to withdrawal seizures and cravings, the alcohol withdrawal syndrome can consist of a period of tremulousness, with hallucinations, psychomotor agitation, confusion and disorientation, sleep disorders, and a variety of associated discomforts. This syndrome is sometimes referred to as *delirium tremens* (DTs).

Fadda and Rossetti (1998) reviewed withdrawal as a sign of alcohol-induced neuroadaptation and the neurodegeneration that may play a role in the persistent cognitive deficits that result from alcohol dependence. Markianos and coworkers (2000) assessed dopamine receptor responsiveness in alcoholic patients during their usual alcohol consumption and after detoxification. Detoxification was characterized by slow recovery of dopamine receptor responsiveness. The Markianos team postulated that the dopamine system is involved in alcohol dependence and withdrawal.

Side Effects and Toxicity

Many side effects and toxicities associated with alcohol have already been mentioned; following is a summary and expansion. In acute use, a *reversible drug-induced dementia* is induced. This syndrome is manifested as a clouded sensorium with disorientation, impaired insight and judgment, anterograde amnesia (blackouts), and diminished intellectual capabilities. Some mental impairments begin at low levels of alcohol. As levels approach about 0.20 grams%, memory becomes severely affected, and by a BAC of about 0.25–0.30 grams%, the ability to form memory diminishes markedly. Perry and coworkers (2006) noted that subjects with a BAC of 0.31 grams% or higher have a greater than 50 percent probability of having an alcoholic blackout. John and Prichep (2005) discuss the different mechanisms probably involved at doses of sedatives required to produce amnesia; loss of consciousness occurs at much higher doses, and "anesthesia" occurs only following very much larger doses. In other words, a person who has ingested a large quantity of alcohol can be amnestic in the presence of consciousness, a concept that was discussed in Chapter 7. Indeed, with alcohol and maintenance of an awake state, these BACs "disrupt limbic areas to prevent consolidation of encoded stimuli into lasting memory traces" (Hartzler and Fromme, 2003, p. 547). In other words, alcohol (and other sedatives capable of inducing memory loss) likely block memory protein formation that is essential for the formation of memory (Gold, 2008).

With increasing doses (or blood levels) of alcohol, a person's affect may be labile, with emotional outbursts precipitated by otherwise innocuous events. With high doses of alcohol, delusions and hallucinations may occur. In social functioning, these alterations result in unpredictable states of disinhibition (drunkenness), alterations in driving performance, and uncoordinated motor behavior. As stated earlier, only at very high doses (perhaps at BACs of 0.4 grams% and greater) is consciousness lost and a state of "anesthesia" with immobilization begun. At this point, respiration becomes shallow and death can result.

Liver damage is a serious physiological long-term consequence of excessive alcohol consumption. Irreversible changes in both the structure and the function of the liver are common. For example, ethanol produces active oxidants during its metabolism by hepatocytes, which results in oxidative stress on liver cells. The significance of alcohol-induced liver dysfunction is illustrated by the fact that 75 percent of all deaths attributed to alcoholism are caused by cirrhosis of the liver, and cirrhosis is the seventh most common cause of death in the United States.

Long-term alcohol ingestion may irreversibly cause the *destruction of nerve cells,* producing a permanent brain syndrome with dementia

(Korsakoff's syndrome). More subtle and persistent cognitive deficits may be present whether or not a diagnosis of Korsakoff's syndrome is made. This condition is termed *alcohol dementia*, and it can involve long-term problems with memory, learning, and other cognitive skills. The *digestive system* may also be affected. *Pancreatitis* (inflammation of the pancreas) and *chronic gastritis* (inflammation of the stomach), with the development of peptic ulcers, may occur.

A great deal of epidemiological evidence now shows that chronic excessive alcohol consumption is a major risk factor for *cancer* in humans. Although ethanol alone may not be carcinogenic, it is a cocarcinogen, or a tumor promoter. The metabolism of ethanol leads to the generation of acetaldehyde and free radicals. Acetaldehyde has been shown to promote tumor growth, promoting cancers of the oral pharynx, stomach, and intestine. Statistically, heavy drinking increases a person's risk of developing cancer of the tongue, mouth, throat, voice box, and liver. The risk of head and neck cancers for heavy drinkers who smoke is 6 to 15 times greater than for those who abstain from both. The risk of throat cancer is 44 times greater for heavy users of both alcohol and tobacco than for nonusers.

Although the finding is controversial, ethanol may increase the risk for breast and other cancers by still unidentified means, perhaps exerted through actions of acetaldehyde (Seitz and Becker, 2007). Alcohol-associated breast cancers appear with highest frequency in postmenopausal women who report regular consumption of alcohol before the age of 40. The increased risk of breast cancer may offset the beneficial effects of moderate alcohol consumption on cardiovascular disease.

Teratogenic Effects

For years we have known that alcohol is both a physical and a behavioral teratogen. Drug-induced alterations occur in brain structure and/or function. *Fetal alcohol syndrome* (FAS) is a devastating developmental disorder that occurs in the offspring of mothers who have high blood levels of alcohol during critical stages of fetal development; it affects as many as 30 to 50 percent of infants born to alcoholic women. Clearly, a relatively large number of otherwise biologically normal infants may be irreversibly damaged by maternal alcohol abuse during pregnancy, and alcohol abuse during pregnancy appears to be the most frequent known teratogenic cause of mental retardation.

Sayal and coworkers (2009) noted that binge drinking in the absence of regular ingestion increased the risk of child mental health problems, primarily related to hyperactivity and inattention problems. Kot-Leibovich and Fainsod (2009) noted that alcohol competes with the biosynthesis of retinoic acid, which is required for normal brain development. Because subtle intellectual and behavioral effects of low-level alcohol consumption may go unnoticed, no safe level of alcohol intake during pregnancy has been established. Features of the full fetal alcohol syndrome include the following:

- CNS dysfunction, including low intelligence and microcephaly (reduced cranial circumference), mental retardation, and behavioral abnormalities (often presenting as hyperactivity and difficulty with social integration)
- Retarded body growth rate (fetal growth retardation)
- Facial abnormalities (short palpebral fissures, short nose, wide-set eyes, and small cheekbones)
- Other anatomical abnormalities (for example, congenital heart defects and malformed eyes and ears).

In the United States, an estimated 2.6 million infants are born annually following significant in utero alcohol exposure. Many display the full features of FAS, and about one newborn out of every hundred live births displays a "lesser degree of damage, termed *fetal alcohol effects,*" perhaps more correctly termed *alcohol-related neurodevelopmental disorder* (ARND). Taken together, the combined rate of FAS and ARND is estimated to be at least 9 per 1000 live births. Alcohol ingestion is thus the third leading cause of birth defects with associated mental retardation; it is the only one that is preventable.

Perhaps a new term should be coined to encompass the full spectrum of fetal damage that can follow ingestion of ethanol by pregnant women. "Fetal alcohol spectrum disorder" would include both fetal alcohol syndrome and fetal alcohol effects, covering that gray area between infants with facial abnormalities and infants with "milder" effects, such as hyperactivity and aggressive behaviors.

Although the structural abnormalities and growth retardation of FAS are well described, the behavioral and cognitive effects of alcohol exposure are less appreciated. Intelligence (IQ), attention, learning, memory, language, and motor and visuospatial activities are affected and subject to deficit in children prenatally exposed to varying amounts of alcohol (Sayal et al., 2009). Also present can be sensory problems involving ocular, auditory, vestibular, and speech and language development. Carmichael and coworkers (1997) studied a cohort of 500 children, 250 of whom were born to "heavier" drinkers who typically drank at "social drinking levels." The other 250 children were born to infrequent drinkers and abstainers. There were significant alcohol-related differences in behavioral and learning difficulties during adolescence. Exposure to alcohol during pregnancy was associated "with a profile of adolescent antisocial behavior, school problems, and self-perceived learning difficulties" (p. 1187). Thus, brain function can be markedly affected in offspring of alcohol-drinking mothers in the absence of the observable structural abnormalities.

In a study in Finland, Autti-Ramo (2000) followed 70 children with fetal alcohol exposure (42 with recognized cognitive and other deficits, 10 with physical growth restrictions only, and 18 classified as normal). They were assessed at age 12 for psychosocial well-being. The longer the alcohol exposure during pregnancy, the more likely the child was to have significant cognitive and social impairments. Of the 42 children with early recognition of cognitive deficits, 29 (69 percent) were in permanent foster or institutional care. Even among the children in the normal and growth-restricted groups, 10 (36 percent) were temporarily or permanently in alternative care. Behavioral problems were significant. Thus, alcohol exposure in utero can be associated with social disadvantages, including alternative care and behavioral problems.

Baer and coworkers (2003) reported results of a 21-year longitudinal study in which they followed offspring of 500 women who, in 1974–1975, drank during their pregnancy (30 percent were binge drinkers). Offspring of 2 women displayed FAS, and 31 offspring were identified as having components of ARND. When these offspring attained the age of 21, 21 percent of their fathers and 11 percent of their mothers were identified as having had a history of alcohol problems. The offspring of mothers who were binge drinkers during pregnancy exhibited three times the likelihood of at least mild alcohol dependence than did offspring of mothers who did not drink alcohol during their pregnancy (14.1 percent versus 4.5 percent).

The prevention of FAS and ARND obviously involves abstinence from alcohol by women who are, plan to become, or are capable of becoming pregnant. Screening questionnaires may be effective in helping to protect not only the unborn infant but also the long-term health of the mother. Because alcohol screening can effectively identify women and infants at risk, it is recommended for women during prenatal visits.

Alcoholism and Its Pharmacological Treatment

Why is it necessary to recognize alcoholism as a major medical problem? Schuckit (2009) stated:

> Alcohol dependence and alcohol abuse or harmful use cause substantial morbidity and mortality. Alcohol-use disorders are associated with depressive episodes, severe anxiety, insomnia, suicide, and abuse of other drugs. Continued heavy alcohol use also shortens the onset of heart disease, stroke, cancers, and liver cirrhosis, by affecting the cardiovascular, gastrointestinal, and immune systems. Heavy drinking can

also cause mild anterograde amnesias, temporary cognitive deficits, sleep problems, and peripheral neuropathy; cause gastrointestinal problems; decrease bone density and production of blood cells; and cause fetal alcohol syndrome. Alcohol-use disorders complicate assessment and treatment of other medical and psychiatric problems. (p. 492)

The recognition of alcoholism as a multifaceted disease and behavioral process is relatively recent. In 1935, Alcoholics Anonymous was founded on a *moral model* of alcoholism; it offered a spiritual and behavioral framework for understanding, accepting, and recovering from the compulsion to use alcohol. In the late 1950s, the American Medical Association recognized the syndrome of alcoholism as an illness. In the mid-1970s, alcoholism was redefined as a *chronic, progressive, and potentially fatal disease.* In 1992, the description was expanded as follows:

Alcoholism is a primary, chronic disease with genetic, psychosocial, and environmental factors influencing its development and manifestations. The disease is often progressive and fatal. It is characterized by impaired control over drinking, preoccupation with the drug alcohol, use of alcohol despite adverse consequences, and distortions in thinking, most notably denial. Each of these symptoms may be continuous or periodic. (Morse and Flavin, 1992, p. 1012)

In this definition, "adverse consequences" involve impairments in physical health, psychological functioning, interpersonal functioning, and occupational functioning as well as legal, financial, and spiritual problems. "Denial" refers broadly to a range of psychological maneuvers that decrease awareness of the fact that alcohol use is the cause of problems rather than a solution to problems. Denial becomes an integral part of the disease and is nearly always a major obstacle to recovery.

As with other addictions, human alcoholism is characterized as a chronically relapsing condition. It contributes to the risk of bodily harm, relationship troubles, problems in meeting obligations, and run-ins with the law. Consequently, the therapeutic goal is the development of clinically effective, safe medications that promote high adherence rates and prevent relapse. These drugs can then be used in conjunction with psychosocial approaches (Lawrence, 2007).

It is now obvious that the *age of onset* of drinking behaviors markedly affects long-term outcomes and societal functioning. Heavy users of alcohol at early ages have, as might be predicted, the poorest outcomes as adults. Heavy drinking as early as age 13 predicts a high risk for subsequent alcohol dependency, low levels of academic achievement, and poor interactions in family and social activities. Binge drinking at age 15 and continuing through age 18 results in an even higher rate of alcohol dependency.

Rohde and coworkers (2001) followed a large cohort of adolescents (14 to 18 years old) through age 24. Approximately three-quarters of the adolescents at initial interview had tried alcohol; those who drank often consumed large quantities of alcohol. Problematic alcohol use occurred in 23 percent. Of the latter group, 80 percent had some form of comorbidity with alcohol use: increased rates of depression, disruptive behavior, drug use disorders, and daily tobacco use. By age 24, problem-drinking adolescents exhibited increased rates of substance abuse disorders, depression, and antisocial and borderline personality disorders. Therefore, excessive alcohol use in early adolescence is not a benign condition that resolves over time.

In many cases, alcohol may (at least at first) be ingested in an attempt at *self-medication* of psychological distress. A person who, before drinking alcohol, experiences anxiety, depression, bipolar, or other responsive psychological disorder may find the symptomatology alleviated by ethanol. This relief then leads to unregulated and unmonitored drug ingestion (the drug is not taken under a physician's supervision). Either the positive reinforcing effects of the drug or drinking to avoid the unpleasantness of withdrawal then trap the person. In support of this concept, Goodwin and Gabrielli (1997) state:

> A good deal of evidence now indicates that many and perhaps most alcoholics do not have primary alcoholism. Their alcoholism is associated with other psychopathology, including addiction to other drugs, depression, manic-depressive illness, anxiety disorder, or antisocial personality. (p. 144)

Goodwin and Gabrielli further state that 30 to 50 percent of alcoholics meet criteria for major depression, 33 percent have a coexisting anxiety disorder, many have antisocial personalities, some are schizophrenic, and many (36 percent) are addicted to other drugs. Some, if not many, alcoholics may have first used alcohol and become psychologically dependent on the drug as a self-prescribed medication to treat their primary disorder. Fergusson and coworkers (2009) discuss the association between alcohol misuse and depression.

Lapham and coworkers (2001) studied psychiatric diagnoses in over 1000 males and females aged 23 to 54 who were convicted of driving while impaired. Eighty-five percent of female and 91 percent of male offenders reported a lifetime alcohol use disorder; 32 percent of female and 38 percent of male offenders had a drug use disorder. Fifty percent of female and 33 percent of male offenders had at least one additional psychiatric disorder, mainly posttraumatic stress disorder or major depression. We obviously need to implement treatment interventions for these offenders. Court and diversionary programs focus on alcohol use, not on drug use and other psychological problems. The costs of treatment are high, and most offenders are unwilling to enter treatment (usually denial is present). Psychological assessments are rare, and education is ineffective. Rearrest rates are high. New incentives are needed, including biweekly urine and blood tests as a condition for driving.

As many as 38 percent of alcohol-dependent patients demonstrate impulse-control problems. The co-occurrence of pathologic gambling (one type of impulse-control disorder) was associated with a younger age of onset of alcohol dependence, a higher number of detoxifications, and a longer duration of dependence. Both alcohol dependence and pathologic gambling are pleasure-seeking dependencies, and alcohol use may provide much the same reinforcement as gambling. Frye and Salloum (2006) discuss the co-occurrence of alcoholism and bipolar disorder. An overwhelmingly positive association exists between alcohol use disorder and personality disorders, especially antisocial, histrionic, and dependent disorders (Grant et al., 2004). *Dual diagnosis* (or *comorbid illness*) must always be considered (Tiet and Mausbach, 2007).

Dawson and coworkers (2007) studied the relationship between early-onset drinking (age 14 or younger) and life's stressors. They found that initiation of drinking at age 14 or younger increased the association between the number of stressors and the average daily volume of alcohol ingested. Early-onset drinking thus appears to increase stress-reactive alcohol consumption. In other words, early-onset ethanol drinkers are more likely to use alcohol as a "stress reducer" than are drinkers who begin drinking at a later age. For example, early-onset drinkers increase their alcohol consumption (even in later life) 19 percent with each stressful event, compared with only a 3 percent increase by older-onset drinkers. Thus, early-onset drinkers grow into adults who rely on alcohol to cope more than do older-onset drinkers of similar age.

Alcoholism is a major public health problem. Of the 160 million Americans who are old enough to drink legally, 112 million do so. As many as 14 million Americans may have serious alcohol problems, and about half that number are considered to be alcoholic. Alcoholism costs about 100,000 Americans lives each year and in excess of $166 billion annually in direct and indirect health and societal costs. Older people who drink are at risk for their own set of problems.

In 2005, the National Institute on Alcohol Abuse and Alcoholism published a clinician's guide asking all clinicians and mental health workers to screen for alcohol use patterns that place a person at risk for alcohol-related problems. This guide, titled *Helping Patients Who Drink Too Much*, was updated in 2007 (National Institute on Alcohol Abuse and Alcoholism, 2007). Men who drink 5 or more standard drinks in a day (or 15 or more per week) and women who drink 4 or more in a day (or 8 or more per week) are at increased risk for alcohol-related problems. The guide asks practitioners to utilize a simple, single question prescreen: "Do you sometimes drink beer, wine, or other alcoholic beverages?" A "yes" answer leads to two additional questions to determine the weekly average number of drinks ingested as well as a maladaptive pattern of alcohol use. This guide can be downloaded at www.niaaa.nih.gov.

Although widely recommended, brief interventions have proven efficacy in decreasing alcohol consumption only in unhealthy drinkers in outpatient settings who do not have alcohol dependence. Saitz and coworkers (2007) demonstrated that brief interventions are insufficient for the treatment of persons with alcohol dependence. More extensive, tailored interventions are necessary. Schuckit (2009) stated that "treatment can include motivational interviewing to help people to evaluate their situations, brief interventions to facilitate more healthy behaviors, detoxification to address withdrawal symptoms, cognitive-behavioral therapies to avoid relapse, and judicious use of drugs to diminish cravings or discourage relapses" (p. 492).

Pharmacotherapies for Alcohol Abuse and Dependence

Because alcoholism involves the ingestion of alcohol, eliminating such ingestion is an obvious therapeutic strategy. Achieving success, however, is an extremely difficult task. Vaillant (1996) performed a remarkable 50-year follow-up of two cohorts of men who began abusing alcohol at an early age. One group consisted of university undergraduates; the second consisted of nondelinquent inner-city adolescents. By 60 years of age, 18 percent of the college alcohol abusers had died, 11 percent were abstinent, 11 percent were controlled drinkers, and 60 percent were still abusing alcohol. By 60 years of age, 28 percent of the inner-city alcohol abusers had died, 30 percent were abstinent, 12 percent were controlled drinkers, and 30 percent were still abusing alcohol. Because alcohol abuse after age 60 can be devastating, the greater levels of abuse by college-educated males need to be addressed. The ideal goals of pharmacotherapy for alcohol dependence and abuse include the following:

1. Reversal of the acute pharmacologic effects of alcohol
2. Treatment and prevention of withdrawal symptoms and complications
3. Maintenance of abstinence and prevention of relapse with agents that decrease craving for alcohol or the loss of control over drinking or make it unpleasant to ingest alcohol
4. Treatment of coexisting psychiatric disorders that complicate recovery
5. Limitation of neuronal injury during detoxification by blocking withdrawal-induced glutaminergic activation and glutamate receptor up regulation (Krupitsky et al., 2007)

Can these goals be met? First, at this time, no agent that can reverse the acute pharmacologic effects of alcohol is available. Some feel that caffeine can antagonize alcohol intoxication and increase alertness. Indeed, 16- to 24-ounce drinks that combine ethanol (usually 9 to 12 percent ethanol) with caffeine and other stimulants have recently been marketed. Caffeine does not reverse the intoxicating effects of alcohol. In fact, as a behavioral stimulant, caffeine can only increase activity, not reverse the motor, cognitive, or other dysfunctions induced by alcohol. Therefore, acute alcohol intoxication is usually treated with supportive care to protect both the intoxicated person and others placed at risk of injury.

Pharmacotherapies are available for four interventions:

1. To treat and prevent withdrawal symptoms
2. To reduce relapse to drinking behaviors
3. To treat complications in alcohol-dependent people who are decreasing or discontinuing alcohol consumption
4. To reduce glutamate release and glutamate receptor up regulation with subsequent neuronal damage

Medications can also effectively prevent and treat the symptoms, seizures, and DTs associated with withdrawal. In addition, medications are available to help address and treat the comorbidities observed in alcohol-dependent people. Medications include anxiolytics, antidepressants, and mood stabilizers. However, pharmacological agents are less effective in reducing the rates of relapse to renewed drinking.

Currently, three oral medications (naltrexone, acamprosate, and disulfiram) and one injectable medication (extended-release injectable naltrexone) have been approved by the FDA for treating alcohol dependence (Johnson, 2008) (Table 13.1). In addition, the cannabinoid receptor antagonists *rimonabant* and *taranabant*; Chapter 14) have been shown to reduce drinking behaviors, presumably by blocking cannabinoid-facilitated alcohol-reinforcing pathways in the mesolimbic dopamine pathways in the brain (Malinen and Hyytia, 2008). Initial optimism, however, has been tempered by disappointingly low levels of efficacy (George et al., 2010; Alen et al., 2009). Use has also been limited by clinically significant side effects that include anxiety reactions as well as major depression with melancholic features (deMattos et al., 2009).

In addition, the mood-stabilizing anticonvulsants currently available have therapeutic efficacy as both detoxification and antirelapse agents. Examples include topiramate (Topamax), gabapentin (Neurontin) (Kenna et al., 2009a; Myrick et al., 2009), and pregabalin (Lyrica) (Martinotti, et al., 2010). Finally, in isolated and novel studies the alpha-1 adrenergic antagonist prazosin (Minecin) yielded positive results (Simpson et al., 2009), as did both the atypical antipsychotic quetiapine (Seroquel) (Kampman et al., 2007) and a novel antidepressant that blocks neurokinin-2 receptors (discussed in Chapter 5) (George et al., 2008).

TABLE 13.1 Drugs used to decrease alcohol consumption, reduce craving, maintain abstinence, or prevent relapse in alcohol-dependent individuals

Drug	Mechanism	Comments
Disulfiram	Inhibits aldehyde dehydrogenase to allow acetaldehyde accumulation	Clinical efficacy in question as a result of controlled trials. Effective in special situations.
Calcium carbimide	Same as disulfiram	May have fewer side effects than disulfiram. Available in Canada, not in USA.
Naltrexone	Endogenous opioid antagonist	Approved by FDA for treating alcohol dependence. Reduces consumption in heavy drinkers.
Acamprosate	NMDA and GABA receptor modulator	Reduces unpleasant effects of alcohol abstinence; reduces craving. May have adverse fetal effects.
Fluoxetine and other serotonin antidepressants	SSR-type serotonin agonists	Reduce depression and anxiety comorbid with alcohol dependency.
Buspirone	Serotonin 5-HT1$_A$ agonist	Little demonstrable efficacy may be due to inadequate amounts in blood.
Ondansetron,	Serotonin 5-HT$_3$ antagonist	May reduce craving. Modest efficacy.
Oxcarbazepine topiramate gabapentin	Mood stabilizers, anticonvulsants	Can reduce unpleasant withdrawal effects and reduce relapse.
Rimonabant and other cannabinoid antagonists	Cannabinoid receptor antagonists	Reduce desire to drink.

Pharmacotherapies for Management of Alcohol Withdrawal

At its simplest, if ingesting alcohol reduces glutamate activity and increases GABA activity in the brain, alcohol withdrawal results in the opposite: reduced GABA activity and increased glutamate activity. These changes result in uncontrolled excitation and can damage cognitive functioning (Duka et al., 2003). The major therapeutic goal of managing acute alcohol withdrawal or detoxification is to prevent uncontrolled excitation by either reducing glutamate activity or increasing GABA activity. Classically this has been achieved through use of either benzodiazepines (Chapter 7) or anticonvulsant medications (Chapter 6).

Benzodiazepines. Increasing GABA activity is the mechanism underlying the classical use of the benzodiazepines for the treatment of acute alcohol withdrawal; they ameliorate the symptoms of withdrawal and also prevent seizures and DTs (Hughes, 2009). It may not seem logical to substitute one potentially addictive drug (a benzodiazepine) for another (ethanol). Here is the explanation: the short duration of the action of alcohol and its narrow range of safety make it an extremely dangerous drug from which to withdraw. When alcohol ingestion is stopped, withdrawal symptoms begin within a few hours. Substituting a long-acting drug prevents or suppresses the withdrawal symptoms. The longer-acting benzodiazepine is then either maintained at a level low enough to allow the person to function or is withdrawn gradually. Preferred drugs are the benzodiazepines with long-acting active metabolites—chlordiazepoxide (Librium) or diazepam (Valium). Acute seizure activity can be controlled with the faster-onset, shorter-acting benzodiazepine lorazepam. The pharmacology of the benzodiazepines is discussed in Chapter 7.

Anticonvulsant Mood Stabilizers. The benzodiazepines have important limitations when used for the treatment of alcohol withdrawal: sedation, psychomotor impairments, additive interactions with alcohol, and the potential for abuse and dependence. Since seizures are common in acute alcohol withdrawal, use of an antiepileptic drug seems intuitively appropriate. Although older anticonvulsants have significant limitations that can be deleterious in alcoholics (contributing to liver and pancreatic problems, for example), they have historically been demonstrated to be effective. For example, carbamazepine (Tegretol) and valproic acid (Depakote) have been used successfully in place of benzodiazepines despite potentially significant adverse side effects (Hughes, 2009). Newer anticonvulsants—for example, gabapentin (Neurontin), pregabalin (Lyrica), oxcarbazepine (Trileptal), lamotrigine (Lamictal), and topiramate (Topamax)—have significant potential and are less toxic than carbamazepine and valproic acid, which may make them a better choice than benzodiazepines for the treatment of alcohol withdrawal. Leggio and coworkers (2008) recently reviewed such use. Rubio and coworkers (2006) and Krupitsky and coworkers (2007) reported on the efficacy of lamotrigine (Lamictal) to improve mood, decrease alcohol craving, and decrease alcohol consumption while reducing glutamate release and presumably exerting "brain protection" during alcohol withdrawal in patients with alcoholism. The pharmacology of anticonvulsants is presented in Chapter 6, where they are discussed as mood stabilizers for the treatment of bipolar disorder.

Pharmacotherapies to Help Maintain Abstinence and Prevent Relapse

Numerous drugs to decrease daily consumption of ethanol and prevent clinical relapse to continued drinking have been tried; many are listed in Table 13.1. Some have been successful and many are of limited use.

Alcohol-Sensitizing Drugs. Disulfiram (Antabuse) and calcium carbimide (Temposil, available in Canada only) are two medications used to deter a patient from drinking alcohol by producing an aversive reaction if the patient drinks. These drugs alter the metabolism of alcohol, allowing acetaldehyde to accumulate. If the patient ingests alcohol within several days of taking the aversive drug, the accumulation results in an acetaldehyde syndrome, characterized by flushing, throbbing headache, nausea, vomiting, chest pain, and other severe symptoms. It is thought that calcium carbimide may have fewer side effects than does disulfiram. If taken daily, aversive agents can result in total abstinence in many patients. However, controlled trials of disulfiram therapy to reduce alcohol consumption have been disappointing. This topic is reviewed by Elbreder and coworkers (2010).

Opioid Antagonists. Naltrexone, an opioid antagonist (Chapter 10), was approved in oral formulation by the FDA in 1994 for use in the treatment of alcohol dependence to reduce the craving for alcohol, even though the effect was small. The hypothesis of action is that the reinforcing properties of alcohol involve the opioid system; blockade of the opioid system by naltrexone should reduce craving by reducing the positive reinforcement associated with alcohol use, blocking the rewards of alcohol or stabilizing systems dysregulated by chronic alcohol intake (Garbutt, 2009). Initial studies with naltrexone were encouraging; however, subsequent studies determined that the efficacy of orally administered naltrexone in the prevention of alcohol relapse is much more modest (Pettinati et al., 2006).

Preparations of naltrexone available for clinical use include oral naltrexone (ReVia), with once-daily dosing, and an extended-release injectable naltrexone (Vivitrol), given as a once-per-month injection

(Swainstron-Harrison et al., 2006). Compliance has always been a problem with naltrexone therapy. It is hoped that the long-acting injectable formulation will facilitate patient compliance by providing therapy over a period of one month per injection (Lobmaier et al., 2008). The pharmacology of naltrexone and other opioid antagonists is discussed further in Chapter 10.

Acamprosate. Acamprosate (Campral) has been approved by the FDA for use in the treatment of alcoholism, as it has been in many other countries. Acamprosate was the first pharmacologic agent specifically designed to maintain abstinence in ethanol-dependent people after detoxification. With a chemical structure similar to that of GABA (see Figure 13.5), acamprosate is thought to exert both a GABA-agonistic action at GABA receptors and an inhibitory action at glutaminergic NMDA receptors. It appears to act in the CNS to restore the normal activity of glutaminergic neurotransmission altered by chronic alcohol exposure (Mason and Heyser, 2010). Acamprosate is poorly absorbed orally and therefore is given in relatively high doses (about 2 grams per day). It has a half-life of about 18 hours and is excreted unchanged by the kidneys; it is not metabolized before excretion.

In early human studies, acamprosate was thought to be about three times as effective as placebo, with drinking frequency reduced by 30 to 50 percent. Today, it is thought perhaps to be comparable to naltrexone, with efficacy increased by adding the drug to established, abstinence-based, cognitive-behavioral rehabilitation programs (Feeney et al., 2002) or by combining the drug with naltrexone (Kiefer et al., 2003) (Figure 13.8). In both situations, naltrexone and acamprosate, although less than impressive individually, can be effective when used together and/or added to intensive psychotherapies. Therefore, combination therapy may be important. Indeed, coadministration of acamprosate and naltrexone significantly increased the rate and extent of absorption of acamprosate, as indicated by a 33 percent increase in acamprosate blood level and a 33 percent reduction in time to peak blood level. Acamprosate did not affect the pharmacokinetics of naltrexone. Thus, when using the two drugs in combination, the dose of acamprosate, although poorly absorbed orally, can be reduced by 33 percent. Used alone in the treatment of alcohol dependence, acamprosate has had unremarkable effects, usually faring little better than placebo (Doggrell, 2006; Morley et al., 2006). This relative lack of efficacy was verified in the COMBINE study discussed later.

Dopaminergic Drugs. *Dopaminergic drugs,* such as *bupropion* (Wellbutrin), have theoretical use in maintaining abstinence because

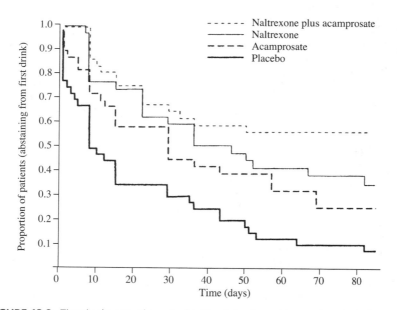

FIGURE 13.8 Time in days to relapse to drinking following a two-week period of detoxification, followed by initiation of therapy with one of four regimens: placebo therapy, acamprosate (2 grams per day), naltrexone (50 milligrams per day), or combined acamprosate/naltrexone. Each group consisted of 40 patients. The three medication groups were significantly different from the placebo group in preventing or delaying relapse. In addition, the effects of combined medication were significantly different from the effects of either medication used alone. [From Kiefer et al. (2003), p. 96.]

(1) the positive reinforcement associated with alcohol attractiveness appears to involve the dopaminergic reward system; (2) withdrawal may be accompanied by hypofunction of this reward system; and (3) depression is often comorbid with alcohol dependency. Since bupropion acts as an antidepressant at least partly through a dopaminergic action, patients with comorbid depression and alcohol dependence might be candidates for treatment with this drug. Further study in this area is probably warranted.

Serotonergic Drugs. Serotonergic drugs have been studied as agents for treating alcohol dependence. The research follows from the concept that there may be a relationship between serotonin function and alcohol consumption. In addition, different subtypes of alcoholics may be differentiated by the type or complexity of their serotonin dysfunction (Pettinati et al., 2003). Beyond excessive drinking, behaviors that are indicators of serotonin dysregulation include depression, anxiety, impulsiveness, and early-onset drinking.

Three classes of drugs that affect serotonin function have been evaluated:

1. Selective serotonin reuptake inhibitors (SSRIs), such as *fluoxetine* (Prozac) and *sertraline* (Zoloft)
2. A serotonin 5-HT$_{1A}$ agonist, *buspirone* (BuSpar)
3. A serotonin 5-HT$_3$ antagonist, *ondansetron* (Zofran)

SSRIs and buspirone have been approved by the FDA for treating depression and anxiety disorders (Chapter 5). SSRIs have also been evaluated for treating alcohol dependence, especially when alcoholic patients exhibit comorbid mood or anxiety disorders. In general, the results have been inconsistent. However, some progress has been made, and efficacy can be differentiated in Type A and Type B alcoholics (Cornelius et al., 2000). Type B alcoholics are characterized by early-age onset of drinking (ages 13 to 14), high levels of premorbid vulnerability, high levels of alcohol and other drug use severity, and high levels of comorbid psychopathology. Type B alcoholics respond poorly to treatment with SSRIs. Type A alcoholics have a later onset of heavy drinking (usually after the age of 20), lower levels of risk/severity of alcoholism, and lower levels of comorbid psychopathology. Type A alcoholics are relatively uncomplicated in their history and clinical presentation, despite high levels of alcohol consumption (Randall et al., 2001). Both drinking behaviors and affective dysregulation (for example, depression) may be positively affected. The efficacy of buspirone has been disappointing.

The serotonin 5-HT$_3$ antagonist ondansetron has been shown to reduce drinking behaviors in patients with early-onset alcoholism. Patients with later-onset alcoholism were less benefited (Dawes et al., 2005). Kenna and coworkers (2009b) discuss the possible genetic basis of this action of ondansetron.

Nicotinic Mechanism.   Chapter 11 discussed a new treatment for cigarette (nicotine) dependence. Varenicline (Chantix) is a "partial nicotinic agonist," reducing the reinforcing effect of nicotine. Crunelle and coworkers (2010) reported that it reduces alcohol consumption, at least in rats. Early data indicate that it reduces the rate of relapse in people with alcohol dependence (Steensland et al., 2007). More should be forthcoming in this interesting area.

Cannabinoid Mechanism.   As discussed, we are learning about a cannabinoid mechanism underlying alcohol craving and relapse. Early data demonstrate that cannabinoid receptor antagonists such as rimonabant (Acomplia) can effectively moderate consumption of alcohol (Fattore et al., 2007; Nowak et al., 2006; Maldonado et al., 2006) and may initiate a new generation of compounds for treating drug and alcohol dependence.

COMBINE Study

Treatment for alcohol dependence may include medications, behavioral therapies, or both. To understand how combining these treatments may impact effectiveness, a large, placebo-controlled study (1383 recently alcohol-abstinent volunteers in 11 treatment sites) was designed—the Combined Pharmacotherapies and Behavioral Interventions for Alcohol Dependence, or COMBINE, study. In different combinations, two medications (oral naltrexone and acamprosate) and two behavioral interventions (medical management, or MM, and combined behavioral intervention, or CBI) were employed. MM employed a series of brief counseling sessions to enhance medication compliance and abstinence from alcohol. CBI was a more intensive treatment similar to that used by trained psychotherapists working in alcoholism treatment facilities.

All treatment groups showed substantial reductions in drinking (Anton et al., 2006). Unexpectedly, acamprosate showed no evidence of efficacy; it reduced drinking no better than placebo. MM with naltrexone, CBI, or both fared better than placebo or acamprosate on drinking outcomes (percent days abstinent from alcohol and time to first heavy drinking day). No combination produced better efficacy than naltrexone or CBI alone in the presence of medical management. Placebo pills and MM had a positive effect above that of CBI alone. Anton and coworkers (2006) concluded that "naltrexone with MM could be delivered in health care settings, thus serving alcohol-dependent patients who might otherwise not receive treatment" (p. 2003).

In a 2008 update, Zarkin and coworkers performed a cost-benefit analysis and concluded:

> Focusing only on effectiveness, MM-naltrexone-acamprosate therapy is not significantly better than MM-naltrexone therapy. However, considering cost and cost-effectiveness, MM-naltrexone-acamprosate therapy may be a better choice, depending on whether the cost of incremental increase in effectiveness is justified by the decision maker. (p. 1214)

Pharmacotherapies to Help Treat Comorbid Psychological Conditions

Relapse to drinking behaviors and untreated comorbid psychological disorders are closely intertwined. Addictive behaviors and cravings as well as affective psychopathology (anxiety, depression, irritability, anger, insomnia, and so on) involve complex and poorly understood interactions among the opioid, dopaminergic, and serotonergic systems. Opioid and dopaminergic systems are probably involved in mechanisms of craving, and serotonergic dysfunction is at a minimum involved in affective dysregulation.

When alcohol abuse and aggressive behaviors occur comorbidly, with or without abuse of other drugs, psychosocial and behavioral therapies are essential. Pharmacological treatments are not (and probably never will be) effective without the addition of intensive psychological therapies in all their various forms. In the treatment of affective disorders that occur comborbidly with alcohol dependence, antidepressants may be useful. Anticonvulsant mood stabilizers (drugs such as pregabalin or topiramate) may be of use in the control of emotional states such as anger, aggression, insomnia, and emotional outbursts.

INHALANTS OF ABUSE

Inhalants are breathable chemical vapors that produce psychoactive (mind-altering) effects. They are among the most toxic and lethal of substances that can be abused.[4] Inhalant abuse (also known as *huffing, sniffing,* or *bagging*) is the intentional inhalation of a volatile substance for the purposes of achieving an altered mental state (Williams et al, 2007). Although other abused substances can be inhaled (for example, nicotine, THC, cocaine, methamphetamine), the term *inhalants* is used to describe a variety of substances whose main common characteristic is that they are rarely, if ever, taken by any route other than inhalation. A variety of products commonplace in the home and the workplace contain substances that can be inhaled. A few were developed as general anesthetics. Examples include nitrous oxide and halothane. These anesthetics were never meant to be used to achieve a "recreational" intoxicating effect. Likewise, other agents were developed for home and industrial use and were never intended to be used to affect the mind. Household inhalants include such products as nail polish remover, spray paint, glues, lighter fluid, hair and deodorant sprays, cleaning fluids, and pressurized whipped cream. Common industrial agents include gasoline, dry cleaning fluids, paint thinner, and paint remover. Table 13.2 lists many of the commonly encountered inhalants of abuse.

Not included in Table 13.2 are the *nitrites*, a special class of inhalants. Although other inhalants are used to alter mood, the nitrites are used primarily as sexual enhancers. Formerly, one nitrite (amyl nitrite) was used to dilate veins and reduce the workload of the heart; it relieved chest pain associated with coronary artery disease. Today, amyl nitrite is infrequently used for this purpose. Other nitrites (isobutyl nitrite and butyl nitrite) are sold as video head cleaners,

---

[4] See www.inhalants.com, sponsored by the National Inhalant Prevention Coalition.

TABLE 13.2 Chemicals commonly found in inhalants

	Inhalant	Chemical
Adhesives	Airplane glue	Toluene, ethyl acetate
	Other glues	Hexane, toluene, methyl chloride, acetone, methyl ethyl ketone, methyl butyl ketone
	Special cements	Trichloroethylene, tetrachloroethylene
Aerosols	Spray paint	Butane, propane (U.S.), fluorocarbons, toluene, hydrocarbons, "Texas shoe shine" (a spray containing toluene)
	Hair spray	Butane, propane (U.S.), CFCs
	Deodorant, air freshener	Butane, propane (U.S.), CFCs
	Analgesic spray	Chlorofluorocarbons (CFCs)
	Asthma spray	Chlorofluorocarbons (CFCs)
	Fabric spray	Butane, trichloroethane
	PC cleaner	Dimethyl ether, hydrofluorocarbons
Anesthetics	Gas	Nitrous oxide
	Liquid	Halothane, enflurane
	Local	Ethyl chloride
Cleaning agents	Dry cleaning	Tetrachloroethylene, trichloroethane
	Spot remover	Xylene, petroleum distillates, chlorohydrocarbons
	Degreaser	Tetrachloroethylene, trichloroethane, trichloroethylene
Solvents and gases	Nail polish remover	Acetone, ethyl acetate
	Paint remover	Toluene, methyl chloride, methanol acetone, ethyl acetate
	Paint thinner	Petroleum distillates, esters, acetone
	Correction fluid and thinner	Trichloroethylene, trichloroethane
	Fuel gas	Butane, isopropane
	Lighter fluid	Butane, isopropane
	Fire extinguisher	Bromochlorodifluoromethane
Aerosol whipped cream canisters		Nitrous oxide
"Room odorizers"	Locker Room, Rush, poppers	Isoamyl, isobutyl, isopropyl or butyl nitrate (now illegal), cyclohexyl

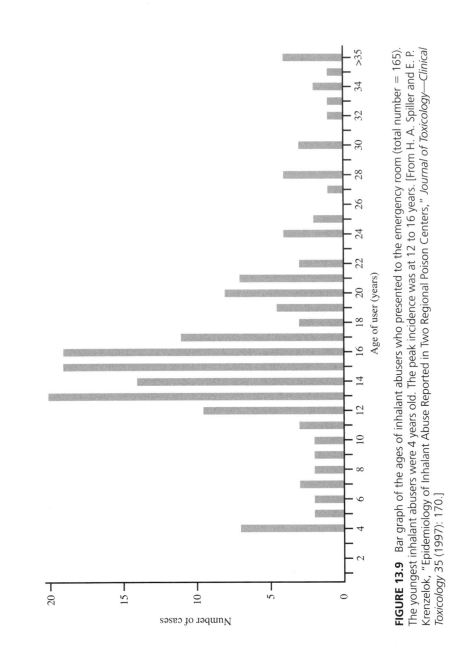

FIGURE 13.9 Bar graph of the ages of inhalant abusers who presented to the emergency room (total number = 165). The youngest inhalant abusers were 4 years old. The peak incidence was at 12 to 16 years. [From H. A. Spiller and E. P. Krenzelok, "Epidemiology of Inhalant Abuse Reported in Two Regional Poison Centers," *Journal of Toxicology—Clinical Toxicology* 35 (1997): 170.]

leather cleaners, and so on. These nitrites produce vasodilatation and a "flush" with reduction in blood pressure that is claimed to increase sexual satisfaction.

Inhalant abuse disproportionately affects young people. Nearly 20 percent of children in middle school and high school have experimented with inhaled substances. Inhalants are frequently the first mind-altering drugs used by children, occasionally as young as 3 or 4 years of age. Inhalant abuse reaches its peak at some point during the seventh to ninth grades, with eighth graders regularly showing the highest rates of abuse (Figure 13.9). Inhalants are popular with youth because of peer influence, low cost, availability, and rapid onset of effect. When inhaled, they produce euphoria, delirium, intoxication, and alterations in mental status, resembling alcohol intoxication or a "light" state of general anesthesia. Users are usually not aware of the potentially serious health consequences that can result. Especially in children, inhalant abuse is an underrecognized form of substance abuse with significant morbidity and mortality.

Why Inhalants Are Abused and Who Abuses Them

Inhalant abuse goes back at least a hundred years, when ether, nitrous oxide, and chloroform were introduced into medicine as general anesthetics. Concomitant with their discovery as anesthetics was their discovery as intoxicating agents, leading to nitrous oxide and ether parties. Today, inhalant abuse is one of the most pervasive yet least recognized drug problems. In a 2010 announcement from the Substance Abuse and Mental Health Services Administration (SAMHSA) more 12 year-olds replaces have used inhalants than have used marijuana, cocaine, and hallucinogens combined (6.7% lifetime use at age 12 compared with 5% nonmedical abuse of prescription drugs, 1.4% use of marijuana, 0.7% use of hallucinogens, and 0.1% use of cocaine.[1]

A few users continue their abuse of inhalants into adulthood, usually as part of a polysubstance abuse pattern (see Figure 13.9). Patterns of abuse resemble patterns seen in abuse of other types of substances: there are experimenters, intermittent users, and chronic abusers. The majority of young inhalant abusers do not view such abuse as being risky (Perron and Howard, 2008), although about 20 percent of abusers will develop an inhalant substance abuse disorder (Perron et al., 2009).

Although injuries are associated with the frequency of use, the so-called sudden sniffing death syndrome can occur in first-time users. Brown and coworkers (1999) reviewed deaths from inhalant abuse in the state of Virginia over the ten-year period 1987–1997. The 39 deaths

[1] See www.samhsa.gov/newsroom/advisories/1013110303.aspx

accounted for 0.3 percent of all deaths in males aged 13 to 22. Age of death ranged from 13 to 42 years; 70 percent of deaths occurred at 22 years of age or younger. Ninety-five percent of deaths occurred in males. Gasoline fuels accounted for 46 percent of the fatalities. Butane and propane sniffing is also associated with "sudden sniffing death" due to production of rapid-onset, potentially fatal cardiac arrhythmias. Alper and coworkers (2008) delineated the probable cause of these sudden deaths.

Medical Consequences of Inhalant Abuse

Most inhaled vapors produce rapid onset of a state of intoxication (or "drunkenness") that resembles alcohol intoxication, with slurred speech, impaired judgment, euphoria, and dizziness. Most inhalants produce intoxication that lasts only a few minutes. Therefore, abusers frequently try to prolong the high by continuing to inhale repeatedly over the course of several hours. This practice can be very dangerous for several reasons, including lack of oxygen (hypoxia) and asphyxiation, as well as the organ toxicities to be discussed. With increasing intoxication, the user experiences ataxia (staggering), dizziness, delirium, and disorientation. With severe intoxication come muscle weakness, lethargy, and signs of light to moderate general anesthesia. Even without hypoxia itself, hallucinations and behavioral changes may occur.

Toluene is a common ingredient in a number of the substances sought out for inhalant abuse, apparently for its euphorigenic, hallucinogenic, and behaviorally rewarding effects. Indeed, toluene is taken up into and activates the central reward centers, including the mesolimbic dopaminergic reward centers and the frontal cortex.

Not all inhalants exert this action on central dopaminergic reward centers, but many do. With some agents (particularly the *nitrites*), vasodilation and muscle relaxant effects appear to underlie use. With anesthetics, such as *nitrous oxide,* a state of light general anesthesia is induced, although reward activation may occur at low doses. With the *volatile solvents* and *fuels,* conclusions are difficult to draw, but their profile of acute behavioral and pharmacological effects is similar to that observed with subanesthetic concentrations of clinically used volatile anesthetics.

Although death is relatively rare during acute intoxication, when it does occur, it usually follows from lack of oxygen to the brain (anoxia), cardiac arrhythmias, aspiration of vomitus, or trauma. *Sudden sniffing death syndrome* may account for 50 percent of fatalities from acute intoxication. Volatile hydrocarbons sensitize the heart to serious arrhythmias when a person is startled or becomes excited during intoxication. The sudden surge of adrenaline acts on the sensitized heart to set off serious and life-threatening arrhythmias. This kind of episode can occur during initial experimentation and during any episode of abuse.

With *chronic abuse* of inhalants, serious complications can include peripheral and central nervous system dysfunction (peripheral neuropathies and encephalopathy), liver and/or kidney failure, dementia, loss of cognitive and other higher functions, gait disturbances, and loss of coordination. In a study of 55 inhalant abusers with an average 10 years of abusing, Rosenberg and coworkers (2002) administered a battery of cognitive tests as well as performing magnetic resonance imaging (MRI). This group was compared with a group of 61 cocaine abusers. Both groups displayed scores below general population averages on tests of cognitive functioning, but inhalant abusers consistently scored even below the cocaine abusers on tests involving working memory, planning, and problem solving. Almost half of the inhalant abusers had abnormalities in their MRI scans (compared to 25 percent of the cocaine abusers). Most marked was diffuse white matter degeneration in several brain areas.

Many people who abuse inhalants for prolonged periods over many days feel a strong need to continue abusing them, implying compulsive abuse. A mild withdrawal syndrome can follow long-term abuse, perhaps similar to withdrawal from any of many sedative-hypnotic drugs. Long-term inhalant abusers exhibit symptoms including weight loss, muscle weakness, disorientation, incoordination, irritability, depression, and neurocognitive deficits.

Treatment of acute inhalant intoxication is primarily supportive with the administration of supplemental oxygen. Treatment of chronic inhalant abuse is much more difficult. Results of a survey of 550 drug treatment program directors indicate that most inhalant abusers have a pessimistic attitude about the treatment effectiveness and hopes for long-term recovery (Beauvais et al., 2002). The surveyed directors perceived that a great deal of neurological damage results from inhalant use and that education, preventive efforts, and treatments are inadequate. Early identification of abusers and rapid intervention are essential in preventing both short-term and long-term consequences.

Standard approaches are generally ineffective for inhalant abusers because of the need for long-term detoxification and adverse effects on cognitive function. Talk therapies are inappropriate for many patients with neurological dysfunction, and the short attention span and poor impulse control of many patients make group therapy a poor choice as well. Instead, special treatment approaches for habitual users might include the following:

- Detoxification
- Medical and neurological evaluation
- Neurocognitive assessment
- Neurocognitive rehabilitation for patients who are impaired

- Academic programs to ensure participation in school
- Team approach with medical, neurological, psychological, occupational, psychomotor rehabilitation, and educational components
- Occupational and physical therapy where indicated
- Restriction or elimination of access to inhalable substances
- Aftercare that takes easy availability of inhalants into account, as well as residual cognitive impairment and poor social functioning

The best treatment is prevention. It must come from everyone involved in a child's life: parents, educators, school nurses, school bus drivers, school cafeteria workers, and any other adults in the child's world.

STUDY QUESTIONS

1. Pharmacologically, what is ethyl alcohol?

2. Describe the metabolism of alcohol. What enzymes are involved? What drug blocks one of these enzymes?

3. How do women and men differ in their metabolism of alcohol?

4. How does the kinetics of alcohol metabolism differ from that of most other drugs?

5. How long does it take for an adult to metabolize the alcohol in a 1-ounce glass of 80 proof whiskey? A 4-ounce glass of wine? A 12-ounce bottle of beer? A pint of 7 percent microbrew?

6. What BAC is defined in most states as "intoxication"?

7. Describe what effects alcohol exerts on the CNS.

8. Why might a person who has developed a physical dependence on alcohol be treated with a benzodiazepine as a substitute for the alcohol?

9. Summarize some of the drugs and techniques used in treating alcoholism. What medications might be used to ameliorate alcohol withdrawal? Discuss in terms of the COMBINE report.

10. Describe the disease concept of alcoholism. Discuss the comorbidity of alcohol dependence with other psychological disorders.

11. Describe some of the fetal effects of alcohol. Is there a "safe" level of drinking during pregnancy?

12. Summarize some of the problems associated with inhalant abuse.

REFERENCES

Abbey, A., et al. (2002). "How Does Alcohol Contribute to Sexual Assault? Explanations from Laboratory and Survey Data." *Alcoholism: Clinical and Experimental Research* 26: 575–581.

Alen, F., et al. (2009). "Cannabinoid-Induced Increase in Relapse-Like Drinking Is Prevented by the Blockade of the Glycine-Binding Site of N-methyl-D-Aspartate receptors." *Neuroscience* 158: 465–473

Alper, A. T., et al. (2008). "Glue (Toluene) Abuse: Increased QT Dispersion and Relation with Unexplained Syncope." *Inhalation Toxicology* 20: 37–41.

Anton, R. F., et al. (2006). "Combined Pharmacotherapies and Behavioral Interventions for Alcohol Dependence: The COMBINE Study: A Randomized Controlled Trial." *Journal of the American Medical Association* 295: 2003–2017.

Autti-Ramo, I. (2000). "Twelve-Year Follow-Up of Children Exposed to Alcohol in Utero." *Developmental Medicine and Child Neurology* 42: 406–411.

Baer, J. S., et al. (2003). "A 21-Year Longitudinal Analysis of the Effects of Prenatal Alcohol Exposure on Young Adult Drinking." *Archives of General Psychiatry* 60: 377–385.

Ballenger, J. C., and Post, R. M. (1978). "Kindling as a Model for Alcohol Withdrawal Syndromes." *British Journal of Psychiatry* 133: 1–14.

Beauvais, F., et al. (2002). "A Survey of Attitudes Among Drug Use Treatment Providers Toward the Treatment of Inhalant Users." *Substance Use and Abuse* 37: 1391–1410.

Becker, H. C., et al. (2006). "Pregabalin Is Effective Against Behavioral and Electrographic Seizures During Alcohol Withdrawal." *Alcohol and Alcoholism* 24: 399–406.

Boehm, S. L., et al. (2002). "Ventral Tegmental Area Region Governs GABA(B) Receptor Modulation of Ethanol-Stimulated Activity in Mice." *Neuroscience* 115: 185–200.

Bowen, S. E., et al. (1999). "Deaths Associated with Inhalant Abuse in Virginia from 1987 to 1996." *Drug and Alcohol Dependence* 53: 239–245.

Brown, S. A., et al. (2000). "Neurocognitive Functioning of Adolescents: Effects of Protracted Alcohol Use." *Alcoholism: Clinical and Experimental Research* 24: 164–171.

Carmichael, H., et al. (1997). "Association of Prenatal Alcohol Exposure with Behavioral and Learning Problems in Early Adolescence." *Journal of the American Academy of Child and Adolescent Psychiatry* 36: 1187–1194.

Cornelius, J. R., et al. (2000). "Fluoxetine versus Placebo in Depressed Alcoholics: A 1-Year Follow-Up Study." *Addiction Behavior* 25: 307–310.

Crunelle, C. L., et al. (2010). "The Nicotinic Acetylcholine Receptor Partial Agonist Varenicline and the Treatment of Drug Dependence: A Review." *European Neuropsychopharmacology* 20: 69–79.

Dawes, M. A., et al. (2005). "A Prospective, Open-Label Trial of Ondansetron in Adolescents with Alcohol Dependence." *Addictive Behaviors* 30: 1077–1085.

Dawson, D. A., et al. (2005). "Quantifying the Risks Associated with Exceeding Recommended Drinking Limits." *Alcoholism: Clinical and Experimental Research* 29: 902–908.

Dawson, D. A., et al. (2007). "Impact of Age at First Drink on Stress-Reactive Drinking." *Alcoholism: Clinical and Experimental Research* 31: 69–77.

de Mattos, V. B., et al. (2009). "Melancholic Features Related to Rimonabant." *General Hospital Psychiatry* 31: 583–585.

Doggrell, S. A. (2006). "Which Treatment for Alcohol Dependence: Naltrexone, Acamprosate, and/or Behavioral Intervention?" *Expert Opinion in Pharmacotherapy* 7: 2169–2173.

Duka, T., et al. (2003). "Impairment in Cognitive Functions After Multiple Detoxifications in Alcoholic Inpatients." *Alcoholism: Clinical and Experimental Research 27:* 1563–1572.

Elbreder, M. F., et al. (2010). "The Use of Disulfiram for Alcohol-Dependent Patients and Duration of Outpatient Treatment." *European Archives of Psychiatry and Clinical Neuroscience* 260: 191–195.

Fadda, F., and Rossetti, Z. L. (1998). "Chronic Ethanol Consumption: From Neuroadaptation to Neurodegeneration." *Progress in Neurobiology* 56: 385–431.

Fattore, L., et al. (2007). "An Endocannabinoid Mechanism in Relapse to Drug Seeking: A Review of Animal Studies and Clinical Perspectives." *Brain Research Brain Research Review* 53: 1–16.

Feeney, G. F., et al. (2002). "Cognitive Behavioural Therapy Combined with the Relapse-Prevention Medication Acamprosate: Are Short-Term Treatment Outcomes for Alcohol Dependence Improved?" *Australian and New Zealand Journal of Psychiatry* 36: 622–628.

Fergusson, D. M., et al. (2009). "Tests of Causal Links Between Alcohol Abuse or Dependence and Major Depression." *Archives of General Psychiatry* 66: 260–266.

Frezza, M., et al. (1990). "High Blood Alcohol Levels in Women: The Role of Decreased Gastric Alcohol Dehydrogenase Activity and First-Pass Metabolism." *New England Journal of Medicine* 322: 95–99.

Frye, M. A., and Salloum, I. M. (2006). "Bipolar Disorder and Comorbid Alcoholism: Prevalence Rate and Treatment Considerations." *Bipolar Disorder* 8: 677–685.

Garbutt, J. C. (2009). "The State of Pharmacotherapy for the Treatment of Alcohol Dependence." *Journal of Substance Abuse Treatment* 36: S15–S23.

George, D. T., et al. (2008). "Neurokinin-1 Receptor Antagonism as a Possible Therapy for Alcoholism." *Science* 319: 1536–1539.

George, D. T., et al. (2010). "Rimonabant (SR141716) Has No Effect on Alcohol Self-Administration or Endocrine Measures in Nontreatment-Seeking Heavy Alcohol Drinkers." *Psychopharmacology* 208: 37–44.

Gold, P. E. (2008). "Protein Synthesis Inhibition and Memory: Formation vs Amnesia." *Neurobiology of Learning and Memory* 89: 201–211.

Goodwin, D. W., and Gabrielli, W. F. (1997). "Alcohol: Clinical Aspects." In J. H. Lowinson, P. Ruiz, R. B. Millman, and J. G. Langrod, eds., *Substance Abuse: A Comprehensive Textbook*, 3rd ed. (pp. 142–148). Baltimore: Williams & Wilkins.

Grant, B. F., et al. (2004). "Co-Occurence of 12-Month Alcohol and Drug Use Disorders and Personality Disorders in the United States." *Archives of General Psychiatry* 61: 361–368.

Hartzler, B., and Fromme, K. (2003). "Fragmentary and En Bloc Blackouts: Similarity and Distinction Among Episodes of Alcohol-Induced Memory Loss." *Journal of Studies on Alcohol* 64: 547–550.

Heinz, A., et al. (2009). "Identifying the Neural Circuity of Alcohol Craving and Relapse Vulnerability." *Addiction Biology* 14: 108–118.

Hindson, R., et al. (2001). "Age of Drinking Onset and Involvement in Physical Fights After Drinking." *Pediatrics* 108: 872–877.

Hoiseth, G., et al. (2008). "Comparison Between the Urinary Markers EtG, EtS, and GTOL/5-HIAA in a Controlled Drinking Experiment." *Alcohol and Alcoholism* 43: 187–191.

Hoiseth, G., et al. (2009). "Serum/Whole Blood Concentration Ratio for Ethyl Glucuronide and Ethyl Sulfate." *Journal of Analytical Toxicology* 33: 208–211.

Hughes, J. R. (2009). "Alcohol Withdrawal Seizures." *Epilepsy and Behavior* 15: 92–97.

Hungund, B. L., et al. (2003). "Cannabinoid CB1 Receptor Knockout Mice Exhibit Markedly Reduced Voluntary Alcohol Consumption and Lack Alcohol-Induced Dopamine Release in the Nucleus Accumbens." *Journal of Neurochemistry* 84: 698–704.

John, E. R., and Prichep, L. S. (2005). "The Anesthetic Cascade: A Theory of How Anesthesia Suppresses Consciousness." *Anesthesiology* 102: 447–471.

Johnson, B. A. (2008). "Update on Neuropharmacological Treatments for Alcoholism." *Biochemical Pharmacology* 75: 34–56.

Johnson, B. A., et al. (2005). "Safety and Efficacy of GABAergic Medications for Treating Alcoholism." *Alcoholism: Clinical and Experimental Research* 29: 248–254.

Junghanns, K., et al. (2009). "Urinary Ethyl Glucuronide (EtG) and Ethyl Sulfate (EtS) Assessment: Valuable Tools to Improve Verification of Abstention in Alcohol-Dependent Patients During In-Patient Treatment and at Follow-Ups." *Addiction* 104: 921–926.

Kampman, K. M., et al. (2007). A Double-Blind, Placebo-Controlled Pilot Trial of Quetiapine for the Treatment of Type A and Type B Alcoholism." *Journal of Clinical Psychopharmacology* 27: 344–351.

Kenna, G. A., et al. (2009a). "Review of Topiramate: An Antiepileptic for the Treatment of Alcohol Dependence." *Current Drug Abuse Reviews* 2: 135–142.

Kenna, G. A., et al. (2009b). "A Within-Group Design of Nontreatment-Seeking 5-HTTLPR Genotype Alcohol-Dependent Subjects Receiving Ondansetron and Sertraline." *Alcoholism: Clinical and Experimental Research* 33: 315–323.

Kerr, W. C., et al. (2008). "Alcohol Content Variation of Bar and Restaurant Drinks in Northern California." *Alcoholism: Clinical and Experimental Research* 32: 1623–1629.

Kiefer, F., et al. (2003). "Comparing and Combining Naltrexone and Acamprosate in Relapse Prevention of Alcoholism: A Double-Blind, Placebo-Controlled Study." *Archives of General Psychiatry* 60: 92–99.

Kohnke, M. D. (2008). "Approach to the Genetics of Alcoholism: A Review Based on Pathophysiology." *Biochemical Pharmacology* 75: 160–177.

Kot-Leibovich, H., and Fainsod, A. (2009): "Ethanol Induces Embryonic Malformations by Competing for Retinaldehyde Dehydrogenase Activity During Vertebrate Gastrulation." *Disease Models and Mechanisms* 2: 295–305.

Krupitsky, E. M., et al. (2007). "Antiglutamatergic Strategies for Ethanol Detoxification: Comparison with Placebo and Diazepam." *Alcoholism: Clinical and Experimental Research* 31: 604–611.

Kushner, M. G., et al. (1996). "The Effects of Alcohol Consumption on Laboratory-Induced Panic and State Anxiety." *Archives of General Psychiatry* 53: 264–270.

Lapham, S. C., et al. (2001). "Prevalence of Psychiatric Disorders Among Persons Convicted of Driving While Impaired." *Archives of General Psychiatry* 58: 943–949.

Lawrence, A. J. (2007). "Therapeutics for Alcoholism: What's the Future?" *Drug and Alcohol Reviews* 26: 3–8.

Lee, H., et al. (2009). "Alcohol-Induced Blackout." *International Journal of Environmental Research and Public Health* 6: 2783–2792

Leggio, L., et al. (2008). "New Developments for the Pharmacological Treatment of Alcohol Withdrawal Syndrome. A Focus on Non-Benzodiazepine GABA-ergic Medications." *Progress in Neuro-Psychopharmacology and Biological Psychiatry* 32: 1106–1117.

Lobmaier, P., et al. (2008). "Sustained-Release Naltrexone for Opioid Dependence." *Cochrane Database Systematic Reviews* 16: CD006140.

Malcolm, R., et al. (2000). "Recurrent Detoxification May Elevate Alcohol Craving as Measured by the Obsessive Compulsive Drinking Scale." *Alcohol* 20: 181–185.

Maldonado, R., et al. (2006). "Involvement of the Endocannabinoid System in Drug Addiction." *Trends in Neuroscience* 29: 225–232.

Malinen, H., and Hyytia. P. (2008): Ethanol Self-Administration Is Regulated by CB1 Receptors in the Nucleus Accumbens and Ventral Tegmental Area in Alcohol-Preferring AA Rats." *Alcoholism: Clinical and Experimental Research* 32: 1976–1983.

Mann, K., et al. (2008). "Acamprosate: Recent Findings and Future Research Directions. *Alcoholism: Clinical and Experimental Research* 32: 1105–1110.

Markianos, M., et al. (2000). "Dopamine Receptor Responsivity in Alcoholic Patients Before and After Detoxification." *Drug and Alcohol Dependence* 57: 261–265.

Martin, S. E., and Bryant, K. (2001). "Gender Differences in the Association of Alcohol Intoxication and Illicit Drug Abuse Among Persons Arrested for Violent and Property Offenses." *Journal of Substance Abuse* 3: 563–581.

Martinotti, G., et al. (2010). "Pregabalin, Tiapride and Lorazepam in Alcohol Withdrawal Syndrome: A Multi-Centre, Randomized, Single-Blind Comparison Trial." *Addiction* 105: 288–299.

Mason, B. J., and Heyser, C. J. (2010). "The Neurobiology, Clinical Efficacy and Safety of Acamprosate in the Treatment of Alcohol Dependence." *Expert Opinion on Drug Safety* 9: 177–188.

Matsuzawa, S., and Suzuki, T. (2002). "Psychological Stress and Rewarding Effect of Alcohol." *Nihon Arukor Yakubutsu Igakkai Zasshi* 37: 143–152.

Morley, K. C., et al. (2006). "Naltrexone versus Acamprosate in the Treatment of Alcohol Dependence: A Multi-Centre, Randomized, Double-Blind, Placebo-Controlled Trial." *Addiction* 101: 1451–1462.

Morse, R. M., and Flavin, D. K. (1992). "The Definition of Alcoholism." *Journal of the American Medical Association* 268: 1012–1014.

Myrick, H., et al. (2009). "A Double-Blind Trial of Gabapentin versus Lorazepam in the Treatment of Alcohol Withdrawal." *Alcoholism: Clinical and Experimental Research* 33: 1582–1588.

National Institute on Alcohol Abuse and Alcoholism. (2007). "Helping Patients Who Drink Too Much." NIAAA Publications Distribution Center, P. O. Box 10686, Rockville, MD 20849-0686. Downloadable at www.niaaa.nih.gov.

Noel, X., et al. (2001). "Supervisory Attentional System in Nonamnestic Alcoholic Men." *Archives of General Psychiatry* 58: 1152–1158.

Nowak, K. L., et al. (2006). "Pharmacological Manipulation of CB1 Receptor Function Alters Development of Tolerance to Alcohol." *Alcohol and Alcoholism* 41: 24–32.

Oscar-Berman, M., and Marinkovic, K. (2007): "Alcohol: Effects on Neurobehavioral Functions and the Brain." *Neuropsychology Review* 17: 239–257.

Palmer, R. B. (2009). "A Review of the Use of Ethyl Glucuronide as a Marker for Ethanol Consumption in Forensic and Clinical Medicine." *Seminars in Diagnostic Pathology* 26: 18–27.

Perron, B. E., and Howard, M. O. (2008). "Perceived Risk of Harm and Intentions of Future Inhalant Use Among Adolescent Inhalant Users." *Drug and Alcohol Dependence* 97: 185–189.

Perron, B. E., et al. (2009). "Prevalence, Timing, and Predictors of Transitions from Inhalant Use to Inhalant Use Disorders." *Drug and Alcohol Dependence* 100: 277–284.

Perry, P. J., et al. (2006). "The Association of Alcohol-Induced Blackouts and Grayouts to Blood Alcohol Concentrations." *Journal of Forensic Science* 51: 896–899.

Pettinati, H. M., et al. (2003). "The Status of Serotonin-Selective Pharmacotherapy in the Treatment of Alcohol Dependence." *Recent Developments in Alcoholism* 16: 247–262.

Pettinati, H. M., et al. (2004). "Gender Differences in Responses to Sertraline Pharmacotherapy in Type A Alcohol Dependence." *American Journal of the Addictions* 13: 236–247.

Pettinati, H. M., et al. (2006). "The Status of Naltrexone in the Treatment of Alcohol Dependence: Specific Effects on Heavy Drinking." *Journal of Clinical Psychopharmacology* 26: 610–625.

Randall, C. L., et al. (2001). "Paroxetine for Social Anxiety and Alcohol Use in Dual-Diagnosed Patients." *Depression and Anxiety* 14: 255–262.

Rohde, P., et al. (2001). "Natural Course of Alcohol Use Disorders from Adolescence to Young Adulthood." *Journal of the American Academy of Child and Adolescent Psychiatry* 40: 83–90.

Rosenberg, N. L., et al. (2002). "Neuropsychologic Impairment and MRI Abnormalities Associated with Chronic Solvent Abuse." *Journal of Toxicology— Clinical Toxicology* 40: 21–34.

Rubio, G., et al. (2006). "Effects of Lamotrigine in Patients with Bipolar Disorder and Alcohol Dependence." *Bipolar Disorder* 8: 289–293.

Saitz, R., et al. (2007). "Brief Intervention for Medical Inpatients with Unhealthy Alcohol Use: A Randomized, Controlled Trial." *Annals of Internal Medicine* 146: 167–176.

Sayal, K., et al. (2009). "Binge Pattern of Alcohol Consumption During Pregnancy and Childhood Mental Health Outcomes: Longitudinal Population-Based Study." *Pediatrics* 123: e289–e296.

Schuckit, M. A. (2009). "Alcohol-Use Disorders." *Lancet* 373: 492–501.

Schweizer, T. A., et al. (2004). "Fast, but Error-Prone, Responses During Acute Alcohol Intoxication: Effects of Stimulus-Response Mapping Complexity." *Alcoholism: Clinical and Experimental Research* 28: 643–649.

Seitz, H. K., and Becker, P. (2007). "Alcohol Metabolism and Cancer Risk." *Alcohol Research and Health* 30: 38–41.

Serra, S., et al. (2002). "Blockade by the Cannabinoid CB(1) Receptor Antagonist, SR 141716, of Alcohol Deprivation Effect in Alcohol-Preferring Rats." *European Journal of Pharmacology* 443: 95–97.

Simpson, T. L., et al. (2009): "A Pilot Trial of the Alpha-1-Adrenergic Antagonist, Prazosin, for Alcohol Dependence." *Alcoholism: Clinical and Experimental Research* 33: 255–263.

Solfrizzi, V., et al. (2007). "Alcohol Consumption, Mild Cognitive Impairment, and Progression to Dementia." *Neurology* 68: 1790–1799.

Steensland, P., et al. (2007). "Varenicline, an α4β2 Nicotinic Acetylcholine Receptor Partial Agonist, Selectively Decreases Ethanol Consumption and Seeking." *Proceedings of the National Academy of Sciences* 104: 12518–12523.

Swainstron-Harrison, T., et al. (2006). "Extended-Release Intramuscular Naltrexone." *Drugs* 66: 1741–1751.

Tiet, Q. Q., and Mausbach, B. (2007). "Treatments for Patients with Dual Diagnosis: A Review." *Alcoholism: Clinical and Experimental Research* 31: 513–536.

Vaillant, G. E. (1996). "A Long-Term Follow-Up of Male Alcohol Abuse." *Archives of General Psychiatry* 53: 243–249.

van der Zwaluw, C. S., et al. (2007). "Polymorphisms in the Mu-Opioid Receptor Gene (OPRM1) and the Implications for Alcohol Dependence in Humans." *Pharmacogenomics* 8: 1427–1436.

Vengeliene, V., et al. (2008). "Neuropharmacology of Alcohol Addiction." *British Journal of Pharmacology* 154: 299–315.

Wand, G. S., et al. (1998). "Family History of Alcoholism and Hypothalamic Opioidergic Activity." *Archives of General Psychiatry* 55: 1114–1119.

Wang, L., et al. (2003). "Endocannabinoid Signaling via Cannabinoid Receptor 1 Is Involved in Ethanol Preference and Its Age-Dependent Decline in Mice." *Proceedings of the National Academy of Sciences* 100: 1393–1398.

Williams, J. F., et al. (2007). "Inhalant Abuse." *Pediatrics* 119: 1009–1017.

Zarkin, G. A., et al. (2008). "Cost and Cost-Effectiveness of the COMBINE Study in Alcohol-Dependent Patients." *Archives of General Psychiatry* 65: 1214–1221.

CHAPTER 13 APPENDIX

What Is a Drink? How Much Alcohol Is in My Drink?

One drink equivalent is the amount of alcohol that contains 10 cubic centimeters (1/3 ounce) of 100 percent ethanol. This is the amount of ethanol that the body metabolizes in 1 hour and that reduces the blood alcohol concentration (BAC) by 0.015 grams%.

This amount of alcohol is contained in about 1 to 1.5 ounces of 40 percent (80 proof) liquor, 4 ounces of 12 percent wine, or a 12-ounce bottle of 5 percent beer.

The following beverages are converted to their calculated drink equivalents and the number of drink equivalents can be used with Figure 13.4 to estimate your BAC.

If you consume	You have consumed about
One 12-oz Budweiser (5% alcohol)	1.5 drink equivalents
One 6-pack of 12-oz Budweiser	9 drink equivalents
Short case (12 bottles) of 12-oz Budweiser	18 drink equivalents
One 16-oz Budweiser	1.9 (about 2) drink equivalents
One 24-oz Budweiser	3 drink equivalents
One 40-oz Budweiser	5 drink equivalents
One 12-oz Bud Light (4.2%)	1.25 drink equivalents
One 12 oz Bud-Ice (5.5%)	1.9 (almost 2) drink equivalents
One 16-oz Old English 800 (8%)	3.8 (almost 4) drink equivalents
One 40-oz Old English 800	9 drink equivalents
Two 40-oz Old English 800	18 drink equivalents (2/3 pint of whiskey)
One 16-oz Rainier Ale (7.2%)	3.5 drink equivalents
One 40-oz St. Ides Malt (7.3%)	8 drink equivalents
One 16-oz microbrew (5% to 7%)	2.2 to 3.4 drink equivalents
One 64-oz pitcher of microbrew	9.5 to 13 drink equivalents
One 12-oz Hornsby Draft Cider (6%)	2 drink equivalents
One 16-oz barley wine (10%)	4.8 drink equivalents
One 12-oz Zima cooler (4.6%)	1.6 drink equivalents
One 12-oz Mike's Hard Lemonade (5%)	1.8 drink equivalents

Comments

Budweiser and the other brand names are used for illustration only. Other beers are similar, with modest differences. Their alcohol concentration may or may not be listed on the label or package. Coors beer, another popular beer, is 4.9 percent alcohol; Coors Light is 4.2 percent. Busch beer is 4.5 percent; Henri Weinhard Private Reserve is 4.6 percent; Red Dog is 5 percent alcohol.

Ice beers are made by slightly freezing the brew and removing some of the ice, increasing the alcohol content. Most are 5.9 percent alcohol (12-oz bottle = 2 drink equivalents).

Wine coolers are classified as malt beverages and have alcohol contents from 4.6 percent to 7 percent. They are considered to be 1.5 to 2 drink equivalents per bottle.

A tavern can sell beer, ale, and malt liquor up to 14 percent alcohol, hard cider up to 10 percent alcohol, and wine up to 14 percent alcohol. Taverns and pubs often serve beer and ale in pitchers that contain from 60 to 72 ounces. If the pitcher contains regular draft beer at about 5 percent alcohol, a 64-ounce pitcher contains about 9.5 drink equivalents of ethanol.

Chapter 14

Cannabinoid Agonists
and Antagonists

The hemp plant *Cannabis sativa*, commonly called marijuana, grows throughout the world and flourishes in most temperate and tropical regions. Although *cannabinol* and *cannabidiol*, among other components, are present in lesser amounts in cannabis, the major psychoactive ingredient of the marijuana plant is *delta-9-tetrahydrocannabinol* (THC; Figure 14.1). THC is probably also responsible for the side effects, the pleasurable effects, and the therapeutic effects associated with smoking marijuana.

Names for cannabis products include marijuana, hashish, charas, bhang, ganja, and sinsemilla. *Hashish* and *charas,* which consist of the dried resinous exudates of the female flowers, are the most potent preparations, with a THC content averaging between 10 and 20 percent. *Ganja* and *sinsemilla* refer to the dried material found in the tops of the female plants, where the THC content averages about 5 to 8 percent. *Bhang* and *marijuana* are lower-grade preparations taken from the dried remainder of the plant, and their THC content varies from 2 to 5 percent, although improved growing, harvesting, and processing techniques have boosted this content considerably; indeed, from about the mid-1970s to 2007, the THC content in cannabis samples has increased from about 4 percent to over 9.0 percent.

Until about 1990, marijuana was classified according to its behavioral effects, usually as a mild sedative-hypnotic agent with effects similar to low doses of alcohol. Like alcohol, THC can produce disruption in attention mechanisms, impairment of short-term memory,

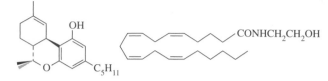

FIGURE 14.1 Structures of delta-9-tetrahydrocannabinol (THC) and anandamide, the endogenous ligand (neurotransmitter) of the cannabinoid receptor.

altered sensory awareness, and altered control of motor movements and postural control. Unlike alcohol, very high doses of THC do not depress respiration and are not lethal.

Since the early 1990s, extensive evidence has accumulated to demonstrate that THC binds to specific *cannabinoid receptors* in both the brain (*cannabinoid-1 receptors*) and the peripheral nervous system (*cannabinoid-2 receptors*). THC mimics the actions of an endogenous cannabinoid (a fatty acid called *anandamide*), which exerts important biological effects of its own. In addition, cannabinoid receptors exist in the brain in quantities that surpass most other G-protein-coupled receptors, approaching or exceeding levels observed for the amino acid receptors glutamate and GABA. This endogenous endocannabinoid system is becoming more clearly elucidated (Onaivi, 2009); is under genetic control; and has been associated with multiple health disorders, including osteoporosis, attention deficit/hyperactivity disorder (ADHD), posttraumatic stress disorder (PTSD), drug dependency, obesity, and depression.

History

The use of *C. sativa* dates from several thousand years ago, when it was used as a mild intoxicant; it is somewhat milder than alcohol. It is much less useful for religious and psychedelic experiences than other naturally occurring psychedelic drugs because it produces much less sensory distortion. Over the years, products from *C. sativa* have been claimed to have a wide variety of medical uses, although few persist in native cultures.

C. sativa was introduced into Western cultures probably in the 1850s. During the early 1920s, marijuana was portrayed as being an underground evil and a menace. Because it was claimed that an association existed between marijuana and crime, laws were passed to outlaw its use. By the mid-1930s, marijuana was looked on as a "narcotic" and as a drug responsible for crimes of violence. By 1940, the public was convinced that marijuana was a "killer drug" that (1) induced people to commit crimes of violence, (2) led to heroin addiction, and (3) was a social menace. The emotional campaign against marijuana persists even today, limiting research into the possible medical uses of cannabinoid agonists and antagonists.

Several facts associated with cannabis abuse are disquieting. First, marijuana is the most widely used illicit drug in the United States and the western hemisphere. The vast majority of America's 15 million illicit drug users use marijuana either alone or in conjunction with other drugs. In 2009, 25 percent of teenage Americans had smoked marijuana in the past month (Partnership for a Drug-Free America, 2010). Perhaps 5 percent of high-school-age people smoke marijuana daily. Second, it now appears that early onset of heavy use (by about 12 years of age) is associated with more severe psychopathology in later years (Hall and Degenhardt, 2009). Combined alcohol and marijuana use often serves as a marker for later pathology, probably because the substances are used early to self-medicate for psychological distress. Third, use of marijuana may increase rates of relapse to the use of other drugs such as alcohol, opioids, and stimulants, although few would call it a "gateway drug" (Degenhardt et al., 2009, 2010), with the "gateway" better conceptualized as a "genetically influenced developmental trajectory" (Cleveland and Wiebe, 2008).

In recent years, voters in fourteen states have approved ballot initiatives to permit the legal use of marijuana for medical purposes. Several other states are considering legalizing marijuana for medical purposes or lessening the penalties for possessing small amounts for personal consumption. Finally, scheduled for public vote on November 2, 2010, is a ballot measure in California (Proposition 09-0024) to legalize (and therefore impose taxes on) marijuana for recreational consumption, similar to treatment of alcohol. Approval of these initiatives would signal the first time since the repeal of the alcohol prohibition amendment some 70 years ago that the public has approved a pullback in the "war on drugs," and these initiatives would place state laws in conflict with federal statutes. The medical efficacy of marijuana is being clarified, and evidence is accumulating that marijuana does have medical uses, perhaps most prominently in the relief of several types of painful conditions (Guindon and Hohmann, 2009). Canada had originally made medical marijuana available, placing the Canadian law in direct conflict with federal statutes in the United States. More recently, Canada approved the use of a product called Sativex (discussed later), the world's first natural marijuana extract pharmaceutical, to relieve neuropathic pain, cancer pain, and pain associated with multiple sclerosis. In the United States, Sativex oromucosal spray is in late-stage (Phase III) study for the treatment of pain in patients with advanced cancer that has not been adequately relieved by opioid medications. It is also under study in the United States for the relief of neuropathic pain. These advances raise several questions:

- Should marijuana (or a Sativex-type medicine) be made available for medical use throughout the United States, and for what medical uses is THC (or crude marijuana) efficacious?

- Should marijuana (or the active drug THC) be made available for recreational use by adults in the United States? If approved for recreational use in California, what standards would be established for driving under the influence (DUI), workplace job testing, and other situations? What standards should be used to determine legal amounts of combined blood alcohol and THC in DUI arrests?
- How should society deal with the use of marijuana by those under the age of 21?

Mechanism of Action: Cannabinoid Receptor

THC was isolated from marijuana as its pharmacologically active ingredient (see Figure 14.1) in 1964. Evidence gathered from then until the mid-1980s led to the hypothesis that THC and other cannabinoids act via a pharmacologically distinct set of receptors. In 1986 it was shown that THC inhibits the intracellular enzyme adenylate cyclase and that the inhibition requires the presence of a G protein complex, similar to the opioid receptors discussed in Chapter 10. In about 1990, it was shown that THC does not directly inhibit adenylate cyclase; rather, it acts on a specific receptor in such a way that the enzyme is ultimately inhibited. In 1990 the THC receptor was isolated, sequenced, and cloned. The receptor is a specific G-protein-coupled receptor that both inhibits adenylate cyclase and binds THC and other cannabinoids. CB-1 receptors are primarily found on presynaptic nerve terminals and act to inhibit calcium ion flux and facilitate potassium channels. As a result, activation of cannabinoid receptors inhibits the release of other neurotransmitters, primarily the excitatory neurotransmitter glutamate, from presynaptic nerve terminals.

Physically, the cannabinoid receptor is a continuous chain of 473 amino acids with seven loops through the cell membrane (Figure 14.2). When THC (or an endogenous endocannabinoid) binds to the cannabinoid receptors, it activates G proteins that act on various effectors, including the second-messenger enzyme adenylate cyclase, to ultimately inhibit glutamate release. Until 1990, the existence of a naturally occurring ligand (an endocannabinoid) that binds to the cannabinoid receptor and thus might function as a natural THC remained to be demonstrated. In the search for this ligand, Devane and coworkers (1992) first isolated an arachidonic acid derivative called *anandamide* (see Figure 14.1), which not only binds to the cannabinoid receptor but also produces cannabinoidlike pharmacological effects.

Many additional reports since then demonstrated that anandamide produces behavioral, hypothermic, and analgesic effects that parallel those caused by psychotropic cannabinoids. Anandamide is a weaker agonist than is THC and has a shorter half-life. It exhibits the essential criteria required to be classified as the endogenous ligand at cannabinoid receptors. Shen and Thayer (1999) demonstrated that THC acts as a

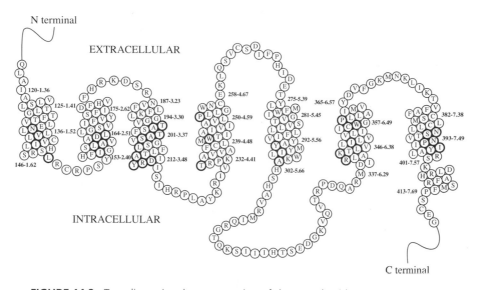

FIGURE 14.2 Two-dimensional representation of the anandamide receptor, a protein consisting of a chain of more than 450 amino acids (the first letter of each amino acid is shown). Like the opioid receptors, the anandamide receptor is a G-protein-linked, seven-membrane-spanning structure with three extracellular loops.

partial agonist at hippocampal glutamate-releasing neurons to "reduce, but not totally block, excitatory transmission" (p. 8). From this statement, we can conclude that both THC and anandamide function as partial agonists that are unable to fully activate cannabinoid receptors at maximally effective concentrations.

There are huge numbers of cannabinoid receptors in the brain, perhaps 10 to 20 times the number of opioid receptors and perhaps more than any other type of receptor. Anandamide, as a partial agonist, activates perhaps only 50 percent of available receptors; THC activates only about 20 percent. In fact, THC is probably effective not because of any inherent efficacy but because of the tremendous number of receptors for it in the brain. Even in the spinal cord, cannabinoid receptors are expressed in sensory nociceptive cells located in the dorsal horn and dorsal root ganglion, where they play important roles in pain-controlling circuits (Pernia-Andrade et al., 2009; Drew et al., 2009).

As can be seen in Figure 14.1, anandamide is structurally dissimilar to THC. Thomas and coworkers (1996) constructed three-dimensional pharmacological models of THC and anandamide and demonstrated that in this conformation the molecules are actually quite similar (Figure 14.3) and would be predicted to interact with the same receptor. As the 1990s ended, the first cannabinoid antagonist was synthesized, and mice lacking the cannabinoid receptor were bred and demonstrated no response to cannabinoid drugs. A marijuana discontinuation syndrome

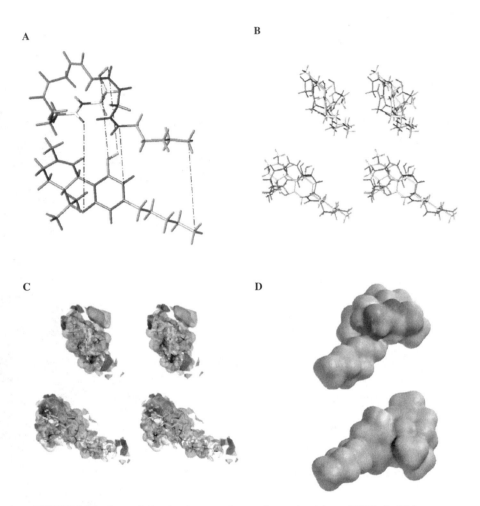

FIGURE 14.3 Several structural comparisons of anandamide and THC. **A.** Stick model showing alignment of the two molecules with dashed lines signifying the five atoms used for superpositioning. **B.** Views of the overlaid structures that predict three-dimensional similarity and thus affinity for the same receptor. **C.** Stereoviews of overlaid structures show nonoverlapping molecular volumes. **D.** Another view of the steric shape and bulk of anandamide (*top*) and THC (*bottom*). [From Thomas et al. (1996), p. 474.]

has been described (Cooper and Haney, 2008), and cannabinoid antagonists are being used to study the discontinuation syndrome and to develop clinical uses in treating obesity and drug craving (discussed later).

Cannabinoid receptors are located throughout the brain (Figures 14.4 and 14.5). They are most dense in the cortex, hippocampus, basal ganglia, cerebellum, and spinal cord. This distribution is consistent with the effects of cannabinoids on memory, cognition, movement, and nociception (pain relief; Felder et al., 2006). The large numbers in the basal

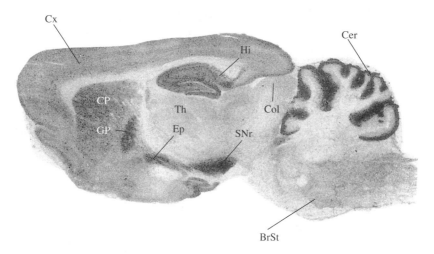

FIGURE 14.4   Autoradiographic binding of potent cannabinoid-to-cannabinoid receptors in the rat brain. BrSt = brain stem; Cer = cerebellum; Col = colliculi; CP = caudate putamen; Cx = cerebral cortex; Ep = entopeduncular nucleus; GP = globus pallidus; Hi = hippocampus; SNr = substantia nigra; Th = thalamus. [Autoradiograph courtesy of Miles Herkenham, NIMH.]

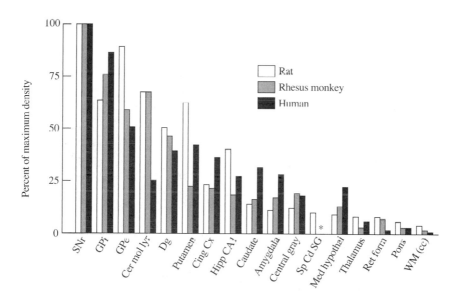

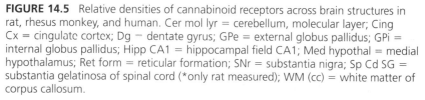

FIGURE 14.5   Relative densities of cannabinoid receptors across brain structures in rat, rhesus monkey, and human. Cer mol lyr = cerebellum, molecular layer; Cing Cx = cingulate cortex; Dg = dentate gyrus; GPe = external globus pallidus; GPi = internal globus pallidus; Hipp CA1 = hippocampal field CA1; Med hypothal = medial hypothalamus; Ret form = reticular formation; SNr = substantia nigra; Sp Cd SG = substantia gelatinosa of spinal cord (*only rat measured); WM (cc) = white matter of corpus callosum.

ganglia and cerebellum reflect the movement and postural controls that are affected by smoking marijuana. Binding of THC to receptors in the cerebral cortex, especially the frontal cortex, probably mediates at least some of the psychoactive effects of the drug, including distortions of the sense of time, sound, color, and taste; alterations in the ability to concentrate; and production of a dreamlike state. Cannabinoid receptors in the hippocampus may account for THC-induced disruption of memory, memory storage, and coding of sensory input. Because brain-stem structures do not bind cannabinoids, THC does not affect basal body functions, including respiration. The absence of cannabinoid–anandamide receptors in the brain stem explains the relative nonlethality of THC.

Cannabinoid receptors outside the brain are of a slightly different type (cannabinoid-2 receptors) than those found in the brain (cannabinoid-1 receptors). Originally thought to be located only on specific components of the lymphoid system, they are also located in the heart and in body tissues involved in inflammatory and pain responses.

Farquhar-Smith and Rice (2003) reported on the effects of anandamide on inflammatory responses mediated by the cannabinoid-2 receptors and immune cells. They noted that in the periphery, certain immune cells coexpress cannabinoid-2 receptors as well as a receptor for a protein called nerve growth factor. The researchers found that anandamide (and another synthetic cannabinoid agonist) blocked nerve growth-factor-induced painful and inflammatory responses and that this peripheral analgesic/anti-inflammatory response of anandamide is independent of central nervous system (CNS) effects involving cannabinoid-1 receptors (which have additional and independent analgesic involvement).

Pharmacokinetics

Most marijuana available in the United States has a THC content that does not exceed 10 percent, although some products contain much higher amounts. THC is usually administered in the form of a hand-rolled marijuana cigarette. Thus, if a marijuana cigarette contains 1.5 grams of plant material with a THC content of about 5 percent, the cigarette contains approximately 75 milligrams of THC. In general, about one-fourth to one-half of the THC present in a marijuana cigarette is actually available in the smoke. Thus, if a cigarette contains 75 milligrams of THC, about 25 milligrams are available in the smoke. In practice, the amount of THC absorbed into the bloodstream as a result of the social smoking of one marijuana cigarette is probably in the range of 5 to 10 milligrams. The absorption of THC from the smoking of marijuana is rapid and complete.

Besides administration by smoking, marijuana can be taken orally, and one THC preparation, dronabinol (Marinol), has been available for

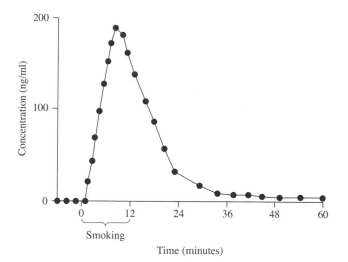

FIGURE 14.6 Expected plasma concentrations of THC following smoking of a single marijuana cigarette containing 3.5 percent THC. Smoking was over a period of 12 minutes, with peak plasma concentration occurring at the cessation of smoking.

oral use since the mid-1980s. Taken orally, onset is delayed and "first-pass metabolism" prevents the drug from reaching significant plasma concentration (Huestis, 2005). When taken orally in therapeutic amounts (for appetite stimulation), plasma concentrations of both THC and its active metabolite (11-hydroxy-delta 9 THC) never exceeded 6.1 nanograms of drug per milliliter of plasma and never persisted beyond 15 hours after oral intake (Goodwin et al., 2006). The levels of inactive metabolite (carboxy-THC, or THCCOOH) were detectable for about 40 hours in plasma, longer in urine (Gustafson et al., 2004).

The behavioral effects of THC in smoked marijuana occur almost immediately after smoking begins and correspond with the rapid attainment of peak concentrations in plasma (Figure 14.6). A "high" is experienced with plasma concentrations of THC of about 5 to 10 nanograms of drug per milliliter of plasma. Unless more is smoked, the effects seldom last longer than 2 to 3 hours. Peak blood levels of THC of 50 to 100 nanograms per milliliter occur about 10 minutes after initiation of smoking cigarettes containing 1.75 percent and 3.55 percent THC, respectively (Huestis, 2007). Within 2 hours, levels fall below 5 nanograms per milliliter and then decline slowly.

Once THC is absorbed, it is distributed to the various organs of the body, especially those that have significant concentrations of fatty material. Thus, THC readily penetrates the brain; the blood-brain barrier does not appear to hinder its passage. Similarly, THC readily crosses the placental barrier and reaches the fetus. THC is almost completely metabolized by hepatic cytochrome P450 enzymes to its active

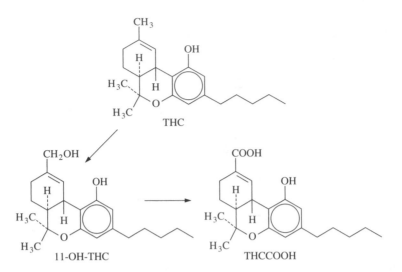

FIGURE 14.7 Major metabolic route for delta-9-tetrahydrocannabinol (THC), including its active metabolite (11-OH-THC) and its primary inactive metabolite (11-nor-9-carboxy-delta-9-tetrahydrocannabinol, or "carboxy-THC").

metabolite, 11-hydroxy-delta-9-THC, which is subsequently converted to the inactive metabolite carboxy-THC (COOH-THC), which is then excreted in the urine (Figure 14.7).

Much of the THC taken into the body is stored in body fat, from which it is slowly released; thus, very low amounts in blood are maintained for a considerable time after drug use ceases. The levels achieved with slow release from fat stores are thought to be very low and clinically without significant effect. In frequent users, THC can be detected in plasma for up to 6 days after smoking cannabis, usually less than 1 day in infrequent users (Huestis, 2005). Therefore, THC can actually persist in the body for several days to about two weeks, longer in chronic smokers and obese smokers. Such a delay tends to prolong and intensify the activity of subsequently smoked marijuana, forming a type of "reverse tolerance" to the drug, where the persistent low levels are potentiated by subsequently smoked THC cigarettes.

As with most psychoactive drugs, only minute quantities of active THC are found in the urine of people who use the drug. Therefore, urine testing for THC focuses on identification of its inactive metabolite, carboxy-THC. Carboxy-THC is only slowly excreted; its half-life in urine varies. In infrequent smokers (less than twice per week), urine samples will generally be positive for 1 to 3 days. In regular smokers (several times per week), urine specimens can test positive for 7 to 21 days. In chronic smokers, daily use for prolonged periods of time can yield positive results for 30 days or longer. If one does not personally smoke marijuana but is exposed to secondhand smoke, such exposure will usually not result in a positive result for cannabinoid metabolites in urine. Thus, a positive urine test does not necessarily mean that a person was under the influence of marijuana at the time the urine specimen was collected; there is little or no correlation between the presence of carboxy-THC in urine and the presence of a pharmacologically significant amount of THC in the blood. This can become quite important in certain legal situations, such as charges of driving while under the influence of marijuana.

Pharmacological Effects

THC produces a unique syndrome of behavioral effects, including analgesia, cognitive alterations, and euphoria. Mice lacking the cannabinoid receptor have increased mortality rates, lose body weight, are less active, and have lower than normal pain thresholds. THC and anandamide are analgesic at spinal, brain-stem, and peripheral sites, especially against the pain resulting from persistent inflammation or neuropathic pain, an action similar to but distinct from the action of the opioids such as morphine (Welch, 2009; Karst and Wippermann, 2009). This effect would be classified as an opioid-sparing action.

Effects on the Central Nervous System

In rodents, THC is analgesic, and this action is blocked by cannabinoid antagonists. As stated earlier, Sativex has been reported to relieve the pain associated with multiple sclerosis. Sativex is a cannabis-based pharmaceutical product containing THC and cannabidiol in a 1:1 mixture, delivered in an oromucosal (mouth) spray containing 2.7 milligrams of THC and 2.5 milligrams of cannabidiol.[1]

At a daily dose of 8 to 12 sprays, a total daily intake of about 22 to 32 millligrams per day of THC and 20 to 30 milligrams per day of cannabidiol is achieved. The efficacy of this product in treating the pain associated with multiple sclerosis is still under study (Perez and Ribera, 2008; Pertwee, 2009; Iskedjian et al., 2009; Centonze et al., 2009; Selvarajah et al., 2010).

It has been known for many years that THC and opioids share actions such as analgesia, sedation, hypothermia, and hypotension. We now know that the cannabinoid and opioid systems interact and that their "cross-talk" may be a target for interventions in the treatment of pain and addiction. A recent issue of the journal *Current Drug Targets* (volume 11, number 4, April 2010) contains six review articles devoted to this important topic.

---

[1] Cannabidiol will be discussed later in this chapter as a naturally occuring nonpsychoactive cannabinoid.

Besides analgesia, THC also exerts a variety of other effects in humans and other animals. THC decreases body temperature, calms aggressive behavior, potentiates the effects of barbiturates and other sedatives, blocks convulsions, and depresses reflexes. In primates specifically, THC decreases aggression, decreases the ability to perform complex behavioral tasks, seems to induce hallucinations, and appears to cause temporal distortions. THC causes monkeys to increase the frequency of their social interactions. High doses can depress ovarian function, lower the concentration of female sex hormones, decrease ovulation, and possibly decrease sperm production. Finally, THC can affect appetite regulation, activating cannabinoid-1 receptors in the hypothalamic nuclei and the limbic system, areas that are involved in the regulation of feeding behavior, especially in the control of the intake of sweet and fattening foods. Intake of THC can thus result in significant weight gain (Tibirica, 2010). Clinically, THC can be used as an appetite stimulant, useful in wasting diseases such as cancer and AIDS (Costiniuk et al., 2008).

The CNS effects of THC vary with dose, route of administration, experience of the user, vulnerability to psychoactive effects, and the setting in which administration occurs. In general, the senses may be enhanced and the perception of time is usually altered. Users report an increased sense of well-being, mild euphoria, relaxation, and relief from anxiety. The subjective effects include dissociation of ideas. Illusions and hallucinations occur infrequently. The effect sought by most users is the "high" and "mellowing out." This effect is described as different from the stimulant high and the opioid high. The effects vary with dose, but the typical marijuana smoker experiences a "high" that lasts about two hours.

THC-induced impairments in cognitive functioning, learning, and memory are currently attracting significant attention. Indeed, THC impairs all stages of memory, including encoding, consolidation, and retrieval. These memory-disrupting effects appear to follow from activation of cannabinoid-1 receptors in the hippocampus, a brain region implicated in spatial learning, episodic memory, and memory consolidation that contains a high concentration of cannabinoid-1 receptors (Puighermanal et al., 2009; Wise et al., 2009). Therefore, THC in the blood can be detrimental to optimal cognitive abilities, especially at higher blood concentrations. These adverse cognitive deficits can persist for at least one month following discontinuation of heavy use, but only minimal effects are likely to persist following a 30-day period of abstinence. THC is certainly not a "dementing drug" as are ethanol or the benzodiazepines.

Also attracting attention are the impairments of coordination, perception, reaction time, and divided attention that persist for several hours beyond one's perception of the "high." These impairments have obvious implications for the operation of a motor vehicle and performance in the workplace or at school. Indeed, THC concentrations in

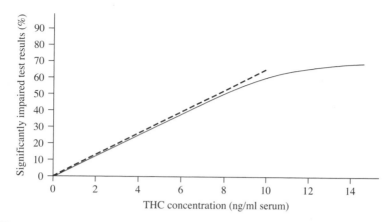

FIGURE 14.8 Percentage of performance decrements (percent) observed in the total number of psychomotor tests applied in 87 experimental studies as a function of THC concentration in blood serum (plasma) after eating (dashed line) and smoking (solid line). [From Ramaekers et al. (2004), p. 114, Figure 1.]

blood in excess of about 2 to 5 nanograms/milliliter are associated with driving impairments (Figure 14.8). Recent use of cannabis, especially with blood concentrations in excess of 5 to 10 nanograms/milliliter, increases accident risk by about three to seven times more than is seen in nonintoxicated persons (Ramaekers et al., 2006). This increased risk is greatly potentiated by concomitant use of alcohol (Sewell et al., 2009). How this knowledge will be put to use in California, should legislation approving recreational use be passed in November 2010, is unclear.

At very high doses, acute depressive reactions, acute panic reactions, and mild paranoia have been observed, probably brought on by drug-induced alterations in perception; some panic responses may follow the feeling of a loss of mental control. Several surveys indicate that 50 to 60 percent of marijuana users have reported at least one anxiety experience. Only at massive doses of THC do delusions, paranoia, hallucinations, confusion and disorientation, depersonalization, altered sensory perception, and loss of insight occur; these reactions are unusual, however, and generally do not last long.

Marijuana can impair the ability to focus attention and filter out irrelevant information. Users demonstrate weakness in attention and synthetic skills, difficulty making subtle distinctions in relevance and memory, decreased psychospatial skills, poor mental representations of the environment, and poor routines of daily life. These impairments are associated with feelings of alienation and a sense that life is not under control and lacks meaning. With cessation of drug use and initiation of psychological treatment, users demonstrate improvement in cognitive functioning within 14 days of abstinence and function normally at the end of 6 weeks of therapy.

To understand the behavioral attractiveness of marijuana, Gardner and Lowinson, as early as 1991, reviewed marijuana's interactions with brain reward systems, particularly in the dopamine-mediated, medial forebrain bundle projection. They stated:

> Acute enhancement of brain reward mechanisms appears to be the single essential commonality of abuse-prone drugs, and the hypothesis that recreational and abused drugs act on these brain mechanisms to produce the subjective reward that constitutes the "high" or "rush" or "hit" sought by drug users is, at present, the most compelling hypothesis available on the neurobiology of recreational drug use and abuse. (p. 571)

More recently, other authors have expanded on the behavioral rewarding effects of both anandamide and THC, concluding that both substances activate the mesolimbic dopaminergic reward system, including the nucleus accumbens (Zangen et al., 2006; Gardner, 2005; Cooper and Haney, 2009). Filbey and coworkers (2009) demonstrated that in abstinent marijuana users, marijuana cues would activate the reward neurocircuitry associated with the neurobiology of addiction, and the magnitude of activation was associated with the severity of problems related to marijuana use. The implication is an involvement of the cannabinoid system in drug dependence (discussed later).

Finally, it has been hypothesized that cannabis use in susceptible adolescents and young adults may be a contributory cause of schizophreniform psychosis, and a large literature is developing in this area. Recent conclusions include the following:

> Cannabis abuse is a risk factor for psychosis in predisposed people; it can affect neurodevelopment during adolescence leading to schizophrenia, and a dysregulation of the endocannabinoid system can participate in schizophrenia. (Fernandez-Espejo et al., 2009, p. 531)

> Only a very small proportion of the general population exposed to cannabinoids develop a psychotic illness. It is likely that cannabis exposure is a "component cause" that interacts with other factors to cause schizophrenia or a psychotic disorder, but is neither necessary nor sufficient to do so alone. (D'Souza et al., 2009, p. 413)

> At present, there is insufficient evidence to support or refute the use of cannabis/cannabinoid compounds for people suffering with schizophrenia. (Rathbone et al., 2008, p. 1)

> Cannabis use is considered a contributory cause of schizophrenia and psychotic illness. However, only a small proportion of cannabis users develop psychosis. (Henquet et al., 2008, p. 1111)

This contributory causal relation is biologically plausible because psychotic disorders involve disturbances in the dopamine neurotransmitter systems with which the cannabinoid system interacts. (Degenhardt and Hall, 2006, p. 556)

It is most plausible that cannabis use precipitates schizophrenia in individuals who are vulnerable because of a personal or family history of schizophrenia. (Degenhardt and Hall, 2006, p. 556)

Cannabis use in adolescence increases the risk of later schizophrenia-like psychosis, especially in genetically vulnerable individuals. (DiForti et al., 2007 p. 228)

From these statements, it appears that the association between cannabis use and psychosis is complex. As stated by D'Souza (2007):

There is renewed interest in the long-recognized association between cannabinoids and psychosis. . . . Cannabinoids can induce acute transient psychotic symptoms or an acute psychosis in some individuals. What makes some individuals vulnerable to cannabinoid-induced psychosis is unclear. Cannabinoids can also exacerbate psychosis in individuals with an established psychotic disorder, and these exacerbations may last beyond the period of intoxication. . . . On the other hand, the large majority of individuals exposed to cannabinoids do not experience psychosis or develop schizophrenia and the rates of schizophrenia have not increased commensurate with the increase in rates of cannabis use. Similar to smoking and lung cancer, it is more likely that cannabis exposure is a component cause that interacts with other factors, for example, genetic risk, to "cause" schizophrenia. . . . Further work is necessary to identify those factors that place individuals at higher risk for cannabinoid-related psychosis, to identify the biological mechanisms underlying the risks and to further study whether CB1 receptor dysfunction contributes to the pathophysiology of psychotic disorders. (p. 289)

Henquet and coworkers (2008) reviewed this association with emphasis on possible sites of genetic alterations that might result in cannabis-associated schizophrenia. They stated that "multiple variations within multiple genes—rather than single genetic polymorphisms—together with other environmental factors (e.g., stress) may interact with cannabis to increase the risk of psychosis" (p. 1111). An example of a possible stress-cannabis-psychosis interaction was first demonstrated by Houston and coworkers in 2008 (Figure 14.9). However, it should be noted that the small numbers in this study limit more generalized conclusions.

Muller-Vahl and Emrich (2008) review a new concept—a "cannabinoid hypothesis of schizophrenia"—that suggests a complex interaction between dopaminergic and cannabinoid receptors, postulating

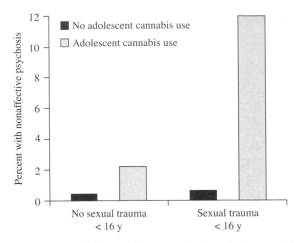

FIGURE 14.9 Cannabis use during adolescence significantly increased the risk of developing nonaffective psychosis later in life (after age 16, right-hand bar), but only in people who experienced sexual trauma during childhood. [From Henquet et al. (2008), p, 1117, Figure 3. Based on data from Houston et al. (2008), p, 583, Table 2.]

that the nonpsychoactive cannabinoid (cannabidiol, a component in Sativex discussed above) might be beneficial in the treatment of psychosis. Future reseach will hopefully further dissect this complex interaction among environmental stressors, genetic predisposition, early cannabis exposure, and proness to future psychosis.

Effects on the Cardiovascular System

A marked increase in heart rate and a mild increase in blood pressure are two commonly observed physiological effects of THC. During periods of intoxication, the combined effect can increase the workload (increasing oxygen requirements) of the heart and simultaneously reduce blood flow to the heart muscle. Ischemia of the heart can follow, perhaps similar to that seen during exercise. Although the increased heart rate could be a problem for people with cardiovascular disease, dangerous physical reactions to marijuana are exceedingly rare. There is no association of marijuana use with cardiovascular disease hospitalizations or mortality. By extrapolation from animal experiments, the ratio of lethal to effective (intoxicating) dose is estimated to be on the order of thousands to one. Interestingly, peripheral cannabinoid-2 receptors in the heart function in an intrinsic defense of the heart against potentially fatal ischemic attacks (Bouchard et al., 2003). This protective effect of cannabinoids may eventually provide an important therapeutic intervention in the prevention of heart attacks.

Blood vessels of the cornea can dilate, which results in bloodshot eyes that can be observed in someone who has just smoked marijuana.

Pulmonary Effects

The gaseous and particulate components of both marijuana and to-bacco smoke provide some insights into the potential for marijuana to cause pulmonary damage. With the exception of the presence of THC in marijuana and nicotine in tobacco, both inhalants are remarkably similar; marijuana smoke contains more tars and many of the same carcinogenic compounds identified in tobacco smoke. A single mari-juana cigarette may be more harmful than a single tobacco cigarette because more tar is inhaled and retained from marijuana. Also, mole-cular alterations of lung tissues can be demonstrated, showing evi-dence of bronchial irritation and inflammation. A recent study demonstrated an associations between marijuana smoking and lung cancer after adjusting for tobacco use, with the risk of lung cancer in-creasing 8 percent for each joint-year of cannabis smoking (Aldington et al., 2008). This increase was comparable to that seen in chronic cig-arette smoking. Fortunately, few marijuana smokers smoke marijuana with anywhere near the frequency that chronic cigarette smokers smoke cigarettes.

Effects on the Immune System

As noted earlier, cannabinoid-2 receptors are found primarily in the immune system and appear to exert a regulatory action on this system. Long-term marijuana use is associated with a degree of immuno-suppression, which might be thought to potentially render the smoker susceptible to infections or disease. Although data in this area are con-troversial and implications have not been proved, marijuana smoking in some circumstances may partially suppress immunity. The clinical significance of this occurrence is not known, but it should be noted that other depressant drugs, such as alcohol, barbiturates, benzodi-azepines, and anticonvulsants, share this immunosuppressive action (Cabral, 2006).

Because both the spleen and the lymphocytes (white blood cells) are important to the body's immune response, they have been investigated to determine how they are affected by cannabinoids. While cannabinoids suppress immunity through activation of cannabinoid-2 receptors, the implications remain unclear. To put the immunosuppressive action of marijuana in perspective, in humans marijuana-induced immune sup-pression is subtle and in most cases insignificant. At this time, little evi-dence points to cannabinoid-induced immunosuppression as a causative agent in disease.

Cannabinoids seem to also exert antitumor effects (Pisanti et al., 2009). While much remains to be learned, Alexander and coworkers (2009) postulate a role for cannabinoid agonists in the treatment of estrogen receptor-negative breast cancer.

Effects on the Reproductive System

Evidence of THC-induced suppression of sexual function and reproduction is controversial. The chronic use of marijuana by males can reduce levels of the hormone testosterone and at the same time reduce sperm formation. Reductions in male fertility and sexual potency, however, have not been reported. In females, the levels of follicle-stimulating hormone and luteinizing hormone are reduced by the use of marijuana. Menstrual cycles can be affected and anovulatory cycles have been reported. All these actions reverse when drug use is discontinued. Wang and coworkers (2006) review this complex topic of endocannabinoids in both male and female fertility (one of the few articles to address the endocannabinoid system in the regulation of male fertility).

Marijuana freely crosses the placenta, so the developing brain is susceptible to marijuana products during the prenatal period when a pregnant female smokes marijuana. It now appears that such exposure induces subtle rather than gross effects on later functioning in offspring, including cognitive deficits especially in visuospatial function, impulsivity, inattention and hyperactivity, depressive symptoms, and substance use disorders (Sundram, 2006). Because the endocannabinoid neurotransmitter system develops during gestation, it is not surprising that THC and other products in marijuana affect this developing system. Fride and coworkers (2009) suggest that fetal exposure to marijuana is "similar to many effects of prenatal stress, which may suggest that prenatal stress impacts on the endocannabinoid system and that, vice versa, prenatal cannabinoid exposure may interfere with the ability of the fetus to cope with stress" (p. 139).

One of the greatest risks appears to be the high probability that a pregnant female who smokes marijuana may also use other, more fetotoxic drugs (including nicotine cigarettes). Infants born of marijuana-smoking mothers display mild withdrawal signs, including tremulousness, abnormal responses to stimuli, and neurobehavioral performance deficits (DeMoraes-Barros et al., 2006). These signs appear to be transient in nature. These data strongly argue against the use of marijuana, as well as cigarettes and alcohol, during pregnancy.

Tolerance and Dependence

Consequences of chronic marijuana use include behavioral tolerance and withdrawal symptoms on drug cessation. Tolerance appears to result from a cannabinoid-induced down regulation and desensitization of brain cannabinoid receptors; dependence is determined by the presence of a withdrawal syndrome upon drug discontinuation.

Until recently, it was generally thought that physical dependence on THC probably did not develop, and if it did, any symptoms were mild and transient. Today, a more extensive literature more clearly defines a marijuana withdrawal syndrome that, by definition, implies that body functioning is altered by marijuana use and that uncomfortable symptoms occur when the drug is withdrawn (Elkashef et al., 2008; Benyamina et al., 2008; Cooper and Haney, 2008, 2009; Vandrey and Haney, 2009). Originally thought to be a relatively benign and infrequent occurrence, cannabis dependence occurs in about one of every ten persons who start smoking cannabis, and marijuana is now the second most common reason for admission to a drug treatment program (Copeland and Swift, 2009). As reported by Elkashef, and coworkers (2008):

> When cannabis users were asked to rate the effects of their own cannabis use as positive, neutral, or negative, they gave overwhelmingly negative ratings of the effects that cannabis had on their social life (70%), their physical health (81%), their cognition (91%), their memory (91%), and their career (79%). (p. 17)

Many of these negative effects seem to be due to being acutely intoxicated every day. With these adverse perceptions of their own use, why does one not just quit? Simply put, quitting is associated with almost universal relapse, with withdrawal symptoms contributing the most to relapse. These symptoms include irritability, anxiety, marijuana craving, disrupted sleep and strange dreams, anger and aggression, depressed mood, restlessness, decreased appetite, and weight loss. Less common symptoms include chills, headache, physical tension, sweating, stomach pain, and general physical discomfort (Vandrey and Haney, 2009). Reinstituting marijuana use ameliorates withdrawal discomfort (as would be expected). Symptoms begin within 48 hours after cessation of drug administration and last at least 2 days, more usually about 7 to 10 days and perhaps longer; EEG changes associated with withdrawal persist for at least 28 days.

Treatment Issues

Early initiation and regular adolescent use are risk factors for later problematic cannabis (and other drug) use, impaired mental health, delinquency, lower educational achievement, risky sexual behavior, and criminal offenses (Copeland and Swift, 2009). However society moves toward or away from marijuana availability for medical or recreational use, availability to youths must be restricted.

There are as yet no evidence-based pharmacotherapies available for the management of cannabis withdrawal and craving (Vandrey and Haney, 2009). Indeed, this area lags far behind development of pharmacological strategies for treating withdrawal and craving for such drugs as alcohol, psychostimulants, nicotine, and opioids.

The usefulness of behavioral therapies, however, is better demonstrated. Psychotherapeutic strategies including cognitive-behavioral therapy, contingency management, family-based interventions, and motivational enhancement interventions have proved to be effective (Elkashef et al., 2008). Medication therapies have been less successful. It is even unclear whether cannabinoid agonist or cannabinoid antagonist therapies might be successful.

Six different pharmacotherapies have been studied in cannabis withdrawal. Of these, only oral THC and mirtazepine (Remeron; Chapter 5) have shown some promise (Benyamina et al., 2008). The medication that has proven most effective in reducing cannabis withdrawal is dronabinol, a synthetic formulation of THC intended for oral use (Vandrey and Haney, 2009). Use of dronabinol would be similar to the use of nicotine replacement products to reduce withdrawal during tobacco abstinence. Other investigated medicines include bupropion (Welbutrin, a dopaminergic agonist), buspirone (BuSpar, a serotonergic antidepressant), rimonabant (a cannabinoid antagonist, discussed below), and mirtazepine. Naltrexone (an opioid antagonist; Chapter 10) can be modestly effective in specific circumstances, but its effects can be overcome with higher doses of cannabis (Vandrey and Haney, 2009). Other possible agents have been too little studied to discuss here; the review by Vandrey and Haney (2009) is recommended.

Therapeutic Uses of Cannabinoid Agonists

The medical applications of marijuana have been a focus of public and scientific interest for a long time, but until recently there was little scientific basis for establishing medical uses. This situation is now changing. Dronabinol (Marinol), which is synthetic THC, has been available for more than 10 years for use as an appetite stimulant in patients with AIDS and for use in the treatment of nausea and vomiting associated with chemotherapy in cancer patients. In general, traditional medical antiemetic (antivomiting) medications are conceded to be superior. Cannabinoids may prove effective only for refractory nausea or as an adjunct to other antiemetics. Smoked marijuana is not superior to orally administered drug.

As discussed earlier, cannabinoids have very specific analgesic properties; analgesic actions have been well described in animals and employed clinically in Canada in the treatment of multiple sclerosis and the pain associated with advanced cancer. The problem has been to separate the therapeutic analgesic effects from the intoxicating effects. Russo and Guy (2006) discuss the fact that cannabidiol antagonizes some of the adverse effects of THC, including intoxication, sedation, and tachycardia (increased heart rate), while contributing analgesic, antiemetic, and antitumor properties of its own. This property of cannabidiol provides a rational basis for combining cannabidiol with THC for clinical efficacy and safety in the treatment of spasticity, pain, and lower urinary tract symptoms in people with multiple sclerosis. This combination appears to increase clinical efficacy while reducing adverse side effects. To date, this product (Sativex) is not available in the United States. Perhaps this will change.[2]

THC increases appetite in patients with AIDS-related wasting disease. Cannabinoids do stimulate appetite, especially for sweet and palatable foods. In fact, one physiological role of the endogenous cannabinoid system is to maintain the stimulus of appetite; a role for endocannabinoids in obesity can be postulated in reward processes that stimulate appetite (Fong et al., 2007).

Cannabinoids and their derivatives have been postulated to possess neuroprotective effects following brain injury. This action is based on the ability of THC to inhibit glutaminergic transmission and reduce reactive oxygen intermediates, which are factors in causing neuronal injury after head injury. One synthetic cannabinoid derivative, dexanabinol, underwent trials as a protective agent after head trauma. Preliminary data were positive, but one double-blind trial found that it was not efficacious in the treatment of traumatic brain injury in humans (Maas et al., 2006). Other potential uses of cannabinoids are discussed by Pertwee (2009).

Finally, not all of the pharmacologically active compounds in the marijuana plant exert the psychotropic actions of THC. One of these is cannabidiol, the main nonpsychotropic component of the glandular hairs of *C. sativa*. It does, however, display a plethora of other actions, including anticonvulsive, sedative, hypnotic, antipsychotic, anti-inflammatory, and neuroprotective properties (Scuderi et al., 2009; Izzo et al., 2009). Currently it is the nonpsychoactive component of Sativex, cannabidiol, used alone, that may be a promising therapeutic agent for many inflammatory, autoimmune, and neurodegenerative diseases (Ignatowska-Jankowska et al., 2009). Cannabidiol lacks intrinsic activity on the cannabinoid-1 receptor and therefore has a potential for therapeutic use in the absence of psychedelic actions. More will certainly be written on cannabidiol and its therapeutic potential in coming years.

Synthetic Cannabinoid Agonists of Abuse

A new generation of recreational, synthetic psychoactive drugs appeared in 2007 with the arrival of a smoking blend of herbals called "spice,"

---

[2] Perhaps, at least for the present, recreational use of marijuana should fall under a Schedule I category, while Sativex, given for neuropathic pain, should be classified as a Schedule II medication. This would be similar to the treatment of gamma-hydroxy butyrate, which is classified as Schedule I when used recreationally and Schedule III when used in the treatment of narcolepsy.

"mojo" (in Louisiana), "K2," and "legal weed." The products are routinely labeled and marketed as "incense," not intended for human consumption. However, they are widely sold on the Internet, in "head-shops," and now even in convenience stores. The herbals in this preparation appear not to be psychoactive; however, synthetic drugs that stimulate the cannabinoid receptor have been added to the products. These synthetic *cannabinomimetics* have greater affinity for the cannabinoid receptors than does THC, and they exert effects similar to or even more intense than those of THC. Structurally distinct from THC, these synthetic cannabinoid agonists so far have been undetectable in chemical analysis of blood and urine routinely tested for cannabinoids and other drugs of abuse (Lindigkeit et al., 2009; Sobolevsky et al., 2010; Uchiyama et al., 2010). In addition, at the time of writing, these synthetic cannabinoid agonists are not detectable with field drug-testing kits used by law enforcement personnel.

Recently, some of the cannabinoid agonists that have been added to this herbal preparation have been identified and called JWH-018 [1-pentyl-3-(1-naphthoyl)-indole] and CP 47,497. Both compounds exert cannabinoid agonist effects at cannabinoid-1 and cannabinoid-2 receptors, producing actions similar to those induced by THC. Several European countries have banned these compounds. In the United States, JWH-018 and CP 47,497 are not yet federally controlled, although Kansas and Kentucky have banned the products, and in several other states (such as Louisiana) legislation is pending. Unfortunately, as legislation and laboratory testing catch up with JWH-018 and CP 47,497, manufacturers can change the chemicals used to mimic THC, and each combination would have to be both outlawed and traceable for prohibitive laws to be enforced.

Cessation of use of spice has been followed by a classic cannabinoid withdrawal syndrome (Zimmermann et al., 2009). It is feared that spice and future compounds of similar effect may herald a new era in difficult-to-detect psychoactive drugs of abuse of unknown safety and toxicity (Erowid and Erowid, 2009).

Cannabinoid Antagonists

As discussed, activation of cannabinoid receptors underlies the psychological effects of THC and other cannabinoid agonists. However, a hyperactive endocannabinoid system appears to contribute to the etiology of several disease states that constitute significant global threats to human health and well-being (Janero and Makriyannis, 2009). Such diseases include obesity, nicotine dependence, obesity-related cardiovascular disorders, lipid-related vascular disorders, and substance abuse. Therefore, there has been great interest in the development of medications that might block cannabinoid receptors (cannabinoid antagonists) or otherwise modify the effects of either a hyperactive endocannabinoid system or administration of exogenous cannabinoid agonists (such as THC). Representative agents have included rimonabant, taranabant, otenabant, surinabant, rosonabant, and others.

Huestis and coworkers (2001) demonstrated for the first time in humans that a specific antagonist for cannabinoid receptors would produce a dose-dependent blockade of marijuana-induced intoxication and tachycardia. This demonstration led to speculation that cannabinoid antagonists might be used to reverse cannabinoid intoxication in people who experience unpleasant reactions to marijuana (for example, panic and psychosis), similar to the use of intravenous naloxone to reverse the effects of opioids. This use, however, would probably be infrequent and often unpleasant because it would precipitate a cannabinoid withdrawal syndrome. Antagonists, however, might be useful in people who wish to stop using marijuana, blocking any positive effects should marijuana be used, analogous to the use of oral naltrexone to prevent the effects of subsequently taken opioids (Chapter 10).

Because cannabinoid receptor activation also reduces learning, reduces memory formation, and enhances food intake, other potential uses of cannabinoid antagonists might include enhancement of learning and memory as well as the treatment of obesity. It is important to note that cannabinoid receptors and opioid receptors are intimately related and overlap in function. Also, cannabinoid receptors have been implicated in opioid-induced reward, suggesting a possible role of cannabinoid antagonists in the treatment of addiction to opioids, psychostimulants (such as cocaine), and nicotine.

Since THC stimulates appetite, especially for sweet and palatable food (Cota et al., 2003), cannabinoid antagonists might be used in the therapy of obesity and other eating disorders to inhibit the reward processes that stimulate appetite. In multiple studies, the cannabinoid antagonist *rimonabant*, when combined with a low-calorie diet, promoted loss of body weight, loss in waist circumference, reduced desire for sweet and fattening foods, and improvements in blood cholesterol and lipid levels (Leite et al., 2009). Indeed, at a dose of 20 milligrams per day, rimonabant significantly reduced body weight and lowered blood glucose levels, cholesterol, and adverse blood lipids in obese patients with type 2 diabetes (Scheen, 2008; Wright et al., 2008; Mach et al., 2009). Other demonstrated uses include the following:

- Reducing the desire to smoke cigarettes, doubling a smoker's success at quitting cigarettes (Gelfand and Cannon, 2006)
- Reducing alcohol ingestion and reducing relapse (Economidou et al., 2006; Lopez-Moreno et al., 2007)
- Reducing opioid and stimulant use (Fattore et al., 2005, 2007)
- Reducing overall aspects of drug abuse (Beardsley et al., 2009)

Rimonabant (Acomplia) was approved for clinical use in several European countries in 2006. In mid-2007, however, an advisory panel of the U.S. Food and Drug Administration concluded that, despite unquestioned efficacy, adequate safety had not been demonstrated. Indeed, evolving problems with rimonabant included nausea and potentially serious psychiatric consequences (anxiety and depression). Because of these side effects, the manufacturer of rimonabant removed the drug from the world market. Consequently, other research programs developing cannabinoid antagonists as antiobesity agents were terminated (Lee et al., 2009). This now leaves a void in the "single largest market for drugs of its kind" (Samat et al., 2008, p. 187).

However, other researchers have concluded that, despite problems with rimonabant, abandonment of research effort has been premature. Indeed, an array of cannabinoid antagonists are being identified that have modifications of rimonabant's action (Lee et al., 2009). These efforts are aimed at reducing the side effect potential. Such mechanisms might include "partial agonists," "inverse agonists," or "weak antagonists" of the receptor (Fong et al., 2007); non-brain-penetrating and peripherally acting antagonists; or "neutral antagonists" of the cannabinoid receptor (Lee et al., 2009; Janero and Makriyannis, 2009). Other options include the testing of nonpsychotropic products from *C. sativa* and the development of antagonists with an acceptable side effect profile. Even with the removal of rimonabant from the marketplace, these options offer an exciting translational frontier on the critical path to developing cannabinoid receptor modulators as medicines.

STUDY QUESTIONS

1. How are the effects of THC similar to those of the nonselective depressants? How are they dissimilar?

2. Compare and contrast the effects of THC and cannabidiol.

3. How does the half-life of THC reflect a person's ability to become intoxicated more easily and with a smaller amount of drug after its repeated use?

4. Discuss some of the concerns and side effects that are associated with varying degrees of THC use by young people.

5. What does THC do to cognition?

6. Are there any long-term effects of marijuana on the brain? The body? Society?

7. Are there any potential long-term effects that might be associated with chronic use of marijuana?

8. Does dependence on marijuana develop? Discuss both views.

9. Discuss the cannabinoid receptor, its location, and its endogenous neurotransmitter.

10. How might a treatment program be organized for people who become dependent on marijuana?

11. What do you think society's response should be to the continued illicit use of marijuana? Should marijuana be legalized for either medical or recreational use? If so, how should it be regulated or restricted?

12. If states approve marijuana for recreational use, what safeguards should be put in place in the workplace (for urine drug testing) and on the highways?

13. Discuss evidence for or against medical uses of marijuana. If it has medical uses, how might efficacy and societal acceptance be improved?

14. How do you see the future of marijuana and cannabinoid research? What are some of the potential therapeutic uses of cannaboid agonists? Antagonists?

REFERENCES

Aldington, S., et al. (2008). "Cannabis Use and Risk of Lung Cancer: A Case-Control Study." *European Respiratory Journal* 31: 280–286.

Alexander, A., et al. (2009). "Cannabinoids in the Treatment of Cancer." *Cancer Letters* 285: 6–12.

Beardsley, P. M., et al. (2009). "Cannabinoid CB1 Receptor Antagonists as Potential Pharmacotherapies for Drug Abuse Disorders." *International Reviews in Psychiatry* 21: 134–142.

Benyamina, A., et al. (2008). "Pharmacotherapy and Psychotherapy in Cannabis Withdrawal and Dependence." *Expert Reviews in Neurotherapy* 8: 479–491.

Bouchard, J. F., et al. (2003). "Contribution of Endocannabinoids in the Endothelial Protection Afforded by Ischemic Preconditioning in the Isolated Rat Heart." *Life Sciences* 72: 1859–1870.

Cabral, G. A. (2006). "Drugs of Abuse, Immune Modulation, and AIDs." *Journal of Neuroimmune Pharmacology* 1: 280–295.

Centonze, D., et al. (2009). "Lack of Effect of Cannabis-Based Treatment on Clinical and Laboratory Measures in Multiple Sclerosis." *Neurological Sciences* 30: 531–534.

Cleveland, H. H., and Wiebe, R. P. (2008). "Understanding the Association Between Adolescent Marijuana Use and Later Serious Drug Use: Gateway Effect or Developmental Trajectory?" *Developmental Psychopathology* 20: 615–632.

Cooper, Z. D., and Haney, M. (2008). "Cannabis Reinforcement and Dependence: Role of the Cannabinoid CB1 Receptor." *Addiction Biology* 13: 188–195.

Cooper, Z. D., and Haney, M. (2009). "Actions of Delta-9-Tetrahydrocannabinol in Cannabis: Relation to Use, Abuse, Dependence." *International Review of Psychiatry* 21: 104–112.

Copeland, J., and Swift, W. (2009). "Cannabis Use Disorder: Epidemiology and Management." *International Review of Psychiatry* 21: 96–103.

Costiniuk, C. T., et al. (2008). "Evaluation of Oral Cannabinoid-Containing Medications for the Management of Interferon and Ribavirin-Induced Anorexia, Nausea, and Weight Loss in Patients Treated for Chronic Hepatitis C Virus." *Canadian Journal of Gastroenterology* 22: 376–380.

Cota, D., et al. (2003). "Endogenous Cannabinoid System as a Modulator of Food Intake." *International Journal of Obesity and Related Metabolic Disorders: Journal of the International Association for the Study of Obesity* 27: 289–301.

Degenhardt, L., and Hall, W. (2006). "Is Cannabis Use a Contributory Cause of Psychosis?" *Canadian Journal of Psychiatry* 51: 556–565.

Degenhardt, L., et al. (2009). "Does the 'Gateway' Matter? Associations Between the Order of Drug Use Initiation and the Development of Drug Dependence in the National Comorbidity Study Replication." *Psychological Medicine* 39: 157–167.

Degenhardt, L., et al. (2010). "Evaluating the Drug Use 'Gateway' Theory Using Cross-National Data: Consistency and Associations of the Oreder of Initiation of Drug Use Among Participants in the WHO World Mental Health Surveys." *Drug and Alcohol Dependence* 108: 84–97.

DeMoraes-Barros, M. C., et al. (2006). "Exposure to Marijuana During Pregnancy Alters Neurobehavior in the Early Neonatal Period." *Journal of Pediatrics* 149: 781–787.

Devane, W. A., et al. (1992). "Isolation and Structure of a Brain Constituent That Binds to the Cannabinoid Receptor." *Science* 258: 1946–1949.

DiForti, M., et al. (2007). "Cannabis Use and Psychiatric and Cognitive Disorders: The Chicken or the Egg?" *Current Opinion in Psychiatry* 20: 228–234.

Drew, G. M., et al. (2009). "Substance P Drives Endocannabinoid-Mediated Disinhibition in a Midbrain Descending Analgesic Pathway." *Journal of Neuroscience* 29: 7220–7229.

D'Souza, D. C. (2007). "Cannabinoids and Psychosis." *International Review of Neurobiology* 78: 289–326.

D'Souza, D. C., et al. (2009). "Cannabis and Psychosis/Schizophrenia: Human Studies." *European Archives of Psychiatry and Clinical Neuroscience* 259: 413–431.

Economidou, D., et al. (2006). "Effect of the Endocannabinoid CB1 Receptor Antagonist SR-141716A on Ethanol Self-Administration and Ethanol-Seeking Behaviour in Rats." *Psychopharmacology* 183: 394–403.

Elkashef, A., et al. (2008). "Marijuana Neurobiology and Treatment." *Substance Abuse* 29: 17–29.

Erowid, E., and Erowid, F. (2009). "Spice & Spin-Offs: Prohibition's High-Tech Cannabis Substitutes." *Erowid Extracts* 16: 12–16.

Farquhar-Smith, W. P., and Rice, A. S. C. (2003). "A Novel Neuroimmune Mechanism in Cannabinoid-Mediated Attenuation of Nerve Growth Factor-Induced Hyperalgesia." *Anesthesiology* 99: 1391–1401.

Fattore, L., et al. (2005). "Endocannabinoid System and Opioid Addiction: Behavioural Aspects." *Pharmacology Biochemistry and Behavior* 81: 343–359.

Fattore, L., et al. (2007). "An Endocannabinoid Mechanism in Relapse to Drug Seeking: A Review of Animal Studies and Clinical Perspectives." *Brain Research Reviews* 53: 1–16.

Felder, C. C., et al. (2006). "Cannabinoid Biology: The Search for New Therapeutic Targets." *Molecular Interventions* 6: 149–171.

Fernandez-Espejo, E., et al. (2009). "Role of Cannabis and Endocannabinoids in the Genesis of Schizophrenia." *Psychopharmacology* 206: 531–549.

Filbey, F. M., et al. (2009). "Marijuana Craving in the Brain." *Proceedings of the National Academy of Sciences USA* 106: 13016–13021.

Fong, T. M., et al. (2007). "Anti-Obesity Efficacy of a Novel Cannabinoid-1 Receptor Inverse Agonist MK-0364 in Rodents." *Journal of Pharmacology and Experimental Therapeutics* 321: 1013–1022.

Fride, E., et al. (2009). "The Endocannabinoid System During Development: Emphasis on Perinatal Events and Delayed Effects." *Vitamins & Hormones* 81: 139–158.

Gardner, E. L. (2005). "Endocannabinoid Signaling System and Brain Reward: Emphasis on Dopamine." *Pharmacology Biochemistry and Behavior* 81: 263–284.

Gardner, E. L., and Lowinson, J. H. (1991). "Marijuana's Interaction with Brain Reward Systems: Update 1991." *Pharmacology Biochemistry and Behavior* 40: 571–580.

Gelfand, E. V., and Cannon, C. P. (2006). "Rimonabant: A Selective Blocker of the Cannabinoid CB1 Receptors for the Management of Obesity, Smoking Cessation, and Cardiometabolic Risk Factors." *Expert Opinions on Investigational Drugs* 15: 307–315.

Goodwin, R. S., et al. (2006). "Delta-9-Tetrahydrocannabinol, 11-Hydroxy-Delta(9)-Tetrahydrocannabinol and 11-nor-9-Carboxy-Delta(9)-Tetrahydrocannabinol in Human Plasma After Controlled Oral Administration of Cannabinoids." *Therapeutic Drug Monitoring* 28: 545–551.

Guindon, J., and Hohmann, A. G. (2009). "The Endocannabinoid System and Pain." *CNS and Neurological Disorders—Drug Targets* 8: 403–421.

Gustafson, R. A., et al. (2004). "Urinary Pharmacokinetics of 11-nor-9-Carboxy-Delta9-Tetrahydrocannabinol After Controlled Oral Delta9-Tetrahydrocannabinol Administration." *Journal of Analytical Toxicology* 28: 160–167.

Hall, W., and Degenhardt, L. (2009). "Adverse Health Effects of Non-Medical Cannabis Use." *Lancet* 374: 1383–1391.

Henquet, C., et al. (2008). "Gene-Environment Interplay Between Cannabis and Psychosis." *Schizophrenia Bulletin* 34: 1111–1121.

Houston, J. E., et al. (2008). "Childhood Sexual Abuse, Early Cannabis Use, and Psychosis: Testing an Interaction Model Based on the National Comorbidity Survey." *Schizophrenia Bulletin* 34: 580–585.

Huestis, M. A. (2005). "Pharmacokinetics and Metabolism of the Plant Cannabinoids, Delta9-Tetrahydrocannabinol, Cannabidiol, and Cannabinol." *Handbook of Experimental Pharmacology* 168: 657–690.

Huestis, M. A. (2007). "Human Cannabinoid Pharmacokinetics." *Chemistry and Biodiversity* 4: 1770–1804.

Huestis, M. A., et al. (2001). "Blockade of Effects of Smoked Marijuana by the CB1 Selective Cannabinoid Receptor Antagonist SR141716." *Archives of General Psychiatry* 58: 322–328.

Ignatowska-Jankowska, B., et al. (2009). "Cannabidiol-Induced Lymphopenia Does Not Involve NKT and NK Cells." *Journal of Physiology and Pharmacology* 60, Supplement 3: 99–103.

Iskedjian, M., et al. (2009). "Willingness to Pay for a Treatment for Pain in Multiple Sclerosis." *Pharmacoeconomics* 27: 149–158.

Izzo, A. A., et al. (2009). "Non-Psychotropic Plant Cannabinoids: New Therapeutic Opportunities from an Ancient Herb." *Trends in Pharmacological Sciences* 30: 515–527.

Janero, D. R., and Makriyannis, A. (2009). "Cannabinoid Receptor Antagonists: Pharmacological Opportunities, Clinical Experience, and Translational Prognosis." *Expert Opinion on Emerging Drugs* 14: 43–65.

Karst, M., and Wippermann, S. (2009). "Cannabinoids Against Pain. Efficacy and Strategies to Reduce Psychoactivity: A Clinical Perspective." *Expert Opinion on Investigational Drugs* 18: 125–133.

Lee, H. K., et al. (2009). "The Current Status and Future Prospects of Studies of Cannabinoid Receptor 1 Antagonists as Anti-Obesity Agents." *Current Topics in Medicinal Chemistry* 9: 482–503.

Leite, C. E., et al. (2009). "Rimonabant: An Antagonist Drug of the Encocannabinoid System for the Treatment of Obesity." *Pharmacological Reviews* 61: 217–224.

Lindigkeit, R., et al. (2009). "Spice: A Never Ending Story?" *Forensic Science International* 191: 58–63.

Lopez-Moreno, J. A., et al. (2007). "The CB1 Cannabinoid Receptor Antagonist Rimonabant Chronically Prevents the Nicotine-Induced Relapse to Alcohol." *Neurobiological Diseases* 25: 274–283.

Maas, A. I., et al. (2006). "Efficacy and Safety of Dexanabinol in Severe Traumatic Brain Injury: Results of a Phase III Randomized, Placebo-Controlled, Clinical Trial." *Lancet Neurology* 5: 38–45.

Mach, F., et al. (2009). "Effect of Blockage of the Endocannabinoid System by CB(1) Antagonism on Cardiovascular Risk." *Pharmacological Reports* 61: 13–21.

Muller-Vahl, K. R., and Emrich, H. M. (2008). "Cannabis and Schizophrenia: Towards a Cannabinoid Hypothesis of Schizophrenia." *Expert Review of Neurotherapeutics* 8: 1037–1048.

Onaivi, E. S. (2009). "Cannabinoid Receptors in Brain: Pharmacogenetics, Neuropharmacology, Neurotoxicology, and Potential Therapeutic Applications." *International Reviews in Neurobiology* 88: 335–369.

Partnership for a Drug-Free America. (2010). "2009 Parents and Teens Attitude Tracking Study Report." See www.drugfree.org/Portal/DrugIssue/Research/Teen_Study_2009

Perez, J., and Ribera, M. V. (2008). "Managing Neuropathic Pain with Sativex: A Review of Its Pros and Cons." *Expert Opinion on Pharmacotherapeutics* 9: 1189–1195.

Pernia-Andrade, A. J., et al. (2009). "Spinal Endocannabinoids and CB1 Receptors Mediate C-Fiber-Induced Heterosynaptic Pain Sensitization." *Science* 325: 760–764.

Pertwee, R. G. (2009). "Emerging Strategies for Exploiting Cannabinoid Receptor Agonists as Medicines." *British Journal of Pharmacology* 156: 397–411.

Pisanti, S., et al. (2009). "Use of Cannabinoid Receptor Agonists in Cancer Therapy as Palliative and Curative Agents." *Best Practice & Research Clinical Endocrinology & Metabolism* 23: 117–131.

Puighermanal, E., et al. (2009). "Cannabinoid Modulation of Hippocampal Long-Term Memory Is Mediated by mTOR Signaling." *Nature Neuroscience* 12: 1152–1158.

Ramaekers, J. G., et al. (2004). "Dose Related Risk of Motor Vehicle Crashes After Cannabis Use." *Drug and Alcohol Dependence* 73: 109–119.

Ramaekers, J.G., et al. (2006). "Cognition and Motor Control as a Function of Delta9-THC Concentration in Serum and Oral Fluids: Limits of Impairment." *Drug and Alcohol Dependence* 85: 114–122.

Rathbone, J., et al. (2008). "Cannabis and Schizophrenia." *Cochrane Database of Systematic Reviews* 16: CD004837.

Russo, E. B., and Guy, G. W. (2006). "The Tale of Two Cannabinoids: The Therapeutic Rationale for Combining Tetrahydrocannabinol and Cannabidiol." *Medical Hypotheses* 66: 234–246.

Samat, A., et al. (2008). "Rimonabant for the Treatment of Obesity." *Recent Patterns in Cardiovascular Drug Discovery* 3: 187–193.

Scheen, A. J. (2008). "CB1 Receptor Blockade and Its Impact on Cardiometabolic Risk Factors: Overview of the RIO Programme with Rimonabant." *Journal of Neuroendocrinology* 20, Supplement 1: 139–146.

Scuderi, C., et al. (2009). "Cannabidiol in Medicine: A Review of Its Therapeutic Potential in CNS Disorders." *Phytotherapeutic Research* 23: 597–602.

Selvarajah, D., et al. (2010). "Randomized Placebo-Controlled Double-Blind Clinical Trial of Cannabis-Based Medicinal Product (Sativex) in Painful Diabetic Neuropathy: Depression Is a Major Confounding Factor." *Diabetes Care* 33: 128–130.

Sewell, R. A., et al. (2009). "The Effect of Cannabis Compared with Alcohol on Driving." *American Journal on Addictions* 18: 185–193.

Shen, M., and Thayer, S. A. (1999). "Delta9-Tetrahydrocannabinol Acts as a Partial Agonist to Modulate Glutamatergic Synaptic Transmission Between Rat Hippocampal Neurons in Culture." *Molecular Pharmacology* 55: 8–13.

Sobolevsky, T., et al. (2010). "Detection of JWH-018 Metabolites in Smoking Mixture Post-Administration Urine." *Forensic Science International* 200: 141–147.

Sundram, S. (2006). "Cannabis and Neurodevelopment: Implications for Psychiatric Disorders." *Human Psychopharmacology* 21: 245–254.

Thomas, B. F., et al. (1996). "Structure-Activity Analysis of Anandamide Analogs: Relationship to a Cannabinoid Pharmacophore." *Journal of Medicinal Chemistry* 39: 471–479.

Tibiriça, E. (2010). "The Multiple Functions of the Endocannabinoid System: A Focus on the Regulation of Food Intake." *Diabetology & Metabolic Syndrome* 2: 5.

Uchiyama, N., et al. (2010). "Chemical Analysis of Synthetic Cannabinoids as Designer Drugs in Herbal Products." *Forensic Science International* 198: 31–38.

Vandrey, R., and Haney, M. (2009). "Pharmacotherapy for Cannabis Dependence: How Close Are We?" *CNS Drugs* 23: 543–553.

Wang, H., et al. (2006). "Jekyll and Hyde: Two Faces of Cannabinoid Signaling in Male and Female Fertility." *Endocrinology Reviews* 27: 427–448.

Welch, S. P. (2009). "Interaction of the Cannabinoid and Opioid Systems in the Modulation of Nociception." *International Review of Psychiatry* 21: 143–151.

Wise, L. E., et al. (2009). "Hippocanpal CB1 Receptors Mediate the Memory Impairing Effects of Delta-9-Tetrahydrocannabinol." *Neuropsychopharmacology* 34: 2072–2080.

Wright, S. M., et al. (2008). "Rimonabant: New Data and Emerging Experience." *Current Atherosclerosis Reports* 10: 71–78.

Zangen, A., et al. (2006). "Two Brain Sites for Cannabinoid Reward." *Journal of Neuroscience* 26: 490–497.

Zimmermann, U. S., et al. (2009). "Withdrawal Phenomena and Dependence Syndrome After the Consumption of 'Spice Gold'." *Deutsches Ärzteblatt International* 106: 464–467.

Chapter 15

Psychedelic Drugs

This chapter introduces a class of drugs that act on various neurotransmitters in the central nervous system (CNS) to produce visual hallucinations and out-of-body experiences. Their actions are also characterized by marked alterations in cortical functioning, including cognition, perception, and mood (Davis et al., 2002). Because of the wide range of psychological and physiological effects they produce, the single term that might best be used to classify these agents has been debated for a long time. The term *hallucinogen* is used because these agents can, in high enough doses, induce hallucinations. However, that term is somewhat inappropriate because illusory phenomena and perceptual distortions are more common than are true hallucinations. The term *psychotomimetic* has also been used because of the alleged ability of these drugs to mimic psychoses or induce psychotic states. However, most of these drugs do not produce the same behavioral patterns that are observed in people who experience psychotic episodes. Descriptive terms, such as *phantasticum* or *psychedelic*, have also been used to imply that these agents all have the ability to alter sensory perception. In this chapter the term *psychedelic* is used because it allows for more flexibility in grouping together a disparate array of effects into a quantifiable and recognizable syndrome.

A psychedelic drug can be defined as any agent that causes alterations in perception, cognition, and mood as its primary psychobiological actions in the presence of an otherwise clear sensorium. This definition separates the pure psychedelic drugs from other substances that can cause altered states of thinking and perception, such as *poisons*, which affect the mind (not discussed in this book), and *intoxicants* (such as ethyl alcohol and the inhalants of abuse; Chapter 13), which primarily produce clouding of consciousness, impaired cognition, and amnesia. This chapter covers the true psychedelics, mixed psychedelic-stimulant drugs ("club drugs"), and certain other abused deliriants such as scopolamine, phencyclidine, ketamine, and dextromethorphan.

Many psychedelic agents occur in nature; others are synthetically produced. Naturally occurring psychedelic drugs have been inhaled, ingested, worshipped, and reviled since prehistory, and many are available in the United States and throughout the world (Halpern, 2004). Many are viewed as having magical or mystical properties. Prior to the 1960s, most Americans were barely aware of their existence. During the late 1960s and the 1970s, however, some people advocated their use to enhance perception, expand reality, promote personal awareness, and stimulate or induce comprehension of the spiritual or supernatural. These drugs heighten awareness of sensory input, often accompanied by both an enhanced sense of clarity and diminished control over what is experienced. Frequently, there is a

---

TABLE 15.1 Classification of psychedelic drugs

ANTICHOLINERGIC PSYCHEDELIC DRUG
  Scopolamine

CATECHOLAMINELIKE PSYCHEDELIC DRUGS
  Mescaline
  DOM, MDA, DMA, MDMA (ecstasy), TMA, MDE
  Myristicin, elemicin

SEROTONINLIKE PSYCHEDELIC DRUGS
  Lysergic acid diethylamide (LSD)
  Dimethyltryptamine (DMT), AMT, 5-MeO-DIPT
  Psilocybin, psilocin, bufotenine
  Ololiuqui
  Harmine

GLUTAMINERGIC NMDA RECEPTOR ANTAGONISTS
  Phencyclidine (Sernyl)
  Ketamine (Ketalar)
  Dextromethorphan

OPIOID KAPPA RECEPTOR AGONIST
  Salvinorin A

feeling that one part of the self seems to be a passive observer, while another part of the self participates and receives the vivid and unusual sensory experiences. In this state, the slightest sensation may take on profound meaning. With the advent of organic chemistry, many of these psychedelic drugs have been chemically identified and many derivatives synthesized.

Most psychedelic drugs structurally resemble one of four neurotransmitters: acetylcholine, two catecholamines (norepinephrine and dopamine), and serotonin. These structural similarities lead to three of the five classes for categorizing psychedelic drugs (Table 15.1): *anticholinergic*, *catecholaminelike*, and *serotoninlike psychedelics*. The fourth and fifth classes of psychedelic drugs are the *glutaminergic NMDA receptor antagonists* (the two psychedelic anesthetics as well as dextromethorphan) and the *opioid kappa receptor agonist* salvinorin A.

Scopolamine: An Anticholinergic Psychedelic

Scopolamine (Figure 15.1), an acetylcholine receptor blocker (antagonist), is the classic example of an anticholinergic drug with psychedelic properties. Because it binds to acetylcholine receptors but is devoid of intrinsic activity, scopolamine blocks the access of acetylcholine to its receptors—hence the term *anticholinergic*. This term implies a constellation of effects, including dry mouth, blurred vision, increased heart rate, and urinary retention. Because scopolamine easily crosses the blood-brain barrier, it causes sedation, cognitive impairments, amnesia,

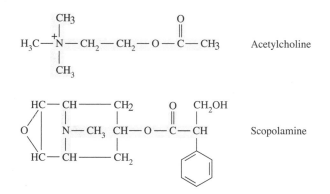

FIGURE 15.1 Structural formulas of acetylcholine (a chemical transmitter) and the anticholinergic psychedelic scopolamine, which acts by blocking acetylcholine receptors. The shaded portion of each molecule illustrates structural similarities, which presumably contribute to receptor fit.

and delirium. Medically, scopolamine is found in some travel-sickness products including motion-sickness skin patches.[1]

Historical Background

The history of scopolamine is long and colorful (Holzman, 1998). The drug is distributed widely in nature, found in especially high concentrations in the plants *Atropa belladonna* (belladonna, or deadly nightshade), *Datura stramonium* (Jamestown weed, jimsonweed, stinkweed, thorn apple, or devil's apple), *Mandragora officinarum* (mandrake), and *Datura inoxia* (moonflower). Both professional and amateur poisoners of the Middle Ages frequently used deadly nightshade as a source of poison. In fact, the plant's name, *Atropa belladonna*, is derived from Atropos, one of the three Fates, who supposedly cut the thread of life. *Belladonna* means "beautiful woman," which refers to the drug's ability to dilate the pupils when it is applied topically to the eyes (eyes with widely dilated pupils were presumably a mark of beauty). Accidental ingestion of berries from *Datura* has even been associated with the incapacitation of whole armies, for example, the defeat of Marc Antony's army in 36 B.C. and the defeat of British soldiers by settlers in the rebellion known as Bacon's Revolution near Jamestown, Virginia, in 1676 (hence the name Jamestown weed).

Scopolamine-containing plants have been used and misused for centuries. For example, the delirium caused by scopolamine may have persuaded certain people that they could fly—and that they were witches (associated with the Halloween customs involving flying witches). Marijuana and opium preparations from the Far East were once fortified with material from *Datura stramonium*. Today, cigarettes made from the leaves of *D. stramonium* and *A. belladonna* are smoked occasionally to induce intoxication. Throughout the world, leaves of plants that contain atropine or scopolamine are still used to prepare intoxicating beverages.

Pharmacological Effects

Scopolamine acts on the peripheral nervous system to produce an anticholinergic syndrome consisting of dry mouth, reduced sweating, dry skin, increased body temperature, dilated pupils, blurred vision, tachycardia, and hypertension. Scopolamine in the CNS functions as a deliriant and intoxicant. Low doses produce drowsiness, mild euphoria, profound amnesia, fatigue, delirium, mental confusion, dreamless sleep,

---

[1] Certain medicines also have anticholinergic properties and can cause similar effects. Examples include antihistamines (such as diphenhydramine, or Benadryl), the tricyclic antidepressants (such as imipramine, or Tofranil), and certain medicines used in the treatment of parkinsonism (e.g., Cogentin).

and loss of attention. Rather than expanding consciousness, awareness, and insight, scopolamine clouds consciousness and produces amnesia; it does not expand sensory perception. The amnesia produced is quite intense. As doses of scopolamine increase, psychiatric symptoms include restlessness, excitement, hallucinations, euphoria, and disorientation (DeFrates et al., 2005).

In higher and much more toxic doses, a behavioral state that resembles a toxic psychosis occurs. Delirium, mental confusion, stupor, coma, and respiratory depression dominate. While scopolamine intoxication can convey a sense of excitement and loss of control to the user, the clouding of consciousness and the reduction in memory of the episode render scopolamine rather unattractive as a psychedelic drug. It is probably more appropriate to refer to it as a somewhat dangerous intoxicant, amnestic, and deliriant. Scopolamine is classically stated to make one "hot as a hare, blind as a bat, dry as a bone, red as a beet, and mad as a hen." Typically, sensorium and psychosis usually clear within 36 to 48 hours.

Catecholaminelike Psychedelics

Norepinephrine and dopamine receptors are important sites of action for a large group of psychedelic drugs that are structurally similar to both catecholamine neurotransmitters and the amphetamines (Figure 15.2). They differ structurally from the normal neurotransmitters by the addition of one or more methoxy ($-OCH_3$) groups to the phenyl ring structure. These methoxy groups, varied as they are, confer psychedelic properties on top of their amphetaminelike psychostimulant properties. Methoxylated amphetamine derivatives include mescaline, DOM (also called STP), MDA, MDE, MDMA (ecstasy), MMDA, DMA, and certain drugs that are obtained from nutmeg (myristicin and elemicin). As a group, these drugs that exhibit a blend of stimulant and hallucinogenic actions have classically been referred to as *entactogens*.

As would be predicted from their structures, catecholamine psychedelics exert amphetaminelike psychostimulant actions, presumably on dopaminergic neurons. They can enhance energy, endurance, sociability, and sexual arousal. However, their psychedelic actions are probably ultimately exerted by augmentation of serotonin neurotransmission— probably as agonists at postsynaptic serotonin 5-HT$_{2A}$ receptors (Gonzalez-Maeso and Sealfon, 2009a). This action would account for their LSD-like effects (discussed later). The combination of catecholamine and serotonin actions points to a complex interaction between dopamine and serotonin and explains their combined stimulant and (LSD-like) hallucinogenic actions. These psychedelics can therefore be safely classified as *mixed dopamine and serotonin agonists*. Some of these drugs are found in nature and others are synthetically manufactured.

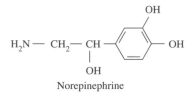

Norepinephrine

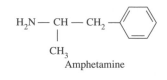

Amphetamine

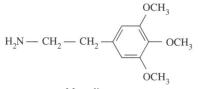

Mescaline

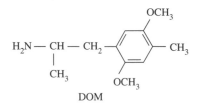

DOM

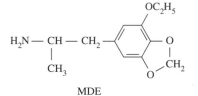

MDA

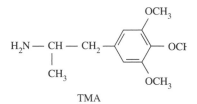

TMA

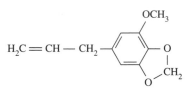

MDE

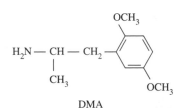

Myristicin

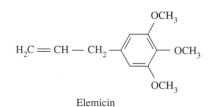

Elemicin

DMA

FIGURE 15.2 Structural formulas of norepinephrine (a chemical transmitter), amphetamine, and eight catecholaminelike psychedelic drugs. These eight drugs are structurally related to norepinephrine and are thought to exert their psychedelic actions by altering the transmission of nerve impulses at norepinephrine and serotonin synapses in the brain.

Mescaline

Peyote (*Lophophora williamsii*) is a common plant in the southwestern United States and in Mexico. It is a spineless cactus that has a small crown, or "button," and a long root. When the plant is used for psychedelic purposes, the crown is cut from the cactus and dried into a hard brown disk. This disk, which is frequently referred to as a "mescal button," is later softened in the mouth and swallowed. The psychedelic chemical in the button is mescaline.

Historical Background. The use of peyote extends back perhaps 5000 years or more in North America; the cactus was used in the religious rites of the Aztecs and other Mexican and North American Indians (el-Seedi et al., 2005). Currently, peyote is legally available for use in the religious practice of the Native American Church of North America, whose members regard peyote as sacramental. The use of peyote for religious purposes is not considered to be abuse, and peyote is seldom abused by members of the Native American Church (Fickenscher et al., 2006). Members of the Native American Church are exempt from federal criminal penalties for religious use of peyote. This exemption predates the Controlled Substances Act.

Pharmacological Effects. Early research on the peyote cactus led in 1896 to the identification of mescaline as its pharmacologically active ingredient. After the chemical structure of mescaline was elucidated in 1918, the compound was produced synthetically. Because of its structural resemblance to norepinephrine, a wide variety of synthetic mescaline derivatives have now been synthesized, and all have methoxy ($-OCH_3$) groups or similar additions on their benzene rings (see Figure 15.2). Methoxylation of the benzene ring apparently adds psychedelic properties to the drug, presumably due to agonist effects at the 5-HT$_{2A}$ receptor.

When taken orally, mescaline is rapidly and completely absorbed, and significant concentrations are usually achieved in the brain within 1 to 2 hours. Between 3.5 and 4 hours after drug intake, mescaline produces an acute psychotomimetic state, with prominent effects on the visual system. The effects of a single dose of mescaline persist for approximately 10 hours. The drug does not appear to be metabolized before it is excreted. In functional brain imaging using SPECT, mescaline produced in healthy volunteers a "hyperfrontal" pattern with an emphasis on the right hemisphere, which was correlated with mescaline-induced psychotomimetic psychopathology.

Interest in mescaline focuses on the fact that it produces unusual psychic effects and visual hallucinations. The usual oral dose (5 milligrams per kilogram body weight) in the average normal subject causes anxiety, sympathomimetic effects, hyperreflexia of the limbs, tremors, and visual hallucinations that consist of brightly colored lights, geometric designs, animals, and occasionally people; color and space perception is often concomitantly impaired, but otherwise the sensorium is normal and insight is retained. The psychotic effects are mainly concerned with the dissolution of ego boundaries, visual hallucinations, and dimensions of boundlessness, often mixed with anxious passivity experiences.

Synthetic Amphetamine Derivatives

DOM, MDA, DMA, MDE, TMA, AMT, 5-MeO-DIPT, and MDMA are structurally related to mescaline and methamphetamine (see Figure 15.2) and, as might be expected, produce similar effects. They have moderate behavioral stimulant effects at low doses, but as with LSD, psychedelic effects dominate as doses increase. These derivatives are considerably more potent and more toxic than mescaline.

DOM, MDA, MDE, and TMA. *DOM* (dimethoxymethamphetamine) has effects that are similar to those of mescaline; doses of 1 to 6 milligrams produce euphoria, which is followed by a 6- to 8-hour period of hallucinations. DOM is 100 times more potent than mescaline but much less potent than LSD. The use of DOM is associated with a high incidence of overdose (because it is potent and street doses are poorly controlled). Acute toxic reactions are common; they consist of tremors that may eventually lead to convulsive movements, prostration, and even death. Because toxic reactions are common, the use of DOM is not widespread.

    MDA (methylenedioxyamphetamine), *DMA* (dimethoxymethylamphetamine), *MDE* (methylenedioxyethylamphetamine), *TMA* (trimethoxyamphetamine), and other structural variations of amphetamine are encountered as "designer psychedelics." MDA is also a metabolite of MDMA, and much of MDMA's effect may be due to the presence of MDA. In general, the pharmacological effects of these drugs resemble those of mescaline and LSD; they reflect the mix of catecholamine and serotonin interactions. Side effects and toxicities (including fatalities) are similar to those of MDMA. MDA is sometimes represented as MDMA; when this occurs, MDA is more lethal in lower doses and its effects are longer lasting than those of MDMA.

AMT and 5-MeO-DIPT. In April 2003, the Drug Enforcement Administration (DEA) designated alpha-methyltryptamine (AMT) and 5-methoxy-diisopropyltryptamine (5-MeO-DIPT, or Foxy) as Schedule I substances under the Controlled Substances Act. This classification for these new "designer" psychedelics implies high abuse potential with no therapeutic usefulness. Administered orally, both drugs cause hallucinations, mood elevation, nervousness, insomnia, and pupilary dilation. AMT is of slow onset (3 to 4 hours) after oral administration and prolonged duration (12 to 24 hours). It is also a potent reuptake inhibitor of norepinephrine, dopamine, and serotonin (Nagai et al., 2007).

Foxy is of more rapid onset (20 to 30 minutes) and shorter duration (3 to 6 hours). It has been reported to induce an acute confusional state for several hours (Itokawa et al., 2007) and to substitute for MDMA. These new drugs are popular at dance raves.

MDMA. MDMA (methylenedioxymethamphetamine, or ecstasy) resembles MDA in structure but may be less hallucinogenic; nevertheless, it induces a sense of disembodiment and visual distortion. MDMA is a potent and selective serotonin neurotoxin both in animals and in humans (Gouzoulis-Mayfrank and Daumann, 2009). The dysfunction is related to dose and duration of use, although today we understand that even low doses may be neurotoxic, resulting in small but significant effects on brain microvasculature, white matter maturation, and possible axonal damage (deWin et al., 2008). It remains unclear whether or not these effects are persistent. Kalant (2001) summarized possible persistent MDMA-induced psychiatric problems:

- Impairments in memory, both verbal and visual
- Impairments in decision making
- Greater impulsivity and lack of self-control
- Panic attacks following withdrawal
- Recurrent paranoia, depersonalization, and flashbacks
- Depression, sometimes resistant to treatment with other than selective serotonin reuptake inhibitor (SSRI) antidepressants

Therefore, repeated use of ecstasy is associated with sleep, mood, and anxiety disturbances, elevated impulsiveness, memory deficits, and attention problems, which may be persisttent. Schilt and coworkers (2007) performed a prospective study on 118 ecstasy-naive volunteers, of whom 58 started using ecstasy and 60 remained ecstasy-naive. They found that even a first low cumulative dose of ecstasy (1.5 tablets) was associated with significant declines in verbal memory. Although theirs was a short-term study, they stated that long-term negative consequences could not be excluded. Certainly, there is abundant suggestion from human studies that MDMA intoxication can result in persistent memory impairment, reduced serotonin transporter binding, and ultimately the destruction of presynaptic serotonin transporter receptors. This reaction can certainly account for the association between ecstasy use and both cognitive difficulties and mood disorders (Fisk et al., 2009; Martin-Santos et al., 2010).

Despite generally positive emotional effects of single uses at raves, "somatic" effects can be significant. Two examples are dramatic increases in blood pressure and body temperature, increases that are generally well tolerated by young users but undesirable in people with cardiovascular disease. Other somatic effects include jaw clenching, suppressed appetite, restlessness, insomnia, impaired gait, and restless legs. Adverse sequelae after 24 hours include lack of energy and appetite, fatigue, restlessness, difficulty in concentrating, and brooding.

Concern about MDMA is increasing as use of this club drug increases around the world, especially at dance clubs and raves. Twenty percent of users have received treatment for an ecstasy-related problem, and 15 percent required formal treatment.[2]

MDMA is potentially a very dangerous drug for human use: abuse of MDMA may lead to severe toxicities, including fatalities. When it is used during periods of intense activity, such as skiing and dancing at raves, symptoms include hyperthermia, tachycardia, disorientation, dilated pupils, convulsions, rigidity, breakdown of skeletal muscle, kidney failure, cardiac arrhythmias, and death (Hall and Henry, 2006). The pathology for these serious effects appears to represent induction of a fatal syndrome called malignant hyperthermia. MDMA may precipitate malignant hyperthermia in susceptible people, and this response could be blocked by a drug called dantrolene (Duffy and Ferguson, 2007). It is hoped that, should an MDMA-intoxicated, hyperthermic patient be taken to an emergency room in time, dantrolene would be administered and a life saved. Despite these consequences, the intense euphoric high promotes continued use.

Occasionally, new MDMA-related drugs emerge. For example, *2,5-dimethoxy-4-propylthiophenethylamine* (Schifano et al., 2005) is known as Blue Mystic, 2C-T-7, T7, Tripstay, and Tweety-Bird Mescaline; *4-bromo-2,5-dimethoxyphenethylamine* is known as 2C-B, Nexus, 2s, Toonies, Bromo, Spectrum, and Venus. These drugs produce hallucinogenic actions with the side effects of nausea, anxiety, panic attacks, and paranoid ideation (Schifano et al., 2005; Fantegrossi et al., 2005). Toxicities specific to these derivatives have not yet been summarized although they may be cause for concern.

---

[2] Ecstasy, gamma hydroxybutyrate (GHB; Chapter 7), ketamine/phencyclidine (discussed later in this chapter), and methamphetamine (Chapter 12) are four examples of club drugs that are increasing in popularity with young people. Ecstasy is a psychostimulant/hallucinogen (an entactogen), GHB is a sedative/amnestic, ketamine and phencyclidine are dissociative anesthetics, and methamphetamine is a psychostimulant.

Myristicin and Elemicin

Nutmeg and mace are common household spices sometimes abused for their hallucinogenic properties. Myristicin and elemicin, the pharmacologically active ingredients in nutmeg and mace, are responsible for the psychedelic action. Ingestion of large amounts (1 to 2 teaspoons—5 to 15 grams—usually brewed in tea) may, after a delay of 2 to 5 hours, induce feelings of unreality, confusion, disorientation, impending doom, depersonalization, unreality, and euphoria as well as visual hallucinations and acute psychotic reactions. Considering the close structural resemblance of myristicin and elemicin to mescaline (see Figure 15.2), these psychedelic actions are not unexpected. Ingestion of nutmeg, however, produces many unpleasant side effects, including vomiting, nausea, and tremors. After nutmeg or mace has been taken to produce its psychedelic action, the side effects usually dissuade users from trying these agents a second time. Extremely unpleasant reactions may occur, but deaths are infrequent.

Serotoninlike Psychedelics

The serotoninlike psychedelic drugs include *lysergic acid diethylamide* (LSD), *psilocybin* and *psilocin*, *dimethyltryptamine* (DMT), and *bufotenine* (Figure 15.3). Serotonin-acting psychedelics produce a characteristic syndrome, with disturbances in thinking, illusions, elementary and complex visual hallucinations, and impaired ego functioning. Because of their structural resemblance to one another and to serotonin, it has been presumed that these agents exert their effects through interactions at serotonin 5-HT$_2$ receptor synapses (Geyer and Vollenweider, 2008).

Almaula and coworkers (1996) first mapped the binding site for LSD on the 5-HT$_{2A}$ receptor and correlated the binding with receptor activation. LSD activation of the medial prefrontal cortex and anterior cingulate cortex is mediated by 5-HT$_{2A}$ receptors, areas involved in the production of hallucinations (see Diederen et al., 2010). In addition to LSD, both DMT and bufotenine act as partial agonists at 5-HT$_{2A}$ receptors. With all this focus of agonist action on serotonin receptors, a major question remains unanswered: Why does serotonin itself not induce psychotomimetic effects? In particular, psychotomimetic effects are seldom seen after administration of SSRI-type antidepressants, although the serotonin syndrome and the behavioral activations that are sometimes seen with SSRI therapy likely are a reflection of such action.

Lysergic Acid Diethylamide

During the mid-1960s and early 1970s, lysergic acid diethylamide (LSD) became one of the most remarkable and controversial drugs known. In doses that are so small that they might even be considered

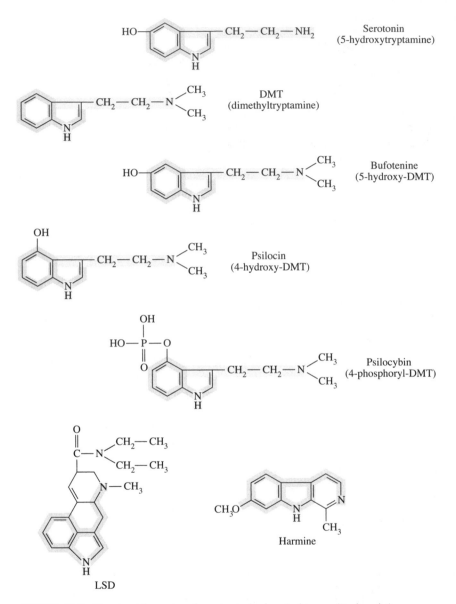

FIGURE 15.3 Structural formulas of serotonin (a chemical transmitter) and six serotoninlike psychedelic drugs. These six drugs are structurally related to serotonin (as indicated by the shading) and are thought to exert their psychedelic actions through alterations of serotonin synapses in the brain. Although LSD is structurally much more complex than serotonin, the basic similarity of the two molecules is apparent.

infinitesimal, LSD induces remarkable psychological change in a person, enhancing self-awareness and altering internal reality, while causing relatively few alterations in the general physiology of the body.

Historical Background. LSD was first synthesized in 1938 by Albert Hofmann, a Swiss chemist, as part of an organized research program to investigate possible therapeutic uses of compounds obtained from ergot, a natural product derived from a fungus (*Claviceps purpurea*). Early pharmacological studies of LSD in animals failed to reveal anything unusual; the psychedelic action was neither sought nor expected. Thus, LSD remained unnoticed until 1943, when Hofmann had an unusual experience:

> In the afternoon of 16 April, 1943, . . . I was seized by a peculiar sensation of vertigo and restlessness. Objects, as well as the shape of my associates in the laboratory, appeared to undergo optical changes. I was unable to concentrate on my work. In a dreamlike state I left for home, where an irresistible urge to lie down overcame me. I drew the curtains and immediately fell into a peculiar state similar to drunkenness, characterized by an exaggerated imagination. With my eyes closed, fantastic pictures of extraordinary plasticity and intensive color seemed to surge toward me. After two hours, this state gradually wore off. (Hofmann, 1994, p. 80)

Hofmann correctly hypothesized that his experience had resulted from the accidental ingestion of LSD. To further characterize the experience, Hofmann self-administered what seemed to be a minuscule oral dose (only 0.25 milligram). We now know, however, that this dose is about ten times the dose required to induce psychedelic effects in most people. As a result of this miscalculation, his response was quite spectacular:

> After 40 minutes, I noted the following symptoms in my laboratory journal: slight giddiness, restlessness, difficulty in concentration, visual disturbances, laughing. . . . Later, I lost all count of time. I noticed with dismay that my environment was undergoing progressive changes. My visual field wavered and everything appeared deformed as in a faulty mirror. Space and time became more and more disorganized and I was overcome by a fear that I was going out of my mind. The worst part of it [was] that I was clearly aware of my condition. My power of observation was unimpaired. . . . Occasionally, I felt as if I were out of my body. I thought I had died. My ego seemed suspended somewhere in space, from where I saw my dead body lying on the sofa. . . . It was particularly striking how acoustic perceptions, such as the noise of water gushing from a tap or the spoken word, were transformed into optical illusions. I then fell asleep and awakened the next morning somewhat tired but otherwise feeling perfectly well. (p. 80)

Dr. Hoffman died in 2008 at the age of 102. The first North American study of LSD in humans was conducted in 1949, and during the 1950s large quantities of LSD were distributed to scientists for research purposes. A significant impetus for research was the notion that the effects of LSD might constitute a model for psychosis, which would provide some insight into the biochemical and physiological processes of mental illness and its treatment (Passie et al., 2008). Some therapists tried LSD as an adjunct to psychotherapy to help patients verbalize their problems and gain some insight into the underlying causes, but it did not prove to be an effective treatment.

Pharmacokinetics. LSD is usually taken orally, and it is rapidly absorbed by that route. Usual doses range from about 25 micrograms to more than 300 micrograms. Because the amounts are so small, LSD is often added to other substances, such as squares of paper, the backs of stamps, or sugar cubes, which can be handled more easily. LSD is absorbed within about 60 minutes, reaching peak blood levels in about 3 hours. It is distributed rapidly and efficiently throughout the body; it diffuses easily into the brain and readily crosses the placenta. The largest amounts of LSD in the body are found in the liver, where the drug is metabolized before it is excreted to 2-oxo-3-hydroxy-LSD. The usual duration of action is 6 to 8 hours.

Because of its extreme potency, only minuscule amounts of LSD can be detected in urine, although the metabolite is present in concentrations 16 to 43 times greater than that of LSD itself. Thus, conventional urine-screening tests are inadequate to detect LSD. When the use of LSD is suspected, urine is collected (up to 30 hours after ingestion) and an ultrasensitive radioimmunoassay is performed to verify the presence of the drug.

Physiological Effects. Although the LSD experience is characterized by its psychological effects, subtle physiological changes also occur. A person who takes LSD may experience a slight increase in body temperature; dilation of the pupils; slightly increased heart rate and blood pressure; increased levels of glucose in the blood; and dizziness, drowsiness, nausea, and other effects that, although noticeable, seldom interfere with the psychedelic experience.

LSD is known to possess a low level of toxicity; the effective dose is about 50 micrograms, while the lethal dose is about 14,000 micrograms. These figures provide a therapeutic ratio of 280, making the drug a remarkably nonlethal compound. This calculation does not include any fatal accidents or suicides that occur when a person is intoxicated by LSD. In fact, most deaths attributed to LSD result from accidents, homicides, or suicide. The use of LSD during pregnancy is certainly unwise, although a distinct fetal LSD syndrome has not been described.

Psychological Effects.   The psychological effects of LSD are intense. At doses of 25 to 50 micrograms, pupillary dilation and a glassy-eyed appearance may be noticed. These effects are accompanied by alterations in perception, thinking, emotion, arousal, and self-image. Time is slowed or distorted, and sensory input is intensified. Cognitive alterations include enhanced power to visualize previously seen or imagined objects and decreased vigilance and logical thought. Visual alterations are the most characteristic phenomenon; they typically include colored lights, distorted perceptions, and vivid and fascinating images and shapes. Colors can be heard and sounds may be seen. The loss of boundaries and the fear of fragmentation create a need for a structuring or supporting environment and experienced companions. During the "trip," thoughts and memories can emerge under self-guidance, sometimes to the user's distress. Mood may be labile, shifting from depression to gaiety, from elation to fear. Tension and anxiety may mount and reach panic proportions. The LSD-induced psychedelic experience typically occurs in three phases:

1. The *somatic phase* occurs after absorption of the drug and consists of CNS stimulation and autonomic changes that are predominantly sympathomimetic in nature.
2. The *sensory* (or *perceptual*) *phase* is characterized by sensory distortions and pseudohallucinations, which are the effects desired by the drug user.
3. The *psychic phase* signals a maximum drug effect, with changes in mood, disruption of thought processes, altered perception of time, depersonalization, true hallucinations, and psychotic episodes. Experiencing this phase is considered a "bad trip."

Tolerance and Dependence.   Tolerance of both the psychological and physiological alterations induced by LSD readily and rapidly develops, and cross-tolerance occurs between LSD and other psychedelics. Tolerance is lost within several days after the user stops taking the drug.

Physical dependence on LSD does not develop, even when the drug is used repeatedly for a prolonged period of time. In fact, most heavy users of the drug say that they ceased using LSD because they tired of it, had no further need for it, or had had enough. Even when the drug is discontinued because of concern about bad trips or about physical or mental harm, few withdrawal signs are exhibited. Laboratory animals do not self-administer LSD.

Adverse Reactions and Toxicity. The adverse reactions attributed to LSD generally fall into five categories:

- Chronic or intermittent psychotic states
- Persistent or recurrent major affective disorder (for example, depression)
- Exacerbation of preexisting psychiatric illness
- Disruption of personality or chronic brain syndrome, known as "burnout"
- Posthallucinogenic perceptual disorder (flashbacks characterized by the periodic hallucinogenic imagery months or even years after the immediate effect of LSD has worn off)

Unpleasant experiences with LSD are relatively frequent and may involve an uncontrollable drift into confusion, dissociative reactions, acute panic reactions, a reliving of earlier traumatic experiences, or an acute psychotic hospitalization. Prolonged nonpsychotic reactions have included dissociative reactions, time and space distortion, body image changes, and a residue of fear or depression stemming from morbid or terrifying experiences under the drug. With the failure of usual defense mechanisms, the onslaught of repressed material overwhelms the integrative capacity of the ego, and a psychotic reaction results.

It appears that LSD-induced disruption of long-established patterns of adapting may be a lasting or semipermanent effect of the drug. In other words, our neocortex modulates awareness of our surroundings and filters a high proportion of incoming information before it can be processed, allowing through only the amount of information that is necessary for survival. LSD works to open this filter, so an increased amount of somatosensory data is processed with a corresponding increase in what is deemed important. Thus, LSD reduces a person's normal ability to control emotional reactions, and drug-induced alterations in perception can become so intense that they overwhelm the ability to cope.

One unique characteristic of LSD and LSD-like substances is the recurrence of some of the symptoms that appeared during the intoxication after the immediate effect of the hallucinogen has worn off. These symptoms are mainly visual and the terms *flashback* and *hallucinogen persisting perception disorder* (HPPD) are used fairly interchangeably. However, a flashback is usually a short-term, nondistressing, spontaneous, recurrent, reversible, and benign condition accompanied by a pleasant affect. In contrast, HPPD is a generally long-term, distressing, spontaneous, recurrent, pervasive, either slowly reversible or irreversible, nonbenign condition accompanied by an unpleasant dysphoric affect (Johnson et al., 2008).

Treatment of flashbacks and HPPD has been symptomatic. Case reports note the success of benzodiazepines as well as other drugs, but there is no consensus on appropriate therapy and no specific treatment. Most commonly, an atypical antipsychotic drug with serotonin-2 blocking activity (Chapter 4) is chosen to treat both acute LSD toxicity and HPPD, although older literature has reported exacerbation of LDS-like panic and visual symptoms. More current data are needed.

Other Serotoninlike Hallucinogens

DMT. DMT (dimethyltryptamine) is a short-acting, naturally occurring psychedelic compound that can be synthesized easily and is structurally related to serotonin. DMT produces LSD-like effects in the user, and like LSD it is a partial agonist at serotonin 5-HT$_2$ receptors. Widely used throughout much of the world, DMT is an active ingredient of various types of South American plants, such as *Virola calophylla* and *Mimosa hostilis.* Used by itself, DMT is snorted or smoked, often in a marijuana cigarette.

Ayahuasca (also called *hoasca*) is a psychoactive beverage that, as a tea, has been drunk for centuries in religious, spiritual, and medicinal contexts by Amazon Indians in the rainforest areas of South America. Two principal ingredients of ayahuasca are harmine (a substance that is a potent monoamine oxidase, or MAO, inhibitor) and DMT. Administered orally to healthy volunteers, DMT produced prominent thought disorders and inappropriate affective reactions (for example, paranoia) rather than the negative schizophrenic reactions characteristic of ketamine (discussed below). Effects have an onset of about 30 to 60 minutes, peak at 1 to 2 hours, and persist for about 3 to 4 hours. In most cases, effects (changes in perceptual, affective, cognitive, and somatic spheres) are well tolerated, but disorientation, paranoia, and anxiety can be displayed. In religious ceremonial use, such reactions are unusual (Gable, 2007). Interestingly, although DMT is commonly thought to exert its psychedelic effect through action of 5-HT$_{2A}$ receptors, Su and coworkers (2009) demonstrated binding to sigma-1 receptors as a possible mode of action.[3]

In 1994, Strassman and coworkers conducted controlled investigations of DMT in "highly motivated," experienced hallucinogen users. When it was administered intravenously (0.04 to 0.4 milligram per kilogram of body weight), onset of action occurred within 2 minutes and was negligible at 30 minutes. DMT elevated blood pressure, heart

---

[3] Formerly thought to be a type of opioid receptor, the sigma-1 receptor is actually an endoplasmic reticulum protein implicated in neuroprotection, neuronal plasticity, anxiety, and depression (Kulkarni and Dhir, 2009; Hashimoto, 2009; Paschos et al., 2009; Maurice and Su, 2009).

rate, and temperature; dilated pupils; and increased body endorphin and hormone levels. The psychedelic threshold dose was 0.2 milligram per kilogram of body weight; lower doses were primarily "affective and somaesthetic." Hallucinogenic effects included a rapidly moving, brightly colored visual display of images. Auditory effects were less common. "Loss of control," associated with a brief but overwhelming "rush," led to a dissociated state, where euphoria alternated or coexisted with anxiety. These effects completely replaced subjects' previously ongoing mental experience and were more vivid and compelling than dreams or waking awareness.

Thus, DMT produces intense visual hallucinations, intoxication, and often a loss of awareness of one's surroundings. When DMT is injected, smoked, or taken as a snuff, after the 30-minute period of effect, the user returns to normal feelings and perceptions—thus the nicknames lunch-hour drug, businessman's lunch, and businessman's LSD. Administered with an MAO inhibitor (such as the ayahuasca tea), it is absorbed orally and has a longer duration of action.

Bufotenine. Bufotenine (5-hydroxy DMT, or dimethylserotonin), like LSD and DMT, is a potent serotonin agonist hallucinogen with an affinity for several types of serotonin receptors, especially the 5-HT$_{2A}$ receptor. The name bufotenine comes from the name for a toad of the genus *Bufo*, whose skin and glandular secretions supposedly produce hallucinogenic effects when ingested. Toad secretions have been used since ancient times for a variety of mythological and medicinal purposes involving magical, shamanic, or occult uses for casting spells and for divination.

After subcutaneous injection to rats, the half-life of bufotenine is about 2 hours, with MAO responsible for metabolism. Bufotenine is not found in the bodies of normal people. However, it can be produced in an alternative and unusual pathway for the metabolic breakdown of serotonin. Indeed, some have attempted to correlate the presence of bufotenine in urine with various psychiatric disorders, although this theory is not generally accepted.

Psilocybin. Psilocybin (4-phosphoryl-DMT) and psilocin (4-hydroxy-DMT) are two psychedelic agents that are found in many species of mushrooms that belong to the genera *Psilocybe*, *Panaeolus*, *Copelandia*, and *Conocybe*. As Figure 15.3 shows, the only difference between psilocybin and psilocin is that psilocybin contains a molecule of phosphoric acid. After the mushroom has been ingested, phosphoric acid is enzymatically removed from psilocybin, thus producing psilocin, the active psychedelic agent.

Psilocybin is a potent hallucinogen that exerts such action through an agonist effect at serotonin 5-HT$_{2A}$ and 5-HT$_{1A}$ receptors, similar to the effects of other serotonin psychedelics. Psilocybin administration (about 0.25 milligram per kilogram of body weight, orally) produces changes in mood, disturbances in thinking, illusions, complex visual hallucinations, and impaired ego functioning, similar to the effects produced by LSD.

Psilocybin-containing mushrooms grow throughout much of the world, including the northwestern United States. Psilocin and psilocybin are approximately 1/200 as potent as LSD; their effects peak in about 2 hours and last about 6 to 10 hours. Unlike DMT, psilocin and psilocybin are absorbed effectively when taken orally; the mushrooms are eaten raw to induce psychedelic effects.

There is great variation in the concentration of psilocybin and psilocin among the different species of mushrooms, as well as significant differences among mushrooms of the same species. For example, the usual oral dose of *Psilocybe semilanceata* (liberty caps) may consist of 10 to 40 mushrooms, while the dose for *Psilocybe cyanescens* may be only 2 to 5 mushrooms. Also, some extremely toxic species of mushrooms are not psychoactive, but they bear a superficial resemblance to the mushrooms that contain psilocybin and psilocin. Because the effects of psilocybin so closely resemble those produced by LSD, the "psilocybin" sold illicitly may *be* LSD, and ordinary mushrooms laced with LSD may be sold as "magic mushrooms."

Although the psychedelic effects of *Psilocybe mexicana* are part of Indian folklore, *Psilocybe* intoxication was not described until 1955, when Gordon Wasson, a New York banker, traveled through Mexico. He mingled with native tribes and was allowed to participate in a *Psilocybe* ceremony, during which he consumed the magic mushroom. Wasson said:

> It permits you to travel backward and forward in time, to enter other planes of existence, even to know God. . . . Your body lies in the darkness, heavy as lead, but your spirit seems to soar and leave the hut, and with the speed of thought to travel where it listeth, in time and space, accompanied by the shaman's singing. . . . At last you know what the ineffable is, and what ecstasy means. Ecstasy! The mind harks back to the origin of that word. For the Greeks, ekstasis meant the flight of the soul from the body. Can you find a better word to describe this state? (Crahan, 1969, p. 17)

Some view psilocybin intoxication as inducing a schizophrenialike psychosis, even capable of inducing a *hallucinogen persisting perceptual disorder* (Espiard et al., 2005). Others have proposed its usefulness in studying the neurobiological basis of cognition and consciousness as well as time perception and timing performance (Wittmann et al., 2007).

Ololiuqui.   Ololiuqui is a naturally occurring hallucinogen in morning glory seeds that is used by Central and South American Indians as an intoxicant and as a hallucinogen. The drug is used ritually for spiritual communication, as are extracts of most plants that contain psychedelic drugs. The use of ololiuqui seeds in Central and South America was first described by the sixteenth-century Spanish explorer Francisco Hernandez de Cordoba, who is said to have reported, "When the priests wanted to commune with their Gods, they ate ololiuqui seeds and a thousand visions and satanic hallucinations appeared to them."

The seeds were analyzed in Europe by Albert Hofmann, the discoverer of LSD, who identified several ingredients, one of which was lysergic acid amide (not lysergic acid diethylamide, LSD). The lysergic acid amide that Hofmann identified is approximately one-tenth as active as LSD as a psychoactive agent. However, considering the extreme potency of LSD, lysergic acid amide is still quite potent.

Side effects of ololiuqui include nausea, vomiting, headache, increased blood pressure, dilated pupils, and sleepiness. These side effects are usually quite intense and serve to limit the recreational use of ololiuqui. Ingestion of a hundred or more seeds produces sleepiness, distorted perception, hallucinations, and confusion. Flashbacks have been reported, but they are infrequent.

Harmine.   Harmine is a psychedelic agent that is obtained from the seeds of *Peganum harmala,* a plant native to the Middle East, and from *Banisteriopsis caapi* of the South American tropics. Intoxication by harmine is usually accompanied by nausea and vomiting, sedation, and finally sleep. The psychic excitement users experience consists of visual distortions that are similar to those induced by LSD. Harmine probably acts through dopaminergic mechanisms as an MAO-A inhibitor (Chapter 5) (Herraiz et al., 2010). Because of the MAO inhibition, harmine appears to have some antidepressant properties (Fortunato et al., 2009). As discussed earlier, harmine is one of the ingredients in ayahuasca.

BZP and TFMPP.   In recent years, a combination "party pill," originating in New Zealand, has appeared as a legal alternative to MDMA, which remains an illegal drug (Wilkins et al., 2008; Antia, 2009). BZP (benzylpiperazine) exerts amphetaminelike stimulant properties, while TFMPP (trifluoromethylphenylpiperazine) exerts hallucinogenlike effects (Yarosh et al., 2007). BZP acts as a norepinephrine- and dopamine-releasing agent, while TFMPP is a serotonergic agonist. Combined, these substances produce effects that resemble those of MDMA (discussed earlier). Side effects include agitation, anxiety, hallucinations, vomiting, insomnia, and migraine headache. Because these two compounds inhibit drug-metabolizing enzymes in the liver, they may potentially increase the toxicity of other drugs (Antia, 2009). Currently, this combination is not controlled by the Food and Drug Administration (FDA).

Glutaminergic NMDA Receptor Antagonists

Phencyclidine and Ketamine

Phencyclidine (PCP, angel dust) and ketamine (Figure 15.4) are referred to as psychedelic anesthetics because they were first developed as amnestic and analgesic drugs for use in anesthesia; later it was found that they also produced a psychedelic or dissociative state of being. These two drugs are structurally unrelated to the other psychedelic agents, and their psychedelic effects are unique: they do not involve actions on serotonin, acetylcholine, or dopamine neurons.

Phencyclidine was developed in 1956 and was briefly used as an anesthetic in humans before being abandoned because of a high incidence of psychiatric reactions, including agitation, excitement, delirium, disorientation, and hallucinatory phenomena. The altered perception, disorganized thought, cognitive dysfunction, suspiciousness, confusion, and lack of cooperation that were exhibited resembled a schizophrenic state that consisted of both positive and negative symptoms. In fact, both phencyclidine and ketamine can induce symptoms that are almost indistinguishable from those associated with schizophrenia (Mouri et al., 2007). Phencyclidine is still used as a veterinary anesthetic, primarily as an immobilizing agent.

Ketamine (Ketalar), which structurally resembles phencyclidine, was developed shortly after the prominent psychedelic properties of phencyclidine were identified. Introduced in 1960, ketamine induces a phencyclidinelike anesthetic state in low doses, with fewer bothersome psychiatric side effects. The anesthetic state is characterized by amnesia and analgesia, combined with maintenance of blood pressure and

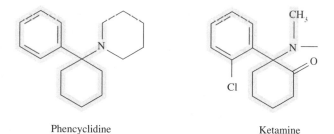

Phencyclidine   Ketamine

FIGURE 15.4 Structural formulas of the psychedelic anesthetic drugs phencyclidine and ketamine.

respiration. Ketamine is occasionally used as anesthesia in patients who cannot tolerate the cardiovascular depressant effects of other anesthetics. Ketamine causes psychiatric reactions similar to but not as severe as those caused by PCP, including brief, reversible positive and negative schizophrenialike symptoms. Both PCP and ketamine can exacerbate psychosis in schizophrenia.

Abuse of phencyclidine and ketamine began in the mid-1960s (Wolff and Winstock, 2006). Today, abuse of phencyclidine and ketamine persists, with periodic resurgences in popularity. Phencyclidine is the more commonly abused of the two and has appeared in the form of powders, tablets, leaf mixtures, and "rock" crystals. It is commonly sold as crystal, angel dust, hog, PCP, THC, cannabinol, or mescaline. When phencyclidine is sold as crystal or angel dust (terms also used for methamphetamine), the drug is usually in concentrations that vary between 50 and 90 percent. When it is purchased under other names or in concoctions, the amount of phencyclidine falls to between 10 and 30 percent; the typical street dose is about 5 milligrams. Phencyclidine can be eaten, snorted, or injected, but it is most often smoked, sprinkled on tobacco, parsley, or marijuana. Frequently, phencyclidine is sold as a club drug, although its pharmacology is entirely distinct from other club drugs such as ecstasy or GHB. As a club drug, PCP is an analgesic/anesthetic/amnestic/psychedelic.

Pharmacokinetics. PCP is well absorbed whether taken orally or smoked. When it is smoked, peak effects occur in about 15 minutes, when about 40 percent of the dose appears in the user's bloodstream. Oral absorption is slower; maximum blood levels are reached about 2 hours after the drug has been taken. The elimination half-life is about 18 hours but ranges from about 11 to about 51 hours. A positive urine assay for PCP is assumed to indicate that PCP was used within the previous week. Because false-positive test results are common, a positive assay requires secondary confirmation.

Mechanism of Action. Phencyclidine and ketamine both exert their psychotomimetic, analgesic, amnestic actions and schizophrenic actions primarily as a result of binding as noncompetitive antagonists of the N-methyl-D-aspartate (NMDA)/glutamate receptors. Several lines of evidence now implicate involvement of NMDA receptor dysfunction in the pathophysiology of schizophrenia (Chapter 4). Adler and coworkers (1999) conducted a neuropsychological comparison of normal volunteers to whom ketamine was administered and patients with schizophrenia (Figure 15.5). As can be seen, the ketamine-induced thought disorder is not dissimilar to that seen in patients with schizophrenia, providing support for the involvement

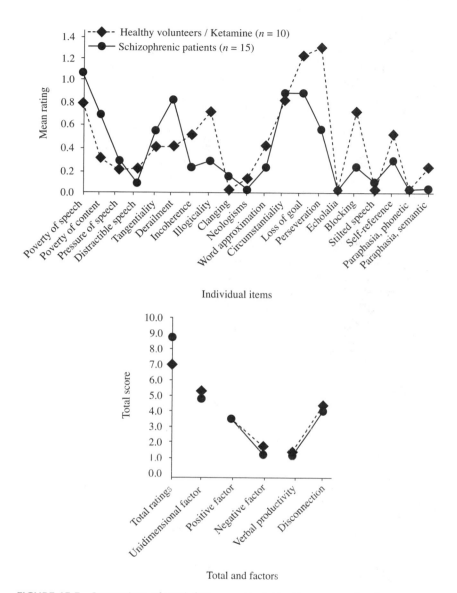

FIGURE 15.5 Comparison of total, factor, and individual item scores for the assessment of thought, language, and communication of 10 healthy volunteers with ketamine-induced thought disorder and 15 patients with schizophrenia (schizophrenic patients were ketamine-free). [From Adler et al. (1999), p. 1647.]

of NMDA receptor dysfunction in the disease.[4] Although acute doses of PCP and ketamine can induce a toxic psychosis, repeated doses induce a more persistent schizophrenic symptomatology, including psychosis, hallucinations, flattened affect, delusions, formal thought disorder, cognitive dysfunction, and social withdrawal.

Phencyclidine and ketamine inhibit NMDA receptors by two mechanisms: (1) blockade of the open channel by occupying a site within the channel in the receptor protein (as discussed earlier for phencyclidine) and (2) reduction in the frequency of NMDA channel opening by drug binding to a second attachment site on the outside of the receptor protein. As noted, PCP and ketamine are powerful analgesic drugs. The mechanism seems to be twofold: these two drugs (1) block NMDA-glutamate receptors in the spinal cord and (2) activate descending analgesic pathways, pathways that appear to involve norepinephrine and dopamine.

More recently, actions of PCP and ketamine on serotonin neurons have been suggested, and a serotonin-glutamate receptor complex has been identified on cortical pyramidal neurons (Gonzalez-Maeso and Sealfon, 2009b).

Psychological Effects. Phencyclidine (and ketamine) dissociates individuals from themselves and their environment. It induces an unresponsive state with intense analgesia and amnesia, although the subject's eyes remain open (with a blank stare); the subject may even appear to be awake. When not used under controlled conditions, phencyclidine in low doses produces mild agitation, euphoria, disinhibition, or excitement in a person who appears to be grossly drunk and exhibits a blank stare. The subject may be rigid and unable to speak. In many cases, however, the subject is communicative but does not respond to pain.

PCP acutely induces a psychotic state in which subjects become withdrawn, autistic, negativistic, and unable to maintain a cognitive set; they manifest concrete, impoverished, idiosyncratic, and bizarre responses to questions. People under the influence of PCP exhibit profound alterations of higher emotional functions affecting judgment and cognition.

High doses of phencyclidine induce a state of coma or stupor. However, abusers tend to titrate their dose to maximize the intoxicant

---

[4] The NMDA/PCP receptor complex is composed of four membrane-spanning polypeptides, which cluster together to form an ion channel that resembles the benzodiazepine-GABA receptor. In the NMDA/PCP receptor complex, however, the drug-binding site (the PCP receptor) is located within the lumen of the ion channel. Attachment of PCP to the receptor occludes the channel and inhibits calcium ion influx when the transmitter (glutamate) attaches to its receptor on the outer surface.

effect while attempting to avoid unconsciousness. Blood pressure usually becomes elevated, but respiration does not become depressed. The patient may recover from this state within 2 to 4 hours, although a state of confusion and cognitive poverty may last for 8 to 72 hours. The disruption of sensory input by PCP causes unpredictable exaggerated, distorted, or violent reactions to environmental stimuli. These reactions are augmented by PCP-induced analgesia and amnesia. Massive oral overdoses, involving up to 1 gram of street-purchased phencyclidine, result in prolonged periods of stupor or coma. This state may last for several days and may be marked by intense seizure activity, increased blood pressure, and a depression of respiration that is potentially lethal. Following this stupor, a prolonged recovery phase, marked by confusion and delusions, may last as long as two weeks. In some people, this state of confusion may be followed by a psychosis that lasts from several weeks to a few months.

Side Effects and Toxicity.   The course of recovery from a PCP-induced psychotic state is variable for reasons that are poorly understood. The intoxicated state may lead to severe anxiety, aggression, panic, paranoia, and rage. A user can also display violent reactions to sensory input, leading to such problems as falls, drowning, burns, driving accidents, and aggressive behavior. Self-inflicted injuries and injuries sustained while physical restraints are applied are frequent, and the potent analgesic action contributes to the absence of response to pain. Respiratory depression, generalized seizure activity, and pulmonary edema have all been reported.

Treatment of Intoxication.   Therapy for PCP intoxication is aimed at reducing the systemic level of the drug, keeping the patient calm and sedated, and preventing any of several severe adverse medical effects. It involves the following:

- Minimization of sensory inputs by placing the intoxicated person in a quiet environment
- Oral administration of activated charcoal, which can bind any PCP present in the stomach and intestine and prevent its reabsorption
- Precautionary physical restraint to prevent self-injury
- Sedation with either a benzodiazepine (such as lorazepam) for agitation or an atypical antipsychotic agent for psychosis.

Hyperthermia, hypertension, convulsions, renal failure, and other medical consequences should be treated as necessary by medical experts. PCP-induced psychotic states may be long-lasting, especially in people with a history of schizophrenia.

Dextromethorphan

Dextromethorphan (DXM) is both an analgesic drug and a drug of abuse. As an analgesic, it potentiates the pain-relieving action of morphine and other opioids (Chapter 10). As a drug of abuse, it is a common ingredient in more than 140 varieties of over-the-counter cough suppressants; high doses produce hallucinations. Because of this effect and ready availability, abuse has rapidly increased, especially in adolescents (Schwartz, 2005; Bryner et al., 2006). The hallucinations follow from high-dose DXM-induced NMDA receptor blockade, an action similar to that produced by PCP and ketamine. DXM and its metabolite dextrorphan (DXO) can substitute for PCP and exert PCP-like effects. Indeed, the active metabolite DXO may be responsible for many of the high-dose effects of DXM (Miller, 2005). In cough and cold preparations, such as various Coricidin products, Robitussin DM, Vicks 44, Tylenol DM (and many others), ingestion of DXM is referred to as roboing, dexing, robo-tripping, or robo-copping. Symptoms associated with intoxication include tachycardia, hypertension, sleepiness, agitation, disorientation, slurred speech, hallucinations, altered mental status, and tremor. Acute psychotic reactions have occasionally been reported.

Salvinorin A

Salvia divinorum (magic mint, diviner's sage, Sally-D), a member of the mint family of perennial herbs, is a psychoactive plant that has been used for curing and for divination in traditional spiritual practices by the Mazatec peoples of Oaxaca, Mexico, for many centuries (Vortherms and Roth, 2006). More recently, young people in Mexico have smoked the dried leaves of the plant as a marijuana substitute. *Salvia* also grows in many parts of the United States as well as in other countries. *Salvia* has been used as a short-acting, legal hallucinogen for several years because neither the "magic mint" nor its active compound are banned.[5] *Salvia* is gaining popularity among adolescents in the United States, and YouTube has received thousands of video posts of people using *Salvia* (Lange et al., 2010).

Salvia is comparable in hallucinogenic efficacy to other hallucinogens such as psilocybin-containing mushrooms. In use, the fresh leaves of the plant are moistened and chewed as a quid and kept in the mouth. Alternatively, the dried leaves are smoked in the manner of marijuana or cocaine freebase. The fresh leaves may also be eaten raw

---

[5] At least four states (Delaware, Missouri, North Dakota, and Illinois) have outlawed *Salvia*, and the DEA lists *Salvia* as a drug of concern.

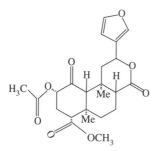

FIGURE 15.6 Structure of salvinorin A, the active drug in *Salvia divinorum.*

or prepared as an aqueous solution. The mint is essentially inactive if taken orally; the compound is effective when smoked in doses of 200 to 500 micrograms of active drug. Hooker and coworkers (2008) stated that "the incredible potency of salvinorin A cannot be underemphasized. We estimate that less than 10 micrograms can account for its psychoactive properties" (p. 1049). Thus, *Salvia* contains the most potent naturally occurring hallucinogen thus far isolated (Vortherms and Roth, 2006).

The main active ingredient of *Salvia divinorum* is a novel compound called *salvinorin A*. The molecular structure (Figure 15.6), mechanism of action, and perhaps clinical effects of salvinorin A are distinct from those of all other naturally occurring hallucinogens or synthetic hallucinogens (Butelman et al., 2010). Salvinorin A is reported to induce an intense hallucinatory experience in humans, with a typical duration of action of several minutes to an hour or so (Hooker et al., 2008). Bucheler and coworkers (2005) describe this state as "a short-lived inebriant state with intense, bizarre feelings of depersonalization" (p. 1). Przekop and Lee (2009) describe a case of persistent (at least four months) psychosis associated with *Salvia* use.

Mechanism of Action

Roth and coworkers (2002) studied the molecular binding profile of salvinorin A at a large number (50) of cloned human G protein receptors, channels, and transporters known to be involved in psychopharmacology. Salvinorin A was active at only one receptor, the kappa opioid receptor, on which it exerted an agonist action. Salvinorin A had no action at the serotonin 5-HT$_{2A}$ receptor, which is the principal molecular target responsible for the actions of classical hallucinogens such as LSD (Figure 15.7). Salvinorin A can therefore now be classified as a *kappa opioid agonist*, the first naturally occurring compound known to exhibit such an action. Roth and coworkers (2002) speculated that because of this action, kappa opioid receptors (see Chapter 10) may play a role in the regulation of human perception, and they suggest that kappa opioid antagonists (the opposite of salvinorin A) could represent

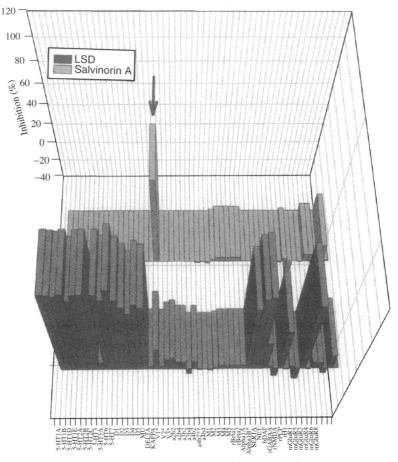

FIGURE 15.7 Large-scale screening of LSD and salvinorin A against many cloned G protein-type receptors. LSD binds to many receptors, especially those involving serotonin. Salvinorin A binds specifically to the kappa opioid receptor and is classified pharmacologically as a specific kappa opioid agonist. [From Roth et al. (2002), p. 11937.]

a novel class of drugs with beneficial activity in diseases in which alterations in perception are predominant. Vortherms and coworkers (2007) expanded on these ideas.

Braida and coworkers (2008) investigated the behaviorally reinforcing effects of salvinorin A. The drug's action was antagonized both by rimonabant (a cannabinoid antagonist; Chapter 14) and by experimental kappa opioid receptor antagonists. Salvinorin A also increased nucleus accumbens dopamine levels by 150 percent.

Potential Therapeutic Uses of Salvinorum Derivatives

In a case report, Hanes (2001) reported on one patient with severe depression unrelieved by traditional antidepressant medications. This person obtained *Salvia* through a mail-order house. She chewed two or three leaves at a time three times per week and claimed total remission of depressive symptoms. Continued use was accompanied by continued effectiveness, "engendering a kind of psychospiritual awakening, characterized by the discovery of her sense of self, greater self-confidence, increased feelings of intuitive wisdom, and connectedness to nature" (p. 634). However, as a kappa agonist, the drug has the potential to induce (rather than relieve) depressivelike reactions. Braida and coworkers (2009) expand on potential antidepressant and anxiolytic effects of salvinorin A.

Historically, *Salvia* preparations have been used to treat gastrointestinal disorders, including diarrhea. Fichna and coworkers (2009) expand on this topic and demonstrate that salvinorin A inhibits colonic contractions and motility through actions on gastric kappa receptors and cannabinoid-2 receptors. The authors postulate use in the treatment of lower intestinal disorders associated with increased intestinal transit and diarrhea.

Currently, derivatives of salvinorin A are being examined for a variety of clinical uses, from GI disorders to analgesic uses and even the treatment of cocaine dependence (Wang et al., 2008; Morani et al., 2009). The occurrence of drug-induced dysphoria, however, has been problematic.

STUDY QUESTIONS

1. What is a psychedelic drug?
2. What differentiates a psychedelic drug from a behavioral stimulant? Discuss from both structural and behavioral viewpoints.
3. List the four classes of psychedelic drugs presented in this chapter.
4. Differentiate between mescaline and LSD.
5. How does LSD exert psychedelic actions?
6. What is the psychedelic syndrome?
7. What are some of the problems associated with LSD use?
8. How does phencyclidine work? Discuss the state of psychosis it produces.
9. What properties characterize the clinical usefulness of phencyclidine and ketamine?
10. Discuss the therapeutic and abuse potentials of dextromethorphan.
11. Compare salvinorin A with other psychedelic drugs.

REFERENCES

Adler, C. M., et al. (1999). "Comparison of Ketamine-Induced Thought Disorder in Healthy Volunteers and Thought Disorder in Schizophrenia." *American Journal of Psychiatry* 156: 1646–1649.

Almaula, N., et al. (1996). "Mapping the Binding Site Pocket of the Serotonin 5-Hydroxytryptamine$_{2A}$ Receptor." *Journal of Biological Chemistry* 271: 14672–14675.

Antia, U. (2009). "'Party Pill' Drugs—BZP and TFMPP." *New Zealand Medical Journal* 122: 55–68.

Antia, U., et al. (2009). "Metabolic Interactions with Piperazine-Based 'Party Pill' Drugs." *Journal of Pharmacy and Pharmacology* 61: 877–882.

Braida, D., et al. (2008). "Involvement of Kappa-Opioid and Endocannabinoid System on Salvinorin A-Induced Reward." *Biological Psychiatry* 63: 286–292.

Braida, D., et al. (2009). "Potential Anxiolytic- and Antidepressant-Like Effects of Salvinorin A, the Main Active Ingredient of *Salvia divinorum*, in Rodents." *British Journal of Pharmacology* 157: 844–853.

Bryner, J. K., et al. (2006). "Dextromethorphan Abuse in Adolescence: An Increasing Trend: 1999–2004." *Archives of Pediatric and Adolescent Medicine* 160: 1217–1222.

Bucheler, R., et al. (2005). "Use of Nonprohibited Hallucinogenic Plants: Increasing Relevance for Public Health? A Case Report and Literature Review on the Consumption of *Salvia divinorum* (Diviner's Sage)." *Pharmacopsychiatry* 38: 1–5.

Butelman, E. R., et al. (2010). "The Discriminative Effects of the Kappa-Opioid Hallucinogen Salvinorin A in Nonhuman Primates: Dissociation from Classic Hallucinogen Effects." *Psychopharmacology* 210: 253–262.

Crahan, M. E. (1969). "God's Flesh and Other Pre-Columbian Phantastica." *Bulletin of the Los Angeles County Medical Association* 99: 17.

Davis, K. L., et al., eds. (2002). *Psychopharmacology—The Fifth Generation of Progress*. Philadelphia: Lippincott, Williams & Wilkins.

DeFrates, L. J., et al. (2005). "Antimuscarinic Intoxication Resulting from the Ingestion of Moonflower Seeds." *Annals of Pharmacotherapy* 39: 173–176.

deWin, M. M. L., et al. (2008). "Sustained Effects of Ecstasy on the Human Brain: A Prospective Neuroimaging Study in Novel Users." *Brain* 131: 2936–2945.

Diederen, K. M. J., et al. (2010). "Deactivation of the Parahippocampal Gyrus Preceding Auditory Hallucinations." *American Journal of Psychiatry* 167: 427–435.

Duffy, M. R., and Ferguson, C. (2007). "Role of Dantrolene in Treatment of Heat Stroke Associated with Ecstasy Ingestion." *British Journal of Anaesthesia* 98: 148–149.

Espiard, M. L., et al. (2005). "Hallucinogen Persisting Perceptual Disorder After Psilocybin Consumption: A Case Study." *European Psychiatry* 20: 458–460.

Fantegrossi, W. E., et al. (2005). "Hallucinogen-Like Actions of 2,5-Dimethoxy-4-(n)-Propylthiophenethylamine (2C-T-7) in Mice and Rats." *Psychopharmacology* 181: 496–503.

Fichna, J., et al. (2009). "Salvinorin A Inhibits Colonic Transit and Neurogenic Ion Transport in Mice by Activating Kappa-Opioid and Cannabinoid Receptors." *Neurogastroenterology and Motility* 21: 1326e–1328e.

Fickenscher, A., et al. (2006). "Illicit Peyote Use Among American Indian Adolescents in Substance Abuse Treatment: A Preliminary Investigation." *Substance Use and Misuse* 41: 1139–1154.

Fisk, J. E., et al. (2009). "The Association Between the Negative Effects Attributed to Ecstasy Use and Measures of Cognition and Mood Among Users." *Experimental and Clinical Psychopharmacology* 17: 326–336.

Fortunato, J. J., et al. (2009). "Acute Harmine Administration Induces Antidepressant-Like Effects and Increases BDNF Levels in the Rat Hippocampus." *Progress in Neuropsychopharmacology and Biological Psychiatry* 33: 1425–1430.

Gable, R. S. (2007). "Risk Assessment of Ritual Use of Oral Dimethyltryptamine (DMT) and Harmala Alkaloids." *Addiction* 102: 24–34.

Geyer, M. A., and Vollenweider, F. X. (2008). "Serotonin Research: Contributions to Understanding Psychosis." *Trends in Pharmacological Sciences* 29: 445–453.

Gonzalez-Maeso, J., and Sealfon, S. C. (2009a). "Agonist-Trafficking and Hallucinogens." *Current Medicinal Chemistry* 16: 1017–1027.

Gonzalez-Maeso, J., and Sealfon, S. C. (2009b). "Psychedelics and Schizophrenia." *Trends in Neuroscience* 32: 225–232.

Gouzoulis-Mayfrank, E., and Daumann, J. (2009). "Neurotoxicity of Drugs of Abuse—The Case of Methylenedioxyamphetamines (MDMA, Ecstasy), and Amphetamines." *Dialogues in Clinical Neuroscience* 11: 305–317.

Hall, A. P., and Henry, J. A. (2006). "Acute Toxic Effects of 'Ecstasy' (MDMA) and Related Compounds: Overview of Pathophysiology and Clinical Management." *British Journal of Anaesthesia* 96: 678–685.

Halpern, J. H. (2004). "Hallucinogens and Dissociative Agents Naturally Growing in the United States." *Pharmacology and Therapeutics* 102: 131–138.

Hanes, K. R. (2001). "Antidepressant Effects of the Herb *Salvia divinorum:* A Case Report." *Journal of Clinical Psychopharmacology* 21: 634–635.

Hashimoto, K. (2009). "Can the Sigma-1 Receptor Agonist Fluvoxamine Prevent Schizophrenia?" *CNS & Neurological Disorders—Drug Targets* 8: 470–474.

Herraiz, T., et al. (2010). "Beta-Carboline Alkaloids in *Peganum harmala* and Inhibition of Human Monoamine Oxidase (MAO)." *Food and Chemical Toxicology* 48: 839–845.

Hofmann, A. (1994). "Notes and Documents Concerning the Discovery of LSD." *Agents and Actions* 43: 79–81.

Holzman, R. S. (1998). "The Legacy of Atropos, the Fate Who Cut the Thread of Life." *Anesthesiology* 89: 241–249.

Hooker, J. M., et al. (2008). "Pharmacokinetics of the Potent Hallucinogen Salvinorin A in Primates Parallels the Rapid Onset, Short Duration of Effects in Humans." *Neuroimage* 41: 1044–1050.

Itokawa, M., et al. (2007). "Acute Confusional State After Designer Tryptamine Abuse." *Psychiatry and Clinical Neurosciences* 61: 196–199.

Johnson, M., et al. (2008). "Human Hallucinogen Research: Guidelines for Safety." *Journal of Psychopharmacology* 22: 603–620.

Kalant, H. (2001). "The Pharmacology and Toxicology of 'Ecstasy' (MDMA) and Related Drugs." *Canadian Medical Association Journal* 165: 917–928.

Kulkarni, S. K., and Dhir, A. (2009). "Sigma-1 Receptors in Major Depression and Anxiety." *Expert Review of Neurotherapeutics* 9: 1021–1034.

Lange, J. E., et al. (2010). "*Salvia divinorum*: Effects and Use Among YouTube Users." *Drug and Alcohol Dependence* 108: 138–140.

Martin-Santos, R., et al. (2010). "5-HTTLPR Polymorphism, Mood Disorders and MDMA Use in a 3-Year Follow-Up Study." *Addiction Biology* 15: 15–22.

Maurice, T., and Su, T. P. (2009). "The Pharmacology of Sigma-1 Receptors." *Pharmacology and Therapeutics* 124: 195–206.

Miller, S. C. (2005). "Dextromethorphan Psychosis, Dependence and Physical Withdrawal." *Addiction Biology* 10: 325–327.

Morani, A. S., et al. (2009). "Effect of Kappa-Opioid Receptor Agonists U69593, U50488H, Spiradoline and Salvinorin A on Cocaine-Induced Drug-Seeking in Rats." *Pharmacology Biochemistry and Behavior* 94: 244–249.

Mouri, A., et al. (2007). "Phencyclidine Animal Models of Schizophrenia: Approaches from Abnormality of Glutamatergic Neurotransmission and Neurodevelopment." *Neurochemistry International* 51: 173–184.

Nagai, F., et al. (2007). "The Effects of Non-Medically Used Psychoactive Drugs on Monoamine Neurotransmission in Rat Brain." *European Journal of Pharmacology* 559: 132–137.

Paschos, K. A., et al. (2009). "Neuropeptide and Sigma Receptors as Novel Therapeutic Targets for the Pharmacotherapy of Depression." *CNS Drugs* 23: 755–772.

Passie, T., et al. (2008). "The Pharmacology of Lysergic Acid Diethylamide: A Review." *CNS Neuroscience & Therapeutics* 14: 295–314.

Przekop, P., and Lee, T. (2009). "Persistent Psychosis Associated with *Salvia Divinorum* Use. *American Journal of Psychiatry* 166: 832.

Roth, B. L., et al. (2002). "Salvinorin A: A Potent Naturally Occurring Nonnitrogenous Opioid Selective Agonist." *Proceedings of the National Academy of Sciences* 99: 11934–11939.

Schifano, F., et al. (2005). "New Trends in the Cyber and Street Market of Recreational Drugs? The Case of 2C-T-7 ("Blue Mystic")." *Journal of Psychopharmacology* 19: 675–679.

Schilt, T., et al. (2007). "Cognition in Novice Ecstasy Users with Minimal Exposure to Other Drugs." *Archives of General Psychiatry* 64: 728–736.

Schwartz, R. H. (2005). "Adolescent Abuse of Dextromethorphan." *Clinical Pediatrics* 44: 565–568.

Seedi, H. R. el-, et al. (2005). "Prehistoric Peyote Use: Alkaloid Analysis and Radiocarbon Dating of Archaeological Specimens of *Lophophora* from Texas." *Journal of Ethnopharmacology* 101: 238–242.

Strassman, R. J., et al. (1994). "Dose-Response Study of N,N-Dimethyltryptamine in Humans. II: Subjective Effects and Preliminary Results of a New Rating Scale." *Archives of General Psychiatry* 51: 98–108.

Su, T. P., et al. (2009). "When the Endogenous Hallucinogenic Trace Amine N,N-Dimethyltryptamine Meets the Sigma-1 Receptor." *Science Signaling* 2: pe12.

Vortherms, T. A., and Roth, B. L. (2006). "Salvinorin A: From Natural Product to Human Therapeutics." *Molecular Interventions* 6: 257–265.

Vortherms, T. A., et al (2007). "Differential Helical Orientations Among Related G Protein-Coupled Receptors Provide a Novel Mechanism for Selectivity: Studies with Salvinorin A and the κ-Opioid Receptor." *Journal of Biological Chemistry* 282: 146–156.

Wang, Y., et al. (2008). "2-Methoxymethyl-Salvinorin B Is a Potent Kappa Opioid Receptor Agonist with Longer Lasting Action *in vivo* than Salvinorin A." *Journal of Pharmacology and Experimental Therapeutics* 324: 1073–1083.

Wilkins, C., et al. (2008). "Patterns of Benzylpiperazine/Trifluoromethyl-phenylpiperazine Party Pill Use and Adverse Effects in a Population Sample in New Zealand." *Drug and Alcohol Review* 27: 633–639.

Wittmann, M., et al. (2007). "Effect of Psilocybin on Time Perception and Temporal Control of Behaviour in Humans." *Journal of Psychopharmacology* 21: 50–64.

Wolff, K., and Winstock, A.R. (2006). "Ketamine: From Medicine to Misuse." *CNS Drugs* 20: 199–218.

Yarosh, H. L., et al. (2007). "MDMA-Like Behavioral Effects of N-Substituted Piperazines in the Mouse." *Pharmacology Biochemistry and Behavior* 88: 18–27.

Chapter 16

Anabolic Steroids

Anabolic steroids and *anabolic-androgenic steroids* are familiar terms for synthetic substances related to the naturally occurring male sex hormone testosterone. Anabolic steroids have both muscle-building (anabolic) and masculinizing effects and are therefore used to enhance athletic performance and appearance (Bahrke and Yesalis, 2004; Rogol, 2010). Illicit use is common among adolescents and adults, both male and female, athletes and nonathletes. It may not be surprising that 55 percent of 27-year-old male and 10 percent of 24-year-old female bodybuilders use anabolic steroids, but it may be surprising that the prevalence of anabolic steroid injection in college athletics may be as high as 20 percent and anabolic steroid use in high schools has been estimated as high as 6 percent for males and 2.5 percent for females. Elliot and coworkers (2007) reported that prior or ongoing anabolic steroid use was reported by 5.3 percent of female high school students—not confined to those in competitive athletics—and was an indicator of a cluster of other health-related behaviors such as illicit drug use, early sexual activity, and daily feelings of hopelessness or sadness.

More than 1 million Americans have used anabolic steroids illicitly either to improve athletic performance or to improve personal appearance, and more than 50 percent are age 26 or older; the prevalence of anabolic steroids use is equal in both athletes and nonathletes. Lifetime use is 4.9 percent for males and 2.4 percent for females, and the numbers are likely to increase.

In both athletes and nonathletes, anabolic steroids promote increased muscle mass and enhance physical strength, endurance, physical appearance, and athletic performance. In 2003, the previously undetectable anabolic steroid *tetrahydrogestrinone* incited a furor in the media when high-profile professional athletes admitted to using this muscle-building, performance-enhancing drug. Subsequently, in March 2004 the U.S. Food and Drug Administration (FDA) classified this drug as an illegal substance. Tests are now available to detect the drug in urine. The use of the testosterone precursor *androstenedione* by baseball home run record holder Mark McGwire focused even more attention on steroid use by athletes.

As well as illicit use, anabolic steroids have well-recognized uses in prescription medicine. Uses of these agents include the treatment of delayed puberty as well as the prevention of weight loss in renal failure patients undergoing hemodialysis and in males with HIV/AIDS-related weight loss. Rabkin and coworkers (2000) studied the effects of weekly injections of testosterone in 70 males with symptomatic HIV illness. The majority reported improved libido and energy, improvements in mood, and increases in muscle mass. More recently, anabolic steroid use has been shown to positively affect mood, muscle mass, and strength, while reducing morbidity and mortality in older men.

Much of the controversy over anabolic steroid use, medical and illicit, involves the documented health risks associated with steroid use as well as the possibly unfair advantage a performance-enhancing drug offers the competitive athlete. Also, adolescent nonathletes who use steroids as cosmetic enhancers place themselves at risk for long-term health problems, and they also may suffer from serious body self-image problems that should be attended to (Kanayama et al., 2006).

Testosterone is the primary male sex hormone. Normally, the levels of testosterone in the body are tightly regulated by a negative feedback system involving the testes (where testosterone is synthesized), the hypothalamus, and the pituitary gland (Figure 16.1). When the plasma level of testosterone falls, cells in the hypothalamus (which has receptors sensitive to the circulating amount of testosterone) sense the decrease and begin producing a releasing factor called *gonadotropin-releasing factor* (GRF). GRF circulates in blood to the pituitary gland and stimulates the pituitary to produce and release *follicle-stimulating hormone* (FSH) and *luteinizing hormone* (LH). In turn, FSH and LH act on the testes to induce both spermatogenesis (the production of sperm) and synthesis and release of testosterone. (A similar process in the female regulates fertility.)

As testosterone levels in blood increase, the hypothalamus decreases its production of GRF, the pituitary decreases production of FSH and LH, the testes decrease production of testosterone and sperm, and the process repeats. Administering anabolic steroids overwhelms this system; abnormally high levels of steroids shut off production of GRF, FSH, LH, and testosterone and shut off the process of

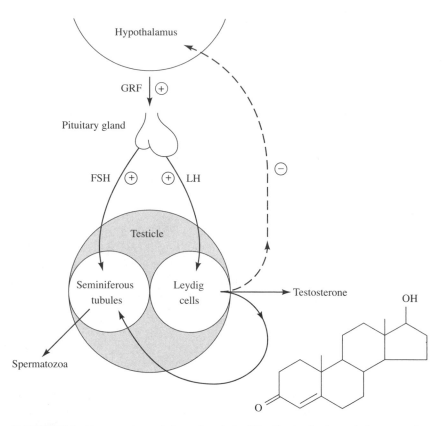

FIGURE 16.1 Hormonal regulation of male fertility. The brain (hypothalamus and pituitary gland) is involved in the control of fertility. However, fertility in the male is not subject to periodic cycling as it is in the female. The structure of naturally occurring testosterone is shown. GRF = gonadotropin-releasing factor; FSH = follicle-stimulating hormone; LH = luteinizing hormone. Solid arrows = stimulation; dashed arrows = inhibition.

spermatogenesis. Therefore, anabolic steroids (1) block the normal process that regulates testosterone, male fertility, and spermatogenesis, (2) exert peripheral hormone actions to increase muscle mass and produce a more masculine appearance, and (3) exert central effects that increase aggression.

Mechanism of Action

The structures of testosterone and several synthetically produced anabolic steroids are illustrated in Figure 16.2. The structures of two related substances, androstenedione, thought to be a precursor to testosterone, and dehydroepiandrosterone (DHEA), an androgen released by the

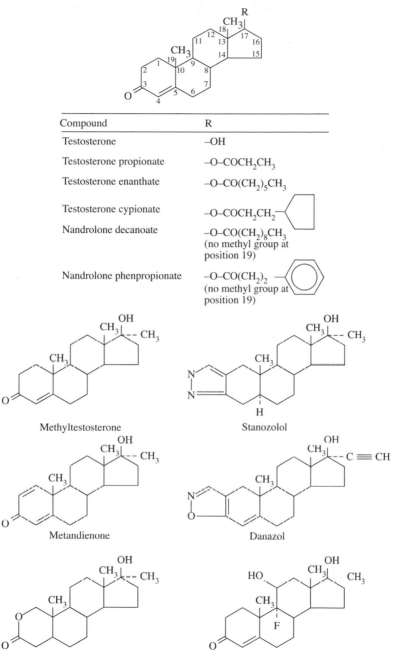

Compound	R
Testosterone	–OH
Testosterone propionate	$-O-COCH_2CH_3$
Testosterone enanthate	$-O-CO(CH_2)_5CH_3$
Testosterone cypionate	$-O-COCH_2CH_2-$
Nandrolone decanoate	$-O-CO(CH_2)_8CH_3$ (no methyl group at position 19)
Nandrolone phenpropionate	$-O-CO(CH_2)_2-$ (no methyl group at position 19)

Methyltestosterone

Stanozolol

Metandienone

Danazol

Oxandrolone

Fluoxymesterone

FIGURE 16.2   Structures of some common parenteral (*left*) and oral (*right*) anabolic-androgenic steroids.

adrenal glands, are not included in Figure 16.2 because, as stated by Yesalis and Bahrke (2002),

> Androstenedione is an anabolic-androgenic steroid used to increase blood testosterone levels for purposes of increasing strength, lean body mass, and sexual performance. However, there is no research indicating androstenedione or its related compounds significantly increase strength and/or lean body mass by increasing testosterone levels. . . . Dehydroepiandrosterone (DHEA) is a weak androgen also used to elevate testosterone levels. DHEA is also advertised as an anti-obesisty and anti-aging supplement capable of improving libido, vitality, and immunity levels. However, research demonstrates that DHEA supplementation does not increase serum testosterone concentrations or increase strength in men and it may have virilizing effects in women. (p. 246)

Bahrke and Yesalis reiterated this statement about DHEA in 2004: "DHEA supplementation does not increase serum testosterone concentrations or increase strength in men, and may actually increase testosterone levels in women, thus producing a virilizing effect" (p. 614).

All anabolic steroids differ from one another not so much in structure as in their resistance to metabolic degradation by liver enzymes. After oral administration, testosterone is effectively absorbed from the intestine. Following absorption, it is rapidly transported in the blood to the liver, where it is immediately metabolized. As a result, little testosterone reaches the systemic circulation. Administered by injection, some of this first-pass metabolism is blunted, and it is the metabolic product androstanolone that is most active as an anabolic substance. Structural modification of the testosterone molecule reduces this rapid metabolic breakdown and thus improves the effectiveness of both oral and intramuscular administration.

The mechanism of action of testosterone and the various anabolic steroids is quite well understood. Testosterone is synthesized principally in a specialized type of cell (the Leydig cell) of the testes (see Figure 16.1) under the influence of GRF released from the hypothalamus, which stimulates the synthesis and release of LH from the pituitary gland; LH acts on the Leydig cells to stimulate testosterone production.

Once in the bloodstream, testosterone (or an anabolic steroid) passes through the cell walls of its target tissues and attaches to steroid receptors in the cytoplasm of the cell (Figure 16.3). This hormone receptor complex is carried into the nucleus of the cell and attaches to the nuclear material (the DNA). A process of genetic transcription follows, and new messenger RNA is produced. Translation of this RNA results in the production of specific new proteins that leave the cell and mediate the biological functions of the hormone. Thus,

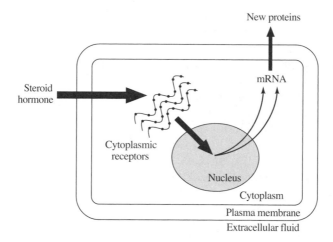

FIGURE 16.3 Mechanism of action of steroid hormones on cells. The hormone passes through the cell wall of its target tissue and binds to steroid receptors in the cytoplasm. The hormone-receptor complex moves into the nucleus and binds to sites on the chromatin, which is transcribed to give specific messenger RNA (mRNA). The mRNA is translated into specific new proteins that mediate the function of the hormone.

the effects of anabolic steroids on target cells are mediated by intracellular receptors and the synthesis of new proteins. The increased levels of circulating testosterone (or anabolic steroid) exert a negative feedback effect on the hypothalamus, inhibiting further stimulation of testosterone release.

Effects

People use anabolic steroids for many reasons. Steroids are used to improve athletic performance because they increase body muscle and reduce body fat. Both competitive bodybuilders and other athletes take advantage of this effect, using either the steroids themselves or their precursors. Nonathletes use anabolic steroids to achieve a desired shape when they have a skewed perception of their body habitus. These people do not recognize the breadth of the effects of these agents on the body, the brain, and behavior.

Not all anabolic steroids are illicit substances. Testosterone and some related steroids have specific therapeutic uses, including testosterone replacement in hypogonadal males; the treatment of certain blood anemias; and the repair of severe muscle loss following trauma, HIV wasting, and renal dialysis. In malnourished males with severe pulmonary disease (chronic obstructive pulmonary disease), prolonged use of oral androgen therapy increases lean body mass and muscle mass even though endurance capacity is little changed. Therefore, in states of malnutrition, anabolic steroid therapy increases muscle mass, an effect that hopefully reduces mortality and improves quality of life (Gullett et al., 2010). In the United States, oxandrolone (Oxandrin) has been approved by the FDA as adjunctive therapy for promotion of weight gain after weight loss following extensive surgery, chronic infection, or severe trauma; for some patients who, without definite pathophysiological reasons, fail to gain or maintain normal weight to offset the protein catabolism associated with long-term use of corticosteroids; and for the relief of the bone pain that frequently accompanies osteoporosis. In these unusual situations, anabolic steroids are clinically indicated.

Effects on Athletic Performance

Because testosterone and anabolic steroids increase protein synthesis, they increase muscle mass and strength and produce a more masculine appearance. The assumption that this is what happens has been around for decades, but a 1996 report by Bhasin and coworkers was the first to demonstrate that supraphysiological doses of testosterone, with or without strength training, increase fat-free mass, muscle size, and strength in normal men. As shown in Figure 16.4, exercise alone or testosterone alone produced increases in strength, triceps and quadriceps size, and fat-free mass. The combination of testosterone and exercise produced additive increases. Despite these beneficial effects of testosterone, the authors concluded:

> Our results in no way justify the use of anabolic-androgenic steroids in sports, because, with extended use, such drugs have potentially serious adverse effects on the cardiovascular system, prostate, lipid metabolism, and insulin sensitivity. Moreover, the use of any performance-enhancing agent in sports raises serious ethical issues. (p. 6)

Hartgens and coworkers (2002) studied the increased muscle fiber size in experienced male athletes. Compared with controls, poly-drug regimens of anabolic steroids at supratherapeutic dosages increased the size of deltoid muscle fibers in experienced strength-trained athletes, while a therapeutic dose of an anabolic steroid (nandrolone) did not exert any effect. Thus, anabolic steroids increase both the size and the strength of the athlete and so improve performance in athletic activities that require size, strength, and endurance. They have no positive effects on aerobic performance (Haupt, 1993). Therefore, athletes who depend on aerobic energy expenditure (for example, long-distance runners) benefit less from anabolic steroids than do athletes who depend on bulk size and short bursts of energy expenditure (football and baseball players and sprint runners, for example).

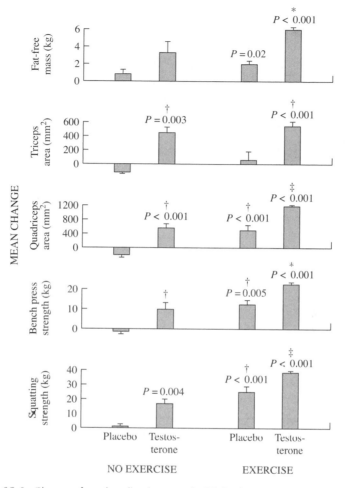

FIGURE 16.4 Changes from baseline in mean ($\pm$SE) fat-free mass, triceps, and quadriceps cross-sectional areas, and muscle strength in the bench press and squatting exercises over 10 weeks of treatment with testosterone. The P values shown are for the comparison between the change indicated and a change of zero. The asterisks indicate that P < 0.05 for the comparison between the change indicated and that in either no-exercise group; the daggers indicate P < 0.05 for the comparison between the change indicated and that in the group assigned to placebo with no exercise; the double daggers indicate that P < 0.05 for the comparison between the change indicated and the changes in all three other groups. [From Bhasin et al. (1996), p. 6.]

Hoffman and coworkers (2009) issued a position stand on androgen and growth hormone use by athletes.

Anabolic steroids have anticatabolic, anabolic, and motivational effects on the athlete. Table 16.1 summarizes the constellation of effects and side effects. In the *anticatabolic effect,* the anabolic steroids block the action of natural cortisone, which normally functions to increase

TABLE 16.1 Effects of anabolic-androgenic steroids

Positive effects
    Transient increase in muscular size and strength
    Treatment of catabolic states
        Trauma
        Surgery
Adverse Effects
    Cardiovascular
        Increase in cardiac risk factors
        Hypertension
        Altered lipoprotein fractions
        Increase in LDL/HDL ratio
        Reported strokes/myocardial infarctions
    Hepatic effects associated with oral compounds
        Elevated liver enzymes
        Peliosis hepatis (greater than 6 months' use)
        Liver tumors
            Benign
            Malignant (greater than 24 months' use)
    Reproductive system effects
        In males
            Decreased testosterone production
                Abnormal spermatogenesis
                Transient infertility
                Testicular atrophy
        In females
            Altered menstruation
    Endocrine effects
        Decreased thyroid function
    Immunological effects
        Decreased immunoglobulins IgM/IgA/IgC
    Musculoskeletal effects
        Premature closure of bony growth centers
        Tendon degeneration
            Increased risk of tendon tears
    Cosmetic
        In males
            Gynecomastia
            Testicular atrophy
            Acne
            Acceleration of male-pattern baldness
        In females
            Clitoral enlargement
            Acne
            Increased facial/body hair
            Coarsening of the skin
            Male-pattern baldness
            Deepened voice
    Psychological
        Risk of habituation
        Severe mood swings
        Aggressive tendencies
        Psychotic episodes
        Depression
        Reports of suicide
    Legislation
        Classified as Schedule III controlled substance

From Haupt (1993), p. 471.

energy stores during periods of stress and training. Cortisone makes energy stores available by breaking down proteins into their constituent amino acids. Carried to excess, muscle wasting can occur. This action is blocked by the anabolic steroids. The anticatabolic action may be the major mechanism by which these drugs increase body mass.

The *anabolic effects* follow both the synthesis of new protein in muscle cells and steroid-induced release of endogenous growth hormone. However, the doses commonly used by athletes are 10 to 200 times the therapeutic dosage for testosterone deficiency. These doses often stack, or pyramid, several drugs, even combining oral and injectable substances, over several weeks.

In the female athlete, anabolic steroids exert the same anabolic and anticatabolic effects found in male athletes. However, these drugs also induce masculinizing and related effects, including increases in facial and body hair, lowered voice, enlarged clitoris, coarser skin, and menstrual cycle cessation or irregularity. Cessation of steroid use results in a variable and often incomplete reversal of the altered functions. Tuiten and colleagues (2000) administered sublingual testosterone to eight healthy females and evaluated its effects on sexual arousal. Testosterone achieved maximal plasma levels in 15 minutes, returning to baseline levels by 90 minutes. At about 4.5 hours, significant increases in arousal and genital responsiveness occurred. Alterations in "central" hormonal mechanisms were postulated to account for the discrepancy between plasma levels and physiological responses.

Effects on Physical Appearance

Anabolic steroids are widely used (and abused) by young male (usually noncompetitive) athletes who take them to develop the muscular physique considered fashionable. As many as 250,000 to 500,000 young adult males may take steroids. Regardless of the exact number, a significant number of teenagers and young adults, primarily male, use supraphysiological doses of anabolic steroids to give them more muscle strength and a more powerful, masculine appearance. Unlike competitive athletes, who often terminate drug use when competition ends, nonathlete youths may continue to take steroids to maintain the cosmetic effect. As stated by Schwerin and coworkers (1996):

> Physique and physical appearance are ever important in how people are viewed in their social environment. With these come the spoils: social acceptance, admiration, and opportunity. To a certain extent, an attractive physique is related to enhanced self-esteem and perceived social competence. . . . Sometimes the drive reaches an unhealthy extreme . . . taking the form of anorexia, bulimia, and anabolic steroid use. (p. 1)

Furthermore,

> Anabolic steroid users present an appearance of healthfulness, strength, "sex appeal," and physical attractiveness. Other illicit drugs do not present such an image of healthfulness. . . . It may be this contradiction of increased steroid use leading to increased appearance of healthfulness and physical attractiveness which may allow the seriousness of steroid use to remain underappreciated. . . . Anabolic steroids are the only addictive substance over the short to middle term that enhances a user's physical appearance and whose purpose is to allow the user to work harder and longer (though stimulants share the latter characteristic). (pp. 6–7)

Effects in Middle-Aged and Elderly Males

Recently, attention has been focused on aging males who use anabolic steroids in an attempt to maintain muscle mass, reduce fat tissue, and delay aging. This group includes aging actors as well as men who use specialized medical clinics to combine steroid use with exercise and weight training. Testosterone levels and muscle mass do decline with age, with loss of muscle mass and absolute numbers of muscle fibers, a doubling of fat mass, and a decrease in bone mineral density by 0.3 percent per year after age 35 (Moretti et al., 2005). Testosterone can inhibit the accumulation of fat tissue, restore the lost muscle mass, and maintain bone mineral density in elderly men.

Bhasin and coworkers (2005) demonstrated that healthy men aged 60 to 75 with normal serum testosterone levels are as responsive to exogenous testosterone as are younger men (Figure 16.5), although high doses were associated with a high frequency of adverse side effects, such as dangerously increased levels of hemoglobin (greater than 54 percent), leg edema, kidney problems, and prostate cancer.

Jankowska and coworkers (2006) studied the levels of testosterone, DHEA, and an insulinlike growth factor in elderly men with moderate to severe chronic heart failure. They noted that age-related decline of these three circulating anabolic hormones is associated with increased morbidity and mortality (Figure 16.6). Three-year survival rates in these patients were 83 percent in those with no hormone deficiencies, 74 percent in those with one hormone deficiency, and 55 percent and 27 percent, respectively, for men with two or three hormone deficiencies. Malkin and coworkers (2006) determined that testosterone replacement in men with chronic heart failure resulted in improved health and functional capacity. Therefore, it appears that in middle-aged and elderly male patients with physical dysfunction associated with chronic illness or aging, testosterone or other anabolic hormones can induce meaningful improvements in physical function and patient-important outcomes (Bhasin et al., 2006). Whether these data

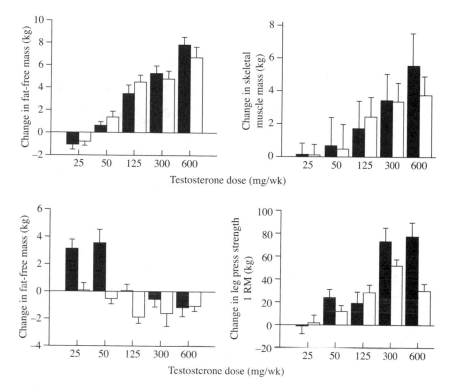

FIGURE 16.5 Changes from baseline in fat-free mass (in kilograms), skeletal muscle mass (in kilograms), total fat mass (in kilograms), and leg press strength (measured as the one-repetition maximum) following weekly intramuscular doses of testosterone enanthate (Delatestryl) at doses of 25, 50, 125, 300, and 600 milligrams per injection. Open bars = results from healthy young men ages 18–35. Dark bars = results from healthy older men ages 60–75. Results demonstrate increased fat-free mass, increased skeletal muscle mass, increased strength, and reduced total body fat mass in both young and older men. The 300- and 600-milligram doses are supraphysiological and the best balance between positive improvements and adverse effects was achieved at the dosage of 125 milligrams per week. [From S. Bhasin et al. (2005), Figure 4.]

should be applied to normally functioning aging males through treatment in "antiaging" clinics is currently the subject of much debate. Positive outcomes may be offset by the side effects to be discussed next, including the possibility of developing steroid-induced cancers and personality changes. Of additional consideration in the elderly taking these substances are increases in hematocrit and in the possibility of developing prostate cancer.

Finally, in 2008, Emmelot-Vonk and coworkers reported that supplemental oral testosterone (80 milligrams twice daily for six months) slightly increased lean body mass and reduced fat mass in 60- to 80-year-old males with low-normal testosterone levels; however, this effect was

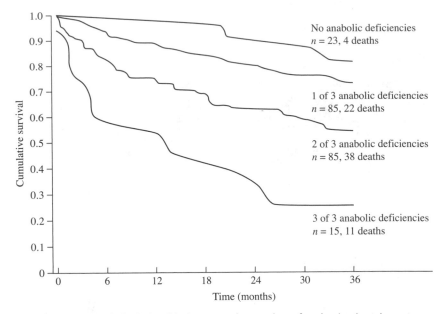

FIGURE 16.6 Graded relationship between the number of endocrine impairments and age-related survival in men (mean age 63) with chronic heart failure. All deaths over the three-year period were cardiovascular in causation (related to the chronic heart failure). See the text for details. [From Jankowska et al. (2006), Figure 3.]

not accompanied by increases in functional mobility or muscle strength. Cognitive functioning was unchanged. Modest increases in cardiovascular risk markers did occur.

Side Effects

Controversies in professional sports such as baseball, football, cycling, and wrestling clearly demonstrate that not only is the use of anabolic steroids beneficial in promoting muscle growth, it also entails significant risks. The risks include aggressive behaviors, cancers, gonadal atrophy, and early onset of atherosclerosis (Basaria, 2010; van Amsterdam et al., 2010).

Endocrine Effects

Males taking anabolic steroids experience a hypogonadal state, which is characterized by atrophy of the testicles, impaired production of sperm, and infertility, causing reduced libido and impotence (Torres-Calleja et al., 2001). In addition, gynecomastia (enlargement of the breasts in males) may occur and may require surgical treatment. In females, puberty is delayed and estrous cyclicity is adversely affected.

These effects are usually reversible within a few months after cessation of drug use.

Cardiovascular Effects

Adverse effects of anabolic steroids on the cardiovascular system have been of concern, and reports of fatal myocardial infarctions (heart attacks) occurring in users of anabolic steroids implicate arteriosclerosis-induced coronary artery disease as a cause of death. Thus, analysis of the potential correlation between anabolic steroids and arteriosclerosis is important. The effect of these steroids on blood cholesterol as a predisposing factor to atherosclerotic coronary artery disease must be considered. Cholesterol is of two types: "bad" cholesterol (low-density lipoprotein cholesterol, or LDL) and "good" cholesterol (high-density lipoprotein cholesterol, or HDL). Decreasing HDL and increasing LDL are strongly correlated with an increased risk of coronary artery disease.

All anabolic steroids induce a reduction in serum HDL cholesterol and an elevation in LDL cholesterol. This effect suggests that people taking these drugs are at greater risk of developing atheromatous plaques within arteries, which places them at increased risk of coronary artery disease. This condition can be expressed as myocardial infarctions, thromboembolic disease (blood clots and emboli), strokes, and hypertension. The actual risk of cardiovascular disease is unknown, largely because of the young age of users, their relatively lean or muscular physiques, and the intermittent pattern of drug use. Once young users become adults, it can be determined whether using anabolic steroids during their earlier years harmed them. Vanberg and Atar (2010) recently reviewed the cardiovascular effects of the anabolic steroids, including alterations in lipid and cholesterol metabolism, increases in coronary heart disease, and even life-threatening, potentially fatal, cardiac arrhythmias.

Effects on the Liver

The use of oral anabolic steroid preparations has been associated with a risk of liver disorders, especially jaundice and tumors. Increases in the blood levels of liver enzymes, indicative of possible liver dysfunction, are quite common among steroid users. Such adverse effects appear to resolve within a year after cessation of drug use. Hepatitis is also common, perhaps as a result of reusing needles (Parkinson and Evans, 2006). In addition, several dozen cases of liver carcinomas of unusual types have been reported. The incidence of developing these potentially fatal carcinomas is estimated to be 1 to 3 percent within two to eight years of exposure to drugs.

Psychological Effects

Anabolic steroids are centrally acting drugs, involved in the regulation of sexuality, aggression, cognition, emotion, and personality. Thus, drug-induced increases in aggression, competitiveness, and combativeness can be predicted in people who use large doses of these drugs. It is now well established that areas of the brain that influence mood and judgment contain steroid receptors and that sharp fluctuations in the levels of steroid hormones have important psychological effects, including depression (Matrisciano et al., 2010).

The *motivational* and *behavioral effects* are profound: athletes taking anabolic steroids often develop very aggressive personalities, a condition nicknamed "roid rage." For some sports, such as football, the enhancement of combativeness can be desirable. But for most purposes, the adverse behavioral effects associated with anabolic steroids are detrimental. These effects include anger, violent feelings, irritability, forgetfulness, and distractibility (Daly et al., 2003). Clearly, users of anabolic steroids tend to be less in control of their aggression, and increases in aggression are reported by 60 percent of steroid users. Until recently, it has been unclear whether steroid use causes aggression or whether aggressive people are attracted to steroid use. Beaver and coworkers (2008), in the National Longitudinal Study of Adolescent Health, found that compared with young persons who had not used anabolic steroids, young adult males who had used steroids reported greater involvement in violent behaviors. The authors urged that young persons with histories of violent behavior be screened for anabolic steroid use.

Pope and colleagues (2000) conducted a six-week trial of testosterone in 56 males, increasing the weekly dose to 600 milligrams. Their goal was to assess drug effects on mood and aggression. Doses of up to 300 milligrams per week produced few psychiatric effects; doses of 500 to 600 milligrams per week produced prominent effects in some of the men. Under these "laboratory" conditions, 84 percent exhibited minimal psychiatric effects, 12 percent became mildly hypomanic, and 4 became markedly hypomanic or manic. Two participants withdrew when they became "alarmingly" hypomanic and aggressive. From these results it appears that in small and unpredictable numbers of users, high doses of anabolic steroids may produce marked signs of mania and/or aggression.

Kanayama and coworkers (2003) interviewed 223 male substance abusers admitted to a substance abuse program. Twenty-nine men (13 percent) reported prior steroid use (only 4 of these men were identified on the physicians' referral forms). Among 88 men who listed opioids as their drug of choice, 22 (25 percent) acknowledged steroid use. Only 7 of the remaining 135 men in the program admitted to steroid use. Many of the opioid-dependent men (who were also steroid abusers) received their opioids from the same person who sold them the injectable steroids. Four of the 29 men with steroid abuse histories (17 percent) reported severe aggressiveness or violence during their periods of steroid use.

Pagonis and coworkers (2006) studied 320 athletes, 50 percent of whom were active users of anabolic steroids. In this well-controlled, 13-month study, extent of steroid use was tightly correlated with increases in all psychometric measures of hostility. As early as 1993, Haupt had stated:

> Athletes taking anabolic steroids suffer some degree of personality change that may range from simple mood swings to a psychosis requiring hospitalization for treatment. A Jekyll-and-Hyde personality is common, where even the slightest provocation can cause an exaggerated, violent, and often uncontrolled response. The users of anabolic steroids often suffer disturbed personality relationships that may include separations from family and friends and even divorce. Arrest records are not uncommon. Fortunately these psychological effects are reversible when the steroids are discontinued, but the social scars may be permanent. (p. 470)

Klotz and coworkers (2006, 2007) updated these earlier findings of steroid-induced aggression and concluded that use of anabolic steroids in certain predisposed people might increase the commission of violent crimes, especially if the use of the steroids is combined with the use of other illicit substances. Recently, Bos and coworkers (2010) demonstrated that a single dose of testosterone decreased trust, making a person more prone to being deceived. Whether this decreased trust relates to outbursts of violence is unclear.

Physical Dependence

Physical dependence is characterized by withdrawal symptoms when a drug is removed. Withdrawal from large doses of anabolic steroids can be accompanied by moderate to severe psychological depression, fatigue, restlessness, insomnia, loss of appetite, and decreased libido. Other withdrawal symptoms that have been reported include drug craving, headache, dissatisfaction with body image, and suicidal ideation (Brower, 2009). Such "muscle dysmorphia" may lead to dependence in these substances (Kanayama et al., 2010). Further, long-term use may cause hypogonadism that may require hormonal therapy or, if associated with endocrine-related depression, may require both endocrine and antidepressant therapies. Despite these observations, no defined psychiatric withdrawal syndrome has been described; neither withdrawal psychosis nor bipolar illness has been reported, although depression is certainly commonplace.

Abuse and Treatment

The use of anabolic steroids for athletic or cosmetic purposes constitutes drug abuse because abuse persists despite recognized, unavoidable side effects and negative consequences for the physical and psychological health of the user. The mechanisms responsible for dependence are largely unknown and may be psychological and/or physiological.

Testosterone is the most potent hormonal determinant of physical and behavioral masculinization. It has been implicated for decades in the stimulation of sexual behavior as well as in the activation of dominance and aggressive behaviors in male primates, including humans. The attraction to the use of supraphysiological doses of testosterone derivatives is strong, with significant numbers of young people succumbing to their attractiveness.

As with all other psychoactive drugs, treatment of steroid dependence requires drug abstinence, treatment of any signs of withdrawal, and maintenance of abstinence. Behavioral and cognitive approaches are possible treatment tools (Kanayama et al., 2010). Supportive therapy, including reassurance, education, and counseling, remains the mainstay of treatment.

One societal response to the use of anabolic steroids has been to ban their use in athletics and institute antidoping testing procedures (Green, 2006; Hoffman et al., 2009). Since the beginning of organized competition, athletes have tried to gain every possible advantage over their competitors. Sometimes this competitive edge is gained fairly by training harder or developing new and improved methods. Sometimes, however, athletes seek an advantage by using substances that affect the body in ways that can improve athletic performance.

The National Collegiate Athletic Association (NCAA) and the United States Olympic Committee (USOC) have declared the use of anabolic steroids illegal, not only because of their ability to artificially increase muscle mass and competitiveness but also because of their serious and sometimes permanent side effects. As early as 1996, Olivier argued in favor of the ban, stating that these drugs not only harm the user but also create a climate of subtle coercion toward their use by others, as well as placing others (for example, partners of steroid users) at risk of violence from users while they are on the drug. Olivier concluded:

> I have argued that prohibition of harmful practices is justified by potential harm to others (rather than just to one's self). One must bear in mind the powerful effects of subtle coercion and influence and the consequent limitations placed on choice. So, on the grounds that it is wrong to harm others or to coerce them into potentially harmful situations, this paper takes issue with sports libertarians who claim that

banning performance-enhancing substances is an unjustified pater-
nalistic action that violates the principle of autonomy. (p. S45)

Education by coaches and teachers has to be the mainstay in the
prevention of anabolic steroid abuse, especially since the drugs initially promote a healthier, more masculine appearance as well as increasing muscle mass and strength. But simply telling young people
about the harmful effects of steroids is not enough; in fact, scare tac-
tics are not only ineffective but can be counterproductive, since young
people know about professional athletes who have used them successfully. Some programs that have had demonstrable success use a combination of approaches.

Goldberg and coworkers (2000), for example, first designed and
tested a team-based, educational interventional program to reduce the
intent of male adolescent athletes to use steroids. Termed the
Adolescents Training and Learning to Avoid Steroids (ATLAS) program,
it was initially conducted with 702 football players in 31 high schools.
Seven weekly classroom sessions, seven weekly weight-room sessions,
and one evening parent session led to increased understanding of anabolic steroid effects, greater belief in personal vulnerability to the adverse
consequences of steroids, improved drug refusal skills, less belief in
steroid-promoting media messages, increased belief in the team as an information source, improved perception of athletic abilities and strength-
training self-efficacy, improved nutritional and exercise behaviors, and
reduced intentions to use steroids.

In 2004 and 2006, the same researchers (Elliot et al., 2004, 2006)
developed and evaluated a similar program, the Athletes Targeting
Healthy Exercise and Nutrition Alternatives (ATHENA), to prevent
young female high school athletes from disordered eating and body-
shaping drug use. This intervention is a scripted, coach-facilitated,
peer-led, eight-session program incorporated into a team's usual training activities. The ATHENA program has reduced ongoing and new use
of diet pills and body-shaping substance use (amphetamines, anabolic
steroids, and sport supplements). As a result of these programs, the
Anabolic Steroid Control Act of 2004 made available monetary grants
to combat steroid abuse. The bill called for $15 million per year from
2005 to 2010 to be spent on anabolic steroid prevention with preference given to programs based on the ATLAS and ATHENA models. The
ATHENA research found that twice as many female nonathletes as female athletes used steroids; the researchers attributed this finding to a
desire to look thin yet fit. This observation deserves additional research and treatment recommendations.

The abuse of anabolic steroids by athletes, bodybuilders, and body-
conscious people poses a special challenge to society. Perhaps the desire
of adolescents and young adults to take steroids has been fostered
largely by our societal fixations on winning and physical appearance.

Thus, successful intervention must go beyond education, counseling, law enforcement, and drug testing to changing the social environment that subtly encourages steroid abuse. Recently, the National Strength and Conditioning Association (NSCA) released a position stand on the use of anabolics by athletes, rejecting their use on the basis of ethics, the ideals of fair play in competition, and concerns for the athletes' health (Hoffman et al., 2009).

Professional sports have certainly fostered the notion that steroid use may be acceptable as long as the goal is to win athletic competitions. Perhaps most notorious is major league baseball, which only in 2004 began testing for anabolic steroid use (many baseball players have since acknowledged steroid use); however, penalties are less than stringent and allow for some positive tests. Testing in professional basketball is more stringent (perhaps because anabolic steroids are of less use for athletes who need prolonged endurance). Professional football bans steroid use. Professional hockey does not have a mandatory drug-testing policy and tests only players already in the league's substance abuse aftercare program. Players who seek help the first time are neither exposed nor suspended. As long as professional athletics "allows" the abuse of anabolic steroids, the example will pass to both fans and younger athletes.

STUDY QUESTIONS

1. What are androgenic-anabolic steroids?
2. How do androgenic-anabolic steroids affect body functions?
3. How do steroids increase muscle mass?
4. Describe the similarities and differences between dependence on anabolic steroids and dependence on the more traditional drugs of abuse.
5. Describe the two groups of people who are the most frequent users of anabolic steroids. How are they similar? How are they different?
6. Describe the anticatabolic, anabolic, and motivational effects of anabolic steroids.
7. What are the side effects associated with use of anabolic steroids?
8. What are the psychological effects associated with use of anabolic steroids?
9. How might the misuse of anabolic steroids be prevented?

REFERENCES

Bahrke, M. S., and Yesalis, C. E. (2004). "Abuse of Anabolic Androgenic Steroids and Related Substances in Sport and Exercise." *Current Opinions in Pharmacology* 4: 614–620

Basaria, S. (2010). "Androgen Abuse in Athletes: Detection and Consequences." *Journal of Clinical Endocrinology & Metabolism* 95: 1533–1543.

Beaver, K. M., et al. (2008). "Anabolic-Androgenic Steroid Use and Involvement in Violent Behavior in a National Representative Sample of Young Adults in the United States." *American Journal of Public Health* 98: 2185–2187.

Bhasin, S., et al. (1996). "The Effects of Supraphysiologic Doses of Testosterone on Muscle Size and Strength in Normal Men." *New England Journal of Medicine* 335: 1–7.

Bhasin, S., et al. (2005). "Older Men Are as Responsive as Young Men to the Anabolic Effects of Graded Doses of Testosterone on the Skeletal Muscle." *Journal of Clinical Endocrinology & Metabolism* 90: 678–688.

Bhasin, S., et al. (2006). "Drug Insight: Testosterone and Selective Androgen Receptor Modulators as Anabolic Therapies for Chronic Illness and Aging." *Nature Clinical Practice Endocrinology & Metabolism* 2: 146–159.

Bos, P. A., et al. (2010). "Testosterone Decreases Trust in Socially Naïve Humans." *Proceedings of the National Academy of Science USA* 107: 9991–9995.

Brower, K. J. (2009). "Anabolic Steroid Abuse and Dependence in Clinical Practice." *The Physician and Sports Medicine* 37: 131–140.

Daly, R. C., et al. (2003). "Neuroendocrine and Behavioral Effects of High-Dose Anabolic Steroid Administration in Male Normal Volunteers." *Psychoneuroendocrinology* 28: 317 331.

Elliot, D. L., et al. (2004). "Preventing Substance Use and Disordered Eating: Initial Outcomes of the ATHENA (Athletes Targeting Healthy Exercise and Nutrition Alternatives) Program." *Archives of Pediatrics & Adolescent Medicine* 158: 1043–1049.

Elliot, D. L., et al. (2006). "Definition and Outcome of a Curriculum to Prevent Disordered Eating and Body-Shaping Drug Use." *Journal of School Health* 76: 67–73.

Elliot, D. L., et al. (2007). "Cross-Sectional Study of Female Students Reporting Anabolic Steroid Use." *Archives of Pediatrics & Adolescent Medicine* 161: 572–577.

Emmelot-Vonk, M. H., et al. (2008). "Effect of Testosterone Supplementation on Functional Mobility, Cognition, and Other Parameters in Older Men: A Randomized Controlled Trial." *Journal of the American Medical Association* 299: 39–52.

Goldberg, L., et al. (2000). "The Adolescents Training and Learning to Avoid Steroids Program: Preventing Drug Use and Promoting Health Behaviors." *Archives of Pediatrics & Adolescent Medicine* 154: 332–338.

Green, G. A. (2006). "Doping Control for the Team Physician: A Review of Drug Testing Procedures." *American Journal of Sports Medicine* 34: 1690–1698.

Gullett, N. P., et al. (2010). "Update on Clinical Trials of Growth Factors and Anabolic Steroids in Cachexia and Wasting." *American Journal of Clinical Nutrition* 91: 1143S–1147S.

Hartgens, F., et al. (2002). "Misuse of Androgenic-Anabolic Steroids and Human Deltoid Muscle Fibers: Differences Between Polydrug Regimens and Single Drug Administration." *European Journal of Applied Physiology* 86: 233–239.

Haupt, H. A. (1993). "Anabolic Steroids and Growth Hormone." *American Journal of Sports Medicine* 21: 468–474.

Hoffman, J. R., et al. (2009). "Position Stand on Androgen and Human Growth Hormone Use." *Journal of Strength and Conditioning Research* 23, Supplement 5: S1–S59.

Jankowska, E. A., et al. (2006). "Anabolic Deficiency in Men with Chronic Heart Failure: Prevalence and Detrimental Impact on Survival." *Circulation* 114: 1829–1837.

Kanayama, G., et al. (2003). "Past Anabolic-Androgenic Steroid Use Among Men Admitted for Substance Abuse Treatment: An Underrecognized Problem?" *Journal of Clinical Psychiatry* 64: 156–160.

Kanayama, G., et al. (2006). "Body Images and Attitudes Toward Male Roles in Anabolic-Androgenic Steroid Users." *American Journal of Psychiatry* 163: 697–703.

Kanayama, G., et al. (2010). "Treatment of Anabolic-Androgenic Steroid Dependence: Emerging Evidence and its Implications." *Drug and Alcohol Dependence* 109: 6–13.

Klotz, F., et al. (2006). "Criminality Among Individuals Testing Positive for the Presence of Anabolic Androgenic Steroids." *Archives of General Psychiatry* 63: 1274–1279.

Klotz, F., et al. (2007). "Violent Crime and Substance Abuse: A Medico-Legal Comparison Between Deceased Users of Anabolic Androgenic Steroids and Abusers of Illicit Drugs." *Forensic Science International* 173: 57–83.

Malkin, C. J., et al. (2006). "Testosterone Therapy in Men with Moderate Severity Heart Failure: A Double-Blind, Randomized, Placebo-Controlled Trial." *European Heart Journal* 27: 57–64.

Matrisciano, F., et al. (2010). "Repeated Anabolic Androgenic Steroid Treatment Causes Antidepressant-Reversible Alterations of the Hypothalamic-Pituitary-Adrenal Axis, BDNF Levels and Behavior." *Neuropharmacology* 58: 1078–1084.

Moretti, C., et al. (2005). "Androgens and Body Composition in the Aging Male." *Journal of Endocrinological Investigation* 28, Supplement 3: S56–S64.

Olivier, S. (1996). "Drugs in Sport: Justifying Paternalism on the Grounds of Harm." *American Journal of Sports Medicine* 24: S43–S45.

Pagonis, T. A., et al. (2006). "Psychiatric Side Effects Induced by Supraphysiological Doses of Combinations of Anabolic Steroids Correlate to the Severity of Abuse." *European Psychiatry* 21: 551–562.

Parkinson, A. B., and Evans, N. A. (2006). "Anabolic Androgenic Steroids: A Survey of 500 Users." *Medicine & Science in Sports & Exercise* 34: 644–651.

Pope, H. C., et al. (2000). "Effects of Supraphysiologic Doses of Testosterone on Mood and Aggression in Normal Men: A Randomized Controlled Trial." *Archives of General Psychiatry* 57: 133–140.

Rabkin, J. G., et al. (2000). "A Double-Blind, Placebo-Controlled Trial of Testosterone Therapy for HIV-Positive Men with Hypogonadal Symptoms." *Archives of General Psychiatry* 57: 141–147.

Rogol, A. D. (2010). "Drugs of Abuse and the Adolescent Athlete." *Italian Journal of Pediatrics* 36: 19–25.

Schwerin, M. J., et al. (1996). "Social Physique Anxiety, Body Esteem, and Social Anxiety in Bodybuilders and Self-Reported Anabolic Steroid Users." *Addictive Behaviors* 21: 1–8.

Torres-Calleja, J., et al. (2001). "Effect of Androgenic Anabolic Steroids on Sperm Quality and Serum Hormone Levels in Adult Male Body Builders." *Life Sciences* 68: 1769–1774.

Tuiten, A., et al. (2000). "Time Course of Effects of Testosterone Administration on Sexual Arousal in Women." *Archives of General Psychiatry* 57: 149–153.

van Amsterdam, J., et al. (2010). "Adverse Health Effects of Anabolic-Androgenic Steroids." *Regulatory Toxicology and Pharmacology* 57: 117–123.

Vanberg, P., and Atar, D. (2010). "Androgenic Anabolic Steroid Abuse and the Cardiovascular System." *Handbook of Experimental Pharmacology* 195: 411–457.

Yesalis, C. E., and Bahrke, M. S. (2002). "Anabolic-Androgenic Steroids and Related Substances." *Current Sports Medicine Report* 1: 246–252.

Chapter 17

Topics in Drug Abuse

Drug abuse has been a societal problem for thousands of years, ever since grain was fermented (ethyl alcohol) and natural substances were found that produced euphoria (cocaine), relieved pain (morphine), or produced altered states of consciousness for divination (psilocybin, mescaline). As history suggests, as long as these drugs persist in society, their use will be associated with compulsive use and abuse as well as with dependency and addiction. This chapter reviews the mechanisms responsible for producing compulsive drug abuse and dependency. It also reviews the literature on the current concepts of treatment of dependency and abuse. The individual drugs discussed in their own chapters are brought together in a chapter devoted to general concepts that apply to all drugs of abuse.

Historical and Current Perspectives

In all of recorded history, every society has used drugs to produce alterations in mood, thought, feeling, or behavior or to provide temporary alterations in reality. Moreover, some people have always digressed from social custom with respect to the time, the amount, and the situation in which drugs are used. Abuse of psychoactive drugs has always produced problems for the person taking the drug, for those in direct contact with the user, and for society at large.

Alcohol is the classic psychoactive drug used throughout history primarily for recreational purposes, but it is not the only such agent. Naturally occurring substances are used to alleviate anxiety, produce relaxation, provide relief from boredom, communicate with the gods, alleviate pain, and/or increase strength or work tolerance. In most cultures, only very few naturally occurring substances have been available and their use has been closely monitored, so just a relatively small minority of people have abused them. Today, patterns of abuse differ considerably from traditional patterns:

- Virtually all the naturally occurring psychoactive and psychedelic drugs ever identified are available at one time (now) and in one culture (ours).
- In most cases, the pharmacologically active ingredient in each natural product has been isolated, identified, often synthesized, and then made available to those who desire it.
- Organic chemistry has made possible synthetic derivatives of naturally occurring drugs. In many cases, the synthetic derivatives magnify the psychoactive potency of the natural substance 100 times or more.
- Users have adopted new methods of drug delivery, starting with the invention of the hypodermic syringe in the 1860s, and new drugs, the most recent of which are crack cocaine, ice methamphetamine, and "designer" derivatives of both fentanyl and mescaline. These developments have markedly increased the delivered dose, decreased the time to onset of drug action, and increased both the potency and the toxicity of these agents compared with their naturally occurring counterparts.

As in past decades, caffeine, nicotine, and ethyl alcohol are the addictive drugs used by the vast majority of people. Caffeine use is nearly universal; 90 percent of Americans over the age of 11 use the drug at least once weekly. Thankfully, little harm seems to follow. Nicotine and alcohol are the next most widely used and abused addictive drugs, and their economic toll on lives, productivity, and health is enormous. In fact, legitimate manufacturers of legal or prescription substances find ways to make them more concentrated and powerful, from increasing the nicotine content in cigarettes and increasing the amount of caffeine in energy drinks to popularizing alcoholic beverages of high alcohol content and making stronger opioid analgesic products without limiting the potential for misuse.

Extent of the Drug Problem

Drug abuse and addiction are a major burden to society. Estimates of the total overall costs of substance abuse in the United States—including health- and crime-related costs as well as losses in productivity—exceed half a trillion dollars annually. This includes approximately $181 billion for illicit drugs, $168 billion for tobacco, and $185 billion for alcohol. Staggering as these numbers are, however, they do not fully describe the breadth of deleterious public health—and safety—implications, which include family disintegration, loss of employment, failure in school, domestic violence, child abuse, and other crimes.

To address the nation's problems in regard to drug abuse and addiction, the president has released the *National Drug Control Strategy—2010*. This document, which can be accessed at www.whitehouse drugpolicy.gov/publications/policy/ndcs10/ndcs2010.pdf, describes the recommendations and proposals of the current administration for reducing the toll of addiction in the United States.

Alcohol

Slightly more than half of Americans aged 12 or older—about 129.0 million people (51.6 percent)—reported being current drinkers of alcohol in the 2008 government survey, which was similar to the 2007 estimate of 126.8 million people (51.1 percent). In 2008, more than one-fifth (23.3 percent, similar to the estimate in 2007) participated in binge drinking, defined as having five or more drinks on the same occasion on at least 1 day in the 30 days prior to the survey. Among young adults aged 18 to 25 in 2008, the rate of binge drinking was 41.0 percent, and the rate of heavy drinking (defined as binge drinking on at least 5 days in the past 30 days) was 14.5 percent. These rates were similar to the rates in 2007. The rate of current alcohol use among youths aged 12 to 17 was 14.6 percent in 2008, which is lower than the 2007 rate (15.9 percent). Youth binge and heavy drinking rates in 2008 were 8.8 percent (lower than the 9.7 percent rate in 2007) and 2.0 percent, respectively. In 2008, an estimated 31 million people (12.4 percent) aged 12 or older reported driving under the influence of alcohol at least once in the past year. Although this reflects a downward trend from 14.2 percent in 2002, it remains a cause for concern. Overall, the prevalence of underage (ages 12–20) alcohol use and binge drinking has been in a long-term, gradual decline.

Tobacco

According to the annual survey by the National Institute on Drug Abuse (NIDA), smoking rates are at their lowest point in the history of the survey. Another encouraging trend is the decline in cigarette use by young adults aged 18 to 25—from 40.8 percent in 2002 to 35.7 percent in 2008. However, from 2008 to 2009, smoking prevalence among all three grades of high school students was unchanged.

Illicit and Prescription Drugs

The decline in illicit drug use by the nation's adolescents since the mid- to late-1990s has leveled off. The trend for illicit drug use has been driven largely by reported use of marijuana.

- Marijuana prevalence rates were the same in 2009 as they were in 2004.
- Between 2004 and 2009, a drop in past-year use of methamphetamine was reported for all grades.

- Cocaine use gradually declined between 2003 and 2008 among people aged 12 or older (from 2.3 million to 1.9 million).
- Both past-year and past-month use rates of hallucinogens among twelfth graders fell significantly between 2008 and 2009.
- Estimated emergency room visits for nonmedical use of opiates increased by 111% between 2004 and 2008; the highest numbers were recorded for oxycodone, hydrocodone, and methadone.

One currently significant issue is that military experts are concerned that the wars in Iraq and Afghanistan may be precipitating a rise in problems related to substance use and abuse among the military personnel who have been deployed to those fronts. NIDA has joined forces with the Department of Defense, Department of Veterans Affairs, and other federal agencies in a campaign to assess and find solutions to this threat to the health and well-being of our service men and women, veterans, and their families.

Tobacco use is about 50 percent higher among the nation's active-duty military personnel and veterans than in the civilian population.

The rate of Army soldiers enrolled in treatment programs for alcohol dependency or abuse nearly doubled between 2003 and 2009—a sign of the growing stress of repeated deployments in Iraq and Afghanistan. Soldiers diagnosed by Army substance abuse counselors with alcoholism or alcohol abuse, such as binge drinking, increased from 6.1 per 1000 soldiers in 2003 to an estimated 11.4 as of March 31, 2009.

Combat exposure appears to be a primary mediator of the impact of war deployment on substance abuse rates. In one study, one in four veterans of Iraq and Afghanistan reported symptoms of a mental or cognitive disorder; one in six reported symptoms of posttraumatic stress disorder (PTSD). These disorders are strongly associated with substance abuse and dependence, as are other problems experienced by returning military personnel, including sleep disturbances, traumatic brain injury, and violence in relationships.

Nosology and Psychopathology of Substance Abuse

Published in 2000 in its revised fourth edition, the *Diagnostic and Statistical Manual of Mental Disorders* (DSM-IV-TR) (American Psychiatric Association, 2000) presents commonly accepted criteria for what constitutes substance dependence and substance abuse (Table 17.1). The two substance use disorders involve maladaptive patterns of substance use, leading to clinically significant impairments or distress. The distinctions between abuse and dependence are listed in the table.

Approximately one-third of people addicted to an illicit drug or alcohol have a diagnosed *comorbid* (Axis I) psychiatric disorder, a situation

---

TABLE 17.1 DSM-IV criteria for substance dependence or abuse

CRITERIA FOR SUBSTANCE DEPENDENCE:

A maladaptive pattern of substance use, leading to clinically significant impairment or distress, as manifested by three (or more) of the following, occurring at any time in the same 12-month period:

(1) tolerance, as defined by either: (a) need for markedly increased amounts of the substance to achieve intoxication or desired effect; (b) markedly diminished effect with continued use of the same amount of substance

(2) withdrawal, as manifested by either: (a) the characteristic withdrawal syndrome for the substance; (b) the same (or a closely related) substance is taken to relieve or avoid withdrawal symptoms

(3) the substance is often taken in larger amounts or over a longer period than was intended

(4) there is a persistent desire or unsuccessful efforts to cut down or control substance use

(5) a great deal of time is spent in activities necessary to obtain the substance, use the substance, or recover from its effects

(6) important social, occupational, or recreational activities are given up or reduced because of substance use

(7) the substance use is continued despite knowledge of having a persistent or recurrent physical or psychological problem that is likely to have been caused or exacerbated by the substance

CRITERIA FOR SUBSTANCE ABUSE:

A. A maladaptive pattern of substance use leading to clinically significant impairment or distress, as manifested by one (or more) of the following occurring within a 12-month period:

(1) recurrent substance use resulting in a failure to fulfill major role obligations at work, school, or home

(2) recurrent substance use in situations in which it is physically hazardous

(3) recurrent substance-related legal problems

(4) continued substance use despite having persistent or recurrent social or interpersonal problems caused or exacerbated by the effects of the substance

B. The symptoms have never met the criteria for Substance Dependence for this class of substance.

Adapted from American Psychiatric Association (2000), pp. 181–183.

---

covered by the term *dual diagnosis*. Among people with a lifetime diagnosis of schizophrenia, 47 percent have met criteria for substance abuse or dependence; those with an anxiety disorder, 23.7 percent; those with obsessive-compulsive disorder, 32.8 percent; those with bipolar disorder, 50 percent; and those with depression, 32 percent—with distribution equal for males and females.

Neurobiology of Addiction

Until 1969 it was generally believed that addictive behavior was primarily driven by the state of drug dependence. Intravenous administration of drugs alone, as behavioral reinforcers, was not considered to be necessary. However, technological advances made it possible to develop procedures by which nonhuman animals could self-administer addictive drugs. It was then seen that almost all of the drugs abused by humans could also produce self-administration behaviors in animals. Thus, reinforcing effects of drugs were shown to be a property of the drug, not of the person. This observation was revolutionary in that era (Bergman and Paronis, 2006). Subsequently, it was shown that the reinforcing effects of drugs (and presumably their "addictive" potentials) were receptor-related phenomena; they were dose-related and could be antagonized by selective receptor blockers, and they did not occur in animals selectively bred to lack certain specific receptors.

However, despite their respective individual pharmacological characteristics, all drugs of abuse have some effects in common. Acutely, the drugs are rewarding, and this effect promotes repeated use. Unfortunately, in vulnerable people, repeated use can lead to addiction—a loss of control over drug use. As a result of chronic use, the addicted nervous system adapts to repeated exposure. If the drug is withdrawn, similar unpleasant emotional reactions and changes in the brain will occur, regardless of the specific drug; it is these effects that are responsible for craving and relapse, even after long periods of abstinence. Even after all traces of the specific abused drug are gone from the body (the process of detoxification), the addicted individual experiences urges to use the drug again and is at risk of relapsing. The development of such cravings indicates that something in the brain has changed as a result of long-term drug use; some process of neuroadaptation has occurred. Appreciation of this phenomenon, which occurs with all abused drugs, has led to increased research into the mechanisms responsible for craving and relapse; the recognition that such processes are similar to other types of learned reactions; and the realization that these mechanisms may be relevant to other types of nondrug addictions, such as gambling, and perhaps other compulsive behaviors as well. Efforts are currently ongoing to develop new treatments for these maladaptive learned responses.

Common Effects of Abused Drugs on Brain Reward Circuits

There is general agreement, from experiments in nonhuman animal models as well as in humans, that almost all drugs of abuse have a common effect on a neural system that serves as a reward circuit. This system consists of one of the major brain pathways for dopamine, called

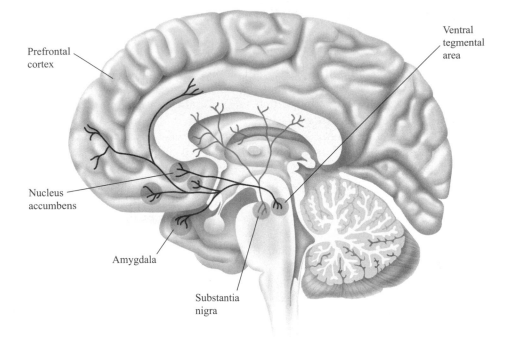

FIGURE 17.1 The reward circuit. The major structures involved in the subjective sensation of pleasure and reward. The pathway starts with dopamine-releasing neurons in the ventral tegmental area. Axons from the VTA neurons release dopamine onto the amygdala, nucleus accumbens, and prefrontal cortex.

the *mesolimbic dopamine pathway* (Figure 17.1). As shown in the figure, this pathway begins with a group of dopamine neurons in the ventral tegmental area (VTA), a structure that is located in the midbrain (Chapter 3). The axons of these dopamine neurons extend to several other brain structures, where they release dopamine when the VTA is activated. The most relevant structures are the nucleus accumbens (NAc), the amygdala, the hippocampus, and the prefrontal cortex. In addition to dopamine neurons, there are also other neurons within the VTA that interact with the dopamine neurons. Some release the neurotransmitter GABA. The release of GABA inhibits dopamine neurons and, under baseline conditions, reduces dopamine release.

During the last few decades, a converging body of evidence has indicated that, regardless of the specific effects of abused drugs, they share a common action with respect to this mesolimbic dopamine pathway. Each drug increases dopamine transmission in this pathway. That is, most abused drugs increase the amount of dopamine that is released from the VTA onto the NAc, amygdala, hippocampus, and frontal lobe. However, they don't all increase dopamine activity in the same way. In some cases the dopamine increase is direct; in others, dopamine is increased indirectly. Some drugs may increase dopamine by more than one mechanism, and some may produce other, non-dopaminergic responses as well.

For example, cocaine (and other stimulants; Chapter 12) increases the amount of dopamine on NAc neurons by blocking dopamine reuptake into VTA neurons after the transmitter has been released. Opioids (Chapter 10) act on receptors located on GABA neurons and inhibit GABA release. When GABA release is reduced, there is less inhibition of dopamine neurons, and dopamine release increases. Alcohol (Chapter 13) may also increase dopamine by inhibiting GABA release as well as by other actions. Nicotine (Chapter 11) may stimulate the dopamine neurons directly and cause them to release dopamine.

How do we know that the effect of drugs on dopaminergic activity is related to their pleasurable subjective effects? Compelling and extensive evidence from studies done for over 30 years in nonhuman animals supports this relationship. However, in 1997 a particularly relevant observation was made in cocaine addicts, which showed that dopamine was also related to the sensation of pleasure in humans. In this study, methylphenidate (Ritalin; Chapter 18) was given to cocaine addicts while they underwent a brain scan. Methylphenidate, like cocaine, blocked the dopamine transporter and increased the amount of dopamine in the synapse. The addicts rated the "high" they experienced after receiving methylphenidate, while the brain scans showed the percent of transporters blocked by each dose. There was an excellent correlation—the greater the subjective rating of the "high," the greater the proportion of transporters blocked, which meant the greater the increase in the amount of dopamine in the brain (Volkow et al., 1997).

Evidence suggests that the VTA-NAc pathway and the other limbic regions are also responsible, at least in part, not only for the positive effect of drugs but also for the pleasurable effects of natural rewards, such as food, sex, and other enjoyable activities. Consequently, these same regions have also been implicated in the so-called natural addictions (that is, compulsive behaviors in regard to natural rewards), such as pathological overeating, pathological gambling, and sexual addictions (Nestler, 2005).

Research indicates that long-term, chronic exposure to any of several drugs of abuse will impair this dopamine pathway such that eventually the system becomes less responsive. In other words, excessive drug use alters the response to naturally rewarding stimuli such that they are not as enjoyable as they once were. Essentially, tolerance develops within the pathway (Nestler, 2005), and naturally rewarding stimuli don't increase dopaminergic activity as much as they used to.

These changes may contribute to the unpleasant emotional state that develops between drug exposures or when drugs are withdrawn.

In brief, drugs, like other rewarding experiences, cause release of dopamine from VTA neurons to NAc neurons. When released, dopamine causes animals to feel good. This positive emotion teaches them to repeat the pleasurable action, leading to compulsive use and addiction.

But this raises another question. Many people use legal drugs, like alcohol. Yet why do only some drug users become addicted? Is there something different about their brains? Some evidence suggests this might be the case. In one study, normal male subjects were given methylphenidate and asked if they found the experience pleasant, unpleasant, or neutral. At the same time, they underwent a brain scan that allowed measurement of their dopamine receptors. It turned out that the subjects who reported that they found the methylphenidate to be pleasant had lower D_2 receptor levels than those who reported that the drug injection was unpleasant. In fact, the subjects who enjoyed the drug experience had receptor levels similar to those previously reported in cocaine abusers, even though these subjects were not abusing drugs (Volkow et al., 2004).

Does this mean that low receptor density signals a biological vulnerability to drug abuse? In other words, perhaps the normal response to "pleasure" of people at risk for acquiring addictions is not as strong as the response of people who are not as vulnerable because of a dopamine receptor deficiency. Such individuals may require a more powerful stimulus (a drug) to experience a normal pleasurable sensation, while, for others, the same drug experience may actually be too strong to be enjoyable.

Regardless of the mechanism responsible, however, repeated drug use may develop into chronic drug use that can become compulsive and result in addiction.

From Abuse to Addiction

Because the frontal lobe is one of the areas of the brain that is part of the reward circuit, it is also profoundly altered by chronic drug abuse. One common change that occurs after long-term drug use is cortical "hypofrontality." This means that the normal baseline activity of several regions of the frontal cortex is reduced, a phenomenon that has been seen in brain scans of addicts. Normally, the role of these frontal lobe regions is to control our ability to pay attention, plan ahead, and inhibit ourselves from making poor decisions. But as drug use becomes chronic and gradually compulsive, the prefrontal cortex becomes sluggish and is no longer able to perform these functions effectively. Even after three or four months of abstinence, the prefrontal cortex may not recover.

At the same time, even though natural rewards are *less* pleasurable, chronic drug exposure seems to *sensitize* the dopamine system. As a result, in response to drugs and especially to cues that are associated with drugs, there is a *greater increase* in dopaminergic transmission than is normal (Nestler, 2005; Pierce and Kumaresan, 2006; Volkow et al., 2004, 2006). This means that, although the frontal cortex becomes inherently less active and less responsive to normal rewards, it is *overactive* in response to drugs or the stimuli that predict drugs. Thus, the reward circuit is responsible for the initial pleasurable effect of drugs, and this may motivate the individual to repeat the behavior. But as this continues, the ability of the frontal cortex to inhibit the behavior weakens.

However, to repeat the behavior, the brain also has to *remember* what the behavior was. This means that, in addition to the frontal cortex, the reward circuit also interacts with structures that mediate emotion (amygdala) and memory (hippocampus) (Figure 17.2). In fact, stimuli that "predict" drugs or were associated with the environment in which drugs were used seem to have greater control over behavior than stimuli associated with natural rewards. Such conditioned responses elicit powerful craving sensations in the frontal cortex. For example, addicted people frequently relapse after returning to an environment where they have previously taken drugs, even after they have gone through detoxification and recently spent time in a rehabilitation program.

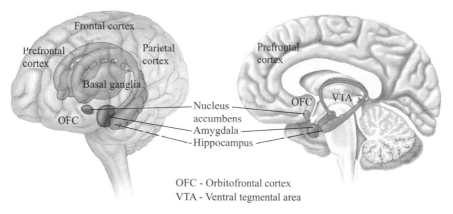

FIGURE 17.2 Major brain structures involved in addiction. The ventral tegmental area (VTA) and nucleus accumbens are key components of the reward system. These, together with the amygdala, hippocampus, and prefrontal cortex (PFC), coordinate drives, emotions, and memories. [Modified from "Imaging the Addicted Human Brain." In J. S. Fowler, N. D. Volkow, C. A. Kassed, and L. Chang, *Science and Practice Perspectives* (2007), p. 5 (NIH Publication No. 07-6171).]

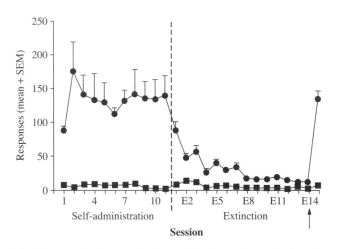

FIGURE 17.3 Variables that promote relapse. This figure illustrates the development, extinction, and relapse phases of addiction in an animal model. Some animals were trained for 12 days to self-administer cocaine in response to a lever press (circles). Control animals (squares) received no cocaine in response to a lever press. At the vertical dashed line, all animals underwent extinction training (lever presses no longer produced the drug) for 14 days. At the end of this phase (arrow at session E14), all animals were presented with either (1) a cue that accompanied the previous cocaine administration in the training stage, (2) a mild stressor, such as a brief electrical stimulus, or (3) a small amount of intravenous cocaine. All three stimuli overcame extinction in animals that had received cocaine before the extinction period (circle at day E14). Cue, stress, or cocaine resulted in resumption of lever pressing in an attempt to obtain cocaine ("reinstatement" of drug seeking). In control animals (squares at days E14 and E15), presentation of a cue at day E14 did not result in drug-seeking behavior. [Modified from Kalivas et al. (2006), p. 340, Figure 1.]

Furthermore, the brain structures involved in addiction are hypersensitive not only to activation by drugs of abuse and drug-associated stimuli but also to environmental *stressors*. In fact, studies in humans and animal models indicate that stress is significantly involved in the vulnerability to develop addiction, in increased drug taking, and in relapse in addicted persons. An example of the importance of stress and learned reactions in triggering relapse is shown in Figure 17.3. This figure is a composite summary of the results of numerous animal experiments. It shows three phases of drug abuse. In the first phase, rats responded on one lever for cocaine infusions but did not respond on a second lever that produced only a saline injection (self-administration). In the second phase, when responding no longer produced cocaine (extinction), the rats eventually stopped pressing the lever. Finally, in the third phase, separate groups of animals were exposed to either (1) direct injection of cocaine, (2) an environmental stimulus previously associated with the drug, or (3) a stressful stimulus (for example, electric shock). Each of these three treatments reinstated responding

on the lever that had previously been associated with cocaine injections. (Although not shown, cocaine responding also increased even
more after a period of abstinence, that is, after drug injections were
stopped but without the extinction responses). This summary figure
shows that even when drug abuse is extinguished, relapse can be readily elicited by three major conditions:

• Reexperience with the drug
• Conditioned drug cues
• Stress (including withdrawal-induced reactions)

Regardless of whether they are triggered by drugs, by conditioning, or by stress, these heightened craving sensations are transmitted
from the frontal cortex through downstream nerve pathways that feed
back onto the reward pathway. A simplified version of this feedback
circuit is illustrated in Figure 17.4. In this case, however, the nerve
fibers that connect the frontal lobe structures with the downstream

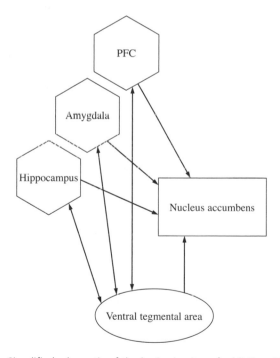

FIGURE 17.4 Simplified schematic of the brain circuitry of addiction. This drawing
indicates that pathways from the hippocampus, amygdala, and prefrontal cortex
(PFC) project to and from the main structures of the reward circuit (the ventral
tegmental area and nucleus accumbens). It is hypothesized that these neural pathways represent the biological basis of cravings, which lead to chronic drug abuse and
addiction.[Modified from C. Pierce and V. Kumaresan (2006), Figure 1.]

reward circuit are not primarily dopaminergic. Rather, they release the transmitter *glutamate* onto the NAc and VTA. Evidence from animal experiments and from human brain scans shows that chronic exposure to any of several drugs of abuse causes complex changes in these frontal cortical regions and their glutamatergic outputs. These changes are believed to be responsible for the profound impulsivity (acting on sudden urges to take a drug) and compulsivity (being driven by irresistible inner forces to take a drug) that define addiction. Therefore, the hypersensitivity of the frontal cortex to drugs or drug cues, which develops in addiction, is the basis of the phenomenon of craving, which is biologically mediated as increased activity of glutamatergic transmission onto the reward circuit.

The increased activation of these pathways also causes some biochemical changes within the neurons of the VTA-NAc and other brain reward regions. One of the most dramatic examples is that chronic exposure to all drugs of abuse, including cocaine, amphetamine, opiates, alcohol, nicotine, cannabinoids, and phencyclidine, increases the amount of a protein, called ΔFosB, which builds up in the NAc. Chronic drive for natural rewards, such as high levels of activity and ingestion of sweets, will produce the same effect in the same sites. There is now considerable data showing that increases in ΔFosB within NAc neurons contribute to a state of sensitization; that is, there are increases in behavioral responses to cocaine and opiates as well as to sucrose and exercise. There are other common biochemical changes that occur in the NAc during the development of addiction, although none are as consistent as the increase in ΔFosB. One of the substances in the brain that is also increased by chronic drug use is the protein BDNF (brain-derived neurotrophic factor, discussed in relation to depression; Chapter 5). When this compound was directly injected into the VTA of drug-naive rats, the rats behaved like opiate-dependent animals. In addition, there was a "switch" in the response of their GABA neurons, from inhibition to excitation (Vargas-Perez et al., 2009).

The fact that common mechanisms seem to contribute to at least some aspects of all drug addictions, and possibly to natural addictions as well, means it might be possible to develop treatments that would be effective for a wide range of addictive disorders. Drugs that target the brain's dopamine, glutamate, or hypothalamic stress systems might help persons addicted to either drugs or natural rewards. Studies are under way in each of these areas. Someday our understanding of common mechanisms for the compulsive use of drugs and natural rewards, involving the BDNF pathway, ΔFosB, or the glutamatergic synapse, might lead to better treatments of all types of compulsive behavior (Briand and Blendy, 2010; Kalivas, 2009; Kalivas et al., 2006; Kalivas and Volkow, 2005; Koob and Volkow, 2010; Feil et al., 2010; Feltenstein and See, 2008).

Pharmacotherapy of Substance Use Disorders

Our current view of the neurobiology of drug abuse broadens the framework for treating addiction. Traditionally, pharmacological treatments for addiction have been relatively specific, focusing on medications that directly affect the biological actions of the primary drug of abuse. However, with a greater appreciation of how stress, learning, and memory influence addiction and relapse, the variety of conceptual targets has increased. This section first describes classic approaches to drug treatment of addiction and then provides examples of some more broadly acting therapies suggested by the recent theoretical developments.

Agonist Substitution Treatment

Prescribing a substitute drug for the abused agent is one of the most well-established pharmacological interventions for addiction. This approach has been most commonly used to treat opioid and nicotine addiction. The method originated with early studies of the opiate methadone, which found that this approach reduced heroin use, crime, and the spread of HIV infections as well as helping to get addicts involved in their treatment (see Lingford-Hughes et al., 2004; NICE, 2007; Nutt and Lingford-Hughes, 2008). It has been estimated that methadone provides substantial economic benefit by reducing the costs of health and social care, reducing criminal activity, and improving crime control. Methadone can substitute for heroin because it is a (relatively) full opioid agonist, but it has a slower onset of effect. Although the oral route produces less of a "rush" than does heroin, its long half-life allows once-daily dosing, which reduces both cravings for and the effect of (and the need to buy) heroin. Nevertheless, because methadone is still a very addictive drug, which can be fatal in overdose and diverted into street use, it is usually given in supervised situations. This practice is expensive; often addicts are allowed to take doses home over the weekend, which leads to diversion and accidental overdoses, often in children.

Agonist substitution has also long been used effectively for treating nicotine addiction. A variety of formulations have been developed, including nicotine lozenges, gum, and patches (Chapter 11). Extended treatment with the patch for up to 24 weeks was shown to improve abstinence rates (Schnoll et al., 2010). Another trial compared five smoking cessation treatments, consisting of different formulations of nicotine, or the dopaminergic reuptake blocker, bupropion, with a placebo condition. All drug treatments were more effective than placebo, but not at a statistical level. However, the combination of the nicotine patch *plus* the lozenge produced significantly greater abstinence outcomes at six months than did placebo (Piper et al., 2009).

A "substitution" approach may also be effective for treating stimulant addiction (Herin et al., 2010). The drug modafinil is a medication currently approved for treating narcolepsy. It is a mild stimulant and enhances glutamate neurotransmission. In three studies with addict patients, modafinil blunted the "high" of a cocaine injection, reduced the subjective state of euphoria attained with a subsequent dose of cocaine, and reduced subjective ratings of cocaine's effects, cocaine self-administration, and increases in heart rate and blood pressure. Modafinil has also improved cocaine abstinence rates in two clinical trials (Kampman, 2008). Again, the dopamine reuptake blocker bupropion has also been found useful in treating stimulant withdrawal (Reichel et al., 2009), which is consistent with the experimental research linking addiction to dopaminergic reward.

Partial Agonist Substitution Treatment

Instead of substituting one full agonist for another, an alternative approach is to use a partial agonist such as buprenorphine for opiate addiction (discussed in Chapter 10). Like methadone, such treatment reduces intravenous injecting, since the addict is exposed to sufficient drug to overcome the effect of additional opiate use. Buprenorphine produces less severe withdrawal than methadone, but that may be due to its long half-life, which may "protect" an addict from heroin use for two to three days. There is still the risk of potentially fatal respiratory depression (overdose death) if buprenorphine is combined with other sedative hypnotics. This risk can be reduced if an opiate antagonist is added to buprenorphine, which has been done (see Chapter 10 for a discussion).

Partial agonists have been successfully developed in nicotine addiction, for which varenicline (an $\alpha_4\beta_2$ partial nicotinic agonist) was approved (Chapter 11). The concept is the same as with buprenorphine for opioid dependence in that the agent provides sufficient stimulation to reduce smoking but does not support self-administration. Interestingly, there is emerging evidence that varenicline may also reduce alcohol consumption (Steensland et al., 2007).

As discussed by Nutt and Lingford-Hughes (2008), dopamine partial agonists would presumably be an interesting target for stimulant addiction. Such drugs should provide enough dopamine activation to reduce the effects of withdrawal yet block the consequences of illicit stimulant use. The antipsychotic aripiprazole is such a drug, and it was reportedly effective in preventing relapse in an animal model of cocaine administration (Feltenstein et al., 2007). However, it was not found effective, in one study, for stimulant abuse in addicts (Tiihonen et al., 2007).

Antagonists as Treatments for Addiction

Another standard approach to treating addiction is to administer an antagonist of the abused drug. By directly blocking the reinforcing effect, an antagonist would eventually reduce the compulsive behavior. The opiate antagonists naloxone, naltrexone, and nalmefene have long been available for such treatment. However, a major difficulty with these agents is compliance—since they offer no positive reinforcement, it is hard to maintain adherence. If the addict continues to take an antagonist, it will be very effective in reducing abuse. But if the patient stops the antagonist and then relapses to heroin, there is a possibility that the opiate will be even more dangerous than it was before the antagonist treatment: the tolerance that developed during prior opiate use (before the antagonist treatment) will have worn off, and renewed opiate use may produce serious problems, such as respiratory depression. Nutt and Lingford-Hughes (2008) discuss the advantages of a long-acting naltrexone implant, although they acknowledge that even this formulation would not eliminate the problems produced by rapid termination of antagonist exposure.

Antagonists of other abused drugs are available, notably the benzodiazepine antagonist flumazenil (Anexate, Romazicon). As yet this approach has not been used for treating benzodiazepine abuse. Naltrexone has been approved for treatment of alcohol addiction (Chapter 13), where it acts indirectly to block the action of endogenous opiates that are stimulated by drinking alcohol.

As Nutt and Lingford-Hughes (2008) note, a similar case could be made in regard to cannabis dependence. A number of potent and selective antagonists have been made for the CB_1 receptor. One of them, rimonabant (Acomplia), was approved for weight loss, but it was subsequently pulled off the market because of reports of depression and suicidality (Chapter 14). Since other cannabinoid antagonists and inverse agonists are currently under development, they may eventually be tested as medications for treating cannabis addiction (Beardsey and Thomas, 2005).

Withdrawal

Stress plays a prominent role in current views of addiction neurobiology, particularly in regard to the influence of withdrawal distress in promoting relapse. In some situations, as with stimulants, symptomatic support of the discomfort during drug termination is sufficient to maintain the patient during withdrawal. In other cases, such as in opiate or alcohol withdrawal, it is common to gradually reduce the substitution medication (methadone, buprenorphine, benzodiazepine) until withdrawal is complete. Specific symptoms such as tachycardia, sweating, runny nose, hair standing on end, and goosebumps (hence the term *going cold turkey*) are reduced by alpha-2-adrenergic agonist medications, such as clonidine or lofexidine, while other medications can be added to deal with insomnia or gastrointestinal (GI) disturbances, such as diarrhea (Nutt and Lingford-Hughes, 2008).

In a similar manner, the beta adrenergic receptor blocker propranolol has been beneficial for severe symptoms of cocaine withdrawal.

Propranolol appears to reduce anxiety and agitation and may lessen some of cocaine's rewarding aspects as well as craving. Several small trials have shown propranolol to improve abstinence rates of cocaine addicts. The main side effect is sedation.

Given the postulated role of prefrontal glutamate overactivity in driving the urge to relapse, it is especially notable that acamprosate (used clinically to maintain alcohol abstinence; Chapter 13) has been found, in animal models, to reduce glutamate overactivity or release in the nucleus accumbens and hippocampus during early ethanol withdrawal and to prevent associated toxicities (Mason and Heyser, 2010).

Targeting the Dopaminergic Mesolimbic System

Evidence from a variety of techniques, such as brain scans of humans (Volkow et al., 2004) and microdialysis of the brains of animals (Di Chiara, 2002), have shown that drugs of abuse such as nicotine, alcohol, and a variety of stimulants increase dopamine levels in the striatum of naive or nondependent subjects. As noted earlier, in some cases the increase in dopamine parallels the "high" experienced from drug ingestion, suggesting a direct effect of this neurotransmitter in mediating the positive effect of these drugs (Volkow et al., 1997). Therefore, clinically, it was hoped that by blocking this dopaminergic effect, the "high" would be reduced and the individual would then stop taking the drug. However, although dopamine antagonists (antipsychotic drugs) can block craving, they did not work clinically and their side effects were not tolerable.

Another option may be to *increase* dopamine as a way to substitute for the loss of the rewarding activation of dopamine. This has been effective in nicotine addiction, where the dopaminergic antidepressant bupropion has been a successful alternative to smoking (Dwoskin, et al., 2006). An alternative approach might be disulfiram (Antabuse), which is a traditional agent for treating alcoholism (Chapter 13). Disulfiram blocks an enzyme that is involved in alcohol metabolism. If alcohol is taken with disulfiram, the substance, acetaldehyde, is not metabolized; it builds up and produces an unpleasant reaction that presumably prevents subsequent alcohol use. However, it has been shown that disulfiram can also block dopamine β-hydroxylase in the brain, thereby increasing dopamine and depleting noradrenaline, both of which changes may be beneficial in stimulant dependence (Gaval-Cruz and Weinshenker, 2009). Disulfiram has shown promise in treating cocaine addiction; it is hypothesized that this may be due to its effects on the dopaminergic system, although clear evidence of this is needed (Preti, 2007). One disadvantage is that disulfiram also blocks the metabolism of cocaine as well as dopamine, which apparently increases the aversive anxiogenic effects of cocaine. If cocaine is abused with disulfiram, the combination could be dangerous (Kampman, 2008).

Targeting Nondopaminergic Neurotransmitter Systems

Pharmacotherapeutic approaches that act directly on the dopaminergic system have not been clinically successful; however, approaches targeting neurotransmitter systems that modulate the dopaminergic system are showing much greater promise.

GABAergic and Glutamatergic Systems. The dopaminergic cell bodies in the ventral tegmental area are under GABAergic control, and the GABA-B receptor is involved in this interaction (Cousins et al., 2002). GABA-B agonists, such as baclofen, can reduce the reinforcing effects of several different classes of abused drugs (for example, heroin, psychostimulants, alcohol) in animal models under a variety of conditions. Studies in humans have also shown baclofen to be promising in treating cocaine addiction and alcoholism (Nutt and Lingford-Hughes, 2008).

Other GABAergic medications being tested as possible agents for preventing cocaine relapse are anticonvulsants. One such drug is gamma-vinyl-GABA (vigabatrin), an anticonvulsant that blocks the enzyme that breaks down GABA. This drug had shown some benefit in small trials and was subsequently found to be effective in a randomized, placebo-controlled clinical trial (Brodie et al., 2009). Because it appears to cause visual field defects, it has not been approved for use in the United States. Tiagabine is an anticonvulsant that blocks one of the GABA transporters. In at least one small trial it also facilitated cocaine abstinence. The anticonvulsant topiramate has been tested in studies of cocaine abstinence and found to be modestly effective. This drug not only facilitates GABA function, it also inhibits glutamate neurotransmission by blocking AMPA receptors. It can cause sedation and memory problems and should not be used in persons with a history of kidney stones (Lingford-Hughes et al., 2004; Sofuoglu and Kosten, 2006; Johnson et al., 2007; Kampman, 2008).

Opioid System. Mu opioid receptors are also located on GABA neurons in the VTA, and they play a key role in modulating ventral tegmental area dopaminergic activity. A link between alcohol use and endogenous opioid activity was suggested by animal models, and the opioid antagonist naltrexone reduced alcohol self-administration by blocking this mu opioid receptor. Naltrexone has now been shown in several clinical trials in alcoholism to reduce the risk of a full-blown relapse (Pettinati et al., 2006). It does not work for everyone and may be most effective for people who are more severely alcohol dependent. Jayaram-Lindström and coworkers (2008) have shown that naltrexone may also promote abstinence from amphetamine. In fact, this drug has also been found to reduce the "rush" in people who have long histories of stealing, that is, kleptomaniacs (Grant et al., 2009). While this was a small study (only 25 people enrolled) and most participants were also on antidepressants, the result is consistent with the current view that both drug and nondrug addictions have a common underlying etiology.

Cannabinoid System. Cannabinoid-opiate interactions are gaining more attention in current concepts of addiction and reward mechanisms. There is increasing research on the role of this system in modulating the addictive properties of MDMA (ecstasy) (Robledo, 2010), nicotine (Maldonado and Berrendero, 2010), and alcohol (López-Moreno et al., 2010). As discussed by Parolaro and coworkers (2010), there are three primary aspects relevant to this model: (1) cannabinoids can release opioid peptides and opioids can release endocannabinoids; (2) when receptors for these two systems are both located on the same cells, there is evidence for direct receptor-receptor interaction; (3) there is an interaction between their intracellular pathways. For example, activation of either of these two systems produces a similar degree of relapse to alcohol in animal models of alcohol addiction. The cannabinoid-opioid relationship in the reward system might also differ from their interaction within other systems, such as the pain pathways. The possibility of differential interactions suggests new therapeutic approaches with cannabinoid or opioid antagonists as treatments for addiction.

New Directions

Vaccines are another promising therapy for relapse prevention. The approach works by stimulating the production of drug-specific antibodies (nicotine, opiates, cocaine, or amphetamine). If the drug is still used, the antibodies bind to the drug molecules in the blood and prevent them from crossing the blood-brain barrier, thereby blocking the euphoria produced in the brain and presumably decreasing further use. Progress has been most advanced with respect to a vaccine for nicotine addiction (Chapter 11), and one agent, NicVAX, is close to approval. Scientists have also created a vaccine against cocaine addiction. After several injections, it changes the body's chemistry so that the drug can't enter the brain and provide a high. One such vaccine, called TA-CD, has shown promise in a few initial trials (Kampman, 2008).

One disadvantage of vaccines is that, although the antibody may prevent drug molecules from reaching the brain and producing the "high," it does not reduce the drug craving that motivates abuse. This was illustrated in the clinical trial of TA-CD (Martell et al., 2009), in which 115 cocaine addicts were treated with the vaccine or placebo. The vaccine did improve abstinence rates over placebo. However, some of the addicts participating in the study started taking massive amounts of cocaine in hopes of overcoming the vaccine's effects. Nobody overdosed, but some of them had 10 times more cocaine coursing through their systems than researchers had encountered before, according to the lead investigator. Some of the addicts reported to researchers that they had gone broke buying cocaine from multiple drug dealers, hoping to find a variety that would get them high. An antibody for methamphetamine is currently in preclinical development (Peterson et al., 2008). Kinsey and coworkers (2009) have reviewed this area of pharmacotherapy for drug abuse.

One area of great interest suggested by the current neurobiological view of addiction is the possibility of using drugs that modify learning and memory to interfere with craving and to block relapse. In other words, if addiction develops from learning the association between drugs and environmental cues, then perhaps another drug could help the addict to *unlearn* addiction. This approach was supported by a study in rats, which were conditioned to go to a specific location for cocaine. When the rats were treated with an experimental drug (called CDPPB) that indirectly stimulated one type of metabotropic glutamate receptor, their preference for the cocaine-associated environment decreased during subsequent tests (Gass et al., 2009).

Neuroscientists have begun to recognize the implications of an impaired prefrontal cortex (which regulates long-term planning, decision making, and moral judgment). Researchers are now searching for ways to make these prefrontal systems more resilient. These approaches raise a question: Is drug use the cause of users' prefrontal problems, or do they have preexisting defects that make them susceptible to addiction? After all, a lot of people might be able to use drugs in a socially controlled manner, but only a certain percentage actually go on to become addicted. Perhaps part of the reason is that such people lack prefrontal-mediated control over behavior. In the protected environment of a rehabilitation center, drugs and other cues associated with drug taking are eliminated and stressful situations that suppress prefrontal activity are minimized. This environment, as much as any medication, provides the context in which prefrontal cortex function can be strengthened. Finally, religion has long been shown to have a strong inverse association with drug addiction. Some religious rituals have been found to provoke enhanced activity in prefrontal regions. It may be that the original insight behind Alcoholics Anonymous, of allowing oneself to be guided by a higher power, has a biological substrate in the frontal lobe (Schnabel, 2009).

However the argument is framed, just as an asthma attack can be triggered by smoke or a diabetic can have a reaction from eating too much sugar, a drug addict can be triggered to return to drug abuse. With other chronic diseases, relapse serves as a signal for returning to treatment. The same response is just as necessary with drug addiction.

As a chronic, recurring illness, addiction may require repeated treatments until abstinence is achieved. Like other diseases, drug addiction can be effectively treated and managed, leading to a healthy and productive life. To achieve long-term recovery, treatment must address specific, individual patient needs and must take the whole person into account. It is not enough simply to get a person off drugs; rather, the many changes that have occurred—physical, social, psychological—must also be addressed to help people stay off drugs, for good.

STUDY QUESTIONS

1. What types of drug abuse problems are currently of most concern, that is, which drugs and which populations?

2. Why might the evaluation of drug-reinforcing properties in animals be valuable in the assessment of human experiences?

3. Is a propensity for abusing drugs caused by a psychopathological process in the user, or is it a property of the particular drug?

4. What is the mechanism that underlies the behavioral reinforcing properties of abused drugs?

5. How does chronic drug use eventually become addiction?

6. What types of receptor-based approaches to the pharmacotherapy of drug abuse have been developed?

7. How has our understanding of the neurobiology of addiction led to new therapies?

REFERENCES

American Psychiatric Association. (2000). *Diagnostic and Statistical Manual of Mental Disorders*, 4th ed., text revision (DSM-IV-TR). Washington, DC: American Psychiatric Association.

Beardsey, P. M., and Thomas, B. F. (2005). "Current Evidence Supporting a Role of Cannabinoid CB1 Receptor (CB1R) Antagonists as Potential Pharmacotherapies for Drug Abuse Disorders." *Behavioral Pharmacology* 16: 275–296.

Bergman, J., and Paronis, C. A. (2006). "Measuring the Reinforcing Strength of Abused Drugs." *Molecular Interventions* 6: 273–284.

Briand, L. A., and Blendy, J.A. (2010). "Molecular and Genetic Substrates Linking Stress and Addiction." *Brain Research* 1314, Special Issue: 219–234.

Brodie, J. D., et al. (2009). "Randomized, Double-Blind, Placebo-Controlled Trial of Vigabatrin for the Treatment of Cocaine Dependence in Mexican Parolees." *American Journal of Psychiatry* 166: 1269–1277.

Cousins, M. S., et al. (2002). "GABA B Receptor Agonists for the Treatment of Drug Addiction: A Review of Recent Findings." *Drug and Alcohol Dependence* 65: 209–220.

Di Chiara, G (2002). "Nucleus Accumbens Shell and Core Dopamine: Differential Role in Behavior and Addiction." *Behavior Brain Research* 137: 75–114.

Dwoskin, L. P., et al. (2006). "Review of the Pharmacology and Clinical Profile of Bupropion, an Antidepressant and Tobacco Use Cessation Agent." *CNS Drug Reviews* 12: 178–207.

Feil, J., et al. (2010). "Addiction, Compulsive Drug Seeking, and the Role of Frontostriatal Mechanisms in Regulating Inhibitory Control." *Neuroscience and Biobehavioral Reviews*. In press.

Feltenstein, M. W., and See, R. E. (2008). "The Neurocircuitry of Addiction: An Overview." *British Journal of Pharmacology* 154: 261–274.

Feltenstein, M. W., et al. (2007). "Aripiprazole Blocks Reinstatement of Cocaine Seeking in an Animal Model of Relapse." *Biological Psychiatry* 61: 582–590.

Gass, J. T., et. al. (2009). "Positive Allosteric Modulation of mGluR5 Receptors Facilitates Extinction of a Cocaine Contextual Memory." *Biological Psychiatry* 65: 717–720.

Gaval-Cruz, M, and Weinshenker, D. (2009). "Mechanisms of Disulfiram-Induced Cocaine Abstinence: Antabuse and Cocaine Relapse." *Molecular Interventions* 9: 175–187.

Grant, J. E., et al. (2009). "A Double-Blind Placebo-Controlled Study of the Opiate Antagonist, Naltrexone, in the Treatment of Kleptomania." *Biological Psychiatry* 65: 600–606.

Herin, D. V., et al. (2010). "Agonist-Like Pharmacotherapy for Stimulant Dependence: Preclinical, Human Laboratory, and Clinical Studies." *Annals of the New York Academy of Sciences* 1187: 76–100.

Jayaram-Lindström, N., et al. (2008). "Naltrexone for the Treatment of Amphetamine Dependence: A Randomized, Placebo-Controlled Trial." *American Journal of Psychiatry* 165: 1442–1448.

Johnson, B. A., et al. (2007) "Topiramate for Treating Alcohol Dependence: A Randomized Controlled Trial." *Journal of the American Medical Association* 298: 1641–1651.

Kalivas, P. W. (2009). "The Glutamate Homeostasis Hypothesis of Addiction." *Nature Reviews Neuroscience* 10: 561–572.

Kalivas, P. W., and Volkow, N. D. (2005). "The Neural Basis of Addiction: A Pathology of Motivation and Choice." *American Journal of Psychiatry* 162: 1403–1413.

Kalivas, P. W., et al. (2006). "Animal Models and Brain Circuits in Drug Addiction." *Molecular Interventions* 6: 339–344.

Kampman, K. M. (2008). "The Search For Medications to Treat Stimulant Dependence." *Addiction Science and Clinical Practice* 4: 28–35.

Kinsey, B. M., et al. (2009). "Anti-Drug Vaccines to Treat Substance Abuse." *Immunology and Cell Biology* 87: 309–314.

Koob, G. F., and Volkow, N. D. (2010). "Neurocircuitry of Addiction." *Neuropsychopharmacology Reviews* 35: 217–238.

Lingford-Hughes, A. R., et al. (2004). "Evidence-Based Guidelines for the Pharmacological Management of Substance Misuse, Addiction and Comorbidity." *Journal of Psychopharmacology* 18: 293–335.

López-Moreno, J. A., et al. (2010). "Functional Interactions Between Endogenous Cannabinoid and Opioid Systems: Focus on Alcohol, Genetics and Drug-Addicted Behaviors." *Current Drug Targets* 11: 406–428.

Maldonado R., and Berrendero, F. (2010). "Endogenous Cannabinoid and Opioid Systems and Their Role in Nicotine Addiction." *Current Drug Targets* 11: 440–449.

Martell, B. A., et al. (2009). "Cocaine Vaccine for the Treatment of Cocaine Dependence in Methadone-Maintained Patients. A Randomized, Double-Blind, Placebo-Controlled Efficacy Trial." *Archives of General Psychiatry* 66: 1116–1123.

Mason, B. J., and Heyser, C. J. (2010). "The Neurobiology, Clinical Efficacy and Safety of Acamprosate in the Treatment of Alcohol Dependence." *Expert Opinion on Drug Safety* 9: 177–188.

Nestler, E. (2005). "Is There a Common Molecular Pathway for Addiction?" *Nature Neuroscience* 8: 1449.

NICE. (2007). Methadone and Buprenorphine for the Management of Opioid Dependence (NICE Technology Appraisal Guidance 114). London: National Institute for Health and Clinical Excellence.

Nutt, D., and Lingford-Hughes, A (2008). "Addiction: The Clinical Interface." *British Journal of Pharmacology* 154: 397–405.

Parolaro, D., et al. (2010). "Cellular Mechanisms Underlying the Interaction Between Cannabinoid and Opiate System." *Current Drug Targets* 11: 393–405.

Peterson, E. C., et al. (2008). "Development and Preclinical Testing of a High-Affinity Single-Chain Antibody Against (+)-Methamphetamine." *Journal of Pharmacology and Experimental Therapeutics* 325: 124–133.

Pettinati, H. M., et al. (2006). "The Status of Naltrexone in the Treatment of Alcohol Dependence: Specific Effects on Heavy Drinking." *Journal of Clinical Psychopharmacology* 26: 610–625.

Pierce, R. C., and Kumaresan, V. (2006). "The Mesolimbic Dopamine System: The Final Common Pathway for the Reinforcing Effect of Drugs of Abuse?" *Neuroscience Biobehavioral Reviews* 30: 215–238.

Piper, M. E., et al. (2009). "A Randomized Placebo-Controlled Clinical Trial of 5 Smoking Cessation Pharmacotherapies." *Archives of General Psychiatry* 66: 1253–1262.

Preti, A. (2007). "New Developments in the Pharmacotherapy of Cocaine Abuse." *Addiction Biology* 12: 133–151.

Reichel, C. M., et al. (2009). "Bupropion Attenuates Methamphetamine Self-Administration in Adult Male Rats." *Drug and Alcohol Dependence* 100: 54–62.

Robledo, P. (2010). "Cannabinoids, Opioids and MNDA: Neuropsychological Interactions Related to Addiction." *Current Drug Targets* 11: 429–439.

Schnabel, J. (2009). "Rethinking Rehab." *Nature* 458: 25–27.

Schnoll, R. A., et al. (2010). "Effectiveness of Extended-Duration Transdermal Nicotine Therapy: A Randomized Trial." *Annals of Internal Medicine* 152: 144–151.

Sofuoglu, M., and Kosten, T. R. (2006). Emerging Pharmacological Strategies in the Fight Against Cocaine Addiction. *Expert Opinion on Emerging Drugs* 11: 91–98.

Steensland, P., et al. (2007). "Varenicline, an $\alpha_4\beta_2$ Nicotinic Acetylcholine Receptor Partial Agonist, Selectively Decreases Ethanol Consumption and Seeking." *Proceedings of the National Academy of Sciences USA* 104: 12518–12523.

Tiihonen, J., et al. (2007). "A Comparison of Aripiprazole, Methylphenidate, and Placebo for Amphetamine Dependence." *American Journal of Psychiatry* 164: 160–162.

Vargas-Perez, H., et al. (2009). "Ventral Tegmental Area BDNF Induces an Opiate-Dependent–Like Reward State in Naïve Rats." *Science* 324: 1732–1734.

Volkow, N. D., et al. (1997). "Relationship Between Subjective Effects of Cocaine and Dopamine Transporter Occupancy." *Nature* 386: 827–830.

Volkow, N. D., et al. (2004). "The Addicted Human Brain Viewed in the Light of Imaging Studies: Brain Circuits and Treatment Strategies." *Neuropharmacology* 47, Supplement 1: 3–13.

Volkow, N. D., et al. (2006). "Cocaine Cues and Dopamine in Dorsal Striatum: Mechanism of Craving in Cocaine Addiction." *Journal of Neuroscience* 26: 6583–6588.

Psychopharmacology for Special Populations

Chapters 4 through 8 of this text covered the pharmacology of medications used to treat psychological disorders such as depression, bipolar disorder, psychosis, insomnia, and the various anxiety disorders. Chapter 12 covered the pharmacology of the amphetamines—medications not only subject to compulsive abuse but also widely used to treat attention deficit/hyperactivity disorder. In the following chapters, we discuss the use of these and other medications in special populations and circumstances.

Chapter 18 discusses use of psychotherapeutic medications in pregnant women, in preschool-aged children, and in older children and adolescents. In recent years, this area of research and therapeutics has increased remarkably. In these as in other populations, pharmacotherapy must be interpreted in light of accurate assessment and diagnosis, combined with appropriate psychotherapeutic interventions.

Chapter 19 discusses the use of psychoactive medications in the geriatric population. Medication therapies are widely employed in the treatment of Parkinson's disease, the dementias, and major depressive disorder. Both the overuse and the underuse of medicines need discussion.

Finally, the text concludes with a discussion of what is currently considered to be the optimal approach to comprehensive therapy of patients with mental health disorders—namely, the combination of pharmacotherapies and psychological therapies in patient care. The pharmacology of psychotherapeutic drugs has been covered in earlier chapters, so Chapter 20 discusses the total needs of patients with mental health disorders. After all, this is what mental health therapeutics is all about: achieving optimal therapy for a given patient to enable the patient to experience the best quality of life that we, as mental health providers, can offer.

Chapter 18

Child and Adolescent Psychopharmacology

The United States is currently experiencing a silent epidemic of mental illness among youth and teenagers. According to the National Comorbidity Survey (Kessler et al., 2005), half of all lifetime serious adult psychiatric illnesses start by 14 years of age, and three-fourths of them are present by 25 years of age. Delays between initial diagnosis and treatment are common. The median delay across disorders is nearly a decade; the longest delays are 20 to 23 years for patients with anxiety disorders, 10 years for patients with mood disorders. However, the majority of mental illnesses in young people go unrecognized and untreated, leaving youth vulnerable to emotional, social, and academic impairments during a critical phase in their lives (Friedman, 2006). In total, about 14 to 25 percent of youths endure a mental disorder during their upbringing; yet among youth and adolescents who need mental health services, 67 percent receive no services, diagnosis, or treatment, at least until the disorder is deeply entrenched and difficult to treat (Costello et al., 2007). According to a recent survey, one in eight children had a mental health disorder at the time of the survey, but only half were being treated (Merikangas et al., 2010). All this despite the fact that mental health disorders are the chronic disorders of young people! Data are quite clear that youth with untreated childhood and adolescent mental health disorders carry the disorder into adulthood and function poorly as adults.

Psychological disorders affecting children and adolescents include anxiety disorders, depression, attention deficit/hyperactivity disorder

(ADHD), schizophrenia, bipolar disorder, eating disorders, disruptive or explosive behavioral disorders, and autism spectrum disorders. Although focus traditionally has been on the effects of prescribed medications on school-aged children and adolescents, today increasing focus is on preschool-aged children and on intrauterine effects when a pregnant female either does or does not take medication for her own mental health disorder. Therefore, this chapter is presented in three parts:

1. Pregnancy and psychotropic drugs
2. Preschool psychopharmacology
3. Child and adolescent psychopharmacology

PREGNANCY AND PSYCHOTROPIC DRUGS

> It should be kept in mind that no psychotropic drug is approved by the FDA for use during pregnancy. Furthermore, no decision (to treat or not to treat) is risk-free and no decision is perfect. (Cohen, 2007, pp. 4–5)

In 2008, the American College of Obstetricians and Gynecologists (ACOG) published a clinical guideline on the use of psychoactive medications during pregnancy and lactation (ACOG Committee on Practice Bulletins–Obstetrics, 2008). They noted that more than 500,000 pregnancies in the United States each year occur in women who have a psychiatric illness that either predates or emerges during pregnancy, and one-third of all pregnant women are exposed to a psychotropic medication at some point during their pregnancy. If the mother takes psychoactive medicines frequently, is there a potential for the medication to injure the fetus (resulting in birth defects or, later in life, in developmental problems)? On the other hand, are there fetal developmental problems that might follow if the mother's mental health disorder goes untreated? Quite a dilemma. By definition, a psychoactive medication crosses the blood-brain barrier and reaches the brain. The blood-brain barrier is the most resistant of all body barriers to drug distribution (Chapter 1), and the placental barrier is the easiest to cross. Therefore, as a general rule, *the fetus will have about the same blood level of drug as does the mother.* Therefore, risks of medication include the following:

- Risk of potential teratogenic (structural) damage if the mother continues medications during pregnancy
- Risk of postnatal behavioral abnormalities resulting from medications administered to the mother during pregnancy
- Risk of perinatal syndromes or neonatal toxicity if a breast-feeding mother continues medications following pregnancy

On the other hand, untreated maternal illness may result in the following:

- Poor compliance with prenatal care
- Inadequate nutrition
- Exposure to undesired drugs, medications, or herbals
- Increased alcohol, caffeine, and tobacco use
- Deficits in mother-infant bonding
- Disruptions in the family environment

Table 18.1 lists some of the complications of a mother's untreated illness on pregnancy outcome.

Certainly, cigarettes (Stroud et al., 2009; U.S. Preventive Services Task Force, 2009a) and alcohol (Sayal et al., 2009) are contraindicated during pregnancy because of adverse fetal outcomes (see also Chapters 11 and 13). Even caffeine is problematic, since intake as low as 100 to

TABLE 18.1 Impact of untreated illness on pregnancy outcome

Disorder	Obstetric	Neonatal	Options
Anxiety disorders	Long labor, fetal distress, preterm labor, spontaneous abortion	Reduced developmental scores, slowed mental development	SSRIs Psychological therapies
Depression and dysthymia	Low birth weight, reduced fetal growth, postnatal complications Hippocampus shrinks	Increased stress hormone levels, reduced bonding, small size and low weight, etc.	SSRIs Psychological therapies Omega-3 fatty acids ECT
Bipolar disorder	Similar to major depression	Similar to major depression	Lithium Anticonvulsants Antipsychotics Omega-3 fatty acids
Schizophrenia	Preterm, low weight, small Placenta abnormalities	Increased rate of postnatal death	Antipsychotics

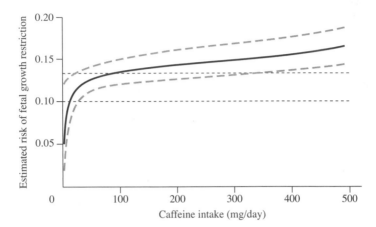

FIGURE 18.1   Relation between the risk of fetal growth restriction and caffeine intake (mg/day) during pregnancy. Horizontal black dashed lines mark the average risk of fetal growth restriction (10 percent) and average risk in the study cohort (13 percent). The solid black line represents the average, with 95 percent confidence levels shown above and below it by the dashed gray lines. [From CARE Study Group (2008), Figure 1.]

200 mg/day (one to three cups of coffee) can result in fetal growth restriction (Figure 18.1) (CARE Study Group, 2008). Sowell and coworkers (2010) demonstrated the neonatal toxicity associated with maternal use of methamphetamine.

Antidepressants in the Pregnant Female and Neonatal Outcomes

Depression, dysthymia, and anxiety disorders are common disorders in women of childbearing age. Many women with these disorders are treated with antidepressant medication, primarily with selective serotonin reuptake inhibitors (SSRIs). Given that 50 percent of pregnancies are unplanned, the effect of these medications on the developing fetus, especially in the first three months of pregnancy, is a potential major public health concern.

In 2009, a collaborative effort by ACOG and the American Psychiatric Association resulted in development of algorithms for the treatment of women with depression who are either contemplating pregnancy or already pregnant (Yonkers et al., 2009). The organizations concluded that adequate treatment is essential, preferably beginning before conception. Women with severe, recurrent depression who stop medication are at high risk for relapse, and depression during pregnancy raises the risk of postpartum depression. As reported by Cohen and coworkers (2006), women who discontinued their

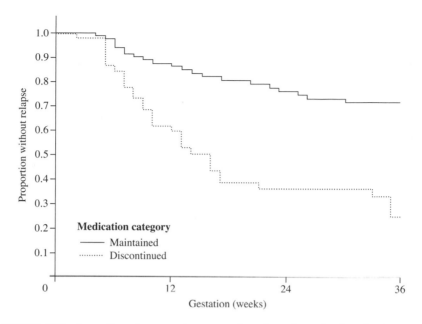

FIGURE 18.2 Proportion of pregnant women who relapsed to episodes of major depression during their pregnancy. Solid line indicates risk of relapse when women remained on their medication. Dotted line indicates relapse in women who discontinued medication during pregnancy. The latter had a fivefold increased risk of relapse over the course of their pregnancy compared with women who maintained their medication. [Adapted from Cohen et al. (2006), p. 505.]

antidepressant medication relapsed significantly more frequently over the course of their pregnancy compared with women who stayed on their medication (Figure 18.2). Pregnancy is not protective against either depression or dysthymia (Parry, 2009; Wisner et al., 2009). Untreated major depression often results in severe depressive disorders as well as substance abuse, both of which can be detrimental to the developing fetus.

In total, about 8 percent of pregnant women will be exposed to antidepressants during their pregnancy. This raises questions as to the teratogenicity of antidepressants as well as the possibility of adverse long-term neurobehavioral outcomes (Buhimschi and Weiner, 2009).[1] By the year 2000, most SSRI-type antidepressants were thought to be nonteratogenic. However, in January 2006, the Food and Drug Administration (FDA) issued a warning that paroxetine (Paxil) used in the first trimester might increase the incidence of congenital malformations, primarily

---

[1]Teratogenicity refers to structural defects in the neonate as a result of maternal drug intake.

cardiac defects. In December 2006, ACOG advised against using paroxetine during pregnancy. Pedersen and coworkers (2009) extended this warning to sertraline (Zoloft) and citalopram (Celexa), although the increase in incidence of congenital malformations attributed to these drugs was small, becoming significant only when the mother was taking more than one antidepressant. Use of fluoxetine resulted in the smallest increase in incidence. Ramos and coworkers (2008), in examining the extensive literature on the teratogenicity of antidepressants, concluded that data "do not support an association between duration of antidepressant use during the first trimester of pregnancy and major congenital malformations in the offspring of women with psychiatric disorders" (p. 344). However, because of a possible association of paroxetine use and heart defects, it might be wise to avoid this drug during the first trimester of pregnancy.

Recent reports have identified the presence of SSRI discontinuation syndrome in the newborn offspring of mothers who used SSRI-type antidepressants in the third trimester of pregnancy (Oberlander et al., 2008; Alwan and Friedman, 2009). Following delivery, classic signs of SSRI withdrawal have been observed: irritability with constant crying, sleep disturbances, hyperactive reflexes, breathing and feeding difficulties, and so on. (This condition is sometimes misdiagnosed as severe colic.) One suggestion is to switch the mother from her SSRI to fluoxetine (Prozac) as soon as pregnancy is confirmed and then stop the fluoxetine at about seven months of gestation, allowing the infant to detoxify in utero. During this period (the seventh to ninth month of pregnancy), the mother can be treated with nonpharmacological psychological interventions and perhaps omega-3 fatty acids (Su et al., 2008).

In sum, as stated by Parry (2009), "from the evidence available to date, the risks of an untreated maternal depression are far greater than the risks of serious adverse sequelae from antidepressant medication" (pp. 512–513).

Mood Stabilizers in the Pregnant Female and Neonatal Outcomes

Freeman (2007) stated:

> Untreated maternal mood disorders during pregnancy are serious risk factors for the fetus. . . . Untreated mania poses clear risks to the individual due to impulsivity and impaired judgment. Mania often results in poor self-care, which is dangerous to both mother and child. (p. 1771)

Untreated bipolar disorder in the pregnant female is associated with relapse to drug and alcohol abuse, manic episodes, and interpersonal life disruptions. Viguera and coworkers (2007a) reported that overall the risk of a bipolar episode during pregnancy is 71 percent, and the risk is two times greater if the woman discontinues medication rather than maintaining it. If medication is stopped, the time to first recurrence is four times shorter than if she stays on medication, and the proportion of weeks spent in bipolar episodes is five times greater (Figure 18.3).

Quite a lot is known about the teratogenicity of mood-stabilizing medications (Chapter 8).

Lithium is recognized as a modest teratogen, with a potential for causing cardiac malformations at a greater rate than the rate in pregnant females not taking lithium (Nguyen et al., 2009). If lithium is absolutely necessary during pregnancy, doses should be minimized and the fetus closely followed by echocardiography. During periods of breast-feeding, some lithium is transferred to the infant. Maternal serum, breast milk, and infant concentrations of lithium averaged 0.76, 0.35, and 0.16 mEq/L, respectively, each lithium level lower than the preceding level by approximately one-half (Viguera et al., 2007b). No significant adverse outcomes were reported.

Valproic acid (Depakote) is associated with the highest rate of major congenital malformations, with a relative risk estimated to be up to 16 percent compared to about 2.9 percent in infants of nonmedicated females (Nguyen et al., 2009; Tomson and Battino, 2009). In addition, use of valproic acid during pregnancy has been associated with

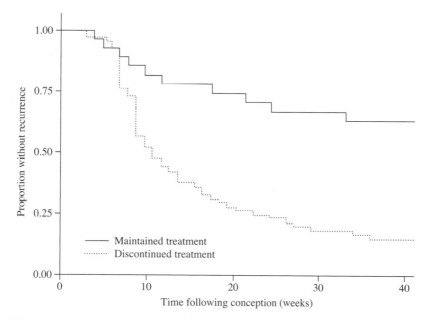

FIGURE 18.3 Proportion of pregnant women with bipolar disorder who relapsed to bipolar episodes during their pregnancy. Solid line indicates risk of relapse when women remained on their medication. Dotted line indicates relapse in women who discontinued medication during pregnancy. Mean time to first recurrence from the date of conception was greater than 41 weeks when treatment was maintained and only 9 weeks when treatment was discontinued. [From Viguera et al. (2007a), p. 1821.]

impaired cognitive functioning at three years of age in offspring, with an IQ 9 points lower than that of children exposed to lamotrigine (Meador et al., 2009; Banach et al., 2010). Recent evidence has been reported that exposure of the fetus to valproic acid increases the risk for autism spectrum disorders (Bromley et al., 2008). Incidence rates for autism spectrum disorders ranged from < 1 percent in control children to 6 percent with valproic acid monotherapy. The FDA has concluded that pregnant women should use valproic acid only if it is essential to manage their medical condition and only if they have been adequately warned of its potential for causing harm. A recent practice parameter reinforces the potential of valproic acid to result in major congenital malformations and adverse cognitive outcomes (Harden et al., 2010).

Carbamazepine (Tegretol, Equitro) is considered to be slightly teratogenic, increasing the incidence of adverse fetal outcomes by about 3 percent more than that seen in nonmedicated females. Interestingly, abnormal effects on postnatal growth and development have not been reported for its close structural derivative oxcarbazepine (Trileptal).

Lamotrigine (Lamictal) is not considered to be a major teratogen, although a slightly increased incidence of cleft lip and cleft palate has been reported. The mean lamotrigine concentration in breast milk was 41 percent of the maternal level; the mean fetal blood concentration was 18 percent of the maternal level and about 50 percent of the concentration in breast milk. No adverse events were observed in breast-fed infants (Newport et al., 2008a). Newport and coworkers (2008b) concluded that "Discontinuing mood stabilizer treatment presents high risks of bipolar recurrence among pregnant women. Lamotrigine may afford protective effects in pregnancy, and its reported fetal safety compares favorably to other agents used to manage bipolar disorder" (p. 432).

Topiramate (Topamax), whether used in the treatment of epilepsy, bipolar disorder, borderline personality disorder, or migraine headache, has been associated with an increase in major congenital malformations, although the number of pregnancies studied is small (Hunt et al., 2008). Oral clefts and penile malformations in male infants occurred at a rate of about 11 times the control rate. Larger sample numbers are needed before broader interpretations can be made.

Limited data to date on *gabapentin* (Neurontin) and *pregabalin* (Lyrica) do not indicate that they are major teratogens (Einarson, 2009).

Atypical Antipsychotics in the Pregnant Female and Neonatal Outcomes

As detailed in Chapter 4, atypical antipsychotic drugs are used to treat schizophrenia, bipolar disorder, posttraumatic stress disorder, borderline personality disorder, and other mental health disorders, many of which occur in women of childbearing years who might be exposed to these drugs during their pregnancy.

Typical antipsychotics have long been used in early pregnancy to treat pregnancy-associated nausea and vomiting. These drugs were not associated with major teratogenic consequences, although a few infants were born with cardiac defects (Reis and Kallen, 2008). The mother's increased risk of developing gestational diabetes was also identified. Einarson and Boskovic (2009), performing a separate analysis, concluded that "to date, no definitive association has been found between use of (typical) antipsychotic drugs during pregnancy and an increased risk of birth defects or other adverse outcomes" (p. 183). The authors concluded that these drugs should not be discontinued in the treatment of major psychiatric disorders in pregnant women because the risks of discontinuation may outweigh any risks of medication continuation.

Newham and coworkers (2008) compared offspring of mothers who ingested either *clozapine* (Clozaril) or *olanzapine* (Zyprexa) during pregnancy with offspring of mothers who ingested traditional antipsychotic medicines during their pregnancy. Thirty-one percent of infants exposed to clozapine or olanzapine were large for gestational age and had birth weights heavier than those exposed to traditional agents. These infants were thought to be at risk of or predisposed to heavy weight and perhaps to diabetes later in life.

Coppola and coworkers (2007) studied the delivery outcome of infants exposed to *risperidone* (Risperdol) during pregnancy. The incidence of congenital malformations and spontaneous abortions paralled the rates in control infants. When exposed to risperidone in the third trimester of pregnancy, the majority of the infants displayed tremor, jitteriness, irritability, feeding problems, and somnolence. These symptoms may represent a withdrawal syndrome. The authors concluded that risperidone should be used during pregnancy only if the benefits outweigh the potential risks.

Newport and coworkers (2007) examined placental passage of several atypical antipsychotics from maternal to placental blood. Placental passage was highest for *olanzapine* (72 percent), followed by *haloperidol* (65 percent), *risperidone* (49 percent), and *quetiapine* (24 percent). There was a trend toward lower birth weights in newborns whose mothers were treated with quetiapine (Seroquel).

In a case report, Werremeyer (2009) reported that a male infant was born without complication to a mother who took *ziprasidone* (Geodon) and citalopram (Celexa) during pregnancy and that his development to age six months was normal. This, to date, is the only report of ziprasidone use in pregnancy. Lutz and coworkers (2010) reported successful neonatal outcome in a single case report of a woman who took aripiprazole (Abilify) during her pregnancy and throughout breast-feeding.

Gentile (2008) reviewed the issue of safety in infants who breast-fed from mothers who were taking atypical antipsychotic medicines. The ACOG clinical guideline on the use of psychoactive medications during pregnancy and lactation (ACOG Committee on Practice Bulletins–Obstetrics, 2008) concluded:

> There is little evidence to suggest that atypical antipsychotics are associated with elevated risks for neonatal toxicity or somatic teratogenesis. No long-term neurobehavioral studies of exposed children have yet been conducted. Therefore, their routine use during pregnancy and lactation cannot be recommended.

PRESCHOOL PSYCHOPHARMACOLOGY

Prior to 2007, there were scant research or practice guidelines for the use of psychopharmacology for very young children. In late 2007, Gleason and coworkers (2007) reviewed the topic and described recommended algorithms for medication use in children aged five and younger. The goal was "to promote responsible treatment of young children, recognizing that this will sometimes involve the use of medication" (p. 1532). This review was followed in 2009 by the first textbook relevant to the topic (Luby and Riddle, 2009) and an updated review of what is currently known about mental health disorders in preschoolers (Fanton and Gleason, 2009). Preschool children with severe mental health problems present a dilemma for prescribers when they do not respond to nonmedication interventions (Luby, 2010). A professional must weigh the potential risks of medication with the risks of not intervening. The focus is on young children with moderate to severe symptoms and functional impairments. Psychopharmacological interventions are not indicated for preschoolers with only mild or single-content symptoms or impairment. In the algorithms presented in the review by Gleason and coworkers (2007), step 1 of each algorithm begins with a diagnostic assessment, step 2 is diagnosis (which generally drives treatment planning), step 3 is development of nonpharmacological treatments, and step 4 is consideration of pharmacological treatment. Tandon and Luby (2010) have also presented algorithms for the psychopharmacological treatment of preschool children with mental health issues.

Medications for Treating Attention Deficit/Hyperactivity Disorder in Very Young Children

Attention deficit/hyperactivity disorder has been well studied in school-aged children, adolescents, and adults. Only recently has there been focus on ADHD in preschoolers (Maayan et al., 2009). ADHD can present during the preschool years and persist into adulthood (Vaughan et al., 2008). Accurate diagnosis requires adaptation of the current diagnostic criteria to account for differences in symptomatology across the life span. Indeed, in a study of 303 preschoolers (3 to 5.5 years of age) with moderate to severe ADHD, 70 percent experienced comorbid disorders, with oppositional defiant disorder, communication disorders, or anxiety disorders being most common (Posner et al., 2007). The differential diagnosis of ADHD and the pattern of psychiatric comorbidity vary with each age group and complicate diagnosis and management. To maximize outcomes, clinicians must be able to accurately identify ADHD in preschoolers and develop comprehensive, collaborative treatment plans.

The Preschool ADHD Treatment Study (PATS) first demonstrated the potential utility of methylphenidate for treating ADHD in preschoolers (Greenhill et al., 2006). At an average daily dose of 14 milligrams (range = 7.5 to 30 mg/day, divided into three daily increments), immediate-release methylphenidate produced significant reductions on ADHD symptom scales, although efficacy was less than that cited for school-aged children (see also Abrikoff et al., 2009). If effective, a discontinuation trial should be initiated after 6 months for reassessment. If ineffective, a trial of d-amphetamine or Adderall should be considered, although few controlled trials are available to show efficacy. In a 10-month continuation phase of the PATS study, with gradual dose increases, efficacy could be maintained, but significant variability was observed, with many participants dropping out of the study because of adverse effects or the worsening of behavior (Vitiello et al., 2007). As an alternative to immediate-release methylphenidate, Maayan and coworkers (2009) studied "beaded methylphenidate" (discussed below) as an alternative. The authors noted that although the prolonged-action preparation was quite effective in reducing symptoms, dosing flexibility was limited (a common 10-mg oral dose being either too low, thus failing to achieve good results, or too high, thus leading to adverse effects in this population).

Although data on the preschool population is lacking, it is generally concluded that if a child does not respond to one stimulant class (e.g., methylphenidate), then switching to another class (e.g., amphetamines) is recommended (Ghuman et al., 2008). If stimulants result in a lack of efficacy or the emergence of undesirable side effects, a trial of atomoxetine (Strattera) (Ghuman et al., 2009) or an alpha-agonist medication such as guanfacine (Intuniv) should be considered.

Medications for Treating Disruptive Behaviors in Very Young Children

Hirshfeld-Becker and coworkers (2007) studied behavioral disinhibition in preschoolers and described it as a temperamental antecedent of disruptive behavioral disorders and their comorbidity with mood disorders in middle childhood, which may be targeted for preventive intervention. Pharmacological interventions were not addressed. Currently, there is a complete absence of evidence (no controlled trials) for the efficacy of medication in preschoolers with obsessive-compulsive disorder, conduct disorder, or disruptive behavioral disorders (DBD) who do not have comorbid mental retardation or a pervasive developmental disorder (including autism). Risperidone can be considered in preschoolers with DBD with severe aggression without ADHD. The use of antipsychotic drugs in very young children was reviewed by Olfson and coworkers (2010), with an editorial by Egger (2010). Not endorsed are medication without accompanying psychotherapy, use of medications as chemical restraints, or use of medication "as needed." In discussing their results, Olfson and coworkers (2010) stated:

> It is widely recommended that children presenting for mental health care receive comprehensive and developmentally sensitive mental health assessments and trials of relevant psychosocial treatments before consideration is given to psychotropic medications. . . . However, most very young children in the present study did not receive a mental health assessment, a psychiatrist visit, or a single session of psychotherapy during the year in which they received antipsychotic medications. (p. 21)

Medications for Treating Depression in Very Young Children

Childhood depression is a serious and relapsing psychiatric disorder. However, until recently, studies have focused on school-aged children and adolescents. In a study of 306 preschoolers, aged three to six, depression symptoms were common, and in 40 percent of the children persisted for the 24 months of follow-up study (Luby et al., 2009a, 2009b). Depression was most common in children with a depressed mother, a mother who had another mood disorder, or a mother who had experienced a traumatic event. Young children were not too emotionally immature to experience depression. Depressed children appear sad even when playing; games may have themes of death or other somber topics; appetite loss, sleep problems, temper tantrums, grumpiness, and high levels of shame and maladaptive guilt are present (Figure 18.4). The authors did not address treatment: psychotherapy rather than medication is usually the first choice (Luby, 2009).

Chapter 5 presented current concepts of brain pathology underlying depression, including hippocampal damage resulting from the lack of neurotropic proteins. Rao and coworkers (2010) reported that similar pathology occurs in youths and places a person at risk of developing a depressive disorder. The authors concluded that "early-life adversity

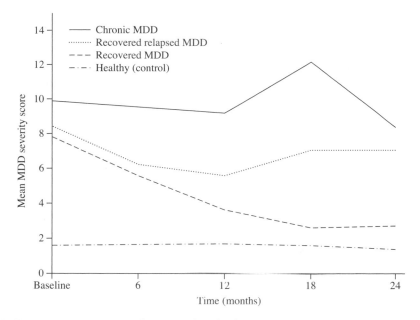

FIGURE 18.4 Mean major depressive disorder (MDD) severity scores in three groups of youth with MDD (chronic; recovered, then relapsed; and recovered) compared with healthy, nondepressed control youths; 24-month time scale is from age 3 to age 5. [Modified from Luby et al. (2009a), p. 903, Figure 3.]

may interact with genetic vulnerability to induce hippocampal changes, potentially increasing the risk for depressive disorder" (page 357).

Medications for Treating Bipolar Disorder in Very Young Children

Bipolar disorder is well described in school-aged children and adolescents; there is no clear consensus that it occurs in preschoolers. Clinically, it tends to be associated with aggressive medication therapies, often with poor diagnosis when not accompanied by psychotherapeutic/social assistance. Chief features are elation, grandiosity, and hypersexuality with impaired functioning. Safest are psychotherapeutic interventions such as parent-child interaction therapy (Luby et al., 2008; Luby et al., 2009c).

Psychopharmacological interventions might be considered in cases of significant impairment and distress associated with signs of serious mood and behavioral dysregulation. However, the literature is scant, and there have been no controlled studies in preschoolers. Generally, the medications used to treat bipolar disorder in older children and adolescents (discussed later) may be tried as treatment for preschool bipolar disorder.

Medications for Treating Anxiety Disorders in Very Young Children

Guidelines for treating preschool anxiety disorders tend to group together situational anxiety disorder, generalized anxiety disorder, selective mutism, and specific phobias. Guidelines deal with posttraumatic stress disorder (PTSD) and obsessive-compulsive disorder (OCD) individually. There are no guidelines for panic disorder because of insufficient evidence that it even exists in preschool children. For non-PTSD, non-OCD anxiety disorders in preschoolers, behavioral therapy techniques and cognitive therapies are valuable. Treatment is continued for at least three months before considering medication. Parental psychiatric assessment may be valuable and necessary. For non-PTSD, non-OCD anxiety disorders in preschoolers, the entire pharmacological literature comprises only three case reports. Fluoxetine may be the first choice for pharmacological treatment of preschool anxiety (empirical evidence only). A trial of discontinuation after six to nine months of therapy has been suggested. Benzodiazepines are not recommended (because of cognitive impairments) except for short-term medical/dental procedures. It is essential to concurrently examine parental psychopathology (Kennedy et al., 2009; Schechter and Willheim, 2009).

PTSD is common in preschoolers and difficult to treat. There is strong evidence in support of psychotherapeutic intervention in preschool PTSD. Medication is not endorsed by the experts; however, according to surveys, only 11 percent of providers reported that they *do not* use medication for preschool PTSD (thus, 89 percent did). Here, experts differ from practitioners. Again, benzodiazepines are not recommended.

There is little research on *OCD* in preschoolers. It can present with extremely rigid behavior patterns, which can cause much functional distress and impairment. Psychoeducation, cognitive therapies, and exposure therapies are useful. In the section of this chapter on school-aged children and adolescents, we will discuss the Pediatric Obsessive-Compulsive Treatment Study (POTS) and extrapolate from it that SSRIs are efficacious and can be combined with cognitive therapies. However, SSRIs should be considered as the treatment of last resort, and SSRI treatment should always occur in the context of ongoing cognitive and/or behavioral interventions.

Medications for Treating Pervasive Developmental Disorders in Very Young Children

Autism must present before age three, and other pervasive developmental disorders (PDDs) are also typically recognized by 3 years of age. Treatment is multimodal and multidisciplinary. A 40-child study

(2 to 9 years of age) with risperidone showed a 63 percent positive response rate in controlling irritability and behaviors associated with autism. Risperidone has been approved by the FDA for children age 5 and over for behaviors associated with autism. The FDA has similarly approved aripiprazole for the treatment of irritability associated with autism in children ages 6 to 17.

PSYCHOPHARMACOLOGY FOR SCHOOL-AGED CHILDREN AND ADOLESCENTS

In September 2009, the American Academy of Child and Adolescent Psychiatry published a clinical practice guideline on the use of psychotropic medication in children and adolescents (Walkup and the American Academy of Child and Adolescent Psychiatry, 2009). Following are some of the principles delineated:

- Before initiating psychotherapy, complete a psychiatric evaluation.
- When appropriate, include a history and medical evaluation in the treatment.
- Communicate with other professionals to obtain a history and set the stage for monitoring outcome and side effects.
- Before prescribing, develop psychosocial and medication plans.
- Develop a plan for outcome monitoring, both short and long term.
- Proceed with caution if no monitoring is involved.
- Educate all about the treatment plan.
- Document assent of the child and consent of the parents.
- Focus on risks and benefits of medications as well as alternatives to medication.
- Implement a medication trial using an adequate dose for an adequate duration.
- Reassess the treatment plan if there is no response to the initial trial of medication.
- Develop a specific plan if there is a medication discontinuation trial.

Medications for Treating Autism Spectrum Disorders

Autism is a pervasive developmental disorder characterized by severe impairment in several areas of development, including deficits in social interactions and communication skills as well as the presence of stereotyped behavior, interests, and activities. The incidence of diagnosed cases of autism is increasing, affecting about 1 percent of children.

The use of psychotropic drugs targeted to possible neurochemical systems involved in the pathophysiology of autism has often been shown to reduce aggression, self-injurious behaviors, anxiety, repetitive behaviors, mood dysregulation, hyperactivity, impulsiveness, and other maladaptive behaviors. Physical aggression and self-injurious behaviors are especially problematic in adolescents, whose large size and physical strength create additional danger. Medications can be quite useful in reducing the intensity and frequency of these behaviors.

Historically, antidepressants were used in attempts to reduce the anxiety and agitation associated with autism. Indeed, until recently, SSRIs were a mainstay of treatment. However, two reports (King et al., 2009; Volkmar, 2009) of large, well-controlled studies demonstrated the lack of efficacy of citalopram (Celexa) accompanied by a high incidence of side effects, such as behavioral activation and agitation.

Atypical antipsychotic drugs are clinically the most effective drugs for reducing aggression, irritability, and severe tantrums in youth with autism (Propper and Orlik, 2009). Indeed, risperidone and aripiprazole are currently considered first-line therapies in child and adolescent autism. However, serious side effects include weight gain, glucose intolerance, and hyperlipidemia, making it necessary to monitor prolactin levels, blood glucose, and body weight. These changes are resistant to treatment, even with stimulant medications (Penzner et al., 2009). However, risperidone and aripiprazole can reduce the behavioral scores for irritability associated with autism (Figure 18.5).

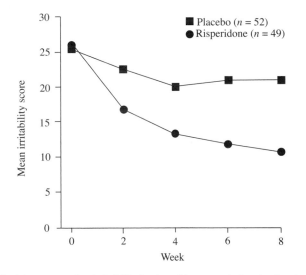

FIGURE 18.5 Mean score for irritability in risperidone- and placebo-treated children with autism. Total number of subjects studied = 101. Higher scores on the irritability subscale of the Aberrant Behavior Checklist indicate greater irritability. [From C. J. McDougle et al. (2003), "Treatment of Aggression in Children and Adolescents with Autism and Conduct Disorder," *Journal of Clinical Psychiatry* 64, Supplement 4: 17.]

Aripiprazole appears to have fewer metabolic and sedating side effects than does risperidone. Whether aripiprazole improves the core symptomatology of autistic disorders (rather then just behaviors) remains to be elucidated.

As a result of the efficacy of risperidone and aripiprazole, in 2007 the FDA formally approved risperidone (Risperdol) for the symptomatic treatment of irritability in autistic children and adolescents. This approval was the first for the use of a drug to treat behaviors associated with autism in children: aggression, deliberate self-injury, and temper tantrums. Risperidone improved mood disorders and reduced disruptive behaviors such as hyperactivity, fighting, anger, labile affect, negativity, and uncooperativeness. The risperidone derivative paliperidone (Invega) has also been shown to be effective in the treatment of irritability in autistic disorder (Stigler et al., 2010).

The approval of risperidone was followed in 2009 with similar approval for aripiprazole (Abilify). In June 2009, Stigler and coworkers reported results from a 14-week, open-label study of aripiprazole in 25 subjects, ages 5 to 17. They reported positive results and urged larger, placebo-controlled studies. The first two such studies were reported by Marcus and coworkers in November and December 2009 (Marcus et al., 2009; Owen et al., 2009). More than 200 children and adolescents, ages 6 to 17, were studied; they received target doses of 5, 10, or 15 milligrams per day. Aripiprazole was generally efficacious, with modest side effects. Hollander and coworkers (2010) reported similar efficacy of valproic acid; it was particularly effective in autistic youth with abnormal activity on the electroencephalogram.

Improved efficacy of medication treatment and longer-term outcomes likely will involve medication plus parent training and other complementary efforts (Aman et al., 2009). The omega-3 fatty acids are one of the most commonly used complementary medicines; they are used in about 28 percent of children with autism (Bent at al., 2009). Currently, fatty acid deficiencies are being implicated in infant neuronal-development and neurocognitive disorders, such as autism (Schuchardt et al., 2010). Although evidence of efficacy in autism is contradictory, supplemental omega-3 fatty acid therapy might be helpful and can be administered without significant side effects (Meiri et al., 2009).

Medications for Treating Behavioral or Aggressive Disorders

Children whose angry, agitated outbursts are so severe that they pose a danger to themselves and others pose both a diagnostic and therapeutic challenge (Carlson et al., 2009). The outbursts, sometimes called "rages," have been increasingly associated with mania, severe mood dysregulation, and overt, reactive, impulsive aggression. These behaviors cut across many diagnoses, including ADHD, autism, PTSD, and bipolar disorder. Perhaps the most common misdiagnosis is bipolar disorder. In the Carlson and coworkers study, one-third of children with rages had been given a bipolar diagnosis prior to hospitalization. However, only 9 percent of children with rages were given a bipolar diagnosis after careful examination. This finding is consistent with a presumed overdiagnosis of bipolar disorder (Zimmerman et al., 2008). The Children's Agitation Inventory appears to be a useful diagnostic tool (Potegal et al., 2009).

Older literature revealed that 50 percent of youth with behavioral disruptive disorders progressed to antisocial personality disorder as adults. Therefore, early intervention is desirable. Externalizing disruptive symptoms in childhood are a marker for more pervasive psychopathology as adults. These behaviors respond positively to *mood stabilizers* and *atypical antipsychotics*, as adjuncts to psychological (especially family) therapies (Barzman and Findling, 2008).

The pharmacology of *mood stabilizers* was presented in Chapter 6. Agents include *lithium* and the *anticonvulsants*. For many years, lithium has been recommended for the management of severe aggressive behaviors in children. Its use is limited by problems, often severe, with weight gain, cognitive impairment, and potentially fatal elevations of blood ammonia in the face of normal liver function (Perrott et al., 2010). Donovan and coworkers (2000) studied 20 youths (ages 10 to18, 80 percent male) with conduct or oppositional defiant disorder as well as explosive temper and mood lability. Subjects received 6 weeks of valproic acid or placebo: 8 of 10 on valproate responded positively. Zero of 10 responded to placebo. Saxena and coworkers (2006) studied the use of valproic acid in youth (average age 11) who had parents with bipolar disorder and who displayed irritability, rapid mood shifts, and aggression. Valproate (dosed to a blood concentration of 50 to 120 micrograms per milliliter) improved both mood and aggressive symptoms, and over 75 percent of the young people studied were considered "responders." Khanzode and coworkers (2006) reexamined the use of valproic acid in incarcerated youths diagnosed with severe conduct disorders. High doses (500 to 1500 milligrams per day) produced improvements in depression and impulse control but no improvement in other emotional states. The researchers suggested that an integrated approach combining pharmacotherapy with psychotherapy may be needed to achieve overall improvement. Likely, the efficacy of valproic acid in rage disorders is limited; other anticonvulsants have been poorly studied (Ipser and Stein, 2007).

Atypical antipsychotic medications are currently the mainstay in the treatment of aggressive, explosive, and rage disorders in children and adolescents (Staller, 2007; Findling, 2008). Risperidone and olanzapine (Chapter 4) have been used to target aggressive behaviors, but they tend to cause weight gain and other adverse metabolic effects. A better side effect profile has been attributed to aripiprazole. Budman and coworkers (2008) reported efficacy of aripiprazole, but, unexpectedly, weight gain was significant. In a broader meta-analysis of aripiprazole in child and adolescent psychiatry, such prominent weight gain was not noted (Greenaway and Elbe, 2009).

Other medication classes used in the treatment of agitation and irritability in children and adolescents include the following:

- *Psychostimulants* are useful for aggressive and conduct disorder, even in the absence of ADHD. Antisocial behaviors, such as stealing and lying, can also be reduced by psychostimulants.

- *SSRIs* (for example, fluoxetine) can be effective in some adults, but there are too few studies in children to warrant conclusions.

- There is some evidence for efficacy of *clonidine* in pediatric hyperactivity and aggression and perhaps in pervasive developmental disorders, but the evidence for efficacy is weak.

- *Benzodiazepines*—for example, clonazepam (Klonopin) and alprazolam (Xanax)—can reduce agitation and irritability, but they can induce behavioral disinhibition. They must be used with great care in children with pathological aggression.

In summary, although aggressive and rage behaviors are highly prevalent in child and adolescent psychiatry, there are no medications specifically approved by the FDA for treating them. In addition, children and adolescents referred for treatment for behavioral and aggressive disorders are likely to show several other problems (for example, ADHD, pervasive developmental disorders, depression, and substance abuse) that raise their own separate challenges. Parents and siblings of children referred for therapies for conduct disorder often themselves show significant impairment (psychiatric disorder, marital discord, family stress, dysfunctional relationships, abusive parenting, and so on). All these problems need to be addressed when drug prescription is being considered (Shechtman and Birani-Nasaraladin, 2006). Currently, off-label use of atypical antipsychotics, especially aripiprazole, appears to be most promising. As always in child and adolescent psychopharmacology, risks must be weighed against possible benefits. Also, the chronicity of illness may necessitate long-term use of these agents. No studies of long-term use of atypical antipsychotic therapy in children have been reported. Despite this, the severity of disease may necessitate a trial of therapy (Fisher, 2010).

Medications for Treating Attention Deficit/Hyperactivity Disorder

Attention deficit/hyperactivity disorder (ADHD) is the most extensively studied pediatric mental disorder. On average, one in every 10 to 15 children in the United States has been diagnosed with the disorder; about one-half of these are on stimulant medication, often Ritalin, Adderall, or Concerta (Mayes et al., 2009). Behavioral descriptions that lead to diagnosis (often with teachers providing diagnostic information) include inattentiveness, hyperactivity, and impulsiveness. It is still not clear if ADHD is a medical disorder, a behavioral problem mainly manifest in schools, or a disorder of human adaptation (Mayes et al., 2009). Many papers have been published on a possible genetic versus environmental contribution to ADHD behaviors, although it has been hard to find genes underlying the disorder (Coghill and Banaschewski, 2009; Franke et al., 2009).

Biologically, ADHD appears to follow from alterations in dopaminergic activity in the prefrontal cortex (PFC) of the brain. The PFC is critical for the regulation of behavior, attention, and cognition (Arnsten, 2009). It reduces the effect of distraction and divided attention. Lesions to the PFC produce a profile of distractibility, forgetfulness, impulsivity, poor planning, and locomotor hyperactivity (all prominent in ADHD). Optimal levels of norepinephrine and dopamine are essential for proper PFC control of behavior and attention. Genetic alterations in norepinephrine or dopamine receptors or systems contribute to dysregulation of PFC circuits in ADHD. Stimulant medications tend to augment deficient dopaminergic (or norepinephrine) systems, optimizing PFC regulation of behavior and attention (Arnsten, 2006).

In addition to being involved in the PFC, dopamine is a major transmitter in the *nucleus accumbens* (NA), the so-called pleasure center in the brain. Augmentation of dopaminergic activity in the NA by stimulants appears to account for the emotional stimulation, pleasure response, and attractiveness of these drugs that leads to compulsive abuse (Chapter 17).

Medication treatment of ADHD is not new. Amphetamines (such as *Benzedrine* and *dextroamphetamine*) were used to treat ADHD as early as 1937; *methylphenidate* (Ritalin) was introduced in the United States in 1955 and formally approved by the FDA for use in children in 1961. Since then, ADHD diagnosis and stimulant use has increased markedly. As a result, numerous stimulants have been marketed (Table 18.2), and a few nonstimulant products have appeared (such as atomoxetine and guanfacine). Stimulants (methylphenidate and amphetamines) are FDA-regulated drugs that are widely abused in society yet improve attention and concentration in persons both with and without ADHD.

TABLE 18.2 Stimulant medications available for the treatment
of ADHD

Medication (trade name)	Mode of delivery	Generic	Maximum dose per day	Duration of action, hours
Methylphenidate (Ritalin)	Immediate release	Yes	60 mg	4
Methylphenidate (Methylin)	Immediate release	No	Lesser of 2 mg/kg/day or 60 mg	4
d-Methylphenidate (Focalin)	Immediate release	Yes	Lesser of 1 mg/kg/day or 20 mg	4
Mixed amphetamine salts (Adderall)	Immediate release	Yes	Lesser of 1 mg/kg/day or 40 mg	8
Amphetamine (Dexedrine)	Immediate release	Yes	40 mg	8
Amphetamine (Dextrostat)	Immediate release	Yes	40 mg	8
Methylphenidate (Ritalin SR)— pulse	Gradually released from wax matrix	No	60 mg	Up to 8
Methylphenidate (Metadate ER)— pulse	Gradually released from wax matrix	No	Lesser than 2 mg/kg/day or 60 mg	7–8
Methylphenidate (Methylin ER)— pulse	Gradually released from wax matrix	No	60 mg	7–8
Methylphenidate (Metadate CD)— pearls	Beaded delivery system—30% immediate release and 70% 3 h later	No	Lesser than 2 mg/kg/day or 60 mg	8–9
Methylphenidate (Ritalin LA)— pearls	Beaded delivery system—50% immediate release and 50% 4 h later	No	60 mg	7–9
d-Methylphenidate (Focalin XR) pearls	Beaded delivery system—50% immediate release and 50% 4 h later	No	Lesser than 1 mg/kg/day or 30 mg	Up to 12

(continued)

TABLE 18.2 Stimulant medications available for the treatment of ADHD (continued)

Medication (trade name)	Mode of delivery	Generic	Maximum dose per day	Duration of action, hours
Methylphenidate (Concerta)— pump	OROS delivery system—22% immediate release outer coating and 78% gradually released osmotically	No	Lesser than 2 mg/kg/day or 72 mg	Up to 12
Methylphenidate (Daytrana)— patch	Patch worn up to 9 h per day, gradually releasing methylphenidate	No	Lesser than 1 mg/kg/day or 30 mg	12
Mixed amphetamine salts (Adderall XR)—pearls	Beaded delivery system—50% immediate release and 50% 4 h later	No	Lesser than 1.0 mg/kg or 30 mg	10
Amphetamine (Dexedrine Spansule)— pearls	Beaded delivery system—initial dose released immediately and remainder gradually released	No	Lesser than 1.0 mg/kg or 40 mg	10
Lisdexamfetamine (Vyvanse)— prodrug	Amphetamine with lysine attached, activated in gastrointestinal tract when lysine is cleaved	No	Lesser than 1.0 mg/kg or 70 mg	10

Modified from J. M. Daughton and C. J. Kratochvil, "Review of ADHD Pharmacotherapies: Advantages, Disadvantages, and Clinical Pearls," *Journal of the American Academy of Child and Adolescent Psychiatry* 48 (2009): 243–244.

Guidelines for Management of ADHD

In 2007, a clinical practice parameter for the assessment and treatment of children and adolescents with ADHD was published by the American Academy of Child and Adolescent Psychiatry. The guideline is both practical and based on evidence. Diagnostic criteria, behavioral rating assessment scales, and medication options are discussed in detail.

Stimulant Treatment for ADHD

Stimulant drugs improve behavior and learning ability in 60 to 80 percent of children who are correctly diagnosed. Children treated with stimulants show improvements in parent- and teacher-rated ADHD symptoms but unfortunately often make little or no improvements in functional impairment (Epstein et al., 2010). Therefore, use of stimulant medication in isolation may only resolve symptoms, and "collaboration with other mental health or educational services in addition to medication appears warranted" (Epstein et al., 2010, p. 160). Despite this limitation, the treatment of ADHD with psychostimulants has become one of the most broadly effective drug therapies of the twenty-first century.

In December 1999, results of the Multimodal Treatment Study of Children with Attention-Deficit/Hyperactivity Disorder were published (MTA Cooperative Group, 1999). In the study, a cohort of 579 children with ADHD was assigned to 14 months of medication management, intensive behavioral treatment, a combination of the two, or standard community care. Carefully structured medication management resulted in a better outcome than did intensive behavioral treatment, and combined treatment yielded an outcome that was better than the outcome of behavioral treatment but equivalent to the outcome of medication management. The study concluded:

> Carefully crafted medication management was superior to behavioral treatment and to routine community care that included medication. Combined treatment did not yield significantly greater benefits than medication management for core ADHD symptoms, but it may have provided modest advantages for non-ADHD symptoms and positive functioning outcomes. (p. 1073)

Since this study covered a period of only 14 months, longer-term efficacy remained unknown. A 24-month follow-up of the MTA study (MTA Cooperative Group, 2004) revealed that cessation of drug therapy was associated with clinical deterioration, continued drug therapy was associated with only mild deterioration, and stimulant initiation (in the group not receiving stimulants in the early study) was associated with clinical improvements. The 24-month follow-up concluded: "Consistent use of stimulant medication was associated with maintenance of effectiveness but continued mild growth suppression" (p. 762).

The participants in the original MTA study have now been followed for eight years, and the results have been recently published (Molina et al., 2009). At eight years, 33 percent of the original participants were still receiving medication, usually stimulants (83 percent). While improvements seen at the end of the 14-month study were generally maintained, MTA participants were not "normalized" at eight years, with 30 percent still meeting the criteria for ADHD. The study's youths now range in age from 13 to 18. Clinically significant antisocial behavior was present in 25 to 30 percent of MTA participants; 25 percent met criteria for oppositional defiant disorder or conduct disorder; 27 percent had been arrested at least one time; and 30 percent reportedly displayed moderate to serious delinquent behavior. Academically, medicated children with ADHD had significant improvements in mathematics and reading scores compared to untreated children with ADHD, but these improvements were insufficient to eliminate the gap in test scores between children with ADHD and those without (Scheffler et al., 2009). Biederman and coworkers (2010) verified ADHD persistence, stating that 78 percent of subjects met at least one definition of persistence and that "persistence of ADHD is associated with greater psychiatric comorbidity, familiality and functional impairments" (p. 299).

Pappadopulos and coworkers (2009) assessed medication compliance by testing the saliva of youths taking psychostimulants for ADHD. Parents' verbal reports of medication compliance did not correlate with saliva testing: 25 percent were noncompliant and only 53 percent were adherent at all four saliva testings during the 14 months of study. Counseling was essential for medication compliance, especially when benefits were suboptimal.

Stimulant Use and Subsequent Substance Abuse

A persistent question is whether or not there is any association between use of stimulants during childhood and later use of drugs of abuse. First, it is clear that untreated youths with ADHD and comorbid conduct, mood, or anxiety disorders are at increased risk of subsequent substance abuse and development of a substance abuse disorder. Second, childhood and adolescent use of stimulant medication for ADHD is not associated with later substance abuse. Abuse is minimal among patients for whom stimulant medications are appropriately prescribed. Wilens and coworkers (2008a) studied 114 adolescent girls with ADHD medicated with stimulants. They reported no increased risks for cigarette smoking or substance abuse. They did find significant protective effects of stimulant treatment on the development of substance abuse disorders.

Diversion of stimulants remains a serious problem. Wilens and coworkers (2008b) noted that reported rates of nonprescribed stimulant use ranged from 5 to 9 percent in grade school- and high school-aged children and 5 to 35 percent in college-aged youths. Lifetime rates of diversion ranged from 16 to 29 percent of students with stimulant prescriptions asked to give, sell, or trade their medication. Reported reasons for non-ADHD use included the desire to concentrate, improve alertness, get high, or experiment. The authors concluded that it is necessary to educate individuals with ADHD about the pitfalls of the misuse and diversion of their stimulant medication. This caution seems to apply particularly to the amphetamines (Setlik et al., 2009).

Methylphenidate

Currently, methylphenidate preparations account for 90 percent of the prescribed medication for ADHD. Because it is so widely used and because no one dosage regimen is ideal, multiple different dosage forms and methods of delivering the drug to the bloodstream have been devised (see Table 18.2). Methylphenidate (as Ritalin) is of rapid onset and short duration; thus, it must be administered two or three times daily. It is not administered in the evening to permit the blood level to drop, permitting normal sleep. The short half-life is a problem in some children, who experience an end-of-dose rebound in dysfunctional behavior.

Early extended-release preparations of methylphenidate were disappointing. Recently, however, more dependable extended-release preparations have become available. The first of these was Concerta, an osmotic-release preparation that extends duration up to 12 hours. The product is prepared with 22 percent of the drug in a coating on the outside of the capsule (immediate-release drug), with 78 percent delivered by an "osmotic pump" that releases drug over a 10-hour period in gradually increasing serum concentrations. One daily dose of Concerta yields about the same plasma concentrations as three daily doses of immediate-release methylphenidate with essentially equal efficacy. Other new formulations of methylphenidate for oral administration are of two types:

1. Single-pulse, sustained-release formulations (Ritalin-SR, Metadate ER, Methylin CD) use a wax matrix to prolong release. Their duration of action is about 8 hours, but they may be unreliable compared with other preparations.

2. Beaded double-pulse products (Ritalin LA, Focalin XR, Metadate CD) use an extended-release formulation with bimodal release.

   a. Ritalin LA and Focalin XR = 50 percent in immediate release and 50 percent in enteric-coated, delayed-release beads.

   b. Metadate CD = 30 percent in immediate-release beads and 70 percent in delayed-release beads that are released 4 hours later, eliminating the lunchtime dose.

Comparing Concerta and Focalin XR showed the superiority of Focalin XR at 0.5 and 5 hours, but Concerta was superior to Focalin XR at 11

TABLE 18.3 Daytrana—Recommended titration schedule (patients new to methylphenidate)

	Upward titration, if response is not maximized			
	Week 1	**Week 2**	**Week 3**	**Week 4**
Patch size	12.5 cm²	18.75 cm²	25 cm²	37.5 cm²
Nominal delivered dose* (mg/9 hours)	10 mg	15 mg	20 mg	30 mg
Delivery rate*	(1.1 mg/hr)*	(1.6 mg/hr)*	(2.2 mg/hr)*	(3.3 mg/hr)*

*Nominal in vivo delivery rate in pediatric subjects aged 6–12 when applied to the hip, based on a 9-hour wear period.

and 12 hours. Using these data, prescribers and parents can find an appropriate preparation of methylphenidate, depending on the desired time of maximal effect and duration of action.

In 2007, a transdermal methylphenidate delivery system (a skin patch sold under the trade name Daytrana) was introduced. The patch is applied daily, has a clinical onset of effect within 2 hours, and is worn for a maximum of 9 hours. Following its removal, the effects of the methylphenidate continue for another 3 hours. Patches containing 10, 15, 20, and 30 milligrams are available (Table 18.3). If removed before 9 hours, less drug is absorbed. Wilens and coworkers (2008c) describe the flexibility of the patch. In a four-week study of 164 children who received extended-release oral methylphenidate preparations (Ritalin LA, Concerta, or Metadate CD) and then switched to the methylphenidate patch, Bukstein and coworkers (2009) found improvement in ADHD behavior and in quality of life. Caregivers (mostly parents) reported high satisfaction with the patch, improved behavior, and less worry about missed doses.

Also commercially available is *dexmethylphenidate* (d-methylphenidate, or Focalin), the active D-isomer of methylphenidate. This isomer has twice the potency of methylphenidate, so the dose of dexmethylphenidate is one-half the dose of methylphenidate. Focalin is available in an extended-release formulation (Focalin XR).

Amphetamines

Since about 1937, amphetamines have been used for the treatment of ADHD. Available amphetamines include *dextroamphetamine* (Dexedrine), *mixed amphetamine salts* (Adderall), an *extended-release formulation of Adderall* (Adderall XR), and *lisdexamfetamine* (Vyvanse). Adderall is called "mixed amphetamine salts"; it is pharmacologically identical to Benzedrine, introduced in 1937. In lisdexamfetamine, a molecule of dextroamphetamine is bonded to L-lysine, a naturally occurring amino acid, resulting in a molecule lacking biological activity (a prodrug). When taken orally, the bond is broken by gastrointestinal enzymes, releasing the amphetamine, which is then absorbed. If crushed and injected, the bond is only slowly broken; thus, diversion may be reduced. In situations where diversion may be a problem, the preparation may be appropriate. Doses of 10, 30, and 70 milligrams of lisdexamfetamine result in bioavailability of about 5 to 30 milligrams of dextroamphetamine or 10 to 60 milligrams of amphetamine.

Once-daily Adderall appears to be similar to twice-daily methylphenidate and is therapeutically equivalent or even superior to generic methylphenidate for improving a relatively wide range of behavior problems commonly displayed by children with ADHD. Head-to-head comparisons of Concerta and Adderall in treating ADHD have not been reported.

Alternative Medications for Treating ADHD

About 10 to 30 percent of ADHD patients do not respond adequately to stimulants and are considered to be treatment-resistant. In addition, some children and their parents may desire that stimulants not be used. Therefore, there is a need for treatment alternatives.

Atomoxetine (Strattera) was approved by the FDA in 2003 for the treatment of child and adult ADHD. In 2008, the FDA expanded its approval to include indication for the maintenance treatment of ADHD in children and adolescents. This is the first selective norepinephrine reuptake inhibitor (SNRI) approved for use in treating ADHD in children 6 years of age and older as well as in adults. At a daily dose of about 1.4 mg/kg/day, the drug is effective in reducing ADHD symptoms (Maziade et al., 2009; Wietecha et al., 2009). The drug appears to be tolerable and relatively safe when used in children over a period of up to four years (Donelly et al., 2009). A British study of 201 children with ADHD reported that atomoxetine was more effective in treatment-naive patients than in patients who had previously been treated with stimulant medication (Prasad et al., 2007), suggesting a trial of atomoxetine prior to initiation of stimulants.

Two CNS-acting antihypertensive (blood pressure-lowering) dopaminergic agonists—*clonidine* (Catapres) and *guanfacine* (Tenex, Intuniv)—have been reported to have positive effects in the treatment of ADHD. Arnsten (2009) relates this efficacy to increased alpha-2-receptor stimulation in the prefrontal cortex. Guanfacine has a longer half-life than does clonidine and is less sedating (Handen et al., 2008). Several studies of an extended-release formulation of guanfacine—*guanfacine-ER* (Intuniv)—have demonstrated modest efficacy at a dose of 2 to 4 milligrams per day (Biederman et al., 2008; Sallee et al., 2009). Sedation and fatigue were the most common side effects, but these were not limiting, and sedation seems to decrease with increasing duration of treatment (Faraone and Glatt, 2010). Combining guanfacine and a stimulant appears to be associated with improvements in ADHD outcome greater than those seen with either drug alone (Spencer et al., 2009). This combination treatment needs further exploration. In 2009, the FDA formally approved guanfacine extended-release tablets (Intuniv) for the treatment of ADHD in children and adolescents, ages 6 to 17.

Tricyclic antidepressants (especially *nortriptyline;* Chapter 5) have been studied and have occasionally been reported to be effective. However, cognitive impairments, limited efficacy, and rare cases of potentially fatal cardiac toxicities associated with tricyclic antidepressant use in children and adolescents pose considerable limitations.

Initial reports on other antidepressants indicate some usefulness of *fluoxetine* (Prozac) and *buspirone* (BuSpar), although the effects were not robust. Quintana and coworkers (2007), however, demonstrated a more robust effect of fluoxetine in ADHD with comorbid nonbipolar mood disorders in children and adolescents aged 6 to 18. Symptoms of inattention, overactivity, aggression, defiance, and depression were improved in 47 percent of participants. Of additional interest is the dopaminergic antidepressant *bupropion SR* (Wellbutrin-SR); the drug has been reported effective in adults with ADHD and in both adults and adolescents with ADHD comborbid with other disorders such as depression or substance abuse.

Modafinil (Provigil) is a nonstimulant drug that has been approved by the FDA for the maintenance of daytime wakefulness in the treatment of narcolepsy, in shift-work sleep disorders, and in sleep apnea. Although efficacious (Kahbazi et al., 2009), it is not approved for use in child and adolescent ADHD, in part because of potentially serious allergic reactions (Kumar, 2008).

Modafinil has been thought to be distinct from stimulants and has not been classified as a stimulant. It was also thought not to have abuse potential. Recently, however, Volkow and coworkers (2009) demonstrated that modafinil increases dopamine in the nucleus accumbens and may therefore have potential for abuse. This may account for some of the increasing use of the drug.

Side Effects of Stimulant Medications

Common side effects of stimulant medications include nighttime wakefulness (insomnia), elevations in blood pressure and heart rate, reductions in appetite, and possible growth suppression. With proper care, these usually can be well managed (Faraone et al., 2008). Other potential side effects include adverse psychiatric problems, including new or worsening behavioral and thought problems, new or worsening bipolar illness, new or worsening aggressive or hostility problems, and, in children and teenagers, new psychiatric symptoms, including hearing voices, believing things that are not true, increased suspiciousness, and new manic symptoms. All these effects are predictable consequences seen in some people using any psychostimulant, whether for therapeutic purposes or for abuse purposes.

More serious effects of stimulant medications involve cardiac (heart) safety and reports of sudden deaths among children and adolescents receiving these medications for treatment of ADHD. Concerns that stimulants may increase the risk of sudden, unexplained deaths in children have surfaced in case reports since the early 1990s. In 2006, the FDA requested that package inserts of stimulant medications contain a warning that stimulant products generally should not be used in children or adolescents with known serious structural cardiac abnormalities, cardiomyopathy, serious heart rhythm abnormalities, or other serious heart problems that may place them at increased vulnerability to the stimulant effects of the drug.

Current labeling instructions emphasize that children should receive a physical examination and a review of personal and family history for relevant cardiac events prior to starting stimulant treatment. If abnormalities are suspected, a pretreatment electrocardiogram (ECG) should be considered. Some advocate a pretreatment ECG for all children before treatment is initiated (Vitiello and Towbin, 2009). The rarity of sudden, unexplained deaths confounds recommendations. For example, one study found no events in an examination of over 125,000 person-years of use (Gould et al., 2009). Stimulants are not innocuous medications, and all side effects need to be taken into account before prescription.

Recently, Denchev and coworkers (2010) studied the relationship between stimulant medication, sudden cardiac death, and exercise; they concluded that the major benefit of cardiac screening is to "identify children with heart disease and restrict them from engaging in competitive sports" (p. 1329). This recommendation applies to all children, not just those with ADHD.

Medications and Medical Issues in Treating Depression

Perhaps the greatest controversy in child and adolescent psychopharmacology during the current decade is the one surrounding the use of antidepressant medication to treat major depressive disorders in children and adolescents. In essence, controversy surrounds the balance between expected benefits (effectiveness in relieving depression) versus potential risks (possibility of increasing the risk of suicide). To understand this controversy, a bit of history is in order.

First, research conducted in the 1990s demonstrated several important points:

- There was a high prevalence of suicidal ideation and completed suicides among untreated children and adolescents with depressive disorders.
- Not only does depression exist in adolescence, but adolescence is the period of highest risk for onset of depression.
- Adolescent depression has a protracted, longitudinal course with persistence into adult life (adolescents do not "grow out of it"), which results in ongoing disruption of interpersonal relationships, risk for substance abuse, early pregnancy, low educational achievement, poor occupational functioning, unemployment, and continued risk of suicide.
- Untreated childhood and adolescent depression is associated with later development of serious personality disorders in early adulthood, such as dependent, antisocial, passive-aggressive, and histrionic personality disorders.

These data compelled clinicians to intervene aggressively to prevent teenagers from developing into troubled and dysfunctional adults. A partial answer was discovered in 1997 when Emslie and coworkers demonstrated that fluoxetine (Prozac) was superior to placebo treatment in lowering scores on the Children's Depression Rating Scale–Revised (Figure 18.6). This discovery led to widespread off-label use of fluoxetine for child and adolescent depression, culminating in the NIMH-funded TADS (Treatment for Adolescents with Depression Study) research, the first phase of which was published in 2004 [Treatment for Adolescents with Depression Study (TADS) Team, 2004]. In brief, the 12-week TADS study compared usual clinical management with fluoxetine (10 to 40 milligrams per day) alone, cognitive-behavioral therapy (CBT) alone, or the combination of CBT and fluoxetine. Response to combination treatment (71 percent) was significantly greater than to fluoxetine alone (61 percent), CBT alone (43 percent), and placebo (usual clinical management, 35 percent). Fluoxetine monotherapy was superior to placebo and to CBT alone. This study set the standard that the best treatment of child and adolescent depression is a combination of fluoxetine and CBT.

Subsequent to this initial study, results of longer-term phases of the TADS study have appeared. In general, since 2004, combination therapy (CBT plus fluoxetine) has emerged as the therapy of choice, yielding the following observations:

- Patients in all treatment groups tended to improve even more after three years of therapy, although about one-third of patients will be resistant to therapy (Kennard et al., 2009a).
- At least nine months of treatment is likely needed for the average patient (Emslie et al., 2008); longer time of treatment is associated

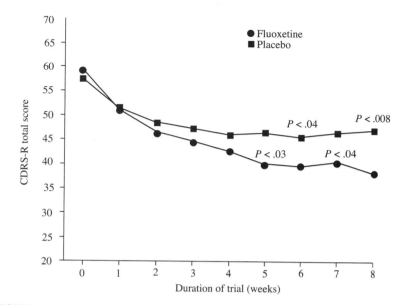

FIGURE 18.6 Weekly Children's Depression Rating Scale in 96 child and adolescent outpatients (aged 7 to 17) with nonpsychotic major depressive disorder treated with fluoxetine or placebo and evaluated weekly for eight consecutive weeks. [From Emslie et al. (1997), p. 1035.]

with persistence of benefits for at least one year following medication discontinuation [Treatment for Adolescents with Depression Study (TADS) Team, 2009].

- About nine months of combination therapy should be the modal treatment from a public health perspective as well as to maximize benefits and minimize harms for individual patients (March and Vitiello, 2009).

- Adding CBT to fluoxetine therapy minimizes persistent suicidal ideation and treatment-emergent suicidal events (discussed below) and enhances treatment safety (March et al., 2009; Vitello, 2009).

- Although combination therapy (CBT plus fluoxetine) is more expensive per year than fluoxetine alone, improved outcomes justify combination therapy as cost effective; CBT alone is not cost effective (Domino et al., 2009).

- The long half-life of fluoxetine seems to account for its superiority over other medications (Smith, 2009).

- Resistance to combination therapy remains a significant problem, indicating that treatment of resistant depression in adolescents (TORDIA) needs addressing (Walkup, 2010).

- Adolescents resistant to fluoxetine alone or to a combination of fluoxetine and CBT may react positively to a combination of CBT and a different SSRI (Brent et al., 2008; Kennard et al., 2009b). Augmentation strategies (such as adding a mood stabilizer to CBT and fluoxetine) improve positive responses (Emslie et al., 2010).

Alternative Medications and Treatments

Until recently, *fluoxetine* was the only drug whose antidepressant effect had been clearly established in a pediatric population and the only drug approved in the United States for the treatment of depression in children and adolescents. In 2009, the FDA gave approval for the use of *escitalopram* (Lexapro) for the treatment of depression in adolescents aged 12 to 17. This approval was based on three studies on citalopram and escitalopram, the last study reporting that scores on the Child Depression Rating Scale were reduced by 22 points compared with a 19-point reduction in the placebo-treated group (Emslie et al., 2009). Whether this is clinically significant is yet unknown. No head-to-head comparisons between fluoxetine and escitalopram have been reported. It does, however, provide clinicians with a second FDA-approved medication.

Emslie and coworkers (2007) performed an open-label trial of extended-release *venlafaxine* (Effexor-XR) in child and adolescent depression (with no placebo group for comparison). Although efficacy was demonstrated, serious side effects occurred in about 8 percent of patients,, including suicide attempts, hostility, and hallucinations. Brent and coworkers (2009) reported that venlafaxine treatment was associated with a higher rate of self-harm events in those with higher suicidal ideation. Since venlafaxine use in adults with bipolar depression is associated with "manic flips," one wonders whether some of this toxicity represents an unmasking of bipolarity in some adolescents suffering these side effects. In a meta-analysis of the literature, Bridge and coworkers (2007) found poor efficacy for venlafaxine. In this same meta-analysis, *paroxetine* (Paxil) was also relatively ineffective in treating child and adolescent depression and was associated with serious side effects, including suicidal ideation.

As discussed earlier, *atomoxetine* (Strattera) is the first commercially available drug in the new class of SNRI-type antidepressants. Atomoxetine is approved for treatment of ADHD in children and adolescents, and it is expected to be effective in child and adolescent depression. Future research will undoubtedly explore this area of use. The drug should certainly be effective in situations of depression comorbid with ADHD or anxiety disorders, especially since, unlike fluoxetine, SNRIs may be better at increasing social functioning; they may improve patient motivation, energy, and self-perception

Finally, adjunctive use of benzodiazepines (in depressed children) was associated with higher rates of both suicidal and nonsuicidal self-harm events (Brent et al., 2009).

Adjuvant Medications. Drugs of two additional pharmacological classes are being evaluated to see whether they can be used as adjuvant medication to improve the efficacy of fluoxetine in child and adolescent depression. First, *lamotrigine* (Lamictal) is now approved by the FDA for the treatment of resistant depression in adults. Pavuluri and coworkers (2009) demonstrated that lamotrigine was very effective in reducing depressive symptomatology in youth (8 to 18 years of age) with bipolar disorder. Similar efficacy in youth with unipolar depressive disease would be predicted.

Second, the atypical antipsychotic drugs *aripiprazole* (Abilify) and quetiapine (Seroquel) have antidepressant properties (Chapter 4) and have been approved by the FDA as augmenting agents in adults with inadequate response to SSRI therapy. Since aripiprazole and quetiapine are widely used in the treatment of various behavioral disorders in children and adolescents, it is likely that they will be studied as augmenting agents for child and adolescent depression only partially responsive or unresponsive to fluoxetine therapy. More on the use of these three medicines in child and adolescent depression should be forthcoming.

Complementary Treatments. Jorm (2006) reviewed evidence of the efficacy of complementary and *self-help treatments* for depression in children and adolescents. Relevant evidence was available for glutamine, S-adenosylmethionine, St John's wort, vitamin C, omega-3 fatty acids, light therapy, massage, art therapy, bibliotherapy, distraction techniques, exercise, relaxation therapy, and sleep deprivation. However, the evidence was limited and generally of poor quality. The only treatment with reasonable supporting evidence was *light therapy* for winter depression.

Antidepressants and Suicidal Ideation

The issue of potential suicidal ideation and behaviors (but rarely completed suicides) has become so contentious that a *PubMed* search by this author in early 2010 using the two words "antidepressant" and "suicide" returned over 2770 separate research article "hits" in the medical literature.[2] Some points relevant to this issue follow:

- In 2002, 264 children and adolescents aged 5 to 14 died by suicide in the United States, the fifth leading cause of death in this age group. The FDA report linked many of these deaths to SSRI treatment and

---

[2] The medical literature can be accessed at www.pubmed.gov.

recommended a black box warning regarding SSRI use and suicidal ideation (Gibbons et al., 2006). The FDA published a warning in 2003 and required a black box warning in 2005. This well-intended warning (to reduce suicide deaths presumably caused by SSRI antidepressants) resulted in reductions in SSRI prescriptions for depression (Libby et al., 2009).

- Unexpectedly, the reduction in antidepressant use (as a result of FDA warnings) resulted not only in reduced prescription for SSRIs but also in *increased* rates of suicide (Gibbons et al., 2007; Nemeroff et al., 2007).
- Vitiello and coworkers (2009) noted that most suicidal events occurred in the context of persistent depression and insufficient improvement without evidence of medication-induced behavioral activation as a precursor. Severity of self-rated suicidal ideation and depressive symptoms predicted emergence of suicidality during treatment.
- As discussed above, adding CBT to fluoxetine therapy enhances the safety of medication therapy.

Therefore, the well-intentioned government effort to reduce suicide rates backfired, with reductions in SSRI use correlating with increases in suicidality. Recognizing this, how does the defensive-oriented prescriber handle this volatile situation? We make the following suggestion for a patient or family handout:

> The FDA requires a warning that antidepressant medications can sometimes increase thoughts of suicide. Studies in children and adolescents have shown that antidepressants can increase suicidal thoughts. However, other studies have shown that this can be blunted with cognitive-behavioral therapies. Also, not taking antidepressants has been shown to increase suicide rates. Therefore, antidepressants seem to help most young persons who take them, but as with any therapy, some people may have negative reactions. Thus, it is important that we initiate psychological therapies along with medication therapy. This offers the best chance for success with minimization of risk. If you have questions about this, please contact me and we can discuss treatment strategies.

Guidelines for Adolescent Depression for Primary Care (GLAD-PC)

In 2007, clinical practice guidelines were published to assist primary care physicians in the treatment of adolescent depression (Cheung et al., 2007; Zuckerbrot et al., 2007). These guidelines emphasize identification of youth at risk, assessment procedures, patient and family psychoeducation, community links, and establishment of a safety plan. They make specific recommendations for collaborative care between prescriber and therapist. These guidelines are essential reading for all who care for these patients.

Calls for Widespread Screening for Youth at Risk

The prevalence of current or recent depression among children is 3 percent and among adolescents is 6 percent. Lifetime prevalence in adolescents may be as high as 20 percent. Child- and adolescent-onset depression is associated with persistent sadness; social isolation; increased risk of death by suicide; suicide attempts; recurrent depression in young adulthood; early pregnancy; poor school and occupational performance; and impaired work, social, and family functioning during young adulthood. Mass screening in schools and primary care offices may help identify missed cases and increase the proportion of depressed youth who might receive appropriate care, hopefully to help prevent the otherwise disastrous long-term effects of untreated depression. Of note, the majority of depressed youth today do not receive any type of treatment, despite the availability of depression-screening tools that are feasible for use in school and clinical settings. Williams and coworkers (2009) reviewed this data, described the commonly used screening tools, and concluded:

> Primary care-feasible screening tools may accurately identify depressed adolescents and treatment can improve depression outcomes. Treating depressed youth with SSRIs may be associated with a small increased risk of suicidality and should only be considered if judicious clinical monitoring is possible. (p. e716)

In a follow-up, the U.S. Preventive Services Task Force (2009b) issued a call to "screen adolescents (12–18 years of age) for major depressive disorder when systems are in place to ensure accurate diagnosis, psychotherapy (cognitive-behavioral or interpersonal), and follow-up." They further stated that "the current evidence is insufficient to warrant a recommendation to screen children (7–11 years of age) for major depressive disorder" (p. 1223).

Table 18.4 summarizes these recommendations. As more data concerning the efficacy of treatment of younger children accumulate, further recommendations will undoubtedly follow.

Medications for Treating Anxiety Disorders

Anxiety disorders are common in children and cause substantial impairment in school, in family relationships, and in social functioning. Such disorders also predict adult anxiety disorders and major depression.

TABLE 18.4 Summary and recommendations from the U.S. Preventive Services Task Force (USPSTF) for broad screening of children and adolescents for depressive disorders[a]

Population	Adolescents (12–18 y)	Children (7–11 y)
Recommendation	Screen (when systems for diagnosis, treatment, and follow-up are in place)	No recommendation
	Grade B[b]	**Grade I**[c]
Risk assessment	Risk factors for major depressive disorder (MDD) include parental depression, having comorbid mental health or chronic medical conditions, and having experienced a major negative life event.	
Screening tests	The following screening tests have been shown to do well in teens in primary care settings: • Patient Health Questionnaire for Adolescents (PHQ-A) • Beck Depression Inventory—Primary Care version (BDI-PC)	Screening instruments perform less well in younger children.
Treatments	Among pharmacotherapies, fluoxetine, a selective serotonin reuptake inhibitor (SSRI), has been found efficacious. However, because of risk of suicidality, SSRIs should be considered only if clinical monitoring is possible. Various modes of psychotherapy, and pharmacotherapy combined with psychotherapy, have been found efficacious.	Evidence on the balance of benefits and harms of treatment of younger children is insufficient for a recommendation.

[a]Also included are the listings of the USPSTF for risk assessment, screening tests, and treatments for depression.
[b]The grade "B" in the recommendation means that the USPSTF recommends the action. Also, there is high certainty that the net benefit is moderate or there is moderate certainty that the net benefit is moderate to substantial. The USPSTF suggests public health workers offer or provide this service.
[c]The grade "I" means that there is insufficient evidence to assess the balances and harms of the service.

Efficacious treatments are available; however, anxiety disorders in childhood remain underrecognized and undertreated. The prevalence of any anxiety disorder in children and adolescents ranges in various studies from 6.0 percent to as high as 17.7 percent. A reasonable estimate is that about 13 percent of 15-year-olds meet diagnostic criteria for having an anxiety disorder. Bridge and coworkers (2007), in their meta-analysis of antidepressant efficacy, found considerable benefit when these drugs were used to treat both OCD and non-OCD anxiety disorders.

A clinical practice parameter for the treatment of children and adolescents with anxiety disorders has been published (Connolly et al., 2007). This practice parameter emphasizes treatment with a combination of pharmacotherapy and psychotherapy. A new six-year study intended to examine the relative efficacy of CBT, sertraline (Zoloft), and their combination for the treatment of generalized anxiety disorder, separation anxiety disorder, and social phobia in children and adolescents is currently under way (Compton et al., 2010). One study using this protocol was published in 2008 (Walkup et al., 2008).

Generalized Anxiety Disorder, Separation Anxiety Disorder, and Social Phobia

In clinical trials, generalized anxiety disorder (GAD), separation anxiety disorder (SAD), and social phobia (SoP) are often grouped together because of the high degree of overlap in symptoms and their distinction from other anxiety disorders (e.g., obsessive-compulsive disorder). GAD, SAD, and SoP are characterized by excessive anxiety, worry, restlessness, fatigue, difficulty in concentrating, irritability, muscle tension, or sleep disturbances of six months' duration or causing functional disturbances. The child may experience tension, apprehension, need for reassurance, and negative self-image as well as having physical complaints. Children with these disorders may appear overly mature, perfectionistic, and sensitive to criticism. They may tend to seek reassurance for worries and self-doubt. Many of youth with GAD, SAD, or SoP have a comorbid depressive disorder (the converse is also true), second anxiety disorder, or ADHD. GAD, SAD, and SoP have a high familial association: 40 percent of parents of children with GAD, SAD, or SoP had the disorder themselves during their childhood.

Treatment of GAD, SAD, and SoP usually involves a combination of pharmacotherapy and psychotherapy (cognitive-behavioral therapy, social skills training, and exposure therapy). In 2008, Walkup and coworkers, in a 12-week study, reported the effects of sertraline, CBT, and a combination of both on GAD, SAD, and SoP in 488 children and adolescents (7 to 17 years of age). The percentage of participants who were rated as much improved or very much improved (on the Clinical Global Impression-Improvement scale) were 80.7 percent for the combination therapy group, 59.7 percent for the CBT group, 54.9 percent for the sertraline group, and 23.7 percent for the placebo drug group. Results on the Pediatric Anxiety Rating Scale were of similar magnitude (Figure 18.7). The authors concluded that CBT alone, sertraline alone, and combination are all efficacious short-term treatments for childhood anxiety disorders. Combination therapy is most efficacious and "provides the best chance for a positive outcome. Any of the three treatments can be recommended, taking into consideration the family's treatment preferences, treatment availability, cost, and time burden" (p. 2764). These results were verified in a second large study of the efficacy of sertraline in the treatment of SAD, GAD, and SoP (Compton et al., 2010).

Keeton and coworkers (2009) expanded on the Walkup study, stating that any SSRI likely would be effective in treating child and adolescent anxiety disorders, with SSRI-CBT therapy likely being most efficacious. They recommend starting doses as follows: fluvoxamine 25 mg/day, fluoxetine 10 mg/day, and sertraline 25 mg/day, though lower starting doses can be used. Doses can be increased as needed and tolerated. They recommend continuation treatment for about one year following remission in symptoms. When discontinuing medication, one should choose a

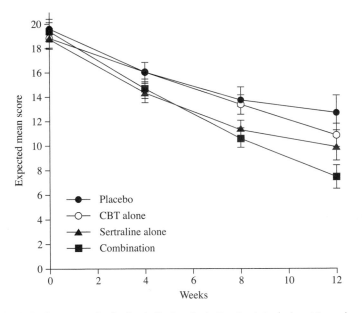

FIGURE 18.7 Scores on the Pediatric Rating Scale For Anxiety during 12 weeks of therapy with placebo, cognitive-behavioral therapy (CBT), sertraline (Zoloft) alone, or a combination of CBT and sertraline. Scores greater than 13 are consistent with moderate levels of anxiety and a diagnosis of an anxiety disorder. Mean scores and confidence levels are shown. [From: Walkup et al. (2008), Figure 2.]

stress-free time of the year. If symptoms return, medication reinitiation should be seriously considered.

Obsessive-Compulsive Disorder

Obsessive-compulsive disorder (OCD) is a disorder of early onset characterized by recurrent obsessions or compulsions that are severe enough to be time-consuming or result in marked distress or significant impairment, especially of social life. In children, the incidence of OCD is thought to be rare, but in adolescents the reported prevalence is estimated at 2 to 3.6 percent. In fact, the majority of adults with OCD had an onset of the disorder during adolescence or earlier. OCD is now estimated as the fourth most common psychiatric disorder in children and adolescents.

Pharmacotherapy is an important component of the multimodal treatment of children and adolescents with OCD. However, treatment of children and adolescents with OCD should begin with the combination of CBT and a single SSRI or CBT alone [Pediatric OCD Treatment Study (POTS) Team, 2004]. Here, the rate for clinical remission was 53.6 percent for combined treatment, 39.3 percent for CBT alone, 21.4 percent for sertraline (Zoloft) alone, and 3.6 percent for placebo (Figure 18.8). A second phase of this study is currently under way (Freeman et al., 2009).

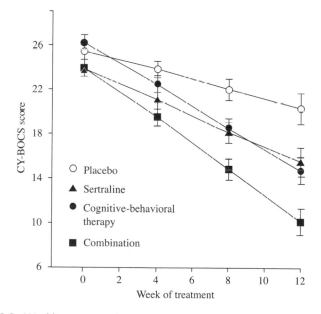

FIGURE 18.8   Weekly scores on the Children's Yale-Brown Obsessive-Compulsive Scale (CY-BOCS) for four treatment groups: treatment with placebo, treatment with sertraline, treatment with cognitive-behavioral therapy, and combined treatment with sertraline plus cognitive-behavioral therapy. [From Pediatric OCD Treatment Study (POTS) Team (2004), Figure 2.]

Despite the efficacy of CBT plus SSRI for treatment of OCD in children and adolescents, perhaps 25 to 30 percent of youth with this disorder do not improve. Augmentation strategies are therefore necessary. One of the most studied and well-documented strategies in adults for treatment-resistant OCD is the addition of an atypical antipsychotic drug to the ongoing SSRI treatment. To date, there has been a paucity of data in young persons regarding the use of aripiprazole in OCD patients who failed to respond to SSRIs. Efficacy in 12 adults was reported by Pessina and coworkers (2009). Storch and coworkers (2007) reported excellent response in a 13-year-old male to a dose of 2.5 milligrams per day of aripiprazole and a reduction in his Yale-Brown OCS score from 30 to 3 when aripiprazole was combined with biweekly CBT.

Panic Disorder

Little is known about the treatment of panic disorder (PD) in children and adolescents. A recent guideline on the subject in adults contained little on pediatric PD (Stein et al., 2009). Small studies suggest SSRI therapy as appropriate medication. CBT and other therapies (for example, exposure therapy) may be efficacious.

Posttraumatic Stress Disorder

PTSD is common in children and adolescents, but scant research has been devoted to pharmacological interventions for this disorder. Recently, the American Academy of Child and Adolescent Psychiatry published a clinical practice parameter for the assessment and treatment of PTSD (Cohen et al., 2010). The practice parameter makes 11 recommendations that support trauma-focused psychotherapy, medications, and combined interventions, with an emphasis on early identification of PTSD, data gathering, and assessment and treatment of comorbidities. Following this practice parameter, Strawn and coworkers (2010) published an extensive review of psychopharmacological treatments for children and adolescents with PTSD.

Medications for Treating Bipolar Disorder

Pediatric bipolar disorder is a chronic and debilitating psychiatric illness associated with many short-term and long-term complications, including poor academic and social performance, legal problems, and increased risk of suicide. In addition, it is often complicated by other serious psychiatric disorders such as ADHD, oppositional defiant disorder (ODD), conduct disorder (CD), and substance abuse disorders. Luby and Navsaria (2010) discuss bipolar prodromal symptoms and early markers for the eventual development of the disorder. Indeed, more than half of children with bipolar disorder experienced a prodromal period of more than one year, and another 44 percent demonstrated a short-lasting, subacute prodrome. Symptoms included agitation, anxiety, stubbornness, bold and bossy behavior, decreased concentration, sleep and mood disturbances, excitability, grandiosity, high energy, mood lability, and somatic complaints. Perhaps early psychotherapeutic prevention programs might address these prodromes and guide early care. Galanter and coworkers (2009) identify these and other clinical characteristics that lead to a diagnosis of bipolar disorder in children.

In 1997, the American Academy of Child and Adolescent Psychiatry published the first clinical practice parameters for the assessment and treatment of bipolar disorder in children and adolescents. This report was updated in 2005 (Kowatch et al., 2005) and again in 2007 (McClellan et al., 2007). In the 2007 edition, the authors state:

> The presentation of bipolar disorder in youth, especially children, is often considered atypical compared with that of the classic adult disorder, which is characterized by distinct phases of mania and depression. Children who receive a diagnosis of bipolar disorder in community settings typically present with rapid fluctuations in mood and behavior, often associated with comorbid ADHD and disruptive behavioral disorders. Thus, at this time it is not clear whether the atypical form of the disorder represents the same illness. The question of diagnostic continuity has important treatment and prognostic implications. Although more controlled trials are needed, mood stabilizers and atypical antipsychotic agents are generally considered the first line of treatment Behavioral and psychosocial therapies are also generally indicated for juvenile mania to address disruptive behavior problems and the impact on family and community functioning. (p. 107)

Smarty and Findling (2007) reviewed the psychopharmacology literature published between 1995 and 2006 and concluded:

> Lithium, some anticonvulsants and second generation antipsychotics may be equally beneficial in the acute monotherapy for youth with mixed or manic states. However, because of limited response to monotherapy, there is increased justification for combination therapy. There is very limited data on the treatment of the depressed phase of bipolar illness in the youth. Also, very few studies have addressed the treatment of comorbidities and maintenance/relapse prevention. (p. 39)

DelBello and coworkers (2006) and Barzman and coworkers (2006) reported on controlled studies comparing valproic acid (Depakote, an anticonvulsant) and quetiapine (Seroquel, an atypical antipsychotic) in pediatric bipolar disorder. Quetiapine was at least as effective as valproic acid and produced a quicker onset of response. Combinations of valproic acid and quetiapine are currently being considered, but valproic acid can reduce the rate of metabolism of quetiapine, and this combination was associated with a 77 percent increase in quetiapine plasma levels (Aichhorn and coworkers, 2006).

Chang and colleagues (2006) report that lamotrigine (Lamictal), either as an adjunct therapy or as monotherapy, may be an effective treatment for adolescents with bipolar disorder. In a study of 20 adolescents, 58 percent were considered to be in remission after eight weeks of therapy. No controls were utilized. Precautions about the side effects of lamotrigine (rash and increased blood levels when combined with valproic acid or certain SSRIs) should be taken. Pavuluri and coworkers (2009) reported that lamotrigine reduced manic symptoms by 72 percent and depressive symptoms by 82 percent; and the remission rate was 54 percent. The average dose was about 200 milligrams after an eight-week upward dose titration; the drug was "safe and tolerable with benign rash in 6.4% of the pediatric bipolar population" (p. 80).

There are as yet no reported clinical trials of antidepressant therapy in pediatric bipolar disorder. SSRIs can alleviate bipolar depression, although the risk of inducing mood destabilization (behavioral activation) is present if the drug is not used with a mood stabilizer.

Wozniak and coworkers (2007) demonstrated that an omega-3 fatty acid supplement high in eicosapentaenoic acid (EPA) was effective for children with ADHD, bipolar disorder, and other educational and behavioral problems. The OmegaBrite D supplement of omega-3 fatty acids was evaluated for efficacy and safety over an eight-week period in 20 boys and girls (ages 6 to 17) with bipolar disorder. Half of the youths experienced a rapid 30 percent reduction in symptoms with no side effects.

Medications for Treating Psychotic Disorders

Schizophrenia and its related conditions are considered quite rare in children, and when it occurs it presents significant challenges to clinicians (Findling et al., 2010). However, schizophrenia is relatively common in adolescents with gray matter deficiencies in frontal and parietal lobes before the onset of first-episode symptoms (Reig et al., 2010). Gray-matter deficiencies may be inheritable (Polanczyk et al., 2010). About one in three patients with schizophrenia develops symptoms of psychosis between 10 and 20 years of age. Since childhood and adolescent schizophrenia are generally associated with a poor long-term outcome, effective treatments are needed for children and adolescents with psychotic disorders or, more hopefully, who are in a prodromal phase that precedes first-episode psychosis (Castro-Fornieles et al., 2007).

In a recent landmark study, Amminger and coworkers (2010) studied the effects of omega-3 polyunsaturated fatty acids (1.2 grams/day) in 81 adolescents and young adults, 13 to 25 years of age, with subthreshold psychosis and at ultra-high risk of psychotic disorder. A 12-week treatment period was followed by a 40-week monitoring period. At cessation of monitoring (12 months), 2 of 41 individuals (4.9 percent) in the omega-3 group and 11 of 40 (27.5 percent) in the placebo group had transitioned to psychotic disorder. The authors concluded that omega-3 fatty acid treatment markedly reduced the risk of progression to psychotic disorder and "may offer a safe and efficacious strategy for indicated prevention in young people with subthreshold psychotic states" (p. 146). This study obviously requires verification and extension.

The current best psychopharmacological agents for the treatment of childhood- and adolescent-onset schizophrenia are the newer atypical antipsychotic drugs (Madaan et al., 2008). While effective, haloperidol and the phenothiazines are best avoided because of their extrapyramidal side effects. Double-blind controlled studies have shown that clozapine (Clozaril), risperidone (Risperdal), olanzapine (Zyprexa), and quetiapine (Seroquel) are all effective for treating children and adolescents with this disorder. In children, no single agent has been shown to be any more or less effective than another (Findling et al., 2010). Clozaril, although effective, is probably a drug of second choice because of unique side effects (Chapter 4). Risperidone and olanzapine are quite effective, but weight gain has been a major problem. Quetiapine has been reported to be effective in limited trials (Kopala et al., 2006). Ziprasidone has been incompletely studied, but initial reports are encouraging (Meighen et al., 2004). However, its use in children and adolescents is limited by adverse electrocardiographic changes (QT interval prolongation) that may require close medical monitoring (Blair et al., 2005). Aripiprazole has been incompletely studied, but initial reports indicate limited effectiveness in treating psychosis in children and adolescents (Rugino and Janvier, 2005); in adults, however, it is comparable to other second-generation agents. In 2008, the FDA approved aripiprazole for the treatment of patients 10 to 17 years old with schizophrenia and bipolar disorder.

STUDY QUESTIONS

1. What is meant by an "off-label" use of a drug?

2. Why are psychotherapeutic drugs usually used "off-label" in children and adolescents?

3. Defend early therapeutic interventions in treating psychological disorders in children.

4. Which classes of psychotherapeutic drugs might be used to treat aggressive disorders in children and adolescents? Which might be of the most benefit?

5. Which classes of psychotherapeutic drugs might be useful in treating autism and other pervasive developmental disorders?

6. How might one of these classes be chosen over another?

7. Besides stimulant medications, what other classes of drugs might be considered for use in treating ADHD? Compare and contrast them with psychostimulants.

8. How does methylphenidate compare and contrast with cocaine?

9. Should depression in children be treated? Defend your answer.

10. Compare and contrast the tricyclic antidepressants and the SSRIs in childhood and adolescent depression.

11. What conditions might be comorbid with generalized anxiety disorder in children? How might this comorbidity affect therapy?

12. Compare and contrast the benzodiazepines and the SSRIs in the treatment of anxiety disorders in children and adolescents.

13. Compare and contrast the neuromodulator mood stabilizers and the atypical antipsychotics in the treatment of bipolar disorder in children and adolescents.

14. Discuss the relevant issues in the treatment of schizophrenia, schizoaffective disorder, and the prodromal phase of schizophrenia in children and adolescents.

REFERENCES

Abikoff, H. B., et al. (2009). "Methylphenidate Effects on Functional Outcomes in the Preschoolers with Attention-Deficit/Hyperactivity Disorder Treatment Study (PATS)." In J. L. Luby and M. A. Riddle, eds., *Advances in Preschool Psychopharmacology* (pp. 141–152*)*. New Rochelle, NY: Mary Ann Liebert, Inc.

ACOG Committee on Practice Bulletins–Obstetrics. (2008). "Use of Psychotropic Medications During Pregnancy and Lactation." *Obstetrics and Gynecology* 92: 1001–1020.

Aichhorn, W., et al. (2006). "Influence of Age, Gender, Body Weight, and Valproate Comedication on Quetiapine Plasma Concentrations." *International Clinical Psychopharmacology* 21: 81–85.

Alwan, S., and Friedman, J. M. (2009). "Safety of Selective Serotonin Reuptake Inhibitors in Pregnancy." *CNS Drugs* 23: 493–509.

Aman, M. G., et al. (2009). "Medication and Parent Training in Children with Pervasive Developmental Disorders and Serious Behavioral Problems: Results from a Randomized Clinical Trial." *Journal of the American Association of Child & Adolescent Psychiatry* 48: 1143–1154.

American Academy of Child and Adolescent Psychiatry. (2007). "Practice Parameter for the Assessment and Treatment of Children and Adolescents with Attention-Deficit-Hyperactivity Disorder." *Journal of the American Academy of Child and Adolescent Psychiatry* 46: 894–921.

American Academy of Child and Adolescent Psychiatry. (2009). "Practice Parameter on the Use of Psychotropic Medication in Children and Adolescents." *Journal of the American Association of Child and Adolescent Psychiatry* 48: 961–973.

Amminger, G. P., et al. (2010). "Long-Chain Omega-3 Fatty Acids for Indicated Prevention of Psychotic Disorders: A Randomized, Placebo-Controlled Trial." *Archives of General Psychiatry* 67: 146–154.

Arnsten, A. F. (2006). "Fundamentals of Attention-Deficit/Hyperactivity Disorder: Circuits and Pathways." *Journal of Clinical Psychiatry* 67, Supplement 8: 7–12.

Arnsten, A. F. (2009). "Toward a New Understanding of Attention-Deficit Hyperactivity Disorder Pathophysiology: An Important Role for Prefrontal Cortex Dysfunction." *CNS Drugs* 23, Supplement 1: 33–41.

Banach, R., et al. (2010). "Long-Term Developmental Outcome of Children of Women with Epilepsy, Unexposed or Exposed Prenatally to Antiepileptic Drugs: A Meta Analysis of Cohort Studies." *Drug Safety* 33: 73–79.

Barzman, D. H., and Findling, R. L. (2008). "Pharmacological Treatment of Pathologic Aggression in Children." *International Reviews in Psychiatry* 20: 151–157.

Barzman, D. H., et al. (2006). "The Efficacy and Tolerability of Quetiapine versus Divalproex for the Treatment of Impulsivity and Reactive Aggression in Adolescents with Co-Occurring Bipolar Disorder and Disruptive Behavior Disorder(s)." *Journal of Child and Adolescent Psychopharmacology* 16: 665–670.

Bent, S., et al. (2009). "Omega-3 Fatty Acids for Autistic Spectrum Disorder: A Systematic Review." *Journal of Autism and Developmental Disorders* 39: 1145–1154.

Biederman, J., et al. (2008). "Long-Term, Open-Label Extension Study of Guanfacine Extended Release in Children and Adolescents with ADHD." *CNS Spectrums* 13: 1047–1055.

Biederman, J., et al. (2010). "How Persistent Is ADHD? A Controlled 10-Year Follow-Up Study of Boys with ADHD." *Psychiatry Research* 177: 299–304.

Blair, J., et al. (2005). "Electrocardiographic Changes in Children and Adolescents Treated with Ziprasidone: A Prospective Study." *Journal of the American Academy of Child and Adolescent Psychiatry* 44: 73–79.

Brent, D. A., et al. (2008). "Switching to Another SSRI or to Venlafaxine with or Without Cognitive Behavioral Therapy for Adolescents with SSRI-Resistant Depression." *Journal of the American Medical Association* 299: 901–913.

Brent, D. A., et al. (2009). "Predictors of Spontaneous and Systematically Assessed Suicidal Adverse Events in the Treatment of SSRI-Resistant Depression in Adolescents (TORDIA) Study." *American Journal of Psychiatry* 166: 418–426.

Bridge, J., et al. (2007). "Clinical Responses and Risk for Reported Suicidal Ideation and Suicide Attempts in Pediatric Antidepressant Treatment: A Meta-Analysis of Randomized Controlled Trials." *Journal of the American Medical Association* 297: 1683–1696.

Bromley, R. L., et al. (2008). "Autism Spectrum Disorders Following *In Utero* Exposure to Antiepileptic Drugs." *Neurology* 71: 1923–1924.

Budman, C., et al. (2008). "Aripiprazole in Children and Adolescents with Tourette Disorder with and Without Explosive Outbursts." *Journal of Child and Adolescent Psychopharmacology* 18: 509–515.

Buhimschi, C. S., and Weiner, C. P. (2009). "Medications in Pregnancy and Lactation: Part I. Teratology." *Obstetrics & Gynecology* 113: 166–188.

Bukstein, O. G., et al. (2009). "Does Switching from Oral Extended-Release Methylphenidate to the Methylphenidate Transdermal System Affect Health-Related Quality-of-Life and Medication Satisfaction for Children with Attention-Deficit Hyperactivity Disorder?" *Child and Adolescent Psychiatry and Mental Health* 3: 39–51.

CARE Study Group. (2008). "Maternal Caffeine Intake During Pregnancy and Risk of Fetal Growth Restriction: A Large Prospective Observational Study." *British Medical Journal* 337: a2332.

Carlson, G. A., et al. (2009). "Rages—What Are They and Who Has Them?" *Journal of Child and Adolescent Psychopharmacology* 19: 281–288.

Castro-Fornieles, J., et al. (2007). "The Child and Adolescent First-Episode Psychosis Study (CAFEPS): Design and Baseline Results." *Schizophrenia Research* 91: 226–237.

Chang, K., et al. (2006). "An Open-Label Study of Lamotrigine Adjunct or Monotherapy for the Treatment of Adolescents with Bipolar Depression." *Journal of the American Academy of Child and Adolescent Psychiatry* 45: 298–304.

Cheung, A. H., et al. (2007). "Guidelines for Adolescent Depression in Primary Care (GLAD-PC): II. Treatment and Ongoing Management." *Pediatrics* 120: e1313–e1326.

Coghill, D., and Banaschewski, T. (2009). "The Genetics of Attention-Deficit-Hyperactivity Disorder." *Expert Review of Neurotherapeutics* 9: 1547–1565.

Cohen, J. A., et al. (2010). "Practice Parameter for the Assessment and Treatment of Children and Adolescents with Posttraumatic Stress Disorder." *Journal of the American Academy of Child and Adolescent Psychiatry* 49: 414–430.

Cohen, L. S. (2007). "Treatment of Bipolar Disorder During Pregnancy." *Journal of Clinical Psychiatry* 68, Supplement 9: 4–9.

Cohen, L. S., et al. (2006). "Relapse of Major Depression During Pregnancy in Women Who Maintain or Discontinue Antidepressant Treatment." *Journal of the American Medical Association* 295: 499–507.

Compton, S. N., et al. (2010). "Child-Adolescent Anxiety Multimodal Study (CAMS): Rationale, Design, and Methods." *Child and Adolescent Psychiatry and Mental Health* 4: 1(5 January).

Connolly, S., et al. (2007). "Practice Parameter for the Assessment and Treatment of Children and Adolescents with Anxiety Disorders." *Journal of the American Academy of Child and Adolescent Psychiatry* 46: 267–283.

Coppola, D., et al. (2007). "Evaluating the Postmarketing Experience of Risperidone Use During Pregnancy: Pregnancy and Neonatal Outcomes." *Drug Safety* 30: 247–264.

Costello, E. J., et al. (2007). "Service Costs of Caring for Adolescents with Mental Illness in a Rural Community, 1993–2000." *American Journal of Psychiatry* 164: 36–42.

DelBello, M. P., et al. (2006). "A Double-Blind, Randomized Pilot Study Comparing Quetiapine and Divalproex for Adolescent Mania." *Journal of the American Academy of Child and Adolescent Psychiatry* 45: 305–313.

Denchev, P., et al. (2010). "Modeled Economic Evaluation of Alternative Strategies to Reduce Sudden Cardiac Death Among Children Treated for Attention-Deficit/Hyperactivity Disorder." *Circulation* 121: 1329–1337.

Domino, M. E., et al. (2009). "Relative Cost-Effectiveness of Treatments for Adolescent Depression." *Journal of the American Academy of Child and Adolescent Psychiatry* 48: 711–720.

Donnelly, C., et al. (2009). "Safety and Tolerability of Atomoxetine over 3 to 4 Years in Children and Adolescents with ADHD." *Journal of the American Academy of Child and Adolescent Psychiatry* 48: 176–185.

Donovan, S. J., et al. (2000). "Divalproex Treatment for Youth with Explosive Temper and Mood Lability: A Double-Blind, Placebo-Controlled Crossover Design." *American Journal of Psychiatry* 157: 818–820.

Egger, H. (2010). "A Perilous Disconnect: Antipsychotic Drug Use in Very Young Children." *Journal of the American Academy of Child and Adolescent Psychiatry* 49: 3–6.

Einarson, A. (2009). "Risks/Safety of Psychotropic Medication Use During Pregnancy." *Canadian Journal of Clinical Pharmacology* 16: e58–e65.

Einarson, A., and Boskovic, R. (2009). "Use and Safety of Antipsychotic Drugs During Pregnancy." *Journal of Psychiatric Practice* 15: 183–192.

Emslie, G. J., et al. (1997). "A Double-Blind, Randomized, Placebo-Controlled Trial of Fluoxetine in Children and Adolescents with Depression." *Archives of General Psychiatry* 54: 1031–1037.

Emslie, G. J., et al. (2007). "Long-Term, Open-Label Venlafaxine Extended-Release Treatment in Children and Adolescents with Major Depressive Disorder." *CNS Spectrums* 12. 223–233.

Emslie, G., et al. (2008). "Fluoxetine versus Placebo in Preventing Relapse of Major Depression in Children and Adolescents." *American Journal of Psychiatry* 165: 459–467.

Emslie, G., et al. (2009). "Escitalopram in the Treatment of Adolescent Depression: A Randomized, Placebo-Controlled Multisite Trial." *Journal of the American Academy of Child and Adolescent Psychiatry* 48: 721–729.

Emslie, G. J., et al. (2010). "Treatment of Resistant Depression in Adolescents (TORDIA): Week 24 Outcomes." *American Journal of Psychiatry* 167: 782–791.

Epstein, J. N., et al. (2010). "Attention-Deficit/Hyperactivity Disorder Outcomes for Children Treated in Community-Based Pediatric Settings." *Archives of Pediatric and Adolescent Medicine* 164: 160–165.

Fanton, J., and Gleason, M. M. (2009). "Psychopharmacology and Preschoolers: A Critical Review of Current Conditions." *Child and Adolescent Psychiatry Clinics of North America* 18: 753–771.

Faraone, S. V., and Glatt, S. J. (2010). "Effects of Extended-Release Guanfacine on ADHD Symptoms and Sedation-Related Events in Children with ADHD." *Journal of Attention Disorders* 13: 532–538.

Faraone, S. V., et al. (2008). "Effect of Stimulants on Height and Weight: A Review of the Literature." *Journal of the American Academy of Child and Adolescent Psychiatry* 47: 994–1009.

Findling, R. L. (2008). "Atypical Antipsychotic Treatment of Disruptive Behavior Disorders in Children and Adolescents." *Journal of Clinical Psychiatry* 69, Supplement 4: 9–14.

Findling, R. L., et al. (2010). "Double-Blind Maintenance Safety and Effectiveness Findings from the TEOSS Study." *Journal of the American Academy of Child and Adolescent Psychiatry* 49: 583–594.

Fisher, C. (2010). "Managing Aggression in Children." *The Carlat Child Psychiatry Report* 1: 1–3.

Franke, B., et al. (2009). "Genome-Wide Association Studies in ADHD." *Human Genetics* 126: 13–50.

Freeman, J. B., et al. (2009). "The Pediatric Obsessive-Compulsive Disorder Treatment Study II: Rationale, Design, and Methods." *Child and Adolescent Psychiatry and Mental Health* 3: 4 (30 January).

Freeman, M. P. (2007). "Bipolar Disorder and Pregnancy: Risks Revealed." *American Journal of Psychiatry* 164: 1771–1773.

Friedman, R. A. (2006). "Uncovering an Epidemic: Screening for Mental Illness in Teens." *New England Journal of Medicine* 26: 2717–2719.

Galanter, C. A., et al., (2009). "Symptoms Leading to a Bipolar Diagnosis: A Phone Survey of Child and Adolescent Psychiatrists." *Journal of Child & Adolescent Psychopharmacology* 19: 641–647.

Gentile, S. (2008). "Infant Safety with Antipsychotic Therapy in Breast-Feeding: A Systematic Review." *Journal of Clinical Psychiatry* 69: 666–673.

Ghuman, J. K., et al. (2008). "Psychopharmacological and Other Treatments in Preschool Children with Attention-Deficit/Hyperactivity Disorder: Current Evidence and Practice." *Journal of Child & Adolescent Psychopharmacology* 18: 413–447.

Ghuman, J. K., et al. (2009). "Prospective, Naturalistic, Pilot Study of Open-Label Atomoxetine Treatment in Preschool Children with Attention-Deficit/Hyperactivity Disorder." *Journal of Child & Adolescent Psychopharmacology* 19: 155–166.

Gibbons, R. D., et al. (2006). "The Relationship Between Antidepressant Prescription Rates and Rate of Early Adolescent Suicide." *American Journal of Psychiatry* 163: 1898–1904.

Gibbons, R. D., et al. (2007). Relationship Between Antidepressants and Suicide Attempts: An Analysis of the Veterans Health Administration Data Sets." *American Journal of Psychiatry* 164: 1044–1049.

Gleason, M. M., et al. (2007). "Psychopharmacological Treatment for Very Young Children: Contexts and Guidelines." *Journal of the American Academy of Child and Adolescent Psychiatry* 46: 1532–1572.

Gould, M. S., et al. (2009). "Sudden Death and Use of Stimulant Medications in Youths." *American Journal of Psychiatry* 166: 992–1001.

Greenaway, M., and Elbe, D. (2009). "Focus on Aripiprazole: A Review of Its Use in Child and Adolescent Psychiatry." *Journal of the Canadian Academy of Child and Adolescent Psychiatry* 18: 250–260.

Greenhill, L. L., et al. (2006). "Efficacy and Safety of Immediate-Release Methylphenidate Treatment for Preschoolers with ADHD." *Journal of the American Academy of Child and Adolescent Psychiatry* 45: 1284–1293.

Handen, B. L., et al. (2008). "Guanfacine in Children with Autism and/or Intellectual Disabilities." *Journal of Developmental and Behavioral Pediatrics* 29: 303–308.

Harden, C. L., et al. (2010). "Practice Parameter Update: Management Issues for Women with Epilepsy—Focus on Pregnancy (an Evidence-Based Review): Teratogenesis and Perinatal Outcomes: Report of the Quality Standards Subcommittee on Therapeutics and Technology Assessment Subcommittee of the American Academy of Neurology and American Epilepsy Society." *Neurology* 73: 133–141.

Hirshfeld-Becker, D. R., et al. (2007). "Clinical Outcomes of Laboratory-Observed Preschool Behavioral Disinhibition at Five-Year Follow-Up." *Biological Psychiatry* 62: 565–572.

Hollander, E., et al. (2010). "Divalproex Sodium vs Placebo for the Treatment of Irritability in Children and Adolescents with Autism Spectrum Disorders." *Neuropsychopharmacology* 35: 990–998.

Hunt, S., et al. (2008). "Topiramate in Pregnancy: Preliminary Experience from the UK Epilepsy and Pregnancy Register." *Neurology* 71: 272–276.

Ipser, J., and Stein, D. (2007). "Systematic Review of Pharmacotherapy of Disruptive Behavioral Disorders in Children and Adolescents." *Psychopharmacology* 191: 127–140.

Jorm, A. F. (2006). "Effectiveness of Complementary and Self-Help Treatments for Depression in Children and Adolescents." *Medical Journal of Australia* 185: 368–372.

Kahbazi, M., et al. (2009). "A Randomized, Double-Blind and Placebo-Controlled Trial of Modafinil in Children and Adolescents with Attention-Deficit/Hyperactivity Disorder." *Psychiatry Research* 168: 234–237.

Keeton, C. P., et al. (2009): "Pediatric Generalized Anxiety Disorder: Epidemiology, Diagnosis, and Management." *Paediatric Drugs* 11: 171–183.

Kennard, B. D., et al. (2009a). "Remission and Recovery in the Treatment for Adolescents with Depression Study (TADS): Acute and Long-Term Outcomes." *Journal of the American Academy of Child and Adolescent Psychiatry* 48: 187–196.

Kennard, B. D., et al. (2009b). "Effective Components of TORDIA Cognitive-Behavioral Therapy for Adolescent Depression: Preliminary Findings." *Journal of Consulting Clinical Psychiatry* 77: 1033–1041.

Kennedy, S. J., et al. (2009). "A Selective Intervention Program for Inhibited Preschool-Aged Children of Parents with an Anxiety Disorder: Effects on Current Anxiety Disorders and Temperament." *Journal of the American Academy of Child and Adolescent Psychiatry* 48: 602–609.

Kessler, R. C., et al. (2005). "Lifetime Prevalence and Age-of-Onset Distributions of DSM-IV Disorders in the National Comorbidity Survey Replication." *Archives of General Psychiatry* 62: 593–602.

Khanzode, L. A., et al (2006). "Efficacy Profiles of Psychopharmacology: Divalproex Sodium in Conduct Disorder." *Child Psychiatry and Human Development* 37: 55–64.

King, B. H., et al. (2009). "Lack of Efficacy of Citalopram in Children with Autism Spectrum Disorders and High Levels of Repetitive Behaviors: Citalopram Ineffective in Children with Autism." *Archives of General Psychiatry* 66: 583–590.

Kopala, L. C., et al. (2006). "Treatment of a First Episode of Psychotic Illness with Quetiapine: An Analysis of 2-Year Outcomes." *Schizophrenia Research* 81: 29–39.

Kowatch, R. A., et al. (2005). "Treatment Guidelines for Children and Adolescents with Bipolar Disorder: Child Psychiatric Workgroup on Bipolar Disorder." *Journal of the American Academy of Child and Adolescent Psychiatry* 44: 213–235.

Kumar, R. (2008). "Approved and Investigational Uses of Modafinil: An Evidence-Based Review." *Drugs* 68: 1803–1839.

Libby, A. M., et al (2009). "Persisting Decline in Depression Treatment After FDA Warnings." *Archives of General Psychiatry* 66: 633–639.

Luby, J. L. (2009). "Early Childhood Depression." *American Journal of Psychiatry* 166: 974–979.

Luby, J. L. (2010). "The Use of Psychotropic Agents in Preschool Children: Issues in Practice, Research and Public Policy." *Child & Adolescent Psychopharmacology News* 14(4): 1–5.

Luby, J. L., and Navsaria, N. (2010). "Pediatric Bipolar Disorder: Evidence for Prodromal States and Early Markers." *Journal of Child Psychology and Psychiatry* 51: 459–471.

Luby, J. L., and Riddle, M. A., eds. (2009). *Advances in Preschool Psychopharmacology.* New Rochelle, NY: Mary Ann Liebert, Inc.

Luby, J. L., et al (2008). "Treatment of Preschool Bipolar Disorder: A Novel Parent-Child Interaction Therapy and Review on Data on Psychopharmacology." In B. Geller and M. P. DelBello, eds., *Treatment of Bipolar Disorder in Children and Adolescents* (pp. 270–286). New York: Guilford.

Luby, J. L., et al. (2009a). "Preschool Depression: Homotypic Continuity and Course over 24 Months." *Archives of General Psychiatry* 66: 897–905.

Luby, J. L., et al. (2009b). "The Clinical Significance of Preschool Depression: Impairment in Functioning and Clinical Markers of the Disorder." *Journal of Affective Disorders* 112: 111–119.

Luby, J. L., et al. (2009c). "Preschool Bipolar Disorder." *Child & Adolescent Psychiatric Clinics of North America* 18: 391–403.

Lutz, U. C. et al. (2010). "Aripiprazole in Pregnancy and Lactation: A Case Report." *Journal of Clinical Psychopharmacology* 30: 204–205.

Maayan, L., et al. (2009). "The Open-Label Treatment of Attention-Deficit/Hyperactivity Disorder in 4- and 5-Year-Old Children with Beaded Methylphenidate." *Journal of Child and Adolescent Psychopharmacology* 19: 147–153.

Madaan, V., et al. (2008). "Child and Adolescent Schizophrenia: Pharmacological Approaches." *Expert Opinion in Pharmacotherapeutics* 9: 2053–2068.

March, J. S., and Vitiello, B. (2009). "Clinical Messages from the Treatment of Adolescents with Depression Study (TADS)." *American Journal of Psychiatry* 166: 1118–1123.

March, J. S., et al. (2009). "The Treatment for Adolescents with Depression Study (TADS): Long-Term Effectiveness and Safety Outcomes." *Archives of General Psychiatry* 64: 1132–1143.

Marcus, R. N., et al. (2009). "A Placebo-Controlled, Fixed-Dose Study of Aripiprazole in Children and Adolescents with Irritability Associated with Autistic Disorder." *Journal of the American Academy of Child and Adolescent Psychiatry* 48: 1110–1119.

Mayes, R., et al. (2009). *Medicating Children: ADHD and Pediatric Mental Health.* Cambridge, MA: Harvard University Press.

Maziade, M., et al. (2009). "Atomoxetine and Neurpsychological Function in Children with Attention-Deficit/Hyperactivity Disorder: Results of a Pilot Study." *Journal of Child and Adolescent Psychopharmacology* 19: 709–718.

McClellan, J., et al. (2007). "Practice Parameter for the Assessment and Treatment of Children and Adolescents with Bipolar Disorder." *Journal of the American Academy of Child and Adolescent Psychiatry* 46: 107–125.

Meador, K. J., et al. (2009). "Cognitive Function at 3 Years of Age After Fetal Exposure to Antiepileptic Drugs." *New England Journal of Medicine* 360: 1597–1605.

Meighen, K. G., et al. (2004). "Ziprasidone Treatment of Two Adolescents with Psychosis." *Journal of the American Academy of Child & Adolescent Psychopharmacology* 14: 137–142.

Meiri, G., et al. (2009). "Omega-3 Fatty Acid Treatment in Autism." *Journal of Child and Adolescent Psychopharmacology* 19: 449–451.

Merikangas, K., et al. (2010). "Prevalence and Treatment of Mental Disorders Among U.S. Children in the 2001–2004 NHANES." *Pediatrics* 125: 75–81.

Molina, B. S., et al. (2009). "The MTA at 8 Years: Prospective Follow-Up of Children Treated for Combined Type ADHD in a Multisite Study." *Journal of the American Academy of Child and Adolescent Psychiatry* 48: 484–500.

MTA Cooperative Group. (1999). "A 14-Month Randomized Clinical Trial of Treatment Strategies for Attention-Deficit/Hyperactivity Disorder." *Archives of General Psychiatry* 56: 1073–1086.

MTA Cooperative Group. (2004). "National Institute of Mental Health Multimodal Treatment Study of ADHD Follow-Up: Changes in Effectiveness and Growth After the End of Treatment." *Pediatrics* 113: 762–769.

Nemeroff, C. B., et al. (2007). "Impact of Publicity Concerning Pediatric Suicidality Data on Physician Practice Patterns in the United States." *Archives of General Psychiatry* 64: 466–472.

Newham, J. J., et al. (2008). "Birth Weight of Infants After Maternal Exposure to Typical and Atypical Antipsychotics: Prospective Comparison Study." *British Journal of Psychiatry* 192: 333–337.

Newport, D. J., et al. (2007). "Atypical Antipsychotic Administration During Late Pregnancy: Placental Passage and Obstetrical Outcomes." *American Journal of Psychiatry* 164: 1214–1220.

Newport, D. J., et al. (2008a). "Lamotrigine in Breast Milk and Nursing Infants: Determination of Exposure." *Pediatrics* 122: e223–e231.

Newport, D. J., et al. (2008b). "Lamotrigine in Bipolar Disorder: Efficacy During Pregnancy." *Bipolar Disorder* 10: 432–436.

Nguyen, H. T., et al. (2009). "Teratogenesis Associated with Antibipolar Agents." *Advances in Therapeutics* 6: 281–294.

Oberlander, T. F., et al. (2008). "Effects of Timing and Duration of Gestational Exposure to Serotonin Reuptake Inhibitor Antidepressants: Population-Based Study." *British Journal of Psychiatry* 192: 338–343.

Olfson, M., et al. (2010). "Trends in Antipsychotic Drug Use by Very Young, Privaterly Insured Children." *Journal of the American Academy of Child and Adolescent Psychiatry* 49: 13–23.

Owen, R., et al. (2009). "Aripiprazole in the Treatment of Irritability in Children and Adolescents with Autistic Disorder." *Pediatrics* 124: 1533–1540.

Pappadopulos, E., et al. (2009). Medication Adherence in the MTA: Saliva Methylphenidate versus Parent Report and Mediating Effect of Concomitant Behavioral Treatment." *Journal of the American Academy of Child and Adolescent Psychiatry* 48: 501–510

Parry, B. L. (2009). "Assessing Risk and Benefit: To Treat or Not to Treat Major Depression During Pregnancy with Antidepressant Medication." *American Journal of Psychiatry* 166: 512–514

Pavuluri, M. N., et al. (2009). "Effectiveness of Lamotrigine in Maintaining Symptom Control in Pediatric Bipolar Disorder." *Journal of Child and Adolescent Psychopharmacology* 19: 75–82.

Pedersen, L. H., et al. (2009). "Selective Serotonin Reuptake Inhibitors in Pregnancy and Congenital Malformations: Population Based Cohort Study." *British Medical Journal* 339: b3569.

Pediatric OCD Treatment Study (POTS) Team. (2004). "Cognitive-Behavior Therapy, Sertraline, and Their Combination for Children and Adolescents with Obsessive-Compulsive Disorder: The Pediatric OCD Treatment Study (POTS) Randomized Controlled Trial." *Journal of the American Medical Association* 292: 1969–1976.

Penzner, J. B., et al. (2009). "Lack of Effect of Stimulant Combination with Second-Generation Antipsychotics on Weight Gain, Metabolic Changes, Prolactin Levels, and Sedation in Youth with Clinically Relevant Aggression or Oppositionality." *Journal of Child and Adolescent Psychopharmacology* 19: 563–573.

Perrott, J., et al. (2010). "L-Carnitine for Acute Valproic Acid Overdose: A Systematic Review of Published Cases." *Annals of Pharmacotherapy* 44: 1287–1293.

Pessina, E., et al. (2009). "Aripiprazole Augmentation of Serotonin Reuptake Inhibitors in Treatment-Resistant Obsessive-Compulsive Disorder: A 12-Week, Open-Label Preliminary Study." *International Clinical Psychopharmacology* 24: 265–269.

Polanczyk, G., et al. (2010). "Etiological and Clinical Features of Childhood Psychotic Symptoms: Results from a Birth Cohort." *Archives of General Psychiatry* 67: 328–338

Posner, K., et al. (2007). "Clinical Presentation of Attention-Deficit/Hyperactivity Disorder in Preschool Children: The Preschoolers with Attention-Deficit/Hyperactivity Disorder Treatment Study (PATS)." *Journal of Child & Adolescent Psychopharmacology* 17: 547–562.

Potegal, M., et al. (2009). "The Behavioral Organization, Temporal Characteristics, and Diagnostic Concomitants of Rage Outbursts in Child Psychiatric Inpatients." *Current Psychiatry Reports* 11: 127–133.

Prasad, S., et al. (2007). "A Multi-Centre, Randomized, Open-Label Study of Atomoxetine Compared with Standard Current Therapy in UK Children and Adolescents with Attention-Deficit/Hyperactivity Disorder." *Current Medical Research and Opinion* 23: 379–394.

Propper, L., and Orlik, H. (2009). "The Use of Psychotropic Drugs in Autism and Other Pervasive Developmental Disorders." *Child & Adolescent Psychopharmacology News* 14(2): 1–8:

Quintana, H., et al. (2007). "Fluoxetine Monotherapy in Attention-Deficit/Hyperactivity Disorder and Comorbid Non-Bipolar Mood Disorders in Children and Adolescents." *Child Psychiatry and Human Development* 37: 241–253.

Ramos, E., et al. (2008). "Duration of Antidepressant Use During Pregnancy and Risk of Major Congenital Malformations." *British Journal of Psychiatry* 192: 344–350.

Rao, U., et al. (2010). "Hippocampal Changes Associated with Early-Life Adversity and Vulnerability to Depression." *Biological Psychiatry* 67: 357–364.

Reig, S., et al. (2010). "Multicenter Study of Brain Volume Abnormalities in Children and Adolescent-Onset Psychosis." *Schizophrenia Bulletin.* In press.

Reis, M., and Kallen, B. (2008). "Maternal Use of Antipsychotics in Early Pregnancy and Delivery Outcome." *Journal of Clinical Pharmacology* 28: 279–288.

Rugino, T. A., and Janvier, Y. M. (2005). "Aripiprazole in Children and Adolescents: Clinical Experience." *Journal of Child Neurology* 20: 603–610.

Sallee, F., et al. (2009). "Guanfacine Extended-Release in Children and Adolescents with Attention-Deficit/Hyperactivity Disorder." *Journal of the American Academy of Child and Adolescent Psychiatry* 48: 155–165.

Saxena, K., et al. (2006). "Divalproex Sodium Reduces Overall Aggression in Youth at High Risk for Bipolar Disorder." *Journal of Child and Adolescent Psychopharmacology* 16: 252–259.

Sayal, K., et al. (2009). "Binge Pattern of Alcohol Consumption During Pregnancy and Childhood Mental Health Outcomes: Longitudinal Population-Based Study." *Pediatrics* 123: e289–e296.

Schechter, D. S., and Willheim, E. (2009). "Disturbances of Attachment and Parental Psychopathology in Early Childhood." *Child and Adolescent Psychiatry Clinics of North America* 18: 665–686.

Scheffler, R. M., et al. (2009). "Positive Association Between Attention-Deficit/Hyperactivity Disorder Medication Use and Academic Achievement During Elementary School." *Pediatrics* 123: 1273–1279.

Schuchardt, J. P., et al. (2010). "Significance of Long-Chain Polyunsaturated Fatty Acids (PUFAs) for the Development and Behavior of Children." *European Journal of Pediatrics* 169: 149–164.

Setlik, J., et al. (2009). "Adolescent Prescription ADHD Medication Abuse Is Rising Along with Prescriptions for These Medications." *Pediatrics* 124: 875–880.

Shechtman, Z., and Birani-Nasaraladin, D. (2006). "Treating Mothers of Aggressive Children: A Research Study." *International Journal of Group Psychotherapy* 56: 93–112.

Smarty, S., and Findling, R. L. (2007). "Psychopharmacology of Pediatric Bipolar Disorder: A Review." *Psychopharmacology* 191: 39–54.

Smith, E. G. (2009). "Association Between Antidepressant Half-Life and the Risk of Suicidal Ideation or Behavior Among Children and Adolescents: Confirmatory Analysis and Research Implications." *Journal of Affective Disorders* 114: 143–148.

Sowell, E. R., et al. (2010). "Differentiating Prenatal Exposure to Methamphetamine and Alcohol versus Alcohol and Not Methamphetamine Using Tensor-Based Brain Morphometry and Discriminant Analysis." *Journal of Neuroscience* 30: 3876–3885.

Spencer, T. J., et al. (2009). "Safety and Effectiveness of Coadministration of Guanfacine Extended Release and Psychostimulants in Children and Adolescents with Attention-Deficit/Hyperactivity Disorder." *Journal of Child and Adolescent Psychopharmacology* 19: 501–510.

Staller, J. A. (2007). "Psychopharmacologic Treatment of Aggressive Preschoolers: A Chart Review." *Progress in Neuro-Psychopharmacology & Biological Psychiatry* 13: 131–135.

Stein, M. B., et al. (2009). "Practice Guideline for the Treatment of Patients with Panic Disorder, Second Edition." *American Journal of Psychiatry* 166, Supplement 2: 42–44.

Stigler, K. A., et al. (2009). "Aripiprazole in Pervasive Developmental Disorder Not Otherwise Specified and Asperger's Disorder: A 14-Week, Prospective, Open-Label Study." *Journal of Child and Adolescent Psychopharmacology* 19: 265–274.

Stigler, K. A., et al. (2010). "Paliperidone for Irritability in Autistic Disorder." *Journal of Child and Adolescent Psychopharmacology* 20: 75–78.

Storch, E. A., et al. (2007). "Aripiprazole Augmentation of Incomplete Treatment Response in an Adolescent Male with Obsessive-Compulsive Disorder." *Depression and Anxiety* 25: 172–174.

Strawn, J. R., et al. (2010). "Psychopharmacological Treatment of Posttraumatic Stress Disorder in Children and Adolescents: A Review." *Journal of Clinical Psychiatry*. In press.

Stroud, L. R., et al. (2009). "Maternal Smoking During Pregnancy and Newborn Neurobehavior: Effects at 10 to 27 Days." *Journal of Pediatrics* 154: 10–16.

Su, K. P., et al. (2008). "Omega-3 Fatty Acids for Major Depressive Disorder During Pregnancy: Results from a Randomized, Double-Blind, Placebo-Controlled Trial." *Journal of Clinical Psychiatry* 69: 644–651.

Tandon, M., and Luby, J. (2010). "Psychopharmacology in Preschoolers: A Brief Guide for Clinicians." *Child & Adolescent Psychopharmacology News* 14(4): 5–7.

Tomson, T., and Battino, D. (2009). "Teratogenic Effects of Antiepileptic Medications." *Neurology Clinics* 27: 993–1002.

Treatment for Adolescents with Depression Study (TADS) Team. (2004). "Fluoxetine, Cognitive-Behavioral Therapy, and Their Combination for Adolescents with Depression: Treatment for Adolescents with Depression Study (TADS) Randomized Controlled Trial." *Journal of the American Medical Association* 292: 807–820.

Treatment for Adolescents with Depression Study (TADS) Team. (2009). "The Treatment for Adolescents with Depression Study (TADS): Outcomes over 1-Year of Naturalistic Follow-Up." *American Journal of Psychiatry* 166: 1141–1149.

U. S. Preventive Services Task Force. (2009a). "Counseling and Interventions to Prevent Tobacco-Caused Disease in Adults and Pregnant Women: U.S. Preventive Services Task Force Reaffirmation Recommendation Statement." *Annals of Internal Medicine* 150: 551–555.

U. S. Preventive Services Task Force. (2009b). "Screening and Treatment for Major Depressive Disorder in Children and Adolescents: U.S. Preventive Services Task Force Reaffirmation Recommendation Statement." *Pediatrics* 123: 1223–1228.

Vaughan, B. S., et al. (2008). "Beyond the 'Typical' Patient: Treating Attention-Deficit/Hyperactivity Disorder in Preschoolers and Adults." *International Reviews of Psychiatry* 20: 143–149.

Viguera, A. C., et al. (2007a): "Risk of Recurrence in Women with Bipolar Disorder During Pregnancy: Prospective Study of Mood Stabilizer Discontinuation." *American Journal of Psychiatry* 164: 1817–1824.

Viguera, A. C., et al. (2007b). "Lithium in Breast Milk and Nursing Infants: Clinical Implications." *American Journal of Psychiatry* 164: 342–345.

Vitiello, B. (2009). "Combined Cognitive-Behavioral Therapy and Pharmacotherapy for Adolescent Depression: Does It Improve Outcomes Compared with Monotherapy?" *CNS Drugs* 23: 271–280.

Vitiello, B., and Towbin, K. (2009). "Stimulant Treatment of ADHD and Risk of Sudden Death in Children." *American Journal of Psychiatry* 166: 955–957.

Vitiello, B., et al. (2007). "Effectiveness of Methylphenidate in the 10-Month Continuation Phase of the Preschoolers with Attention-Deficit/Hyperactivity Disorder Treatment Study (PATS)." *Journal of Child & Adolescent Psychopharmacology* 17: 593–604.

Vitiello, B., et al. (2009). "Suicidal Events in the Treatment of Adolescents with Depression Study (TADS). *Journal of Clinical Psychiatry* 70: 741–747.

Volkmar, F. R. (2009). "Citalopram Treatment in Children with Autism Spectrum Disorders." *Archives of General Psychiatry* 66: 581–582.

Volkow, N. D., et al. (2009). "Effects of Modafinil on Dopamine and Dopamine Transporters in Male Human Brain: Clinical Implications." *Journal of the American Medical Association* 301: 1148–1154.

Walkup, J. T. (2010). "Treatment of Depressed Adolescents." *American Journal of Psychiatry* 167: 734–737.

Walkup, J. T., and the American Association of Child and Adolescent Psychiatry. (2009). "Practice Parameter on the Use of Psychotropic Medication in Children and Adolescents." *Journal of the American Association of Child and Adolescent Psychiatry* 48: 961–973.

Walkup, J. T., et al. (2008). "Cognitive Behavioral Therapy, Sertraline, or a Combination in Childhood Anxiety." *New England Journal of Medicine* 359: 2753–2766.

Werremeyer, A. (2009). "Ziprasidone and Citalopram Use in Pregnancy and Lactation in a Woman with Psychotic Depression." *American Journal of Psychiatry* 166: 1298.

Wietecha, L. A., et al. (2009). "Atomoxetine Treatment in Adolescents with Attention-Deficit/Hyperactivity Disorder." *Journal of Child and Adolescent Psychopharmacology* 19: 719–730.

Wilens, T. E., et al. (2008a). "Impact of Prior Stimulant Treatment for Attention-Deficit Hyperactivity Disorder in the Subsequent Risk for Cigarette Smoking, Alcohol, and Drug Use Disorders in Adolescent Girls." *Archives of Pediatric and Adolescent Medicine* 162: 916–921.

Wilens, T. E., et al. (2008b). "Misuse and Diversion of Stimulants Prescribed for ADHD: A Systematic Review of the Literature." *Journal of the American Academy of Child and Adolescent Psychiatry* 47: 21–31.

Wilens, T. E., et al. (2008c). "Varying the Wear Time of the Methylphenidate Transdermal System in Children with Attention Deficit/Hyperactivity Disorder." *Journal of the American Academy of Child and Adolescent Psychiatry* 47: 700–708.

Williams, S. B., et al. (2009). "Screening for Child and Adolescent Depression in Primary Care Settings: A Systematic Evidence Review for the U.S. Preventive Services Task Force." *Pediatrics* 123: e716–e735.

Wisner, K. L., et al. (2009). "Major Depression and Antidepressant Treatment: Impact on Pregnancy and Neonatal Outcomes." *American Journal of Psychiatry* 166: 557–566.

Wozniak, J., et al. (2007). "Omega-3 Fatty Acid Monotherapy for Pediatric Bipolar Disorder: A Prospective Open-Label Trial." *European Neuropsychopharmacology* 17: 440–447.

Yonkers, K. A., et al. (2009). "The Management of Depression During Pregnancy: A Report from the American Psychiatric Association and the American College of Obstetricians and Gynecologists." *Obstetrics and Gynecology* 114: 703–713.

Zimmerman, M., et al. (2008). "Is Bipolar Disorder Overdiagnosed?" *Journal of Clinical Psychiatry* 69: 935–940.

Zuckerbrot, R. A., et al. (2007). "Guidelines for Adolescent Depression in Primary Care (GLAD-PC): I. Identification, Assessment, and Initial Management." *Pediatrics* 120: e1299–e1312.

Chapter 19

Geriatric Psychopharmacology

This chapter applies the drugs discussed in earlier chapters to specific issues in geriatric psychopharmacology: drug treatment of depression, anxiety disorders, behavioral agitation and aggression, Parkinson's disease, and Alzheimer's disease. First, however, we present several general principles concerning the actions and effects of psychoactive drugs administered to elderly patients:

- Lower doses of medication are often as effective in the elderly as higher doses in younger people.
- When initiating drug therapy in the elderly, it is wise to "start low and go slow."
- Elimination half-lives are often prolonged in the elderly, sometimes to about twice as long as half-lives in younger people. This phenomenon can drastically reduce the total daily dose that may need to be administered.
- Sedative-hypnotic drugs, especially the long-half-life benzodiazepines, can be quite "dementing" in the elderly, causing marked and often prolonged loss of the ability to form memory.
- Sedative-hypnotic drugs can also induce psychomotor incoordination, resulting in an increased incidence of falls, altered driving behaviors, and so on.
- Depression and combined anxiety and depression are common in the elderly and need to be addressed and treated.

- Psychological therapies can be used effectively to treat anxiety disorders, sleep disorders, and other psychological disorders for which drugs are often prescribed.
- Inappropriate drug use in the elderly is a common problem with potentially tragic consequences.
- Underdiagnosis and undertreatment of psychological disorders occur frequently, perhaps most prominently in the treatment of anxious and depressive disorders.

Inappropriate Drug Use in the Elderly

The elderly are frequently prescribed medication that they do not need or that cause them significant problems either because of extensions of expected pharmacological effects or through adverse interactions with other medications. Inappropriate medication use in the elderly is a major functional and safety issue and may cause a substantial proportion of drug-related hospital or care-center admissions (Laroche et al., 2007). To help document inappropriate drug use in the elderly, M. H. Beers in 1997 developed specific criteria for inappropriate use, which included a list of drugs that were either ineffective or posed unnecessarily high risks for people over 65 years of age. In 2003, the list was updated to include 48 individual medicines or classes of medicines to avoid in older adults. Of these drugs, 66 were considered to have adverse outcomes of high severity (Fick et al., 2003).

Since 2003, workers in different health care systems have developed modifications of the Beers criteria; examples are the Medication Appropriateness Index (Steinman et al., 2006), the 2006 Health Plan Employer Data and Information Set (HEDIS) (Pugh et al., 2006), the Zhan modification of the Beers criteria (Barnett et al., 2006), and the Improved Prescribing in the Elderly Tool (Ryan et al., 2009). All attempt to identify medicines commonly considered of more risk than benefit to the elderly. All agree that the extent of inappropriate prescription use is common, with a rate between 20 and 40 percent. In elderly patients taking eight or more medications, the incidence of inappropriate drug use rises to well over 60 percent. Among the psychoactive medicines, long-acting benzodiazepines are most commonly inappropriately prescribed, followed by drugs with anticholinergic side effects (for example, tricyclic antidepressants), then antihistamines, skeletal muscle relaxants, and opioid narcotics. Another problematic situation is concomitant use of two or more psychotropic medicines of the same therapeutic class. Inappropriate drug use can lead to suboptimal care that is not consistent with evidence-based clinical practice.

Considering the medications listed, it is obvious that all the lists of criteria for avoiding inappropriate drug use in the elderly recommend avoiding drugs that produce *cognitive inhibition* (with drug-induced dementia as the most severe manifestation), *unwanted sedation* (leading to falls and hip fractures), or *bizarre behaviors and/or drug-induced delirium*. Long-acting benzodiazepines, tricyclic antidepressants (or other drugs with anticholinergic properties), and sedating antihistamines are prominent drugs of concern. Indeed, discontinuing such medications can lead to improvements in psychomotor and cognitive functioning, including memory and attention (Nishtala et al, 2009; Tsunoda et al., 2010).

Control of Agitated and Aggressive Behaviors in the Elderly

Atypical antipsychotic medications (Chapter 4) have become the standard of care for behavioral and psychological symptoms of dementia (BPSD). These medicines control agitated and aggressive behaviors in the elderly, especially residents of care centers. However, in 2005, the Food and Drug Administration (FDA) issued a public health advisory warning indicating a 1.7-fold risk of all-cause mortality from these medicines compared to placebo. This advisory has been controversial because other studies have failed to verify any increased risk of death (Simoni-Wastila et al., 2009; Elie et al., 2009). Despite this advisory and controversy, the use of atypical antipsychotics to treat elderly persons with BPSD is common, especially in long-term-care settings (Connelly et al., 2009). In many care centers, the rates of residents receiving such medicine have been reported to be 25 to 40 percent, with many residents having no identified clinical indication for such therapy (Chen et al., 2010). Figure 19.1 illustrates the extent of use of these medicines: 29 percent of all residents received antipsychotic medication, and over 16 percent of residents who had no clinical indication for antipsychotic therapy (no psychosis and no dementia) nonetheless received such medication. Recently, Dorsey and coworkers (2010) reported that this use of atypical antipsychotic medicines is decreasing in the elderly with dementia, probably to levels clinically more appropriate.

These medicines help to relieve various core symptoms that arise in the course of dementia (Omelan, 2006):

- Agitation (pacing, wandering, restlessness, inability to sit long enough to eat)
- Aggression (verbal and physical), which might be directed at staff or other residents
- Physical resistance and noncompliance with care
- Psychosis (hallucinations, delusions)

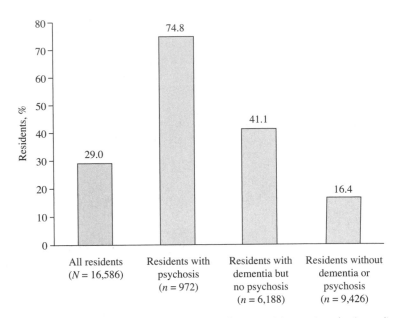

FIGURE 19.1 Percentages of nursing home residents receiving antipsychotic medication in a U.S. nationwide, cross-sectional population of 16,586 newly admitted nursing home residents in 2006. [From Chen et al. (2010), p. 90.]

- Depressive symptoms (apathy, lack of interest)
- Inappropriate sexual behaviors (verbal and physical)
- Sleep disturbances (day/night reversal)

Although agitation and aggression apparently can be reduced through use of an atypical antipsychotic drug, there is little evidence of drug efficacy against the core symptoms of dementia. According to Omelan (2006), certain behaviors should not be expected to improve (wandering, pacing, entering rooms uninvited, disruptive vocalizations). Nevertheless, severe agitation and aggression can be modified. In reviewing early data, the *Medical Letter* (2005) published the following statement:

> Even though controlled clinical trials proving efficacy are lacking, Medical Letter consultants have found atypical antipsychotics such as risperidone and olanzapine beneficial in calming agitated or aggressive elderly patients. The FDA has found a slightly increased risk of mortality with such use, but there are no good alternatives. (p. 62)

Initially, risperidone (Risperdal) and olanzapine (Zyprexa) were used most frequently, but quetiapine (Seroquel) has rapidly gained favor, perhaps because quetiapine seems to cause less undesired weight gain and has less propensity to induce type 2 diabetes. Unfortunately,

Paleacu and coworkers (2008) reported results from a six-week, double-blind, placebo-controlled study of 44 patients with dementia and BPSD showing that quetiapine, in quite large doses, was only modestly more effective than placebo in reducing behavioral symptoms. However, a few patients showed a positive and sustained response.

Streim and coworkers (2008) reported on the efficacy of aripiprazole (Abilify) in the treatment of psychosis in nursing home patients with Alzheimer's disease. The drug did not confer specific benefits for the treatment of psychotic symptoms, but BPSD symptoms—including agitation, anxiety, and depression—were significantly improved, with a low risk of side effects. Although aripiprazole is capable of reducing anxiety and agitation, it can also produce these same symptoms as side effects in about 8 to 10 percent of patients at doses of about 10 milligrams per day (Coley et al., 2009). Further delineation of the usefulness of aripiprazole in BPSD would be welcome.

Finally, it was recently shown that the anti-Alzheimer's medication *donepezil* (Aricept) failed to be effective against agitation in patients with Alzheimer's disease, although it modestly improved cognitive functioning (Howard et al., 2007). Therefore, at this point, despite the FDA's public health advisory, an atypical antipsychotic remains a reasonable choice for the treatment of severe BPSD in the elderly with dementia.

In agitated, aggressive, anxious elderly with dementia, the benefits of behavioral improvement may allow the patient to remain in a less structured and less confining environment than otherwise would be possible. Thus, the humanitarian benefits may outweigh any increase in risk. These agents should be used with discretion and only as part of nonpharmacological, environmental, and behavioral interventions (Omelan, 2006).

Undertreatment of the Elderly: Focus on Depression

Untreated depression in the elderly can seriously reduce both the quality of life and the length of life. However, depression in the elderly remains underdiagnosed and often poorly or inadequately treated. Adults 65 years of age and older account for 20 percent of all suicides in the United States and have the highest suicide completion rate of any age group. In addition, only 8 percent of seniors with depression visit a mental health specialist in any given year. On a positive note, it has been said that a team approach to treating depression in the elderly can be quite successful. One team approach program is called IMPACT (Improving Mood: Promoting Access to Collaborative Treatment). Results from the IMPACT research have recently been updated by Van Leeuwen and coworkers (2009). IMPACT involved a team including a depression case manager (psychologist, social worker or a nurse), a primary care physician, and a consulting psychiatrist. Hunkeler and coworkers (2006) stated:

> Tailored collaborative care actively engages older adults in treatment for depression and delivers substantial and persistent long term benefits. Benefits included less depression, better physical functioning, and an enhanced quality of life. The IMPACT model may show the way to less depression and healthier lives for older adults. (p. 259)

In support of this collaborative care model, Reynolds and coworkers (2006) studied 116 patients over the age of 70 who had been diagnosed with major depression. Here, they compared the efficacy of placebo medication, medication alone, psychological therapy alone, and combined medication and psychological therapy. The medication chosen was paroxetine (Paxil); the psychological therapy chosen was weekly interpersonal psychotherapy. Combination therapy improved the percentage of patients achieving remission from 35 percent with either alone to 58 percent, a remarkable improvement. Results indicated that depression in the elderly can be treated and is best treated by a combination of antidepressant medication and psychological interventions. It is hoped that combined therapy will be more acceptable for the elderly who suffer from major depression than is electroconvulsive therapy, currently a preferred treatment for severe depression in this population (Dombrovski and Mulsant, 2007). Paroxetine was effective in the Reynolds study as well as in a study by Dombrovski and coworkers (2007). Kasper and coworkers (2006) demonstrated the efficacy of escitalopram (Lexapro) in the elderly (mean age 74 years; 82 percent female); escitalopram was later noted to be less efficacious for the treatment of generalized anxiety disorder in the elderly (Lenze et al., 2009).

Nelson and coworkers (2006) reported results on the use of mirtazepine (Remeron) to treat major depression in 50 patients aged 85 and older residing in nursing homes. In 45 percent of patients, mirtazepine (average dose 18 milligrams per day) was effective in decreasing the average Hamilton Rating Scale for Depression score from 17 at baseline to 7 at end point. Sedation and weight gain were prominent side effects. Administering the drug at bedtime made the sedation a positive effect. Weight gain was also seen as a positive effect in this age group, where maintaining adequate body weight is often a concern. Concern is always present when using sedative medication at bedtime in the elderly. In this study, the incidence of falls did not seem to increase; however, a control (placebo) group was not employed, so the incidence of falls could not be determined with certainty.

The presence of an anxiety disorder comorbid with a depressive disorder correlates with poorer outcome for depression treatment (Lenze et al., 2005). Similarly, a high pretreatment level of anxiety increases the risk of nonresponse to antidepressant treatment as well as the risk of recurrence in the first two years of maintenance treatment (Andreescu et al., 2007). These results indicate that depressed elderly patients should be screened for anxiety disorders and treated for them, if they are present, as aggressively as for the depressive disorder.

In a small study of older patients with unipolar depression that was resistant to selective serotonin reuptake inhibitors (SSRIs), Rutherford and coworkers (2007) reported that aripiprazole (Abilify) augmentation of citalopram therapy resulted in a 50 percent rate of remission in formerly resistant elderly. This outcome was recently verified by Lenze and coworkers (2008), who also noted that remission was sustained in all 24 patients during six months of continuation treatment. The authors added:

> Incomplete response in the treatment of late-life depression is a large public health challenge: at least 50% of older people fail to respond adequately to first-line antidepressant pharmacotherapy, even under optimal treatment conditions. Treatment-resistant late-life depression increases risk for early relapse, undermines adherence to treatment for coexisting medical disorders, amplifies disability and cognitive impairment, imposes greater burden on family caregivers, and increases the risk for early mortality, including suicide. (p. 419)

Augmentation studies such as these with aripiprazole may help us advance toward the goal of more personalized and effective treatment of late-life depression.

Parkinson's Disease

Parkinson's disease (PD) is the second most common neurodegenerative disease after Alzheimer's disease. PD occurs in about 0.5 to 1 percent of people 65 to 69 years of age (about 1.5 million Americans and 6 million people worldwide), rising to 1 to 3 percent of people 80 years of age and older. More than 60,000 new cases are diagnosed in the United States each year. Although the cause of PD remains unknown, its symptoms are thought to follow from a deficiency in the number and function of dopamine-secreting neurons located primarily in the substantia nigra (a subthalamic area) of the brain. Progressive loss of these neurons is a feature of normal aging; however, most people do not lose the huge number of dopamine neurons required to cause the symptoms of PD.

Chapter 4 discussed the first-generation, or traditional, antipsychotic agents (haloperidol and the phenothiazines) used to treat schizophrenia. The most prominent side effects of those drugs are movement disorders that resemble those seen in idiopathic Parkinson's disease. Mechanistically, these side effects result from drug-induced blockade of dopamine-2 receptors, resulting in a hypodopaminergic state. PD is similarly associated with a hypodopaminergic state, characterized by a progressive loss of dopamine neurons. Currently there are no effective neuroprotective therapies. Patients are currently treated with a combination of dopamine replacement therapies (discussed here) or receive deep brain electrical stimulation to combat behavioral symptoms (Williams et al., 2010). The ideal candidate therapy would be one that prevents neurodegeneration of dopamine neurons in the brain, and specific neurotropic factors are being researched. Transplantation of dopaminergic stem cells into the brains of persons with PD has not yet met with success (Olanow et al., 2009a). The continuing therapy of PD is dopamine replacement therapy to replace the lost dopaminergic function and (hopefully) slow or reverse the loss of dopamine neurons.

Regardless of the etiology of neuronal loss in PD, the clinical features emerge when dopamine is depleted to about 20 percent of normal. In other words, the disease results when about 80 percent of dopamine neurons are lost. The clinical syndrome of PD has several cardinal features:

- Bradykinesia (slowness and poverty of movement)
- Muscle rigidity (especially a "cogwheel" rigidity)
- Resting tremor, which usually abates during voluntary movement
- Impairment of postural balance, leading to disturbances of gait and falling
- Without treatment, progression over 5 to 10 years to a state of severe rigidity and loss of movement in which patients cannot care for themselves (reminiscent of the movie *Awakenings*)

The availability of effective treatments for the symptoms of PD has radically altered the prognosis of this disease. In most cases, good functional mobility can be maintained for many years, and the life expectancy of an affected person has been greatly extended. Replacement of the dopamine or the administration of either dopaminergic agonists or inhibitors of dopamine breakdown can restore function and ameliorate much of the symptomatology. These three approaches—dopamine replacement therapy, administration of a dopaminergic agonist, and administration of dopamine breakdown inhibitors—underlie today's palliative treatment of the disease. Increasing dopamine in the brain, however, does bring with it some untoward effects, most notably impulse control disorders such as pathological gambling, binge eating, and hypersexuality (Abler et al., 2009; Weintraub et al., 2010).

Levodopa

Levodopa, a precursor drug to dopamine, continues to be the mainstay of therapy for Parkinson's disease, although today it is usually used in combination with other medications. Because a loss of dopamine is the primary problem in patients who have PD, replacement of the dopamine would be expected to ameliorate the symptoms of the disease. It does, but not by itself, because dopamine poorly crosses the blood-brain barrier from plasma into the central nervous system (CNS). However, the precursor compound in the biosynthesis of dopamine from the amino acid tyramine, a substance called *dihydroxyphenylalanine,* or *dopa* (Figure 19.2), crosses the blood-brain barrier and in the CNS is converted into dopamine, replacing the dopamine that is absent. Therefore, today, levodopa (the *levo* isomer being more active than the *dextro* isomer) is the most effective treatment for the motor disability, and many practitioners consider an initial beneficial response an important criterion for the diagnosis of parkinsonism.

Mechanism of Action. Administered orally, levodopa is rapidly absorbed into the bloodstream, where most of it (about 95 percent) is converted to dopamine in the plasma. Although only a small amount (about 1 to 5 percent) of levodopa crosses the blood-brain barrier and is converted to dopamine in the brain, it is enough to alleviate

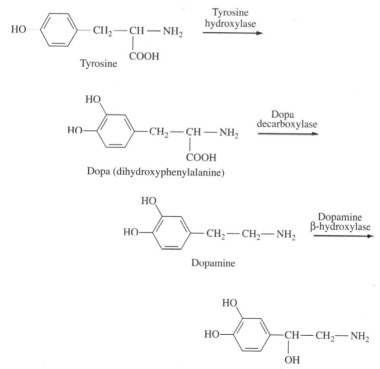

FIGURE 19.2 Synthesis of dopamine from tyrosine.

the symptoms of PD. In the CNS, levodopa is converted to dopamine, primarily within the presynaptic terminals of dopaminergic neurons in the basal ganglia.

One problem with this therapy is that, when levodopa is administered by itself, it is converted to dopamine in the body, resulting in undesirable side effects such as nausea. One approach to solving the problem is to reduce the high levels of dopamine in the systemic circulation while maintaining sufficient quantities in the brain. To do so, the biosynthetic pathway that leads to dopamine (see Figure 19.2) must be examined. Since the enzyme *dopa decarboxylase* is responsible for converting dopa to dopamine by inhibiting this enzyme in the systemic circulation but not in the brain, systemic biotransformation of the drug should be reduced, with a concomitant reduction in blood levels of dopamine and therefore in side effects. The drug would need a unique characteristic: it would have to be active in the body but not cross the blood-brain barrier into the brain. Thus, the metabolic conversion would occur in the CNS but not in the periphery.

An example of such a drug is *carbidopa,* available in combination with levodopa (the combination is marketed as Sinemet). By combining carbidopa with levodopa, the dose of levodopa is reduced by 75 percent, with a concomitant reduction in side effects and no loss of CNS therapeutic effect. The current treatment of PD relies heavily on the use of Sinemet. The combination of levodopa and carbidopa provides near maximal therapeutic benefit with the fewest side effects.

Limitations of Levodopa Therapy. Unfortunately, as time goes on, each dose of levodopa becomes less effective and the patient's symptoms fluctuate dramatically between doses, eventually developing into the "wearing-off" phenomenon. Part of the phenomenon is due to the short half-life of levodopa and can be minimized by increasing the dose and by decreasing the interval between doses. This adjustment, however, risks the development of levodopa-induced movement disorders (for example, dyskinesias), which can be as uncomfortable and disabling as the rigidity and akinesia of parkinsonism. Indeed, within about five years after initiating levodopa treatment, over 50 percent of patients develop these disabling motor disorders. Stocchi and Marconi (2010) discuss a new formulation (Sirio) to reduce this "wearing-off" phenomenon.

Does levodopa therapy adversely accelerate the course of PD? One theory of the disease is that the metabolism of dopamine produces free radicals that contribute to the death of the dopamine-releasing neurons. Oxidative stress may therefore be an important precipitating mechanism, and neuroprotective drugs might eventually be of more use in prevention of the disease. For the present, however, there is continuing concern that by ameliorating symptoms, we may be aggravating the disease. Thus, levodopa therapy is often delayed until the symptoms of PD cause an unacceptable degree of functional impairment.

COMT Inhibitors

A newer advance in the PD therapeutic regimen involves an enzyme called *catechol-o-methyltransferase* (COMT). Even with the Sinemet combination, much of an oral dose of levodopa is wasted. COMT in the vasculature of the gastrointestinal tract and liver converts levodopa to an inactive metabolite with no clinical benefit. The half-life and clinical effects of Sinemet can be increased with the addition of a COMT-inhibitory drug. In 1998, the first of these drugs—*tolcapone* (Tasmar)—was introduced; it blocks the COMT enzyme, increasing the half-life of levodopa and prolonging its effect. Unfortunately, tolcapone caused a few cases of serious liver toxicity, so in late 1998 it was withdrawn from the market in Canada and in Europe. In the United States, its use is restricted to cases where all other adjunctive therapies have failed, and close monitoring of liver function is required.

A second COMT inhibitor, *entacapone*, became available in 2001 under the trade name Comtan; entacapone has not yet been associated with liver toxicity. Like tolcapone, entacapone inhibits peripheral COMT; it does not alter central COMT. Inhibition of peripheral degradation of levodopa increases central levodopa and, therefore, central dopamine concentrations. Coadministration of entacapone with levodopa plus carbidopa potentiates the effects of levodopa in patients with PD and reduces the so-called wearing-off phenomenon. In 15 to 20 percent of patients, the wearing-off phenomenon may be extreme and disabling: doses that originally were effective for 8 hours last for only 1 or 2 hours.

In 2004, the FDA approved a fixed combination product containing levodopa, carbidopa, and entacapone (available under the trade name Stalevo). As noted, the carbidopa increases the amount of dopamine in the brain while the entacapone inhibits the degradation of dopamine through inhibition of its degradative enzyme COMT. The combination provides more dopamine to the brain for a longer period of time, providing more "on" time and less "wearing off" associated with each dose of the drug (Hauser, 2009).

Dopamine Receptor Agonists

Between one and five years after the start of levodopa therapy, most patients gradually become less responsive. One hypothesis for this effect is that the progression of PD may be associated with an increasing inability of dopamine neurons to synthesize and store dopamine. To relieve this problem, attempts have been made to identify drugs that directly stimulate postsynaptic dopamine receptors in the basal ganglia. These drugs do not depend on the ability of existing dopaminergic neurons to synthesize dopamine. In addition, if the free radical theory described in the previous subsection is accepted, these drugs would avoid the biotransformation of dopamine into potentially neurotoxic metabolites. As a result, they are increasingly being advocated for use in early stages of PD, especially in patients younger than about 65. These drugs might also be effective in the later stages of PD, when dopamine neurons are largely absent or nonfunctional.

Several dopamine receptor agonists are available in the United States for the treatment of PD (Figure 19.3): *bromocriptine* (Parlodel),

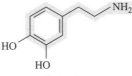

Dopamine

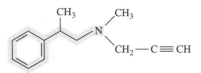

Selegiline

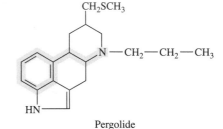

Pergolide

Pramipexole

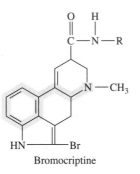

Bromocriptine

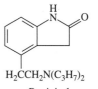

Ropinirole

FIGURE 19.3 Structures of dopamine, selegiline, and four dopamine receptor agonists that are used to treat parkinsonism. The shaded portions, which are shared by selegiline, bromocriptine, and pergolide, resemble dopamine. The two newer dopamine receptor agonists are structurally unique and have greater affinity for dopamine-3 receptors than do older dopamine receptor agonists (which stimulate dopamine-2 receptors).

pergolide (Permax), *pramipexole* (Mirapex), and *ropinirole* (Requip). Others have been introduced and are not clinically used because of side effects (*cabergoline*, or Dostinex) or problems with manufacture (*rotigotine*, or Neupro, developed as a transdermal skin patch).

Bromocriptine has been available since 1978 and pergolide since 1989; both have structures that closely resemble that of dopamine. They are only marginally effective, and they have a number of potentially serious side effects. For example, pergolide has been associated with damage to the heart valves, involving 20 percent of the patients who have taken the drug. In March 2007, the manufacturers of pergolide voluntarily removed the drug from sale in the United States.

Pramipexole and ropinirole were marketed in 1997. Unlike the older two drugs, pramipexole and ropinirole are indicated for use in early-onset PD; their efficacy and safety profile is much better than that of the two older drugs. Both can increase quality of life in the early stages of the disease by improving motor problems and decreasing fluctuations in response to levodopa. Pramipexole also exerts a beneficial antidepressant effect (Fernandez and Merello, 2010). Their long half-lives may at least partially explain the reduction in the wearing-off phenomenon of levodopa therapy. Side effects of dopamine agonists include somnolence, dizziness, nausea, hallucinations, insomnia, and impulse control disorders.

Selective Monoamine Oxidase-B Inhibitors

Selegiline (Eldepryl) (see Figure 19.3) reduces the symptoms of PD through a unique mechanism. The enzyme monoamine oxidase (MAO) exists in two forms (isoenzymes): MAO-A and MAO-B. Both are present in the brain; MAO-A is more closely involved with norepinephrine and serotonin nerve terminals, while MAO-B has preferential affinity for dopamine neurons located in the substantia nigra. Selegiline selectively and irreversibly inhibits MAO-B.[1] As a result, selegiline inhibits the local breakdown of dopamine, thus preserving the small amounts of dopamine that are present. Both actions enhance the therapeutic effect of levodopa. Unlike the older nonselective MAO inhibitors used as clinical antidepressants (Chapter 5), selegiline does not inhibit peripheral metabolism of levodopa; thus, it can safely be taken with levodopa. Selegiline also exhibits fewer drug/food interactions, at least at the lowest dose commercially available (6 mg daily). Unfortunately, in PD, selegiline's usefulness is limited.

Approved by the FDA in May 2006, *rasagiline* (Azilect) is the second selective MAO-B inhibitor for PD. Olanow and coworkers (2009b)

---

[1] In Chapter 5, selegiline was discussed as the antidepressant transdermal skin patch marketed under the trade name Emsam.

reported a possibly beneficial effect of the early use of rasagiline at a 1 mg/day dose, but negative findings at a 2 mg/day dose. Rasagiline may also possess a potential neuroprotective effect against the progression of PD (Malaty and Fernandez, 2009; Naoi and Maruyama, 2009). Recent studies have been consistent with a beneficial effect of rasagiline in the treatment of Parkinson's disease (Leegwater-Kim and Bortan, 2010; Lew et al., 2010).

Muscarinic Receptor Antagonists

Although widely used before the introduction of levodopa, certain anticholinergic agents (muscarinic antagonists) are now used much less and are considered second-tier agents for the treatment of symptoms of PD. Their use was originally postulated on the basis of an unopposed cholinergic system after death of the dopaminergic neurons.

Occasionally, anticholinergic drugs are used as an adjunct to L-dopa in patients with difficult-to-control tremors. Anticholinergic drugs relieve tremor in about 50 percent of patients, but they do not reduce rigidity or motor slowing. Cognitive dysfunction limits their use, especially in the elderly, who may have an underlying cognitive disorder. Representative agents include *trihexyphenidyl* (Artane), *procyclidine* (Kemadrin), *biperiden* (Akineton), *ethopropazine* (Parsidol), and *benztropine* (Cogentin). Occasionally, the antihistaminic drug *diphenhydramine* (Benadryl) is also used (Benadryl has significant anticholinergic properties).

Amantadine and Memantine

Amantadine (Symmetrel) is an antiviral agent (used to treat viral influenza) with modest antiparkinsonian actions. Its mechanism of action in PD is unclear; it may alter dopamine release or reuptake, or it may have anticholinergic properties. Amantadine and a related drug, *memantine*, are active at NMDA-type glutaminergic receptors; this action perhaps offers a degree of "brain protection" that may contribute to its effects. Side effects are usually mild and reversible. A possible cognitive-enhancing effect of memantine might slow the cognitive decline that may accompany PD and Alzheimer's disease in the elderly (Burn, 2010).

Gottwald and Aminoff (2008) discuss new pharmacological horizons for the future treatment of PD.

Alzheimer's Disease

Alzheimer's disease (AD) is the most common neurodegenerative disease and accounts for the majority of all cases of dementia. AD is a progressive neurodegenerative disease that results in the irreversible loss of cholinergic neurons, particularly in the cerebral cortex and hippocampus. Onset occurs generally after 60 years of age but is being increasingly reported in people younger than 65. Upwards of 10 million Americans who are part of the baby-boom demographic will develop AD unless science finds a way to effectively treat and prevent this debilitating and tragic disease (Alzheimer's Association, 2010). By 2030, AD could afflict 7.7 million Americans, increasing to between 11 million and 16 million by 2050. Currently, slightly more than 5 million Americans are living with AD. About 500,000 Americans younger than age 65 have either early-onset AD or another form of dementia.

Time between symptom onset and death may span eight to ten years. The gradual and continuous decline caused by AD is characterized by cognitive deterioration, changes in behavior, loss of functional independence, and increasing requirements for care. Hallmarks of AD include progressive impairment in memory, judgment, decision making, orientation to physical surroundings, and language. Dementia (defined as cognitive impairment with the inability to form recent memory) is the critical feature of AD. Diagnosis is based on neurological examination and the exclusion of other causes of dementia. A definitive diagnosis can be made only at autopsy, where neuronal loss and accumulation of deposits of protein plaques (beta-amyloid) and neurofibrillatory tangles, composed of abnormal microtubules, are observed. It is currently not known whether the plaques and tangles cause AD, are inactive byproducts of the disease process, or may actually be protective. Much research is devoted to this area (Rhein et al., 2009), but, to date, results from studies of potential interventions affecting amyloid have been disappointing (Green et al., 2009).

The drugs currently used for treating AD patients act on brain neurotransmitters, although it is well recognized that they do not alter the course of the disease. The fact that some of the symptoms of AD are thought to be due to a deficiency of acetylcholine neurotransmission has given rise to a cholinergic-deficiency theory of AD. Therefore, reinforcing cholinergic function by inhibiting the enzyme that breaks down acetylcholine in the synapse (Chapter 3) is a widespread therapy. These drugs, called cholinesterase inhibitors, do not alter the course of the dementia, but they can slow cognitive decline. As AD progresses and fewer cholinergic neurons remain functional, the effects of these drugs diminish. The pharmacology of the four available cholinesterase inhibitors was recently reviewed by Shah and coworkers (2010).

Memantine, discussed earlier in the section on Parkinson's disease, is a noncholinesterase inhibitor that has some usefulness in AD (and is approved by the FDA for this use); it may act through effects exerted at specific subtypes of glutamate neurons thought be important for memory formation. Neither the cholinesterase inhibitors nor memantine attack the root cause of AD, which is believed to involve brain proteins and peptides rather than neurotransmitters. Current therapy is therefore discouraging.

AD is associated not only with cognitive impairments but with a myriad of bothersome mood alterations and behavioral symptoms that pose further challenges to treatment:

- Depression associated with AD is common and is usually treated with antidepressant medications that lack anticholinergic side effects. Thus, SSRIs are used rather than the tricyclic agents (Chapter 5).

- Treatment for apathy may be considered. Drugs employed include psychostimulants, the antidepressant bupropion, the dopamine receptor agonist bromocriptine, and the antiparkinsonian agent amantadine and/or memantine.

- Psychosis, agitation, and other behavioral disturbances may require treatment with a newer atypical antipsychotic agent (discussed above) for BPSD.

- Of possible benefit in treating behavioral symptoms are the antiepileptic mood stabilizers, the sedating antidepressants trazodone and mirtazepine, and the SSRIs.

Treatment alternatives to memantine and cholinesterase inhibitors are available. Estrogen replacement (for women), antioxidants (for example, vitamin E), and nonsteroidal anti-inflammatory drugs (NSAIDs) all may have some usefulness. Of these treatments, estrogen has been found to be of little value. Vitamin E, either alone or in combination with an AChE-I, may have a small beneficial effect in some patients with mild cognitive impairment (Isaac et al., 2008). This effect is thought to follow from reductions in oxidative stress markers in a few patients, although it may actually be detrimental (worsening cognition) in nonresponders (Lloret et al., 2009). Ginkgo biloba (Chapter 8) has been shown to be without effect in improving cognitive function in patients with AD (McCarney et al., 2008).

On a positive note, Schaefer and coworkers (2006) demonstrated that a diet rich in fish oils, primarily the omega-3 fatty acid decosahexaenoic acid (DHA), resulted in a 47 percent reduction in the incidence of AD in a large population of British elderly. More recent studies indicate that low blood levels of DHA are related to an increased risk of AD (Pauwels et al., 2009), likely because DHA may be neuroprotective against dementia, reducing the production and accumulation of the beta-amyloid peptide and the microtubule-associated protein tau that may promote production of the neurofibrillatory tangles (Cole et al., 2009). At a minimum, current thought is that it may be wise to increase omega-3 fatty acid (especially DHA) intake as a possible prophylaxis against the age-related cognitive decline that may lead to AD.

Much effort is being directed toward new drugs that may block the formation of amyloid plaques. Hopefully, these agents may lead to disease modification rather than merely symptom reduction. Among these drugs are *tramiprosate* and *tarenflurbil*. Neither of these experimental medicines has demonstrated sufficient efficacy (Sabbagh, 2009), although in a preliminary study, Wilcock and coworkers (2008) reported positive effects in a one-year study of tarenflurbil on global functioning and activities of daily living in patients with mild AD, but not in patients with moderate AD. The drug had no significant effect on cognitive functioning. Less encouraging has been lack of efficacy in further, larger-scale research (unpublished). Panza and coworkers (2009) and Frisardi and coworkers (2010) review research targeting antiamyloid drugs as disease-modifying agents in PD.

In 2008, the American College of Physicians and the American Academy of Family Physicians published a clinical practice guideline for the pharmacological treatment of dementia (Qaseem et al., 2008; Raina et al., 2008).

Acetylcholinesterase Inhibitors (AChE-I)

As discussed, deficits in the functioning of acetylcholine-secreting neurons (cholinergic deficits) are correlated with the cognitive impairments of AD. Originally this idea stemmed from the observation that drugs that block the actions of acetylcholine (for example, scopolamine) are intense cognitive inhibitors. Therefore, drugs that increase acetylcholine levels might be cognitive enhancers and slow the rate of progression of cognitive decline seen in AD. Consistent with this idea is the observation that patients with severe AD show AChE levels that are 60 to 85 percent lower than normal, which implies very little residual AChE in the cortex—a condition that is still compatible with life but no longer optimal for brain function.

The most successful effort to increase cholinergic functioning has targeted the AChE enzyme, inhibition of which increases levels of acetylcholine in the brain. Four of these AChE-I medications have been approved by the FDA for the treatment of AD: *tacrine* (Cognex), *donepezil* (Aricept), *rivastigmine* (Exelon), and *galantamine* (Razadyne). Each improves cholinergic neurotransmission by preventing the synaptic breakdown of acetylcholine in the brain. These drugs can produce modest improvements in cognition and activities of daily living, but their side effects include nausea, diarrhea, abdominal cramping, and anorexia. The side effects result from inhibition of AChE in the periphery, not from the elevations of acetylcholine in the brain. In small numbers of patients receiving AChE-I medication, drug-induced increases in aggressive behaviors may be seen (Coco and Cannizaro, 2010); these behaviors are reversible with drug discontinuation (or dosage reductions), and treatment with antipsychotic drugs (without stopping the AChE-I) is inappropriate. The modest efficacy combined with these side effects tends to limit the therapeutic usefulness of these agents.

Tacrine was the first of these agents to be approved; it is now the least used of the four, primarily because it needs frequent administration and can cause a reversible toxicity in the liver. Liver toxicity has not been associated with donepezil, rivastigmine, and galantamine.

Donepezil appears to be selective for AChE in the brain more than in the periphery. It has a long half-life and produces fewer gastrointestinal side effects. It is much more tolerable than tacrine. Petersen and coworkers (2005) reported that donepezil may slow the progression of cognitive decline in early AD but that the protective effect was lost after 18 months of treatment. Winblad and coworkers (2006) reported that donepezil improved cognitive ability and helped preserve patient functioning. Burns and coworkers (2007) reported that, over 24 weeks of treatment, donepezil produced positive effects on cognition, but that effect was lost over 132 weeks of study. Furthermore, if treatment was discontinued, benefits were not regained after treatment restart. Finally, Doody and coworkers (2009) reported that, in a 48-week study, donepezil was no better than placebo in elderly patients with mild amnestic cognitive impairments. Persons with such mild cognitive impairments are expected to progress to AD within about six years.

Rivastigmine is clinically effective, producing modest improvements in cognitive functioning and activities of daily living (Olin et al., 2010). It is better tolerated than tacrine but somewhat less so than donepezil. In contrast to the other three agents, rivastigmine causes a very slowly reversible inhibition of AChE, prolonging its therapeutic action. Newly available is a rivastigmine transdermal patch (Exelon Patch). Oral administration of cholinesterase inhibitors is limited by wide fluctuations in blood concentrations. With the patch, 24-hour concentrations remain relatively stable. Several recent articles attest to the superiority of the patch over oral administration of capsules (Grossberg et al., 2009; Sadowsky et al., 2010; Darreh-Shori and Jelic, 2010). Caregivers prefer the patch to the capsule (Grossberg et al., 2009); however, to avoid toxicity, only one patch at a time should be used.

Galantamine appears to have a safety and efficacy profile similar to that of rivastigmine in measures of both cognitive functioning and functional ability. In a study of quite elderly patients (average age 84 years) with severe AD, Burns and coworkers (2009) reported that galantamine moderately improved cognitive functioning but failed to significantly improve measures of overall activities of daily living.

These data imply that cholinesterase inhibitors have modest but positive effects compared with placebo in the treatment of AD, affecting cognition, function, and behavioral outcomes. They are effective in mild to moderate disease, and data with galantamine suggest that this effect is mirrored in severe disease as well. Perhaps the rivastigmine patch will provide the stability of blood concentrations that may result in more predictable effects.

There are limitations to these medications, however, because although stabilization occurs, there is typically only a modest improvement from baseline. Additionally, the effects are not sustained indefinitely, and the disease continues to progress even while patients are receiving treatment with cholinesterase inhibitors. Adverse effects are manageable and, with careful titration, patients can tolerate increases quite well; however, side effects can include diarrhea, nausea, vomiting, dyspepsia, asthenia, dizziness, headache, weight loss, and even anorexia—sometimes to such an extreme that patients must discontinue treatment. Hopefully, the patch delivery system may reduce some of these side effects. Additional therapies for AD need to be developed that include highly tolerable agents with alternative mechanisms of action and broader efficacy to delay disease onset, arrest the disease, and even reverse the progression of the disease entirely. Until these new therapies are developed, the cholinesterase inhibitors will remain important treatments for AD.

Recently interest has been expressed in a naturally occurring AChE-I called *huperzine A*. This substance, derived from the moss *Huperzia serrata*, has been used for centuries as a Chinese folk medicine. It has modest AChE-I activity, and it may be useful as an alternative medication for the treatment of AD (Li et al., 2008; Desilets et al., 2009). Early results are modestly positive, but the limited results are too few and the design is too weak to establish its role in the treatment of AD.

Memantine

As discussed in Chapter 3, *glutamate* is the principal excitatory neurotransmitter in the brain. Glutaminergic overactivity may result in neuronal damage, a phenomenon termed *excitotoxicity*. Excitotoxicity ultimately leads to neuronal calcium overload and has been implicated in neurodegenerative disorders. In addition, glutaminergic NMDA receptor activity appears to be important in memory processes, dementia, and the pathogenesis of AD. Glutaminergic overstimulation at NMDA receptors is thought to be toxic to neurons, and prevention of this neurotoxicity affords a degree of brain protection to limit further deterioration.

Memantine (Namenda) is a moderate-affinity noncompetitive NMDA receptor antagonist that has been shown to reduce clinical deterioration in patients with moderate to severe AD, a phase associated with significant distress for patients and caregivers alike and for which no other treatments are available (Aarsland et al., 2009). It appears to have therapeutic potential without the undesirable side effects associated with high-affinity NMDA antagonists such as ketamine (Chapter 15). Available in Germany since 1982, memantine became available for use in the United States in 2004.

Tariot (2006) and Cummings and coworkers (2006) all reported improved cognition, patient functioning, and behaviors, as well as amelioration of agitation and other negative behaviors, in AD patients treated with a combination of an AChE-I and memantine. It is thought that the combination may delay nursing home placement, a step that can be exceedingly distressing to patients with AD and their caregivers.

As with other NMDA antagonists, high brain concentrations of memantine can inhibit glutaminergic mechanisms of synaptic plasticity that are believed to underlie learning and memory. In other words, at high doses, memantine can produce the same amnestic effects as does ketamine. At lower, clinically relevant doses, however, memantine seems to promote cellular plasticity, can preserve or enhance memory, and can protect against the excitotoxic destruction of cholinergic neurons. As a "weak" NMDA antagonist, memantine may reduce overactive NMDA receptor activity that would be neurotoxic while sparing the synaptic responsiveness required for normal behavioral functioning, cognition, and memory.

Principles of Care for Patients with Alzheimer's Disease

In 2006, the American Association for Geriatric Psychiatry outlined minimal care standards and principles for patients with AD and their caregivers. The association issued a position statement calling on clinicians to treat AD as part of their typical practice (Lyketsos et al., 2006). The statement focuses on the following five important areas of therapy:

- Disease therapies for AD, targeting aspects of the current pathophysiological understanding of the disease
- Symptomatic therapies for cognitive symptoms
- Symptomatic therapies for other neuropsychiatric symptoms
- Interventions targeted at and the provision of supportive care for patients
- Interventions targeted at and the provision of supportive care for caregivers

These principles still apply today. Disease therapies (item 1) include therapies aimed at preventing deposits of amyloid plaques and preventing excitotoxic neuronal damage. Therapies for cognitive symptoms include the AChE-I drugs and memantine. Therapies for other symptoms might include treatments for depression, agitation, aggression, and delusions, among other symptoms; therapies can be both nonpharmacological and pharmacological. Supportive care for patients and caregivers should be tailored to the condition, circumstances, and progression of functional and cognitive decline. Caregivers need to be educated about AD and how their services are essential. They especially need to be given emotional support and respite.

STUDY QUESTIONS

1. What is Parkinson's disease?

2. What does Parkinson's disease have in common with traditional neuroleptic drugs? Why?

3. List the various ways that dopaminergic action in the brain might be augmented or potentiated.

4. Explain how carbidopa potentiates the action of levodopa.

5. Explain how a COMT inhibitor potentiates the action of levodopa.

6. Differentiate the newer from the older dopamine receptor agonists.

7. How does selegiline work in the treatment of Parkinson's disease?

8. Besides treatment with drugs, how might parkinsonism be managed? List the nonpharmacological options.

9. What is the currently accepted hypothesis for the genesis of Alzheimer's disease?

10. What are the currently available medications used to treat Alzheimer's disease?

11. Differentiate cholinesterase inhibitors from one another and from memantine.

12. How is glutamate involved in the action of memantine and how does this involvement relate to neuroprotection?

REFERENCES

Aarsland, D., et al. (2009). "Memantine in Patients with Parkinson's Disease Dementia or Dementia with Lewy Bodies: A Double-Blind, Placebo-Controlled, Multicentre Trial." *Lancet Neurology* 8: 613–618.

Abler, B., et al. (2009). "At-Risk for Pathological Gambling: Imaging Neural Reward Processing Under Chronic Dopamine Agonists." *Brain* 132: 2396–2402.

Alzheimer's Association. (2010). "2010 Alzheimer's Disease Facts and Figures." The Alzheimer's Association. *Facts and Figures*. Available at www.alz.org.

Andreescu, C., et al. (2007). "Effect of Comorbid Anxiety on Treatment Response and Relapse Risk in Late-Life Depression: Controlled Study." *British Journal of Psychiatry* 190: 344–349.

Barnett, M. J., et al. (2006). "Comparison of Rates of Potentially Inappropriate Medication Use According to the Zhan Criteria for VA versus Private Sector Medicare HMOs." *Journal of Managed Care Pharmacy* 12: 362–370.

Burn, D. J. (2010). "The Treatment of Cognitive Impairment Associated with Parkinson's Disease." *Brain Pathology* 20: 672–678.

Burns, A., et al. (2007). "Efficacy and Safety of Donepezil over 3 Years: An Open-Label, Multicentre Study in Patients with Alzheimer's Disease." *International Journal of Geriatric Psychiatry* 22: 806–812.

Burns, A., et al. (2009). "Safety and Efficacy of Galantamine (Reminyl) in Severe Alzheimer's Disease (the SERAD Study): A Randomized, Placebo-Controlled, Double-Blind Trial." *Lancet Neurology* 8: 39–47.

Chen, Y., et al. (2010). "Unexplained Variation Across US Nursing Homes in Antipsychotic Prescribing Rates." *Archives of Internal Medicine* 170: 89–95.

Coco, D. L., and Cannizaro, E. (2010). "Inappropriate Sexual Behaviors Associated with Donepezil Treatment: A Case Report." *Journal of Clinical Psychopharmacology* 30: 221–222.

Cole, G. M., et al. (2009). "Omega-3 Fatty Acids and Dementia." *Prostaglandins, Leukotrienes, and Essential Fatty Acids* 81: 213–221.

Coley, K. C., et al. (2009). "Aripiprazole Prescribing Patterns and Side Effects in Elderly Psychiatric Inpatients." *Journal of Psychiatric Practice* 15: 150–153.

Connelly, P. J., et al. (2009). "Fifteen Year Comparison of Antipsychotic Use in People with Dementia Within Hospital and Nursing Home Settings: Sequential Cross-Sectional Study." *International Journal of Geriatric Psychiatry* 25: 160–165.

Cummings, J. L., et al. (2006). "Behavioral Effects of Memantine in Alzheimer's Disease Patients Receiving Donepezil Treatment." *Neurology* 67: 57–63.

Darreh-Shori, T., and Jelic, V. (2010). "Safety and Tolerability of Transdermal and Oral Rivastigmine in Alzheimer's Disease and Parkinson's Disease Dementia." *Expert Opinion on Drug Safety* 9: 167–176.

Desilets, A. R., et al. (2009). "Role of Huperzine-A in the Treatment of Alzheimer's Disease." *Annals of Pharmacotherapeutics* 43: 514–518.

Dombrovski, A. Y., and Mulsant, B. H. (2007). "ECT: The Preferred Treatment for Severe Depression in Late Life." *International Psychogeriatrics* 19: 10–14.

Dombrovski, A. Y., et al. (2007). "Maintenance Treatment for Old-Age Depression Preserves Health-Related Quality of Life: A Randomized, Controlled Trial of Paroxetine and Interpersonal Psychotherapy." *Journal of the American Geriatrics Society* 55: 1325–1332.

Doody, R. S., et al. (2009). "Donepezil Treatment of Patients with MCI: A 48-Week Randomized, Placebo-Controlled Trial." *Neurology* 72: 1555–1561.

Dorsey, E. R., et al. (2010). "Impact of FDA Black Box Advisory on Antipsychotic Medication Use." *Archives of Internal Medicine* 170: 96–103.

Elie, M., et al. (2009). "A Retrospective, Exploratory, Secondary Analysis of the Association Between Antipsychotic Use and Mortality in Elderly Patients with Delirium." *International Psychogeriatrics* 21: 588–592.

Fernandez, H. H., and Merello, M. (2010). "Pramipexole for the Treatment of Depressive Symptoms in Patients with Parkinson's Disease: Can We Kill Two Birds with One Stone?" *Lancet Neurology,* 9: 556-557.

Ferreira, J. J., et al. (2006). "Sleep Disruption, Daytime Somnolence, and 'Sleep Attacks' in Parkinson's Disease: A Clinical Survey in PD Patients and Age-Matched Healthy Volunteers." *European Journal of Neurology* 13: 209-214.

Fick, D. M., et al. (2003). "Updating the Beers Criteria for Potentially Inappropriate Medication Use in Older Adults: Results of a U.S. Consensus Panel of Experts." *Archives of Internal Medicine* 163: 2716-2724.

Frisardi, V., et al. (2010). "Towards Disease-Modifying Treatment of Alzheimer's Disease: Drugs Targeting Beta-Amyloid." *Current Alzheimer's Research* 7: 40-55.

Gottwald, M. D., and Aminoff, M. J. (2008). "New Frontiers in the Pharmacological Management of Parkinson's Disease." *Drugs Today* 44: 531-545.

Green, R. C., et al. (2009). "Effect of Tarenflurbil on Cognitive Decline and Activities of Daily Living in Patients with Mild Alzheimer Disease." *Journal of the American Medical Association* 302: 2557-2564.

Grossberg, G., et al. (2009). "Safety and Tolerability of the Rivastigmine Patch: Results of a 28-Week Open-Label Extension." *Alzheimer Disease & Associated Disorders* 23: 158-164.

Hauser, R. A. (2009). "Levodopa: Past, Present, and Future." *European Neurology* 62: 1-8.

Howard, R. J., et al. (2007). "Donepezil for the Treatment of Agitation in Alzheimer's Disease." *New England Journal of Medicine* 357: 1382-1392.

Hunkeler, E. M., et al. (2006). "Long-Term Outcomes from the IMPACT Randomized Trial for Depressed Elderly Patients in Primary Care." *British Medical Journal* 332: 259-263.

Isaac, M. G., et al. (2008). "Vitamin E for Alzheimer's Disease and Mild Cognitive Impairment." *Cochrane Database of Systematic Reviews* 16: CD002854.

Kasper, S., et al. (2006). "Escitalopram in the Long-Term Treatment of Major Depressive Disorder in Elderly Patients." *Neuropsychobiology* 54: 152-159.

Laroche, M. L., et al. (2007). "Is Inappropriate Medication Use a Major Cause of Adverse Drug Reactions in the Elderly?" *British Journal of Clinical Pharmacology* 63: 177-186.

Leegwater-Kim, J., and Bortan, E. (2010). "The Role of Rasagiline in the Treatment of Parkinson's Disease." *Clinical Interventions in Aging* 5: 149-156.

Lenze, E. J., et al. (2005). "Efficacy and Tolerability of Citalopram in the Treatment of Late-Life Anxiety Disorders: Results from an 8-Week, Randomized, Placebo-Controlled Trial." *American Journal of Psychiatry* 162: 145-150.

Lenze, E. J., et al. (2008). "Incomplete Response in Later-Life Depression: Getting to Remission." *Dialogues in Clinical Neurosciences* 10: 419-430.

Lenze, E. J., et al. (2009). "Escitalopram for Older Adults with Generalized Anxiety Disorder." *Journal of the American Medical Association* 301: 295-303.

Lew, M. F., et al. (2010). "Long-Term Efficacy of Rasagiline in Early Parkinson's Disease." *International Journal of Neuroscience* 120: 404-408.

Li, J., et al. (2008). "Huperzine A for Alzheimer's Disease." *Cochrane Datebase of Systematic Reviews* 16: CD005592.

Lloret, A., et al. (2009). "Vitamin E Paradox in Alzheimer's Disease: It Does Not Prevent Loss of Cognition and May Even Be Detrimental." *Journal of Alzheimer's Disease* 17: 143–149.

Lyketsos, C. G., et al. (2006). "Position Statement of the American Association for Geriatric Psychiatry Regarding Principles for Care of Patients with Dementia Resulting from Alzheimer's Disease." *American Journal of Geriatric Psychiatry* 14: 561–572.

Malaty, I. A., and Fernandez, H. H. (2009). "Role of Rasagiline in Treating Parkinson's Disease: Effect on Disease Progression." *Therapeutics and Clinical Risk Management* 5: 413–419.

McCarney, R., et al. (2008). "*Ginkgo biloba* for Mild to Moderate Dementia in a Community Setting: A Pragmatic, Randomized, Parallel-Group, Double-Blind, Placebo-Controlled Trial." *International Journal of Geriatric Psychiatry* 23: 1222–1230.

Medical Letter. (2005). "Atypical Antipsychotics in the Elderly." *Medical Letter on Drugs and Therapeutics* 47 (August 1): 61–62.

Naoi, M., and Maruyama, W. (2009). "Functional Mechanism of Neuroprotection by Inhibitors of Type B Monoamine Oxidase in Parkinson's Disease." *Expert Reviews in Neurotherapeutics* 9: 1233–1250.

Nelson, J. C., et al. (2006). "Mirtazepine Orally Disintegrating Tablets in Depressed Nursing Home Residents 85 Years of Age and Older." *International Journal of Geriatric Psychiatry* 21: 898–901.

Nishtala, P. S., et al. (2009). "Anticholinergic Activity of Commonly Prescribed Medications and Psychiatric Adverse Effects in Older People." *Journal of Clinical Pharmacology* 49: 1176–1184.

Olanow, C. W., et al. (2009a). "Dopaminergic Transplantation for Parkinson's Disease: Current Status and Future Prospects." *Annals of Neurology* 66: 591–596.

Olanow, C. W., et al. (2009b). A Double-Blind, Delayed-Start Trial of Rasagiline in Parkinson's Disease." *New England Journal of Medicine* 361: 1268–1278.

Olin, J. T., et al. (2010). "Rivastigmine in the Treatment of Dementia Associated with Parkinson's Disease: Effects on Activities of Daily Living." *Dementia and Geriatric Cognitive Disorders* 29: 510–515.

Omelan, C. (2006). Approaches to Managing Behavioural Disturbances in Dementia." *Canadian Family Physician* 52: 191–199.

Paleacu, D., et al. (2008). "Quetiapine Treatment for Behavioural and Psychological Symptoms of Dementia in Alzheimer's Disease Patients: A 6-Week, Double-Blind, Placebo-Controlled Study." *International Journal of Geriatric Psychiatry* 23: 393–400.

Panza, F., et al. (2009). "Disease-Modifying Approach to the Treatment of Alzheimer's Disease: From Alpha-Secretase Activators to Gamma-Secretase Inhibitors and Modulators." *Drugs and Aging* 26: 537–555.

Pauwels, E. K., et al. (2009). "Fatty Acid Facts, Part IV: Docosahexaenoic Acid and Alzheimer's Disease. A Story of Mice, Men and Fish." *Drug News and Perspectives* 22: 205–213.

Petersen, R., et al. (2005). "Vitamin E and Donepezil for the Treatment of Mild Cognitive Impairment." *New England Journal of Medicine* 352: 2379–2388.

Pugh, M. J., et al. (2006). "Assessing Potentially Inappropriate Prescribing in the Elderly Veterans Affairs Population Using the HEDIS 2006 Quality Measure." *Journal of Managed Care Pharmacy* 12: 537–545.

Qaseem, A., et al. (2008). "Current Pharmacologic Treatment of Dementia: A Clinical Practice Guideline from the American College of Physicians and the American Academy of Family Physicians." *Annals of Internal Medicine* 148: 370–378.

Raina, P., et al. (2008). "Effectiveness of Cholinesterase Inhibitors and Mematine for Treating Dementia: Evidence Review for a Clinical Practice Guideline." *Annals of Internal Medicine* 148: 379–397.

Reynolds, C. F., et al. (2006). "Maintenance Treatment of Major Depression in Old Age." *New England Journal of Medicine* 354: 1130–1138.

Rhein, V., et al. (2009). "Amyloid-Beta and Tau Synergistically Impair the Oxidative Phosphorylation System in Triple Transgenic Alzheimer's Disease Mice." *Proceedings of the National Academy of Science* 106: 20057–20062.

Rutherford, B., et al. (2007). "An Open Trial of Aripiprazole Augmentation for SSRI Non-Remitters with Late-Life Depression." *International Journal of Geriatric Psychiatry* 22: 986–991.

Ryan, C., et al. (2009). "Appropriate Prescribing in the Elderly: An Investigation of Two Screening Tools, Beers Criteria Considering Diagnosis and Independent of Diagnosis and Improved Prescribing in the Elderly Tool to Identify Inappropriate Use of Medicines in the Elderly in Primary Care in Ireland." *Journal of Clinical Pharmacy and Therapeutics* 34: 369–376.

Sabbagh, M. N. (2009). "Drug Development for Alzheimer's Disease: Where Are We Now, and Where Are We Headed?" *American Journal of Geriatric Pharmacotherapy* 7: 167–185.

Sadowsky, C. H., et al. (2010). "Safety and Tolerability of Rivastigmine Transdermal Patch Compared with Rivastigmine Capsules in Patients Switched from Donepezil: Data from Three Clinical Trials." *International Journal of Clinical Practice* 64: 188–193.

Schaefer, E. J., et al. (2006). "Plasma Phosphatidylcholine Docosahexaenoic Acid Content and Risk of Dementia and Alzheimer's Disease." *Archives of Neurology* 63: 1545–1550.

Shah, D., et al. (2010). "Medications for Treating Alzheimer's Dementia." *The Carlat Psychiatry Report* 8(4): 1–3.

Simoni-Wastila, L., et al. (2009). "Association of Antipsychotic Use with Hospital Events and Mortality Among Medicare Beneficiaries Residing in Long-Term Care Facilities." *American Journal of Geriatric Psychiatry* 17: 417–427.

Steinman, M. A., et al. (2006). "Polypharmacy and Prescribing Quality in Older People." *Journal of the American Geriatric Society* 54: 1516–1523.

Stocchi, F., and Marconi, S. (2010). "Factors Associated with Motor Fluctuations and Dyskinesia in Parkinson's Disease: Potential Role of a New Melovodopa Plus Carbidopa Formulation (Sirio)." *Clinical Neuropharmacology.* In press.

Streim, J. E., et al. (2008). "A Randomized, Double-Blind, Placebo-Controlled Study of Aripiprazole for the Treatment of Psychosis in Nursing Home Patients with Alzheimer Disease." *American Journal of Geriatric Psychiatry* 16: 537–550.

Tariot, P. N. (2006). "Contemporary Issues in the Treatment of Alzheimer's Disease: Tangible Benefits of Current Therapies." *Journal of Clinical Psychiatry* 67, Supplement 3: 15–22.

Tsunoda, K., et al. (2010). "Effects of Discontinuing Benzodiazepine-Derivative Hypnotics on Postural Sway and Cognitive Functions in the Elderly." *International Journal of Geriatric Psychiatry.* In press.

Van Leeuwen, W. E., et al. (2009). "Collaborative Depression Care for the Old-Old: Findings from the IMPACT Trial." *American Journal of Geriatric Psychiatry* 17: 1040–1049.

Weintraub, D., et al. (2010). "Impulse Control Disorders in Parkinson's Disease: A Cross-Sectional Study of 3,090 Patients." *Archives of Neurology* 67: 589–595.

Wilcock, G. K., et al. (2008). "Efficacy and Safety of Tarenflurbil in Mild to Moderate Alzheimer's Disease: A Randomized Phase II Trial." *Lancet Neurology* 7: 483–493.

Williams, A., et al. (2010). "Deep Brain Stimulation Plus Best Medical Therapy versus Best Medical Therapy Alone for Advanced Parkinson's Disease (PD SURG Trial): A Randomized, Open-Label Trial." *Lancet Neurology,* 9: 681–681.

Winblad, B., et al. (2006). "Donepezil in Patients with Severe Alzheimer's Disease: Double-Blind, Parallel-Group, Placebo-Controlled Study." *Lancet* 367: 1057–1065.

Chapter 20

Integrating Psychopharmacology and Psychological Therapies in Patient Care

In 2003, a U.S. Presidential Commission on Mental Health report noted that care for the mentally ill must go beyond prescribing medication and crisis management of symptoms (U.S. Department of Health and Human Services, 2003). The report called for counselors to help patients lead a fuller life, including (but moving beyond) administering drugs. The commission issued a vision statement as well as goals for treatment, along with recommendations for achieving these goals. The vision statement was as follows:

> We are committed to a future where recovery is the expected outcome and when mental illness can be prevented or cured. We envision a nation where everyone with mental illness will have access to early detection and the effective treatment and supports essential to live, work, learn, and participate fully in their community.

Following are the goals of the commission report:

- *Mental health is essential to health.* Every individual, family, and community will understand that mental health is an essential part of overall health.

- *Early mental health screening and treatment in multiple settings.* Every individual will have the opportunity for early and appropriate mental health screening, assessment, and referral to treatment.
- *Consumer/family-centered care.* Consumers and families will have the necessary information and the opportunity to exercise choice over the care decisions that affect them. Continuous healing relationships will be a key feature of care.
- *Best care science can offer.* Adults with serious mental illness and children with serious emotional disturbance will have ready access to the best treatments, services, and supports leading to recovery and cure. Research will be accelerated to enhance the prevention of, recovery from, and ultimate discovery of cures for mental illnesses.

The commission stated:

> These goals provide a set of ideals toward which to work. Symptom reduction via pharmacological means is only part of the plan: all mental health care should be delivered in an integrated fashion. All mental health personnel should understand their clients' medications well enough to allow them to interact meaningfully with other professionals. These goals require collaborative efforts, mutual respect, and a true heath care team approach.

The commission was calling for a mental health care treatment team, including both a prescriber (usually a physician) and one or more mental health care professionals. Witko and coworkers (2005) discussed a collaborative care model for treating psychological problems in primary care medicine. They begin by stating that physicians do not have enough time to treat psychological issues, that they are inadequately trained to deliver such care, and that 20 percent (minimum) of their patients have serious psychological problems. Often, primary care physicians may treat patients by themselves, usually by prescribing psychotherapeutic medications. Many barriers exist to perpetuate this situation, which only serves to limit effective care of patients with mental health issues. Physicians and psychologists have different training, work styles, language, and theoretical paradigms, and they have different expectations and views of each other's work. Patient resistance to referral (being labeled as having a mental health problem), lack of mutual feedback, lack of collaboration, and lack of respect are additional barriers to collaboration. Cost is considered to be a major factor limiting collaboration, in that two practitioners are more expensive than one.

Gilbody and coworkers (2006) performed a meta-analysis evaluating the efficacy of collaborative care on both the short-term and long-term treatment of depression. Collaborative care involved a role for three distinct professionals working together within the primary care setting: a case manager, a primary care practitioner, and a mental health professional. Meta-analysis involved 37 studies including 12,355 patients with depression who were randomized to receive either collaborative care or usual primary care. Results confirmed the effectiveness of collaborative care in improving short-term outcomes in depression as well as significant long-term benefits (for up to five years). An editorial on the role of collaborative care concluded that "the evidence base is now sufficient for the emphasis to shift from research to dissemination and implementation" (Simon, 2006, p. 250).

Limitations to Pharmacological Therapy

There is a general perception among physicians and their patients that medications alone can alleviate illness, be it physical or psychological. In other words, it is expected that, if taken, the medicine will "work." To be sure, in most cases of bacterial infections, an antibiotic can be prescribed, and if the antibiotic is taken in compliance with directions, the bacterium will be eliminated from the body and the patient's infection will resolve. With chronic physical diseases, however, such as hypertension, diabetes, and elevated cholesterol, the medication will usually not work if life-style changes are not made. The same holds true for the treatment of psychological illnesses. This need to go beyond medication alone has been supported in numerous studies:

- In the STAR*D study (Chapter 5), medication efficacy in treating depression in adults was only 30 percent with the first drug. With multiple medication switches or augmentation, the remission rate increased to about 60 percent. Of course, this leaves about 40 percent without remission, despite intensive medication trials. Recently, Thase and coworkers (2007) demonstrated that in depressed persons who failed to respond to citalopram therapy, an augmentation strategy adding cognitive therapy resulted in the same likelihood of remission and similar symptomatic improvement as did switching from citalopram to either sustained-release bupropion or buspirone.

- In the TADS study (Chapter 18), efficacy in treating depression in children and adolescents was only about 35 percent with medication alone. Adding cognitive-behavioral therapies markedly improved results.

- In the STEP-BD study (Chapter 6), although remission of bipolar symptoms could be achieved in about 60 percent of people with the disorder, 50 percent of responders relapsed frequently.

- In the CATIE and CUtLASS studies (Chapter 4), patients with schizophrenia were relatively noncompliant with medication prescription, regardless of which antipsychotic was prescribed.

- Swartz and coworkers (2007) concluded that medications alone are not sufficient to offer rehabilitative outcomes and that adjunctive psychosocial therapies are needed to make meaningful gains, such as being able to work, attend school, or maintain a home.

In these studies, treatment with medication alone was less effective than anticipated by the prescriber, the client, the client's family, and even mental health practitioners. Therefore, it is important to recognize the limitations to pharmacological therapy.

Developing a Plan to Integrate Pharmacological and Psychological Therapies

Medication alterations can often result in clinical improvement. Currently, many mental health practitioners may not be familiar with methods to integrate pharmacology information into their daily practice. To do so, they must first take a medication history and keep a running record of a client's medications, emphasizing potential side effects. They should follow up with the development of an effective means of communication with the client's prescriber.

Client Medication List

Figure 20.1 is a one-page medication record suggested for use by mental health clinicians for each client seen for therapy.

Medication history for: _____

Date	Drug (generic/ trade)	Currently taking (Y/N)	Class of drug	Indication	Side effects/ Discontinued

FIGURE 20.1 Medication history form. See the text for details.

- Column 2 lists all medications that the client is taking, whether the medicine is psychoactive or administered for another reason (for example, hypertension, diabetes, elevated blood lipids, gastric reflux, and so on); it includes names by which the drugs are easily recognized (for example, Abilify for aripiprazole).

- Column 4 gives the classification of the drug (antipsychotic, anxiolytic, antidepressant, antihypertensive, antidiabetic, and so on).

- Column 6 lists the most prominent or concerning side effects (for example, benzodiazepines = cognitive impairment; olanzapine = weight gain; selective serotonin reuptake inhibitors (SSRIs) = agitation, insomnia, sexual dysfunction; bupropion = worsening anxiety).

With a medication list, the clinician can watch for side effects that might otherwise be missed, perhaps further improving patient care.

Suggested Communication Letter

Communication with a client's prescriber is vital to developing and maintaining a treatment team approach to care. Figure 20.2 is a sample client communication letter. This letter acknowledges the prescriber's referral and lists diagnoses and treatments. Because clients frequently receive medications from more than one prescriber, it lists medications the client claims to be taking. It communicates in one place all diagnoses, services, medications, and concerns for a client. For reference, the appendix to this chapter lists the major psychotherapeutic drugs, their range of usual daily doses, and other data.

Clinical Examples

The following examples illustrate how knowledge about medication side effects and alternatives can benefit a client. These examples are from a *clinical psychologist* who evaluated patients, made clinical diagnoses, determined that problems may have arisen as a result of prescribed medications, and made clinical recommendations that resulted in improvements in the quality of life of the patient. As will become clear, knowledge of psychopharmacology was essential.

Client A is a 45-year-old male who was prescribed lithium for a diagnosis of bipolar II disorder. He presented with complaints of an 80-pound weight gain and an inability to remember names. The psychologist recognized these problems as side effects of lithium therapy. The psychologist identified a study on the efficacy of valproic acid for bipolar II. With this recommendation, the prescribing physician made the medication switch. Thereafter, Client A lost about 40 pounds and his memory function improved, allowing him to continue working.

Date: _____

To: _____ From: _____

My client_____ is your patient.
I saw him/her on _____ (date).

My diagnoses are _____
_____

I have planned the following treatment(s): _____
_____

My client says that he/she is taking the following medications:
1. _____ 4. _____ 7. _____
2. _____ 5. _____ 8. _____
3. _____ 6. _____ 9. _____

I have the following concerns:
1. _____
_____
2. _____
_____
3. _____
_____
4. _____
_____

If you would like to discuss your patient with me, I can be reached at
_____.

Sincerely,

_____

FIGURE 20.2 Patient communication form.

Five years later, Client A presented with complaints of listlessness, lack of energy, and sexual dysfunction. The psychologist learned that a physician had diagnosed the client with depression and had prescribed escitalopram (Lexapro) in addition to the client's valproic acid. The psychologist suggested discontinuation of escitalopram and valproate and initiation of aripiprazole (Abilify) and/or lamotrigine (Lamictal). The prescriber followed the recommendation and replaced the valproate and escitalopram with aripiprazole. About two weeks later, the client reported that the new drug was "intolerable" and complained of aches, myalgias, flulike symptoms, and electric shocks in his head. The psychologist determined that the client had serotonin discontinuation syndrome (rather than side effects of aripiprazole) and counseled the client about serotonin discontinuation syndrome. Three weeks later, the symptoms had ceased, the client was more energized, sexual function was improving, and no bipolar symptoms were reported. Continual progress was made over the next few months.

Clients B and C were two men, both in their late twenties, referred by a physician for evaluation of cognitive difficulties. Testing was performed and diagnosis was made of notable cognitive dysfunction, with the greatest difficulty being with word finding. Medication review revealed that both clients had recently been prescribed topiramate (Topamax). Replacement of the Topamax [prescribed for anxiety and posttraumatic stress disorder (PTSD)] with pregabalin (Lyrica) led to rapid resolution of the cognitive difficulties.

Client D was a 48-year-old woman diagnosed with depression and anxiety. She was prescribed sertraline (Zoloft) and showed some improvement. However, she gradually developed a panic disorder and was referred to a psychologist. Further history-taking revealed that she had recently undergone surgery for breast lesions that were diagnosed as benign breast cysts. It turned out that Client D was a heavy coffee drinker. Sertraline interferes with the metabolism of caffeine, in essence doubling her blood level of caffeine. Caffeinism is associated with increasing anxiety (the panic disorder) and the development of benign breast cysts. Cessation of caffeine drinking (small amounts of caffeinated coffee and the remainder decaffeinated) led to resolution of the panic disorder.

Client E was a 28-year-old Gulf War veteran with severe PTSD presenting with nighttime terror and threatening actions toward his wife. Moreover, he was amnestic for these episodes. Medication review revealed a prescription for zolpidem (Ambien) for sleep. It was determined that the Ambien might be causing the amnesia. Replacement of Ambien with gabapentin at bedtime improved PTSD symptoms, and the amnestic episodes were resolved.

Client F was an 88-year-old female care center resident whose family took her to therapy for increasing dementia. Medication review revealed that she had been receiving imipramine (Tofranil) for depression and diazepam (Valium) for anxiety and sleep difficulties. Because tricyclic antidepressants have anticholinergic difficulties, they can cause cognitive impairments. Benzodiazepines are widely known to worsen dementias. Cessation of these medicines and replacement with quetiapine (Seroquel) and mirtazepine (Remeron) at bedtime led to cognitive improvements, reductions in anxiety, better sleep patterns, and improvements in appetite.

Client G was a 5-year-old girl presenting with rages and aggressive behaviors made worse by psychostimulants and antidepressants. She was prescribed valproic acid (Depakote) and showed marked improvement in behavior. When she was referred to a psychologist, it was decided that with behavioral improvement, family therapy could be instituted to address problems underlying the client's behaviors. The psychologist explained that the medication would not solve the problem but only make it possible to calm the child and thus allow the family to address underlying problems—and that, with family therapy, the valproic acid might eventually be stopped.

Client H was a 28-year-old woman with bipolar I illness. She had experienced multiple bouts of mania and was treated with lithium. However, weight gain and cognitive impairments led to noncompliance, which led to additional manic episodes. These bouts cycled on and off for months. Recommendation was made to her prescriber to consider a switch from lithium to either lamotrigine (Lamictal) or aripiprazole (Abilify). She was stabilized on a modest dose of aripiprazole with excellent results.

What do these cases have in common? First, all clients had been prescribed reasonable medications as therapy. Second, while efficacious, all the medications had significant side effects that limited optimal life functioning. Third, suggestions were made for reasonable modifications in therapy that often resulted in improved compliance, better life functioning, or amenability to the institution of psychological therapies. Keitz and coworkers (2007) demonstrated that physicians usually comply with reasonable requests and are quite amenable to meeting expectations.

To make specific suggestions for a client, it is important to be aware of three important factors that may affect patient compliance. Also, by addressing these three points, long lists of medicines can be drastically narrowed to reasonable therapeutic recommendations that benefit the client:

- *Can the client afford the prescribed medication?* Patients and physicians alike are susceptible to ads for heavily promoted brand-name (expensive!) medications. New medicines often do have significant advantages over older medicines, but they also have their own constellation of side effects. One might reasonably suggest pregabalin (Lyrica), for example, for treatment of symptoms of PTSD or bipolar disorder, but it would hardly make sense to prescribe pregabalin for a client who cannot afford the medication and probably would not fill a prescription once any free sample was exhausted. Generic gabapentin, at much lower cost, would be a reasonable alternative. Thankfully, in the last couple of years, numerous psychotherapeutic drugs have become available in less expensive generic forms.

- *Can the client tolerate any degree of weight gain?* As has become apparent in this text, some medications are associated with weight gain, while others are not. Similarly, some clients can tolerate a degree of weight gain, while undesirable weight gain might lead to noncompliance in others. In choosing an antidepressant, for example, mirtazepine (Remeron) might be appropriate for a client who can tolerate weight gain, while duloxetine (Cymbalta) or bupropion (Wellbutrin) might be appropriate for a client who wants to lose weight. The same considerations apply in the treatment of bipolar disorder and behavioral disorders associated with anger, agitation, and aggressive behaviors.

- *Can the client tolerate any degree of cognitive dysfunction?* Many psychotherapeutic drugs are associated with drug-induced cognitive dysfunction; among them are benzodiazepines, tricyclic antidepressants, lithium, some anticonvulsant mood stabilizers, and some antipsychotic drugs. The young, the elderly, and people suffering from traumatic brain injury (for example) might not tolerate agents that can be detrimental to cognitive functioning. Others, however, might be able to tolerate some degree of cognitive slowing if the therapeutic benefit seems to outweigh the side effect. If these agents are prescribed, professionals need to know that dysfunction may interfere not only with the efficacy of cognitive therapies but also with overall life functioning.

The treatment of chronic pain in this country could use improvement. Too often, patient complaints of pain result in the prescription of opioid narcotics (Chapter 10), commonly a combination of OxyContin and Vicodin for "breakthrough" pain. The classic model of pain management advocated by John Bonica seems to have been forgotten (Loeser et al., 2001). This model seeks to minimize opioid use through a "layering" of medications. Nonsteroidal anti-inflammatory drugs (Chapter 9) form a base for therapy. Norepinephrine-acting antidepressants (Chapter 5) contribute analgesic, anxiolytic, and antidepressant actions. Anticonvulsants such as gabapentin (Neurontin) and pregabalin (Lyrica; Chapter 6) provide additional analgesic and anxiolytic actions. Only after these three drugs are optimized should opioids be considered. Bonica advocates a collaborative approach to the management of chronic pain, with a pain management team of a prescribing physician, a physical therapist, and a psychologist caring for the patient.

A final example involves withdrawal effects on the newborn when a mother takes serotonin-acting antidepressants during pregnancy. Since SSRIs are considered to be relatively safe for a woman to take during her pregnancy and since these medications markedly reduce episodes of major depression during pregnancy, a newborn may have to withdraw from the medication following delivery. Decisions need to be made about whether to prescribe an antidepressant during pregnancy, whether to offer alternative treatments, whether to taper the medication prior to labor and delivery, and how to handle neonatal withdrawal syndrome should it occur. Collaboration between the obstetrician and a mental health professional is important in deciding on an appropriate course of management.

Considerations for Current Practice

In some areas of the country, specially trained psychologists can be licensed to prescribe psychotherapeutic medications, thus adding prescribing privileges to the armamentarium of treatment modalities for DSM-IV diagnoses. Psychologists first obtained prescriptive privileges in the military as a result of a demonstration project implemented through the Department of Defense. At the time of this writing, psychologists, with the required training and credentials, can prescribe psychotropic medications in the states of New Mexico (as of 2002) and Louisiana (as of 2004).

These developments have been accompanied by discussions, often heated, among the professional disciplines. Opinions have ranged from strong arguments against the prescribing of psychotropic drugs by psychologists (Heiby, 2010) to more conciliatory consideration of the reasons behind this development (Muse and McGrath, 2010), such as the substantial unmet need for mental health treatment and the lack of access to appropriate care, either because of financial constraints of patients, profound shortages of psychiatrists, or lack of sufficient expertise among nonpsychiatric medical professionals.

Furthermore, as one psychiatrist noted (Carlat, 2010), most patients do best on both—medication and psychological therapy—but there are disincentives that discourage such integrated care. Insurance companies are more likely to reimburse medications than nondrug therapies, pharmaceutical firms put tremendous resources into marketing their products, and academic research of drug treatments is more likely to be supported than research into alternative approaches. Carlat also states that current medical training does not select for people who are "psychologically minded" and suggests that it may be time to reconsider the medical training curriculum (p. 2). He proposes that the American Psychiatric Association and the American Psychological Association create a working group to discuss a curriculum for "integrative psychiatric practitioners" (p. 3). It will be interesting to hear the reaction to this extraordinarily collaborative viewpoint.

Meanwhile, there have been some dramatic developments within the psychological profession as well. Baker and colleagues (2009) published an extensive, influential critique of the current situation in regard to the status of clinical psychology. They argue that, in the current climate of increasing health care costs, with corresponding demands for evidence of treatment effectiveness, clinical psychologists are "losing the opportunity to play a leadership role" (p. 67). Even though the number of Americans receiving mental health care has almost doubled in the past 20 years, other practitioners, as well as the increasing use of medication, have minimized the role of psychologists in providing theraputic interventions.

Baker and colleagues (2009) further state that, although many types of behavioral therapy are effective, these treatments are not used as much as they should be because psychologists themselves do not practice them and don't support the interventions even when such treatments would benefit patients. Why? According to these authors, clinical psychologists are not adequately trained in science and are ambivalent about the role of science in their profession. Too many practitioners do not think scientific evidence is as important as their own subjective impression of what works.

The authors fault many training programs in clinical psychology for not upholding high academic admission standards and not emphasizing science in their curricula. They propose a new accreditation system, the Psychological Clinical Science Accreditation System (PCSAS), which would raise the standards of scientific quality in doctoral training in clinical psychology.

It remains to be seen whether this argument will reshape clinical training programs for psychologists. But there seems to be increased attention to both the dissemination of evidence-based behavioral therapies and the integration of psychological and psychiatric approaches to mental health treatments. Newnham and Page (2010) address the "status of evidence-based treatments, measurement of change, patient-focused research and the public availability of risk-adjusted outcomes data" (p. 127). It may be that this discussion will revitalize comparisons within psychology of behavioral treatments themselves (see Ehlers et al., 2010, and references therein, for a critical review of psychological treatments for PTSD). One outcome of the Commission on Mental Health report was the development of the Mental Health Strategic Plan of 2004. This plan called for the integration and improvement of mental health care within the Veterans Health Administration, which is the largest organized system of health care in the United States. One of the objectives of this plan was the dissemination of evidenced-based psychological treatments (EBPTs). McHugh and Barlow (2010) review these developments and the difficulties of integrating such interventions within the clinical community.

Of more relevance to this text, the convergence of these economic, public health, academic, and professional developments has perhaps reinvigorated the discussion of collaborative interventions between psychology and primary medical care (Gunn and Blount, 2009; Kessler, 2009). Gunn and Blount, for example, describe the clinical benefits for patients of coordinated comprehensive care. Support for collaboration among practitioners and integration of behavioral and pharmacological treatments should also promote important comparative research. For patients with social anxiety disorder (SAD), the combination of a monoamine oxidase inhibitor (MAOI) antidepressant and phenelzine plus cognitive behavioral group therapy (CBGT) was found to be superior to either of the individual treatments alone. Surprisingly, neither the drug treatment alone nor the behavioral treatment alone differed in outcome from the placebo treatment. Because patients in the combination group had larger average improvements than the patients receiving the monotherapies, it was concluded that the combination produced an additive or synergistic effect (Blanco et al., 2010).

There is now also extensive evidence that psychological treatments have significant effects on depression (Cuijpers et al., 2008) and that combined treatments can be better than psychological therapy (Cuijpers et al., 2009a) or pharmacological treatment alone (Cuijpers et al., 2009b). Nevertheless, for chronic depression (lasting two years or longer) and especially for dysthymia, results of a meta-analysis show that psychotherapy may be less effective than it is in nonchronic depressive disorders and that pharmacotherapy was significantly more effective. Combined treatments were better than pharmacotherapy alone and even more effective than psychotherapy alone (Cuijpers et al., 2010). Such results illustrate the complexity of treatment for psychiatric disorders and the importance of objective, scientific analyses in determining the respective benefits of psychological and pharmacological treatment.

REFERENCES

Baker, T. B., et al. (2009). "Current Status and Future Prospects of Clinical Psychology. Toward a Scientifically Principled Approach to Mental and Behavioral Health Care." *Psychological Science in the Public Interest* 9: 67–103.

Blanco, C., et al. (2010). "A Placebo-Controlled Trial of Phenelzine, Cognitive Behavioral Group Therapy, and Their Combination, for Social Anxiety Disorder." *Archives of General Psychiatry* 67: 286–295.

Carlat D. (2010). "Psychologist Prescribing: The Best Thing That Can Happen to Psychiatry." The Carlat Psychiatry Blog. Retrieved April 5, 2010, from http://carlatpsychiatry.blogspot.com/2010/03/psychologists-prescribing-best-thing.html.

Cuijpers, P., et al. (2008). "Characteristics of Effective Psychological Treatments of Depression: A Meta-Regression Analysis." *Psychotherapy Research* 18: 225–236.

Cuijpers, P., et al. (2009a). "Psychological Treatment versus Combined Treatment of Depression: A Meta-Analysis." *Depression and Anxiety* 26: 279–288.

Cuijpers, P., et al. (2009b). "Adding Psychotherapy to Pharmacotherapy in the Treatment of Depressive Disorders in Adults: A Meta-Analysis." *Journal of Clinical Psychiatry* 70: 1219–1229.

Cuijpers, P., et al. (2010). "Psychotherapy for Chronic Major Depression and Dysthymia: A Meta-Analysis." *Clinical Psychology Review* 30: 51–62.

Ehlers, A., et al. (2010). "Do All Psychological Treatments Really Work the Same in Posttraumatic Stress Disorder?" *Clinical Psychology Review* 30: 269–276.

Gilbody, S., et al. (2006). "Collaborative Care for Depression: A Cumulative Meta-Analysis and Review of Longer-Term Outcomes." *Archives of Internal Medicine* 166: 2314–2321.

Gunn, W. B., and Blount, A. (2009). "Primary Care Mental Health: A New Frontier for Psychology." *Journal of Clinical Psychology* 65 (Special Issue): 235–252.

Gunn, W. B., and Blount, A. (2009). "Primary Care Mental Health: A New Frontier for Psychology." *Journal of Clinical Psychology* 65 (Special Issue): 235–252.

Heiby, E. M. (2010). "Concerns about Substandard Training for Prescription Privileges for Psychologists." *Journal of Clinical Psychology* 66: 104–111.

Keitz, S. A., et al. (2007). "Behind Closed Doors: Management of Patient Expectations in Primary Care Practices." *Archives of Internal Medicine* 167: 445–452.

Kessler, R. (2009). "Across the Great Divide: Introduction to the Special Issue on Psychology in Medicine." *Journal of Clinical Psychology* 65 (Special Issue): 231–234.

Loeser, J. D., et al. (ed.). (2001). *Bonica's Management of Pain*, 3rd ed. Philadelphia: Lippincott Williams & Wilkins.

McHugh, R. K., and Barlow, D. H. (2010). "The Dissemination and Implementation of Evidence-Based Psychological Treatments." *American Psychologist* 65: 73–84.

Muse, M., and McGrath, R. E. (2010). "Training Comparison among Three Professions Prescribing Psychoactive Medications: Psychiatric Nurse Practitioners, Physicians, and Pharmacologically Trained Psychologists." *Journal of Clinical Psychology* 66: 96–103.

Newnham, E. A., and Page, A. C. (2010). "Bridging the Gap Between Best Evidence and Best Practice in Mental Health." *Clinical Psychology Review* 30: 127–142.

Simon, G. (2006). "Collaborative Care for Depression." *British Medical Journal* 332: 249–250.

Swartz, M. S., et al. (2007). "Effects of Antipsychotic Medications on Psychosocial Functioning in Patients with Chronic Schizophrenia: Findings from the NIMH CATIE Study." *American Journal of Psychiatry* 164: 428–436.

Thase, M. E., et al. (2007). "Cognitive Therapy versus Medication in Augmentation and Switch Strategies as Second-Step Treatments: A STAR*D Report." *American Journal of Psychiatry* 164: 739–752.

U.S. Department of Health and Human Services. (2003). *President's New Freedom Commission on Mental Health, Final Report* (Publication SMA 03-3832). National Institute of Mental Health, Bethesda, MD. Available online at www.mentalhealthcommission.gov/. . ./FullReport.htm.

Witko, K. D., et al. (2005). "Care for Psychological Problems." *Canadian Family Physician* 51: 799–801.

CHAPTER 20 APPENDIX

Quick Reference to Psychotropic Medication

This appendix provides several quick-reference medication tables initially prepared by John Preston, Psy.D., ABPP, and reproduced and modified by the authors of this textbook with his permission. The tables present a list of recommended doses and side effects for psychotherapeutic drugs. To the best of our knowledge the information provided is accurate. However, the material is intended for general reference only, not as a guideline for prescribing for individual patients. It supplements the discussion of the pharmacology of these medicines presented in earlier chapters. The tables are designed to answer questions about the average doses of psychotherapeutic medicines encountered in clinical practice. They also detail the effects of therapeutic drugs on production of sedative side effects, potential for inducing weight gain, potential for producing cognitive impairments, and availability in generic (less expensive) formulations. Please check the manufacturer's product information sheet or the PDR for any changes in dosage schedule or contraindications. (Brand names are registered trademarks).

Antidepressants

Names		Usual daily dosage range	Sedation	Weight gain	Cognitive impairment	Generic available
Generic	Brand					
imipramine	Tofranil	150–300 mg	mid	0–low	mid	yes
desipramine	Norpramin	150–300 mg	low	0–low	mid	yes
amitriptyline	Elavil	150–300 mg	high	0–low	mid	yes
nortriptyline	Aventyl, Pamelor	75–125 mg	mid	0–low	low	yes
protriptyline	Vivactil	15–40 mg	mid	0–low	mid	yes
trimipramine	Surmontil	100–300 mg	high	0–low	mid	yes

Antidepressants (continued)

Generic	Brand	Usual daily dosage range	Sedation	Weight gain	Cognitive impairment	Generic available
doxepin	Sinequan, Adapin	150–300 mg	high	0–low	mid	yes
clomipramine	Anafranil	150–250 mg	high	0–low	mid	yes
maprotiline	Ludiomil	150–225 mg	high	0–low	low	yes
amoxapine	Asendin	150–400 mg	mid	0–low	low	yes
trazodone	Desyrel, Oleptro (XR)	150–400 mg	mid	0–low	low–mid	yes
fluoxetine[1]	Prozac, Sarafem	20–80 mg	low	low	0–low	yes
bupropion-XL[1]	Wellbutrin-XL	150–400 mg	low	0	0	yes
sertraline	Zoloft	50–200 mg	low	low	0	yes
paroxetine	Paxil	20–50 mg	low	low	0	yes
venlafaxine-XR[1]	Effexor-XR	75–350 mg	low	low	0	yes
desvenlafaxine	Pristiq	50 mg	mid	low	0	no
fluvoxamine	Luvox	50–300 mg	low	low	0	yes
mirtazapine	Remeron	15–45 mg	mid	low–mid	low	yes
citalopram	Celexa	10–60 mg	low	low	0	yes
escitalopram	Lexapro	5–20 mg	low	low	0	no
duloxetine	Cymbalta	20–80 mg	low	low	0	no
atomoxetine	Strattera	60–120 mg	low	0	0	no
MAO INHIBITORS						
phenelzine	Nardil	30–90 mg	low	0	0	yes
tranylcypromine	Parnate	20–60 mg	low	0	0	yes
selegiline	Emsam (patch)	6–12 mg	low	0	0	no

[1] Available in standard formulation and time release (XR or XL). Prozac available in 90-mg time-release/weekly formulation.

Bipolar Disorder Medications

| Names | | Serum level[1] | Weight gain | Cognitive impairment | Generic available |
Generic	Brand				
lithium carbonate	Eskalith, Lithonate	0.6–1.5	high	high	yes
olanzapine/ fluoxetine	Symbyax	—[2]	high	high	no
carbamazepine	Tegretol, Equetro	4–10+	low	low	yes
oxcarbazepine	Trileptal	—[2]	low	low	yes
valproic acid	Depakote	50–100	mid	mid	yes
gabapentin	Neurontin	—[2]	low	low	yes
lamotrigine	Lamictal	1–5	0	0	yes
topiramate	Topamax	—[3]	0	mid–high	no
tiagabine	Gabitril	—[3]	0	low–mid	no

[1]Lithium levels are expressed in mEq/l, carbamazepine, valproic acid, and lamotrigine levels in mcg/ml.
[2]Serum monitoring may not be necessary.
[3]Not yet established.

Antiobsessional

Name		Daily
Generic	Brand	dosage range[1]
clomipramine	Anafranil	150–250 mg
fluoxetine	Prozac	20–80 mg
sertraline	Zoloft	50–200 mg
paroxetine	Paxil	20–60 mg
fluvoxamine	Luvox	50–300 mg
citalopram	Celexa	10–60 mg
escitalopram	Lexapro	5–20 mg

[1]Often higher doses are required to control obsessive-compulsive symptoms than the doses generally used to treat depress on.

Psychostimulants

Names		Daily
Generic	Brand	dosage range[1]
methylphenidate[2]	Ritalin	5–50 mg
methylphenidate	Concerta[3]	18–54 mg
methylphenidate	Metadate	5–40 mg
methylphenidate[2]	Methylin	10–60 mg
methylphenidate	Daytrana (patch)	15–30 mg
dexmethylphenidate	Focalin	5–40 mg
dextroamphetamine[2]	Dexedrine	5–40 mg
pemoline	Cylert	37.5–112.5 mg
D- and L-amphetamine	Adderall	5–40 mg
modafinil	Provigil, Sparlon	100–400 mg
armodafinil	Nuvigil	150–250 mg
lisdexamfetamine	Vyvanse	30–70 mg

[1]Adult doses.
[2]Available in generic formulation.
[3]Sustained release.

Antipsychotics

Names		Daily	Weight	Cognitive	Generic
Generic	Brand	dosage range[1]	gain	impairment	available
LOW POTENCY					
chlorpromazine	Thorazine	50–800 mg	low	mid	yes
thioridazine	Mellaril	150–800 mg	low	mid	yes
clozapine	Clozaril	300–900 mg	high	low	yes
mesoridazine	Serentil	50–500 mg	low	mid	no
quetiapine	Seroquel (XR)	150–400 mg	low	0	no
HIGH POTENCY					
molindone	Moban	20–225 mg	low	low	no
perphenazine	Trilafon	8–60 mg	low	low	yes
loxapine	Loxitane	50–250 mg	low	low	yes
trifluoperazine	Stelazine	2–40 mg	low	mid	yes
fluphenazine	Prolixin[2]	3–45 mg	low	low	yes
thiothixene	Navane	10–60 mg	low	low	yes
haloperidol	Haldol[2]	2–40 mg	low	low	yes
pimozide	Orap	1–10 mg	low	low	no
risperidone	Risperdal[3]	4–16 mg	mid	low	yes
paliperidone	Invega	3–12 mg	mid	low	no
olanzapine	Zyprexa	5–20 mg	high	low	no
ziprasidone	Geodon	60–160 mg	0	0	no
aripiprazole	Abilify	15–30 mg	0	0	no
iloperidone	Fanapt	12–24 mg	low	low	no
asenapine	Saphris	10–20 mg	low	low	no

[1] Usual daily oral dosage.
[2] Dose required to achieve efficacy of 100 mg chlorpromazine.
[3] Available in time-release IM format.

Hypnotics[1]

Names		Single-dose dosage range
Generic	**Brand**	
flurazepam[2]	Dalmane	15–30 mg
temazepam[2]	Restoril	15–30 mg
triazolam[2]	Halcion	0.25–0.5 mg
estazolam[2]	ProSom	1.0–2.0 mg
quazepam[2]	Doral	7.5–15 mg
zolpidem	Ambien	5–10 mg
zaleplon	Sonata	5–10 mg
eszopiclone	Lunesta	1–3 mg
ramelteon	Rozerem	4–16 mg
diphenhydramine[2]	Benadryl	25–100 mg
doxepin[3]	Silenor	3–6 mg

[1]All hypnotics produce cognitive impairment.
[2]Available in generic formulation.
[3]Also marketed as Sinequan for the treatment of depression (Chapter 5).

Antianxiety (Anxiolytics)

Names		Single-dose dosage range
Generic	**Brand**	
BENZODIAZEPINES[1]		
diazepam	Valium	2–10 mg
chlordiazepoxide	Librium	10–50 mg
prazepam	Centrax	5–30 mg
clorazepate	Tranxene	3.75–15 mg
clonazepam	Klonopin	0.5–2.0 mg
lorazepam	Ativan	0.5–2.0 mg
alprazolam	Xanax, XR	0.25–2.0 mg
oxazepam	Serax	10–30 mg
OTHER ANTIANXIETY AGENTS[2]		
buspirone	BuSpar	5–20 mg
gabapentin	Neurontin	200–600 mg
hydroxyzine	Atarax, Vistaril	10–50 mg
propranolol[3]	Inderal	10–80 mg
atenolol[3]	Tenormin	25–100 mg
guanfacine[3]	Tenex	0.5–3 mg
clonidine[3]	Catapres	0.1–0.3 mg

[1]All benzodiazepines produce cognitive impairment and are available in generic formulation.
[2]All agents listed are available in generic formulation.
[3]Antihypertensive drugs.

Over-the-Counter

Name	Daily dose
St. John's wort[1,2]	600–1800 mg
SAMe[3]	400–1600 mg
Omega-3[4]	1–9 g

[1]Treats depression and anxiety.
[2]May cause significant drug-drug interactions.
[3]Treats depression.
[4]Treats depression, bipolar disorder, and perhaps psychosis.

Common Side Effects

ANTICHOLINERGIC EFFECTS
(block acetylcholine)

- Dry mouth
- Constipation
- Urinary retention
- Blurred vision
- Memory impairment
- Confusional states

EXTRAPYRAMIDAL EFFECTS
(dopamine blockade in basal ganglia)

- Parkinsonlike effects: rigidity, shuffling gait, tremor, flat affect, lethargy
- Dystonias: Spasms in neck and other muscle groups
- Akathisia: Intense, uncomfortable sense of inner restlessness
- Tardive dyskinesia: Often a persistent movement disorder (lip smacking, writhing movements, jerky movements)

Note: These are common side effects. All medications can produce specific or unique side effects.

GLOSSARY

Abstinence syndrome. State of altered behavior that follows cessation of drug administration. See also **Withdrawal syndrome**

Acetylcholine. Neurotransmitter in the central and peripheral nervous systems, which activates two types of receptors, muscarinic and nicotinic. See **Muscarine; Nicotine**

Additive effect. Effect that occurs when two drugs that have similar biological actions are administered. The net effect is the sum of the independent effects exerted by the drugs.

Adenosine. Chemical neuromodulator in the CNS, primarily at inhibitory synapses.

Adenylate cyclase. Intracellular enzyme that catalyzes the conversion of cyclic AMP to adenosine monophosphate.

Affective disorder. Type of mental disorder characterized by recurrent episodes of mania, depression, or both.

Agonist. Drug that attaches to a receptor and produces actions that mimic or potentiate those of an endogenous transmitter.

Aldehyde dehydrogenase. Enzyme that carries out a specific step in alcohol metabolism: the metabolism of acetaldehyde to acetate. This enzyme may be blocked by the drug disulfiram (Antabuse).

Alzheimer's disease. Progressive neurological disease that occurs primarily in the elderly. It is characterized by a loss of short-term memory and intellectual functioning. It is associated with a loss of function of acetylcholine neurons.

Amphetamine. Behavioral stimulant that acts by increasing the amount of biogenic amines in neuronal synapses.

Anabolic steroid. Testosteronelike drug that acts to increase muscle mass and produces other masculinizing effects.

Anandamide. Endogenous chemical compound that attaches to cannabinoid receptors in the CNS and to specific components of the lymphatic system.

Anandamide receptor. Receptor to which anandamide and tetrahydrocannabinol bind.

Anesthetic. Sedative-hypnotic compound used primarily in doses capable of inducing a state of general anesthesia that involves both loss of sensation, amnesia, and loss of consciousness.

693

Antagonist. Drug that attaches to a receptor and blocks the action of either an endogenous transmitter or an agonistic drug.

Anticonvulsant. Drug that blocks or prevents epileptic convulsions. Some anticonvulsants (for example, carbamazepine and valproic acid) are also used to treat certain nonepileptic psychiatric disorders.

Antidepressant. Drug that is useful in treating mentally depressed patients but does not produce stimulant effects in nondepressed persons. Subdivided into several categories.

Antipsychotic. Medication effective in the treatment of psychosis, particularly for reducing the positive symptoms of schizophrenia, such as hallucinations, delusions, and thought disorder.

Anxiolytic. Drug used to relieve the symptoms associated with defined states of anxiety. Classically, the term refers to the benzodiazepines and related drugs.

Attention deficit/hyperactivity disorder (ADHD). Learning and behavioral disorder characterized by reduced attention span, impulsivity, and/or hyperactivity.

Atypical antipsychotic. Drug that alleviates the positive symptoms of schizophrenia (hallucinations, delusions, and thought disorder) without necessarily causing the neurological side effect of abnormal motor movements. Also used in the treatment of mania.

Autonomic nervous system. Portion of the peripheral nervous system that controls, or regulates, the visceral, automatic, usually involuntary functions of the body, such as heart rate and blood pressure.

Barbiturates. Class of chemically related sedative-hypnotic compounds that share a characteristic six-membered ring structure.

Basal ganglia. An anatomical system in the brain consisting of three primary nuclei (the caudate nucleus, the putamen, and the globus pallidus) located at the base of the brain that are primarily responsible for coordinating and organizing smooth, voluntary motor functions. The basal ganglia are abnormal in a number of important neurological conditions including Parkinson's disease and Huntington's disease. This system may also be referred to as the *extrapyramidal system* to distinguish it from the pyramidal component of the motor system, which is responsible for controlling fine motor responses.

Benzodiazepines. Class of chemically related sedative-hypnotic agents of which chlordiazepoxide (Librium) and diazepam (Valium) are examples. Primarily used in the treatment of anxiety and in alcohol withdrawal.

Bipolar disorder. Affective disorder characterized by alternating bouts of mania and either depression or euthymia (normal affective state). Also called *manic-depressive illness.*

Blackout. Period of time during which a person may be awake but memory is not imprinted. It frequently occurs in people who have consumed excessive alcohol or to whom have been administered (or who have taken) large doses of sedative drugs.

Brain syndrome, organic. Pattern of behavior induced when neurons are either reversibly depressed or irreversibly destroyed. Behavior is characterized by clouded sensorium, disorientation, shallow and labile affect, and impaired memory, intellectual function, insight, and judgment.

Brand name. Unique name licensed to one manufacturer of a drug. Contrasts with *generic name*, the name under which any manufacturer may sell a drug.

Caffeine. Behavioral and general cellular stimulant found in coffee, tea, cola drinks, and chocolate. Acts by blocking an adenosine receptor.

Caffeinism. Habitual use of large amounts of caffeine.

Cannabis sativa. Hemp plant; contains marijuana.

Carbidopa. Drug that inhibits the enzyme dopa decarboxylase, allowing increased availability of dopa within the brain. Contained in the medication Sinemet.

Central nervous system (CNS). Brain and spinal cord.

Cirrhosis. Serious, usually irreversible liver disease. Usually associated with chronic excessive alcohol consumption.

Clonidine (Catapres). Antihypertensive drug useful in alleviating the symptoms of narcotic withdrawal.

Cocaine. Behavioral stimulant. Acts primarily by blocking reuptake of the transmitter dopamine into the neuron from which it was released.

Codeine. Sedative and pain-relieving agent found in opium. Structurally related to morphine but less potent; constitutes approximately 0.5 percent of the opium extract.

Comorbid disorder. Psychiatric disorder that coexists with another psychiatric disorder (for example, multisubstance abuse in a patient with major depressive disorder).

Compulsion. Repetitive or ritualistic behaviors or mental acts performed over and over in response to an obsessive thought, such as repeated hand washing.

Convulsant. Drug that produces convulsions (seizures) by blocking inhibitory neurotransmission.

COX inhibitors. Aspirinlike analgesic drugs that produce their actions by inhibiting the enzyme cyclooxygenase. Two variants of the enzyme occur: COX-1 and COX-2. Some drugs are specific for COX-2; others are nonspecific inhibitors.

Crack. Street name for a smokable form of potent, concentrated cocaine.

Cross-dependence. Condition in which one drug can prevent the withdrawal symptoms associated with physical dependence on a different drug.

Cross-tolerance. Condition in which tolerance of one drug results in a lessened response to another drug.

Delirium tremens (DTs). Syndrome of tremulousness with hallucinations, psychomotor agitation, confusion and disorientation, sleep disorders, and other associated discomforts, lasting several days after alcohol withdrawal.

Dementia. Loss of mental ability severe enough to interfere with normal activities of daily living, lasting more than six months, not present since birth, and not associated with a loss or alteration of consciousness.

Detoxification. Process of allowing time for the body to metabolize and/or excrete accumulations of drug. Usually a first step in drug abuse evaluation and treatment.

Differential diagnosis. Listing of all possible causes that might explain a given set of symptoms.

Dimethyltryptamine (DMT). Psychedelic drug found in many South American plants.

Dopamine. One of the monoaminergic (catecholamine) neurotransmitters in the central nervous system, considered to be the primary reward neurotransmitter in the brain, and important in mediating voluntary movement (loss of dopamine neurons produces Parkinson's disease). It is the precursor to norepinephrine.

Dopamine transporter. Presynaptic protein that binds synaptic dopamine and transports the neurotransmitter back into the presynaptic nerve terminal.

Dose-response relation. Relation between drug doses and the response elicited at each dose level.

Drug. Chemical substance used for its effects on bodily processes.

Drug absorption. Mechanism by which a drug reaches the bloodstream from the skin, lungs, stomach, intestinal tract, or muscle.

Drug administration. Procedures through which a drug enters the body (oral administration of tablets or liquids, inhalation of powders, injection of sterile liquids, and so on).

Drug dependence. State in which the use of a drug is necessary for either physical or psychological well-being.

Drug interaction. Modification of the action of one drug by the concurrent or prior administration of another drug.

Drug misuse. Use of any drug (legal or illegal) for a medical or recreational purpose when other alternatives are available, practical, or warranted or when drug use endangers either the user or others with whom he or she may interact.

Drug receptor. Specific molecular substance in the body with which a given drug interacts to produce its effect.

Drug tolerance. State of progressively decreasing responsiveness to a drug.

DSM-IV, DSM-IV-TR. Abbreviation for *Diagnostic and Statistical Manual of Mental Disorders,* Fourth Edition, published by the American Psychiatric Association in 1994. A comprehensive classification of officially recognized psychiatric disorders. The Text Revision of the Fourth Edition was published in 2000.

Dual-action antidepressants. Antidepressant drugs that act by inhibiting the active presynaptic reuptake of more than one neurotransmitter, for example, norepinephrine and serotonin.

Electroconvulsive therapy (ECT). A procedure in which an electric current is passed through the brain to produce controlled convulsions (seizures) to treat patients with depression, particularly for those who cannot take or are not responding to antidepressants, have severe depression, or are at high risk for suicide.

Endorphin. Naturally occurring protein that causes endogenous morphine-like activity.

Enkephalin. Naturally occurring protein that causes morphinelike activity.

Enzyme. Large organic molecule that mediates a specific biochemical reaction in the body.

Enzyme induction. Increased production of drug-metabolizing enzymes in the liver, stimulated by certain drugs (inducers). As a result of induction, drugs that are metabolized by the induced enzyme will be degraded more rapidly. It is one mechanism by which pharmacological tolerance is produced.

Epilepsy. Neurological disorder characterized by an occasional, sudden, and uncontrolled discharge of neurons.

Fetal alcohol syndrome. Symptom complex of congenital anomalies, seen in newborns of women who ingested high doses of alcohol during critical periods of pregnancy.

G protein. Specific intraneuronal protein that links transmitter-induced receptor alterations with intracellular second-messenger proteins or with adjacent ion channels.

Gamma aminobutyric acid (GABA). Inhibitory amino acid neurotransmitter in the brain.

Generic name. Name that identifies a specific chemical entity (without describing the chemical). Often marketed under different brand names by different manufacturers.

Glutamic acid. Excitatory amino acid neurotransmitter. It is the precursor to GABA, the inhibitory neurotransmitter.

Hallucinogen. Psychedelic drug that produces profound distortions in perception.

Harmine. Psychedelic agent obtained from the seeds of *Peganum harmala*.

Hashish. Extract of the hemp plant (*Cannabis sativa*) that has a higher concentration of THC than does marijuana.

Heroin. Semisynthetic opiate produced by a chemical modification of morphine.

Hypothalamus. Brain structure located below the thalamus and above the pituitary gland that regulates bodily temperature, certain metabolic processes, and other autonomic activities.

Hypoxia. State of relative lack of oxygen in the tissues of the body and the brain.

Ice. Street name for a smokable, free-base form of potent, concentrated methamphetamine.

Levodopa. Precursor substance to the transmitter dopamine; useful in alleviating the symptoms of Parkinson's disease.

Limbic system. Group of brain structures involved in emotional responses and emotional expression.

Lithium. Alkali metal effective in the treatment of mania and depression.

Lysergic acid diethylamide (LSD). Semisynthetic psychedelic drug.

Major tranquilizer (archaic). See **Antipsychotic**

Mania. Mental disorder characterized by an expansive emotional state, elation, hyperirritability, excessive talkativeness, flights of ideas, and increased behavioral activity.

MAO. See **Monoamine oxidase**

Marijuana. Mixture of the crushed leaves, flowers, and small branches of both the male and female hemp plant (*Cannabis sativa*).

Mescaline. Psychedelic drug extracted from the peyote cactus.

Minor tranquilizer. Sedative-hypnotic drug promoted primarily for use in the treatment of anxiety.

Mixed agonist-antagonist. Drug that attaches to a receptor, producing weak agonistic effects but displacing more potent agonists, precipitating withdrawal in drug-dependent persons.

Monoamine oxidase (MAO). Enzyme capable of metabolizing norepinephrine, dopamine, and serotonin to inactive products.

Monoamine oxidase inhibitor (MAOI). Drug that inhibits the activity of the enzyme monoamine oxidase. Identifies one category of antidepressant medications.

Mood stabilizer. Drug used in the treatment of bipolar illness. Examples are lithium and any of the neuromodulator anticonvulsants.

Morphine. Major sedative and pain-relieving (analgesic) drug found in opium; makes up approximately 10 percent of the crude opium exudate.

Muscarine. Drug extracted from the mushroom *Amanita muscaria* that directly stimulates acetylcholine receptors.

Myristin. Psychedelic agent obtained from nutmeg and mace.

Neuromodulator. Antiepileptic drug used to treat bipolar illness, aggressive disorders, chronic pain, and a variety of other disorders.

Neuropathic pain. Pain caused by a primary lesion or dysfunction in the nervous system, that is, damage to nerves, to the brain, or the spinal cord.

Neurotransmitter. Endogenous chemical released by one neuron that alters the electrical activity of another neuron.

Nicotine. Behavioral stimulant found in tobacco that directly stimulates acetylcholine receptors.

Norepinephrine (also known as *noradrenaline*). One of the monoaminergic (biogenic) excitatory neurotransmitters, a catecholamine in chemical structure, involved in alertness, concentration, aggression and motivation, among other actions.

Norepinephrine-specific reuptake inhibitor. See **Selective norepinephrine reuptake inhibitor**

Obsession. Intrusive thoughts that produce anxiety and that lead to repetitive behaviors (compulsions) aimed at reducing anxiety.

Off-label. Term applied to the clinical use of a drug for an indication other than that for which the drug was approved by the U.S. Food and Drug Administration. Use is usually justified by medical literature, even though formal USDA approval for the use was not sought by the manufacturer of the drug. The manufacturer is not permitted to promote a drug for an off-label use.

Ololiuqui. Psychedelic drug obtained from the seeds of the morning glory plant.

Opioid. Natural or synthetic drug that exerts actions on the body similar to those induced by morphine, the major pain-relieving agent obtained from the opium poppy (*Papaver somniferum*).

Opium. Crude resinous exudate from the opium poppy. Contains morphine and codeine as active opioids.

Parkinson's disease. Disorder of the motor system characterized by involuntary movements, tremor, and weakness, resulting from the loss of dopamine-producing neurons.

Partial agonist. Drug that binds to a receptor, contributing only part of the action exerted by the endogenous neurotransmitter or producing a submaximal receptor response. Buprenorphine (in Suboxone) is an example.

Peptide. Chemical composed of a chain-link sequence of amino acids.

Peyote. Cactus that contains mescaline.

Pharmacodynamics. Study of the interactions of a drug and the receptors responsible for the action of the drug in the body.

Pharmacokinetics. Study of the factors that influence the absorption, distribution, metabolism, and excretion of a drug.

Pharmacology. Branch of science that deals with the study of drugs and their actions on living systems.

Phencyclidine (Sernyl, PCP). Psychedelic surgical anesthetic; acts by binding to and inhibiting ion transport through the NMDA-glutamate receptors.

Phenothiazine. Class of chemically related antipsychotic neuroleptic medications useful in the treatment of psychosis.

Physical dependence. State in which the use of a drug is required for a person to function normally. Physical dependence is revealed by withdrawing the drug and noting the occurrence of withdrawal symptoms (abstinence syndrome). Characteristically, withdrawal symptoms can be terminated by readministration of the drug.

Placebo. Pharmacologically inert substance that may elicit a significant reaction largely because of the mental set of the patient or the physical setting in which the drug is taken.

Potency. Measure of drug activity expressed in terms of the amount required to produce an effect of given intensity. Potency varies inversely with the amount of drug required to produce this effect—the more potent the drug, the lower the amount required to produce the effect.

Psilocybin. Psychedelic drug obtained from the mushroom *Psilocybe mexicana.*

Psychedelic. Drug that can alter sensory perception.

Psychoactive drug. Chemical substance that alters mood or behavior as a result of alterations in the functioning of the brain.

Psychological dependence. Compulsion to use a drug for its pleasurable effects. Dependence may lead to a compulsion to misuse a drug.

Psychopharmacology. Branch of pharmacology that deals with the effects of drugs on the nervous system and behavior.

Psychopharmacotherapy. Clinical treatment of psychiatric disorders with drugs.

Psychotherapy. Nonpharmacological treatment of psychiatric disorders utilizing a wide range of modalities from simple education and supportive counseling to insight-oriented, dynamically based therapy.

Receptor. Location in the nervous system at which a neurotransmitter or drug binds to exert its characteristic effect. Most receptors are members of genetically encoded families of specialized proteins.

Reye's syndrome. Rare CNS disorder that occurs in children; associated with aspirin ingestion.

Risk-to-benefit ratio. Arbitrary assessment of the risks and benefits that may accrue from administration of a drug.

Schizophrenia. Debilitating neuropsychiatric illness associated with disturbances in thought, perception, emotion, cognition, relationships, and psychomotor behavior.

Scopolamine. Anticholinergic drug that crosses the blood-brain barrier to produce sedation and amnesia; antagonist at the muscarinic receptor.

Second messenger. Intraneuronal protein that, when activated by a G protein, mediates the response that is initiated when neurotransmitter molecules bind to an extracellular receptor.

Sedative-hypnotic. Chemical substance that exerts a nonselective general depressant action on the nervous system.

Selective norepinephrine reuptake inhibitor (SNRI). Drug that blocks the active presynaptic transporter for norepinephrine. Clinically used to treat ADHD, depression, and other disorders, including seasonal affective disorder.

Selective serotonin reuptake inhibitor (SSRI). Second-generation antidepressant drug that blocks the reuptake transporter for serotonin.

Serotonin (5-hydroxytryptamine, 5-HT). Indoleamine neurotransmitter in both the brain and the peripheral nervous system (gut) that is involved in depression, appetite, sleep, and sexual responsiveness, among other functions.

Serotonin syndrome. Clinical syndrome resulting from excessive amounts of serotonin in the brain. The syndrome can follow use of excessive doses of SSRIs, and it is characterized by extreme anxiety, confusion, and disorientation.

Serotonin withdrawal syndrome. Clinical syndrome that can follow withdrawal or cessation of SSRI therapy. The syndrome is characterized by mental status alterations, severe flulike symptoms, and feelings of tingling or electrical shock in the extremities.

Side effect. Drug-induced effect that accompanies the primary effect for which the drug is administered.

Substance P. Protein neurotransmitter that regulates affective behavior, increasing the perception of pain. Substance P antagonists exhibit analgesic and antidepressant actions.

Tardive dyskinesia. Movement disorder that appears after months or years of treatment with neuroleptic (antipsychotic) drugs. It usually worsens with drug discontinuation. Symptoms are often masked by the drugs that cause the disorder.

Teratogen. Chemical substance that induces abnormalities of fetal development.

Testosterone. Hormone secreted from the testes that is responsible for the distinguishing characteristics of the male.

Tetrahydrocannabinol (THC). Major psychoactive agent in marijuana, hashish, and other preparations of hemp (*Cannabis sativa*).

Therapeutic drug monitoring (TDM). Process of correlating the plasma level of a drug with therapeutic response.

Tolerance. Clinical state of reduced responsiveness to a drug; can be produced by a variety of mechanisms, all of which require increased doses of drug to produce an effect once achieved by lower doses.

Toxic effect. Drug-induced effect either temporarily or permanently deleterious to any organ or system of an animal or person. Drug toxicity includes both the relatively minor side effects that invariably accompany drug administration and the more serious and unexpected manifestations that occur in only a small percentage of patients who take a drug.

Unipolar depression (*also known as* clinical depression, major depression, and unipolar disorder). Mental disorder characterized by an all-encompassing low mood accompanied by low self-esteem and loss of interest or pleasure in normally enjoyable activities.

Ventral tegmental area (VTA). Group of neurons, located on the floor of the midbrain (mesencephalon), that contain dopamine and serotonin; the VTA is a major component of the reward pathway in the brain.

Withdrawal syndrome. Onset of a predictable group of symptoms following the abrupt discontinuation or rapid decrease in dosage of a psychoactive substance on which the body has become dependent. May include anxiety, insomnia, delirium tremens, perspiration, hot flashes, nausea, dehydration, tremors, weakness, dizziness, convulsions, and psychotic behavior.

Zero-order metabolism (kinetics). Condition in which the plasma concentration of a drug decreases (is metabolized) at a constant rate; the rate of metabolism does not depend on the amount (concentration) of the drug.

INDEX